T0392384

Vascular Malformations

Advances and Controversies in Contemporary Management

Vascular Malformations
Advances and Controversies in Contemporary Management

Edited by

Byung-Boong Lee MD PhD FACS
Professor of Surgery
Department of Surgery
Division of Vascular Surgery
George Washington University
Washington, District of Columbia, USA

Peter Gloviczki MD FACS
Joe M. and Ruth Roberts Professor of Surgery (Emeritus), Chair, Division of Vascular
and Endovascular Surgery (Emeritus), Director, Gonda Vascular Center (Emeritus)
Mayo Clinic, Rochester, Minnesota, USA
Editor-In-Chief, *Journal of Vascular Surgery*

Francine Blei MD
Director, Vascular Anomalies Program of Lenox Hill Hospital
New York City, New York, USA

Assistant Editor
Jovan N. Markovic MD
Department of Surgery
Division of Vascular Surgery
Duke University School of Medicine
Durham, North Carolina, USA

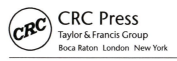

CRC Press
Taylor & Francis Group
Boca Raton London New York

CRC Press is an imprint of the
Taylor & Francis Group, an **informa** business

CRC Press
Taylor & Francis Group
6000 Broken Sound Parkway NW, Suite 300
Boca Raton, FL 33487-2742

© 2020 by Taylor & Francis Group, LLC
CRC Press is an imprint of Taylor & Francis Group, an Informa business

No claim to original U.S. Government works

Printed on acid-free paper

International Standard Book Number-13: 978-0-367-25012-6 (Hardback)

Library of Congress Cataloging-in-Publication Data

Names: Lee, Byung-Boong, editor. | Gloviczki, Peter, editor. | Blei, Francine, editor. | Markovic, Jovan N., editor.
Title: Vascular malformations : advances and controversies in contemporary management / editors, Byung-Boong Lee, Peter Gloviczki, Francine Blei ; assistant editor, Jovan N. Markovic.
Other titles: Vascular malformations (Lee)
Description: Boca Raton : CRC Press, [2020] | Includes bibliographical references and index. | Summary: "This book uses evidence-based chapters to provide clarity and certainty in the clinical management of congenital vascular malformations (CVM). Each chapter written by the world authorities on each topic, reviews in depth the controversial issues in CVM management. Learn the up-to-date answer(s) on each topic"-- Provided by publisher.
Identifiers: LCCN 2019030759 (print) | ISBN 9780367250126 (hardback : alk. paper) | ISBN 9780367255343 (ebook)
Subjects: MESH: Vascular Malformations--therapy | Vascular Malformations--diagnosis
Classification: LCC RC388.5 (print) | LCC RC388.5 (ebook) | NLM WG 220 | DDC 616.8/1--dc23
LC record available at https://lccn.loc.gov/2019030759
LC ebook record available at https://lccn.loc.gov/2019030760

Visit the Taylor & Francis Web site at
http://www.taylorandfrancis.com

and the CRC Press Web site at
http://www.crcpress.com

Contents

Preface

Major advances in recent years in medical genetics and tremendous progress in the fields of imaging and minimally invasive, percutaneous interventions have revolutionized both evaluation and management of vascular malformations. Progress brought hope to many patients previously not treated for their frequently disabling malformation, although it also generated ample controversies about appropriate use of drugs, devices, and new medical, interventional, and surgical technology. This book on vascular malformations brings together more than 65 experts to present advances and discuss controversies in the multidisciplinary management of patients with congenital vascular malformations.

Divided into six major parts, the book starts with general discussion on the latest classifications, new genetic studies, and advantages of interdisciplinary collaboration between vascular specialists. The remining parts focus on advances and controversies of arteriovenous, venous, lymphatic, capillary, and mixed vascular malformations. Diagnostic evaluations that include the latest imaging studies are discussed in detail for each type of malformation. These discussions are followed by presentation of cutting-edge medical, minimally invasive endovascular, and open surgical management. Multiple chapters are devoted to sclerotherapy, embolization, and endovenous thermal ablations of arteriovenous and venous malformations. Primary lymphedema is discussed with the new imaging studies such as magnetic resonance and fluorescent lymphangiography. Compression therapy, manual lymphatic drainage, liposuction, as well as medical, microsurgical, and open surgical treatments are presented. A large section of the book is devoted to combined malformations, including one of the most challenging of all syndromic malformations, Klippel–Trenaunay syndrome.

Beautifully illustrated with color line drawings, numerous photographs, and informative tables, advances and controversies of the full spectrum of vascular malformations are presented in 90 chapters. This book brings new information and unparalleled insights to vascular specialists and physicians, trainees and allied health professionals, and all those who participate in the care of patients with vascular malformations, either in a private practice setting or at a major institution in an interdisciplinary vascular center.

We would like to express our most sincere gratitude to all vascular specialists who contributed to this volume. We are indebted to our publisher, CRC Press, Taylor & Francis Group in England, to Medical Editor Miranda Bromage and Editorial Assistant Samantha Cook for their invaluable assistance, for their expertise, and for producing such a beautiful volume in such a short time. The editors sincerely hope that the information provided in this book will contribute to improve the quality of life and decrease the disability of millions of patients who suffer from vascular malformations worldwide.

Byung-Boong Lee, MD, FACS
Peter Gloviczki, MD, FACS
Francine Blei, MD, MBA
Editors

Jovan N. Markovic, MD
Assistant Editor

Foreword

Vascular malformations: Aspects of historic cross-fertilization (I still remember….)

Byung-Boong Lee is a real master of bringing people together, ending up with books on difficult topics, which are critically examined by experts coming from different countries, disciplines, and schools. Lot of space for controversies indeed.

This time the hot topics are "Advances and Controversies in Vascular Malformations," which are highlighted by specialists presenting nondogmatic exciting overviews on different aspects of this very complex pathology.

As Byung-Boong told me, the process of trying to find a consensus on such topics and to come up with a list of 90 chapters written by international authorities took more than one year and was substantially supported by Leonel Villavicencio by organizing small steering groups and by Peter Gloviczki, who proposed publishing this all in one book.

Anyhow, I know only very few people who have such a tolerant spirit of appreciation of the ideas of other colleagues as Byung-Boong has.

In spite of new classification systems for vascular malformations, trying to ban eponyms connected to the names of historical authors, some of these names seem to be immortal. One example is the Klippel–Trenaunay syndrome (KTS), to which a special section is dedicated in this book and which previously was frequently lumped together with FP Weber syndrome. One of my first publications in which I was involved as a coauthor in 1967 still used the term "Klippel–Trenaunay–Weber."[1]

Reading the original publications, it became clear that actually two different entities presenting with distinct clinical features had been described by these authors. Frederick Parks Weber described congenital pulsating "phlebarteriectasias," obviously due to arteriovenous (AV) fistulae, several decades before angiography was introduced,[2] while the main features of the cases described by M. Klippel and P. Trenaunay are the typical triad of overgrowth, nevus flammeus, and atypical varicose veins.[3] (By the way, "Trenaunay" is written without an "accent aigu" in the original publication, so it is "Trenaunay" and not "Trénaunay".)[4]

The deciding main difference between these entities is the presence of large AV shunts in FP Weber syndrome.

However, the occurrence of AV shunts is an ongoing discussion, not only in patients with KTS but also in those with leg ulcers or even varicose veins, supported by an "early venous filling" phenomenon in angiography.

In 1968, our group published a method of measuring the shunt volume in cases with suspected AV shunts following an intra-arterial injection of radioactively labeled albumin particles (diameters 5–50 micron).[5] Later, microspheres were used. These particles, which are too big to pass normal capillaries, will be trapped in the arterioles of the peripheral circulation. In the presence of AV shunts, a certain number of microspheres penetrate into the veins and are transported into the pulmonary circulation, where the particles are stuck and can be registered by a lung scan. The extent of the increase of radioactivity over the lungs is proportional to the shunt volume, which can be calculated after an intravenous injection of particles (=100%).

My Austrian mentor, Robert May, was happy with this method, because it gave him clear indication for or against surgery, as he wrote me in a letter.

Among 24 patients with vascular malformations of the extremities, three groups of shunt volumes were differentiated[5]:

1. [N]ormal values (0%–4%) 18 patients (15 legs, 3 upper extremities).
2. 11%–18%: 4 patients ("av-microfistulae"?)
3. 45% and 76% in 2 cases with FPW syndrome.

At the invitation of Norman Rich and Leonel Villavicencio, I reported our experiences at the fourth European American Venous Symposium (EAVS) in Bethesda, Maryland, in 1987. This method was used by Byung-Boong Lee under the name of transarterial lung perfusion scintigraphy (TLPS).[6]

In 1994, Byung-Boong had returned to Seoul, South Korea, where he spent a productive decade, setting up a Hopkins-style surgery program at Samsung Medical Center as clinical professor of Johns Hopkins University. When he invited me to a meeting in Seoul in 1996, I had the opportunity to visit his now-legendary Vascular Malformation program, which had been organized with unlimited funds from Samsung. I was deeply impressed by seeing so many cases, more than I have ever seen, along with extensive clinical implementation of TLPS.

In a private discussion with Bob Rutherford at a Hurtigruten boat trip in Norway, organized by Bo Eklof, it turned out that he also had used the same method.[7] Both of us still remembered the satisfaction of treating the first case with a major AV shunt without knowing that this method had been discovered by another group as well.

I met Leonel Villavicencio and his wife, Suzie, for the first time in Acapulco, Mexico, at the third European American Venous Symposium (EAVS). Since the airplane had lost my luggage, he lent me a shirt, a tie, and a jacket, and he was extremely supportive in planning the fifth EAVS meeting scheduled for 1990 in Vienna, Austria, which was the last one after the American Venous Forum had been founded by several illustrious personalities one year before.

Throughout the years, Leonel and I maintained contact, not only discussing scientific agendas (he kindly translated the book I wrote with Robert Stemmer and Eberhard Rabe on compression therapy from German into English[8]) but also sharing updates on family and even sending our children to each other's homes for visits.

Some of my own memories have been presented here, underscoring the fact that international cross-fertilization has enriched our knowledge in the field of vascular malformations. This book gives an impressive testimonial that an interchange also between different disciplines will support better comprehension of a difficult subject if the contributions are carefully selected. Byung-Boong Lee and his editorial team have to be congratulated for reaching this goal in presenting this great work.

Hugo Partsch, MD
Department of Dermatology
University of Wien
Baumeistergasse, Wien, Austria

REFERENCES

1. Lindemayr W, Lofferer O, Mostbeck A, Partsch H. Das Lyphgefäßsystem bei der Klippel–Trenaunay–Weberschen Phakomatose. *Z. Haut-Geschl-Krankh.* 1968,43:183–191.
2. Lofferer O, Mostbeck A, Partsch H. Untersuchungen zur Gefäßregulation der Extremiäten mit besonderer Berücksichtigung arteriovenöser Shunts. In: Fellinger K, Höfer R, eds. *Radioaktive Isotope in Klinik und Forschung, Band VIII.* München, Berlin, Wien: Urban & Schwarzenberg; 1968:454–460.
3. Klippel M, Trenaunay P. Du naevus variqueux ostéo-hypertrophique. *Arch Général.* 1900;3:641–672.
4. Weber FP. Haemangiectatic hypertrophy of limbs – Congenital phlebarteriectasis and so-called congenital varicose veins. *Br J Child Dis.* 1918;15:13–17.
5. Partsch H, Motbeck A, Lofferer O. Zur Diagnostik von arteriovenösen Fisteln bei Angiodysplasien der Extremitäten. (*Kriterien für eine Operationsindkation*) VASA. 1975;4:288–295.
6. Lee BB, Mattassi R, Kim YW, Kim BT, Park JM, Choi JY. Advanced management of arteriovenous shunting malformation with transarterial lung perfusion scintigraphy for follow-up assessment. *Int Angiol.* 2005;24(2):173–184.
7. Rutherford RB, Anderson BO. Diagnosis of congenital vascular malformations of the extremities: New perspectives. *Int Angiol.* 19909(3):162–167.
8. Partsch H, Stemmer Rabe R, Villavicencio JL. *Compression Therapy of the Extremities.* Paris, France: Editions Phlebologiques Francaises; 2000.

Contributors

Claudio Allegra
Angiology Department S. Giovanni Hospital in Rome
UIP
Rome, Italy

Miguel A. Amore
Phlebology and Lymphology Unit
Cardiovascular Surgery Division
Central Military Hospital
and
Buenos Aires University
Buenos Aires, Argentina

Pier Luigi Antignani
International Union of Angiology
Nuova Villa Claudia
Rome, Italy

Michelangelo Bartolo
Telemedicine for Africa, S. Giovanni
    Hospital Rome
Angiology O.U.
Department of Medical Sciences
S. Giovanni Hospital
Rome, Italy

Iris Baumgartner
Division of Angiology
Swiss Cardiovascular Center
University Hospital
University of Bern
Bern, Switzerland

Jean-Paul Belgrado
Faculté des Sciences de Motricité
Unité de Recherche en Lymphologie
    et Réadaptation
Université Libre de Bruxelles
Bruxelles, Belgium

Peter Berlien
Wissenschaft & Forschung
Ev. Elisabeth Klinik Zentrum Lasermedizin
Stuttgart, Germany

Sarah Bernhard
Inselspital, Bern University Hospital
Department of Angiology
Bern, Switzerland

Matteo Bertelli
MAGI Euregio
Bolzano, Italy

Tobias Bertsch
Földi Klinik
Hinterzarten, Germany

Salvino Bilancini
J.F. Merlen Angiology Center
Frosinone, Italy

Francine Blei
Vascular Anomalies Program of Lenox Hill Hospital
New York City, New York

Francesco Boccardo
Department of Cardio-Thoracic-Vascular and
    Endovascular Surgery
Lymphatic Surgery and Microsurgery
San Martino Hospital
University of Genoa
Genoa, Italy

Håkan Brorson
Department of Clinical Sciences
Lund University
Lund, Sweden

and

Lymphedema Center
Plastic and Reconstructive Surgery
Skåne University Hospital
Malmö, Sweden

Corradino Campisi
Department of Surgery—DISC
Section of Lymphatic Surgery and Microsurgery
University School of Medicine and Pharmaceutics
Genoa, Italy

Corrado Cesare Campisi
Department of Plastic and Reconstructive Surgery
Salus Hospital
GVM Care and Research
Reggio Emilia (RE) and ICLAS Hospital
Rapallo, Italy

Justin Chin-Bong Choi
Vascular Surgery Fellow
MedStar Georgetown University Hospital-Washington
    Hospital Center
Fellowship Program in Vascular Surgery
Washington, District of Columbia

Mihai Constantinescu
Department of Plastic and Hand Surgery
Inselspital, Bern University Hospital
University of Bern
Bern, Switzerland

Robert J. Damstra
Department of Dermatology
Expert center for lympho-vascular medicine
Nij Smellinghe Hospital
Drachten, The Netherlands

Sara Dessalvi
Department of Cardio-Thoracic-Vascular and
    Endovascular Surgery
Lymphatic Surgery and Microsurgery
San Martino Hospital
University of Genoa
Genoa, Italy

Pietro Di Summa
Department of Plastic and Reconstructive Surgery
University Hospital of Lausanne
Lausanne, Switzerland

Young Soo Do
Department of Radiology
Sungkyunkwan University School of Medicine
Samsung Medical Center
Seoul, South Korea

David J. Driscoll
Mayo Clinic College of Medicine
Division of Pediatric Cardiology
Department of Pediatrics
Rochester, Minnesota

Alessandro Failla
Department of Vascular Rehabilitation
San Giovanni Battista Hospital
ACISMOM
Rome, Italy

Jawed Fareed
Department of Pathology
Hemostasis and Thrombosis Research Laboratories
Loyola University Medical Center
Maywood, Illinois

Alessandro Fiorentino
Department of Vascular Rehabilitation
San Giovanni Battista Hospital
ACISMOM
Rome, Italy

Isabel Forner-Cordero
Department of Physical Medicine and Rehabilitation
    Service
Hospital Universitari i Politecnic La Fe
University of Valencia
Valencia, Spain

Sabrina Frey
ARTORG Center for Biomedical Engineering Research
University of Bern
Bern, Switzerland

Sergio Gianesini
Department of Morphology Surgery and Experimental
    Medicine
University of Ferrara
Ferrara, Italy

and

Department of Surgery
USUHS University
Bethesda, Maryland

Peter Gloviczki
Division of Vascular and Endovascular
    Surgery (Emeritus)
Gonda Vascular Center (Emeritus)
Mayo Clinic
Rochester, Minnesota

Jamison Harvey
Department of Dermatology
Mayo Clinic
Scottsdale, Arizona

Evi Kalodiki
Josef Pflug Vascular Laboratory
Ealing Hospital and Imperial College London
London, United Kingdom

and

Thrombosis and Hemostasis Research Laboratory
Loyola University Medical Center
Maywood, Illinois

Mina Kang
Department of Dermatology
St. Vincent's Hospital
Sydney, Australia

Vaughan Keeley
Lymphoedema Clinic
Royal Derby Hospital
Derby and University of Nottingham Medical School
Nottingham, United Kingdom

Young-Wook Kim
Department of Vascular Surgery
Kangbuk Samsung Hospital
Sungkyunkwan University School of Medicine
Seoul, South Korea

James Laredo
Division of Vascular Surgery
Department of Surgery
George Washington University Medical Center
Washington, District of Columbia

Byung-Boong Lee
Division of Vascular Surgery
Department of Surgery
George Washington University
Washington, District of Columbia

Xiaoxi Lin
Department of Plastic and Reconstructive Surgery
Shanghai Ninth People's Hospital
Shanghai Jiao Tong University School of Medicine
Shanghai, China

Ningfei Liu
Department of Plastic and Reconstructive Surgery
Shanghai Ninth People's Hospital
Shanghai Jiao Tong University School of Medicine
Shanghai, China

Dirk A. Loose
Section Vascular Surgery and Angiology
Center for the Diagnosis and Treatment of Congenital
Vascular Malformations
Hamburg, Germany

Juan Carlos López Gutiérrez
Department of Pediatric Surgery
La Paz Children's Hospital
University Autonoma of Madrid
Madrid, Spain

Paul Marji
MedStar Georgetown University Hospital
Washington Hospital Center
Washington, DC

Jovan N. Markovic
Department of Surgery
Division of Vascular Surgery
Duke University School of Medicine
Durham, North Carolina

Michele Maruccia
Division of Plastic and Reconstructive Surgery
Department of Emergency and Organ Transplantation
University of Bari
Bari, Italy

Raul Mattassi
Department of Vascular Surgery
Center for Vascular Malformations "Stefan Belov"
Clinical Institute Humanitas Mater Domini
Varese, Italy

Erica Menegatti
Department of Morphology Surgery and Experimental
    Medicine
University of Ferrara
Ferrara, Italy

Sandro Michelini
Department of Vascular Rehabilitation
San Giovanni Battista Hospital
ACISMOM
Rome, Italy

Giovanni Moneta
Department of Vascular Rehabilitation
San Giovanni Battista Hospital
ACISMOM
Rome, Italy

Fabio Nicoli
Department of Plastic and Reconstructive Surgery
Newcastle upon Tyne Hospitals NHS Trust
Newcastle upon Tyne, United Kingdom

Furuzan Numan
Cerrahpasa School of Medicine
Interventional Radiology Department
Istanbul University
Istanbul, Turkey

Dominik Obrist
Division of Angiology
Swiss Cardiovascular Center
University Hospital
University of Bern
Bern, Switzerland

Stefano Paolacci
MAGI'S Lab
Rovereto, Italy

Cristobal M. Papendieck
Angiopediatria
Universidad del Salvador (USAL)
Buenos Aires, Argentina

Kwang Bo Park
Department of Radiology
Sungkyunkwan University School of Medicine
Samsung Medical Center
Seoul, South Korea

Kurosh Parsi
University of New South Wales
and
Dermatology, Phlebology
Fluid Mechanics Research Laboratory
St. Vincent's Centre for Applied Medical Research
Sydney, Australia

Neil Piller
Lymphoedema Clinical Research Unit
Flinders Medical Centre
Adelaide, Australia

Stanley G. Rockson
Center for Lymphatic and Venous Disorders
Lymphatic Research and Medicine
Stanford University School of Medicine
Stanford, California

Jochen Karl Rössler
Department of Pediatric Hematology and Oncology
Inselspital, Bern University Hospital
University of Bern
Bern, Switzerland

Melissa Ryan
Department of Surgery—DISC
Section of Lymphatic Surgery and Microsurgery
University School of Medicine and Pharmaceutics
Genoa, Italy

Jong Sup Shim
Department of Orthopedic Surgery
Samsung Medical Center
Sungkyunkwan University School of Medicine
Seoul, Korea

Cynthia K. Shortell
Department of Surgery
Division of Vascular Surgery
Duke University School of Medicine
Durham, North Carolina

Győző Szolnoky
Department of Dermatology and Allergology
University of Szeged
Szeged, Hungary

Alfonso Tafur
Department of Medicine
Cardiovascular Medicine
NorthShore University Health System
Evanston, Illinois

Megha M. Tollefson
Dermatology and Pediatrics
Mayo Clinic College of Medicine
Vascular Malformation Clinic
Department of Dermatology
Rochester, Minnesota

Aleksandra Tuleja
Inselspital, Bern University Hospital
Department of Angiology
Bern, Switzerland

Massimo Vaghi
Vascular Surgery Department
Ospedale Maggiore
Crema, Italy

Leonel Villavicencio
Department of Surgery
Uniformed Services University
School of Medicine
Bethesda, Maryland

Hendrik von Tengg-Kobligk
Department of Diagnostic, Interventional, and
   Pediatric Radiology
Inselspital, Bern University Hospital
University of Bern
Bern, Switzerland

Takumi Yamamoto
Department of Plastic and Reconstructive Surgery
Supermicrosurgery International Lymphedema
   Center (SILC)
National Center for Global Health and Medicine (NCGM)
Toyama, Japan

Xi Yang
Department of Plastic and Reconstructive Surgery
Shanghai Ninth People's Hospital
Shanghai Jiao Tong University School of Medicine
Shanghai, China

PART 1

Congenital Vascular Malformations (CVMs) in General

Definition and Classification

ISSVA classification: Controversy with the benefit and liability

RAUL MATTASSI

The classification of vascular anomalies of the International Society for the Study of Vascular Anomalies (ISSVA) was approved by the general assembly of the society during the 19th meeting in 2014 in Melbourne, Australia, and updated and approved in 2018 during the general assembly of the society in 2018 in Amsterdam, the Netherlands. This classification is the result of a main job of the French pathologist Michel Wassef, who tried to create a structural basis in which all the different types of vascular anomalies could be included.[1]

The classification has a multilevel structure with a main first step (an overview), which includes all the types of defects and many subgroups in which all the known anomalies are included. One of the main advantages of this classification is the possibility to add different new forms without changing the main base, as this topic is quickly evolving due to active research in the field (Figure 1.1).

One of the main updates of the classification, approved in Amsterdam, was the inclusion in the classification of the

ISSVA classification for vascular anomalies ©
(Approved at the 20th ISSVA Workshop, Melbourne, April 2014, last revision May 2018)

This classification is intended to evolve as our understanding of the biology and genetics
of vascular malformations and tumors continues to grow

Overview table

Vascular anomalies				
Vascular tumors	**Vascular malformations**			
	Simple	Combined °	of major named vessels	associated with other anomalies
Benign Locally aggressive or borderline Malignant	Capillary malformations Lymphatic malformations Venous malformations Arteriovenous malformations* Arteriovenous fistula*	CVM, CLM LVM, CLVM CAVM* CLAVM* others	See details	See list

° defined as two or more vascular malformations found in one lesion
* high-flow lesions

A list of causal genes and related vascular anomalies is available in Appendix 2

The tumor or malformation nature or precise classification of some lesions is still unclear. These lesions
appear in a separate provisional list.

Abbreviations used

For more details, click on
the underlined links

Figure 1.1 International Society for the Study of Vascular Anomalies classification, first overview table, last revision 2018. Available at www.issva.org—by clicking on the underlined links, additional tables open with all subgroups of vascular anomalies.

new genetic data. This rapidly developing field requires a continuous update that is easily possible with such a flexible classification.

To switch over to the new classification from the older one, however, was not quickly achieved by many doctors, as some aspects of the new one were not immediately understood. Old, eponym-/syndrome-based classifications (Klippel–Trenaunay/Parkes Weber syndromes and others) and hemodynamic-/flow-based classifications (fast flow/low flow) remain to cause significant confusion and failed to make a clear distinction between types of malformations (e.g., arteriovenous [AV] malformation and AV fistula).

The most accepted former classification was the Hamburg one (Belov, 1989), which has the advantage of simplicity, only dividing the different types of anomalies in main groups, rendering simple and clear a field that was confusing in the past.[2,3]

The Hamburg classification was an anatomopathological one, with a distinction between defects of the main vessels (truncular forms) and areas of dysplastic vessels in tissues (extra-truncular defects). The distinction is important because extra-truncular defects were considered areas of immature vessels (remnants of primitive vascular tissue) that may recur, while truncular forms may not. The issue is discussed in detail in Chapter 2.

Similar groups (truncular and extra-truncular) exist also in ISSVA classification however in different names. Truncular forms are denominated in ISSVA classification "defects of the main named vessels," an expression a little uncomfortable to use because of its length. Extra-truncular forms are named in ISSVA "simple forms," a term that may be misleading in case of extensive defects.

In the first/original version, ISSVA classification failed to distinguish clearly truncular lymphatic defects, which were included in the "simple" group, but this is now corrected through the latest version.

The general structure of this new updated version, however, is complex, due to the different tables (a total of 19) that cover all types of defects, including some forms that are still not clearly understood. Nevertheless, it can be managed simply by the basic classification on the first overview table (see Figure 1.1), which is roughly similar to the Hamburg classification, with only a new group, the association with other anomalies. To go more in detail, further tables and subclassifications can be consulted (Figure 1.1).

In conclusion, the ISSVA classification is the most modern and complete classification for vascular anomalies. For vascular malformations, it is based on the type of defect, like in the Hamburg classification. The step-by-step structure, from general overview to single groups, allows all known defects to be included and new knowledge to be adapted and expanded. Genetic data inclusion is a further progression.

REFERENCES

1. Wassef M, Blei F, Adams D et al. ISSVA Board and Scientific Committee. Vascular anomalies classification: Recommendations from the International Society for the Study of Vascular Anomalies. *Pediatrics.* 2015;136(1):e203–e214.
2. Belov St, Loose DA, Weber J. *Vascular Malformations.* Reinbeck: Einhorn Presse; 1989: 29 (Editor's comment, classification).
3. Belov St. Anatomopathological classification of congenital vascular defects. *Semin Vasc Surg.* 1993;6(4): 219–224.

Hamburg classification: Controversy with the benefit and liability

PETER GLOVICZKI AND DAVID J. DRISCOLL

Classifications are organized knowledge of a subject. As new information accumulates, updates or entirely new, powerful classifications emerge. The best classifications of diseases and disorders are not only all inclusive, but they also guide us in management.

Vascular malformations have been classified in many ways, some simply based on appearance of the lesions or resemblance to fruits, birds, fish, or insects. More complex classifications were arranged according to morphological features, embryological development, endothelial characteristics, and cell biology, hemodynamics, angiographic appearance, or genetics.[1-7] The classification from the International Society for the Study of Vascular Anomalies (ISSVA) was approved at the 20th ISSVA Workshop in Melbourne, Australia, in 2014 and updated in 2018.[8,9] As presented in Chapter 1, the updated ISSVA classification has been gaining traction, particularly because of major recent progress in genetics. It is used frequently now by scientists and physicians worldwide, since this complex classification, based on anatomy, embryology, and genetics, is helpful in management, particularly when deciding on drug therapy based on genetic information.

The Hamburg classification has had an established role in the classification of vascular malformations; it is simple and easier for clinicians for everyday use than the continuously enlarging, updated, and all-inclusive ISSVA classification with over 120 types of vascular anomalies listed now in 13 tables.[9] Using the updated Hamburg classification, physicians can make rapid assessments of the type and extent of the malformation, which is particularly helpful in selecting interventions for management. Clinical practice guidelines of the International Union of Phlebology,[10] the International Union of Angiology,[11] the Italian Society for Vascular Investigation,[11] the American Venous Forum,[3] and the European Society for Vascular Surgery all recommend at present using the modified Hamburg classification of vascular malformations.[12]

MODIFIED HAMBURG CLASSIFICATION

The Hamburg classification was developed under the leadership of Belov, Loose, and Weber during the seventh Meeting of the International Workshop on Vascular Malformations in Hamburg in 1988.[13] The group working on vascular malformations was formed earlier by Mulliken during their first meeting in Boston, Massachusetts, in 1976. The classification was updated in Seoul, Korea, in 1995, and the currently used modified Hamburg Classification was published in the 2013 Consensus Document of the International Union of Phlebology, by Lee and others.[10] The modified Hamburg classification is primarily an anatomic classification, with an embryological subclassification.

Primary anatomic classification

The primary anatomic classification distinguishes the subgroups based on predominant anatomy. Although the original classification did not include all segments of the circulatory system, in the new, updated classification, the anatomical subclasses are all inclusive, and arterial, venous, arteriovenous, capillary, lymphatic, and mixed vascular malformations are distinguished (Table 2.1). Parts 2, 3, 4, and 6 of this book discuss in detail each anatomic class. Over 70% of the vascular malformations are mixed, and these frequently complex abnormalities may include capillary, venous, arteriovenous, or lymphatic elements. Although the Hamburg classification discourages the use of eponyms, many have been widely accepted and used. The list of some of the clinical syndromes with vascular malformations includes Klippel–Trenaunay (Figure 2.1a through c), Parkes Weber, Servelle–Martorell, Sturge–Weber, Rendu–Osler–Weber, von Hippel–Lindau, Kasabach–Merritt, Proteus, and Maffucci syndromes, among others. Syndromic classifications are presented in detail in Chapter 3 and in Part 5 of this book.

Table 2.1 Modified Hamburg classification of congenital vascular malformations

A. Anatomical classification (predominant vascular bed)
- Arterial malformation
- Venous malformation
- Arteriovenous malformation
- Lymphatic malformation
- Capillary malformation
- Combined vascular malformation

B. Embryological subclassification
1. Extra-truncular forms
   - Infiltrating, diffuse
   - Limited, localized
2. Truncular forms
   - Obstruction (occlusion or stenosis)
     - Agenesis
     - Aplasia
     - Hypoplasia
     - Coarctation
     - Hyperplasia
     - Membranous obstruction
     - Congenital spur
   - Dilatation
     - Aneurysm (localized)
     - Ectasia (diffuse)
   - Persistence of embryonic vessels
   - Anomalies of the origin, course, number, and length of major vessels
   - Anomalies of venous valves
   - Abnormal arteriovenous communication of truncal vessels

Source: Adapted from Lee BB et al. *Int Angiol.* 2015;34:97–149.

Embryological subclassification

Vascular malformations are developmental, congenital abnormalities due to inherited or somatic mutations and activated or inhibited signaling pathways.[14] Aberrant signaling at the molecular level results in dysfunction of normal proliferation, differentiation, maturation, and apoptosis of the vascular cells. The persistence of the primitive embryonic vascular system and/or abnormal cell developments result in vascular malformations. Embryological subclassification, therefore, is of utmost importance, since clinical presentation, complications, treatment, and prognosis of the malformations depend to a great extent on when an arrest or abnormality occurred during the development of the vascular system.

During development, the primitive vascular channels first appear in the embryo in the third week of gestation. Woollard defined three stages in the development of the vascular system:[15] Stage 1 is the *undifferentiated* stage when only a capillary network, a collection of primitive vascular channels, is present. Stage 2 is the *retiform* stage when large plexiform structures are seen, while stage 3, the *maturation* stage, includes development of distinct large channels, named *arteries* and *veins*. The embryological subclassification of the Hamburg classification distinguishes two major groups based on the stages when abnormality in the development of the vascular system occurs.[16] Differentiation of the malformations into the subgroups of *truncular* and *extra-truncular* forms is helpful for establishing the diagnosis, predicting the prognosis, and selecting an intervention, if needed, to treat the vascular lesions.

Extra-truncular malformations are the result of an arrest or a defect in the vascular development either in the *undifferentiated* or in the *retiform* stages. The term *extra-truncular* was coined by Belov et al. to distinguish malformations from angiomas, which are vascular tumors.[13] Extra-truncular lesions are embryonic tissue remnants of mesodermal origin that retain the characteristics of the mesenchymal cells (angioblasts).[7] Microfistulous or macrofistulous *extra-truncular* arteriovenous malformations develop if there is an arrest in stage 2. The *extra-truncular* forms can be diffuse (Figure 2.2a and b) or localized. It is likely that these malformations retain their potential to grow and proliferate when stimulated by menarche, pregnancy, hormones, trauma, or surgery.[7]

Truncular malformations occur due to a defect that occurs later in development, in stage 3, the *maturation* stage. Truncular lesions affect major vascular channels, frequently named *arteries* or *veins*, and no longer exhibit the evolutional potential to grow.[5] Their hemodynamic effects can be significant. These can be persistent embryonic vessels or congenital defects or lesions affecting normal vessel development, presenting with obstruction due to aplasia, hypoplasia, or sometimes hyperplasia or with stenosis due to coarctation, membranous occlusion/stenosis, or congenital spurs. The wall of truncular lesions is frequently weak, causing localized dilations and frank aneurysms. Diffuse dilations present as ectasia, mega-arteries, or veins. A persistent sciatic artery or a persistent sciatic vein is a truncal malformation and so is a persistent lateral embryonic vein, frequently seen in patients with Klippel–Trenaunay syndrome (Figure 2.1).[17–19] These also include arterial malformations like an aberrant left subclavian artery that runs behind the esophagus and causes dysphagia lusoria. Thoracic or abdominal aortic coarctations,[20] anomalies of the aortic arch, or persistence of embryonic mesenteric vessels, are additional examples.

Hemodynamic and angiographic classifications

Although not part of the updated Hamburg classification, it is important to note that vascular malformations are also classified based on hemodynamics and contrast angiographic appearance. Depending on the amount of blood supplying the malformation, *high-flow* and *low-flow* lesions are distinguished in a new, integrated classification proposed by Lee et al. and endorsed by Shortell and Nevidomskyte.[10,21] Arterial and arteriovenous malformations are high-flow lesions, while capillary, venous, and lymphatic malformations

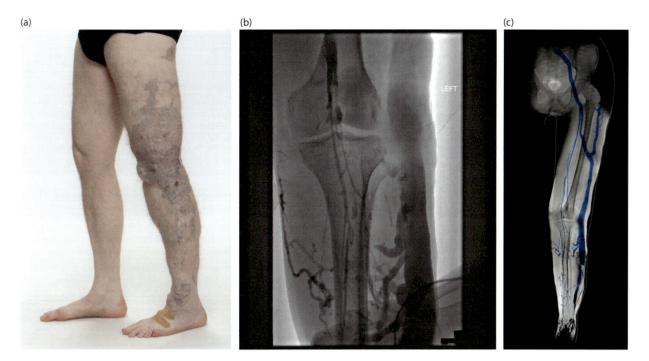

Figure 2.1 **(a)** Thirty-five-year-old male with advanced symptomatic Klippel–Trenaunay syndrome, presenting with a larger and longer left lower extremity, phlebo-lymphedema, extensive capillary malformation, and atypical lateral varicosity with a persistent lateral embryonic vein. **(b)** Venogram shows the huge persistent lateral embryonic vein and a patent, although diminutive deep venous system. **(c)** Venogram of the entire leg and pelvis. (From Rathore A et al. *J Vasc Surg Venous Lymphat Disord*. 2018;6:523–525.)

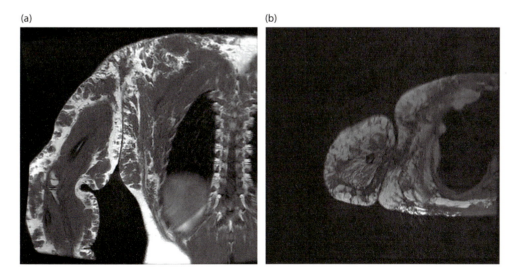

Figure 2.2 Nine-year-old male patient with extra-truncular venous malformation of the right arm, neck, and chest. **(a)** Coronal and **(b)** axial T2-weighted magnetic resonance imaging showing the diffuse low-flow malformation.

are low-flow lesions. The integrated classification is useful to facilitate effective diagnosis and interventional treatment, although it lacks classification of the genetic mutations that occur in vascular malformations.

The angiographic classification of arteriovenous malformations is discussed in detail in Chapter 13. This classification focuses on nidus morphology of arteriovenous malformations, on the number of feeding arteries and draining veins, and on the number of shunts in the lesion, and it is extremely helpful in planning interventional treatment, particularly embolization of these lesions.

CONCLUSIONS

The modified Hamburg classification is an anatomical and embryological classification of vascular malformations that is user friendly, simplified, and enables physicians to make rapid assessment of the type and extent of the malformation that is helpful for management. The classification lacks a genetic basis, but it is particularly useful for selecting interventional treatment. With progress in genetic research and the advent of effective drug therapy of vascular malformations, most elements of the Hamburg classification together with a genetic classification have been incorporated into the complex, all-inclusive ISSVA classification. Controversy over which classification should be used continues, but the benefits of a physician-friendly simple classification for everyday clinical use outweigh the liability that this classification is not all inclusive. The last chapter in the classification of vascular malformations, however, has not been written yet, since new genetic information is rapidly accumulating, new malformations are being described, and new, effective, minimally invasive, catheter-based therapies and drug treatments are introduced with increasing frequency.

REFERENCES

1. Mulliken JB, Glowacki J. Hemangiomas and vascular malformations in infants and children: A classification based on endothelial characteristics. *Plast Reconstr Surg.* 1982;69:412–422.
2. Rutherford RB. Congenital vascular defects or malformations (CVMs). *Semin Vasc Surg.* 1993;6:197–198.
3. Markovic J, Shortell C. The management of venous malformations. In: Gloviczki P, ed. *Handbook of Venous and Lymphatic Disorders.* 4th ed. London, UK: CRC Press, Taylor & Francis Group; 2017:663–673.
4. Puig S, Casati B, Staudenherz A, Paya K. Vascular low-flow malformations in children: Current concepts for classification, diagnosis and therapy. *Eur J Radiol.* 2005;53:35–45.
5. Lee BB, Laredo J. Classification of congenital vascular malformations: The last challenge for congenital vascular malformations. *Phlebology.* 2012;27:267–269.
6. Gloviczki P, Duncan A, Kalra M et al. Vascular malformations: An update. *Perspect Vasc Surg Endovasc Ther.* 2009;21:133–148.
7. Lee BB, Laredo J, Lee TS, Huh S, Neville R. Terminology and classification of congenital vascular malformations. *Phlebology.* 2007;22:249–252.
8. Wassef M, Blei F, Adams D et al. Vascular anomalies classification: Recommendations from the International Society for the Study of Vascular Anomalies. *Pediatrics.* 2015;136:e203–e214.
9. ISSVA classification for vascular anomalies. 2018. https://www.issva.org/UserFiles/file/ISSVA-Classification-2018.pdf. Accessed May 12, 2019.
10. Lee BB, Baumgartner I, Berlien P et al. Diagnosis and treatment of venous malformations. Consensus Document of the International Union of Phlebology (IUP): Updated 2013. *Int Angiol.* 2015;34:97–149.
11. Lee BB, Antignani PL, Baraldini V et al. ISVI-IUA consensus document diagnostic guidelines of vascular anomalies: Vascular malformations and hemangiomas. *Int Angiol.* 2015;34:333–374.
12. Wittens C, Davies AH, Baekgaard N et al. Editor's choice—Management of chronic venous disease: Clinical practice guidelines of the European Society for Vascular Surgery (ESVS). *Eur J Vasc Endovasc Surg.* 2015;49:678–737.
13. Belov S, Loose DA, Weber J. *Vascular Malformations.* Reinbek, Germany: Einhorn-Presse Verlag; 1989.
14. Queisser A, Boon LM, Vikkula M. Etiology and genetics of congenital vascular lesions. *Otolaryngol Clin North Am.* 2018;51:41–53.
15. Gloviczki P. Venous vascular malformations. In: Moore WS, Lawrence PF, Oderich GS, ed. *Vascular and Endovascular Surgery: A Comprehensive Review.* Philadelphia, PA: Elsevier; 2019:146–156.
16. Belov S. Anatomopathological classification of congenital vascular defects. *Semin Vasc Surg.* 1993;6:219–224.
17. Noel AA, Gloviczki P, Cherry KJ, Jr., Rooke TW, Stanson AW, Driscoll DJ. Surgical treatment of venous malformations in Klippel–Trenaunay syndrome. *J Vasc Surg.* 2000;32:840–847.
18. Rathore A, Gloviczki P, Bjarnason H. Management of giant embryonic vein in Klippel–Trenaunay syndrome. *J Vasc Surg Venous Lymphat Disord.* 2018;6:523–525.
19. Malgor RD, Gloviczki P, Fahrni J et al. Surgical treatment of varicose veins and venous malformations in Klippel–Trenaunay syndrome. *Phlebology.* 2016;31:209–215.
20. West CA, Delis KT, Service GJ, Driscoll DJ, McPhail IR, Gloviczki P. Middle aortic syndrome: Surgical treatment in a child with neurofibromatosis. *J Vasc Surg.* 2005;42:1236.
21. Shortell CK, Nevidomskyte D. Congenital arterial malformations. In: Moore WS, Lawrence PF, Oderich GS, ed. *Vascular and Endovascular Surgery: A Comprehensive Review.* Philadelphia, PA: Elsevier; 2019:157–171.

3

Syndromic classification of congenital vascular malformations: How useful is it?

FRANCINE BLEI

Vascular malformations are often misdiagnosed and not generally understood by members of the medical community who do not focus their practices on these disorders. Classification of medical conditions in general affords a framework for more precise diagnoses and management. Syndromes represent clusters of clinical findings. Patients may have mild ("forme fruste") or more elaborate degrees of syndromic expression. Awareness of the components of vascular anomalies syndromes is extremely important when discussing potential complications, presenting realistic precautions and expectations, and considering treatment planning. Syndromic classification provides this framework, which now includes genetic information. As discussed in chapters reviewing genetics (see Chapters 7, 8, and 10), many disorders associated with congenital vascular malformations are not isolated to the blood and/or lymphatic vessels.

Syndromes with vascular malformations can either be (1) syndromes with a vascular malformation as the *predominant* component or (2) syndromes that incidentally have a vascular malformation as one of many constituents of the syndrome.

WHAT IS A SYNDROME, AND WHY DOES IT MATTER?

It is important to first clarify the definition of a syndrome. The traditional definition is "a group of symptoms that consistently occur together, or a condition characterized by a set of associated symptoms" or "a combination of symptoms and signs that together represent a disease process." The word *syndrome* is derived from the Greek *sundromē* (the prefix *sun* ["together"] and the root *dramein* ["to run"]) or "concurrence."

One must possess the clinical acumen to identify phenotypic and genetic features of syndromic conditions, i.e., family history and inheritance pattern, so the appropriate evaluation, management decisions, and possible genetic

studies and counseling can ensue (Table 3.1). This entails examining the entire patient, taking a meticulous history, imaging, and being aware of the constellation of clinical features typifying each of the known syndromes. In fact, novel syndromes have been identified due to the recognition of clinical patterns, and often dedicated workshops focus on establishing criteria/definitions of specific syndromes.[1–3] It is worth emphasizing that evaluation of these patients needs to be performed in a multidisciplinary setting.

In addition to the vascular malformations, there may be coexisting, underlying disorders (i.e., renal, skeletal, cardiac, ophthalmologic, neurological, gastrointestinal, cutaneous, or other abnormalities) in these patients (Table 3.2). The International Society for the Study of Vascular Anomalies (ISSVA) classification is a useful tool for categorizing

Table 3.1 What is a syndrome, and why does it matter?

- Known associated constellation of clinical findings
- Helps guide *appropriate evaluation* and *referral* to proper specialists
- Allows for *proactive approach*—what to expect, how to avoid "surprises"
- May be associated with a *genetic mutation*

Table 3.2 Questions aiding diagnoses of vascular anomaly syndromes

Are there skeletal abnormalities—polydactyly, syndactyly of fingers or toes?
Is the head disproportionately large or small?
Are any other organs abnormally developed (e.g., brain, heart, kidneys, eyes)?
Are there any skin abnormalities (tan spots, flat pink/red lesions, small raised bumps, lipomas)?
Does anyone in the family have the previous symptoms or symptoms similar to the patient?

Table 3.3 Clinical criteria and genetic mutation associated with vascular anomaly syndromes

Syndrome	Components	Mutation
Klippel–Trenaunay syndrome[a]	CM + VM + LM + limb overgrowth	PIK3CA
Parkes Weber syndrome	CM + AVF + limb overgrowth	RASA1
Servelle–Martorell syndrome	Limb VM + bone undergrowth	
Sturge–Weber syndrome	Facial + leptomeningeal CM (leading to seizures) + eye anomalies (leading to glaucoma) ± bone and/or soft tissue overgrowth	GNAQ
Limb capillary malformation and congenital nonprogressive limb growth		GNA11
Maffucci syndrome	VM ± spindle-cell "hemangioma" + enchondroma	IDHH1/IDH2
Macrocephaly-capillary malformation (MCAP/M-CM)[a]		PIK3CA
Microcephaly capillary malformation (MICCAP)		STAMPBP
CLOVES syndrome[a]	LM + VM + CM ± AVM + lipomatous overgrowth	PIK3CA
Proteus syndrome	CM, VM and/or LM + asymmetrical somatic overgrowth	AKT1
Bannayan–Riley–Ruvalcaba syndrome	AVM + VM + macrocephaly, lipomatous overgrowth, malignancies, trichilemmomas	PTEN
CLAPO syndrome[a]	Lower lip CM + face and neck LM + asymmetry and partial/generalized overgrowth	PIK3CA
Blue rubber bleb nevus (Bean) syndrome	Multifocal venolymphatic malformations	PTEK (Tie2)
Capillary malformation/AVM	CM-AVM − cutaneous + CNS/spine AVM	RASA1, EPHB4
Gorham syndrome	LM + osteolysis	
Heritable lymphedema syndromes	Various	Many

Abbreviations: AVM, arteriovenous malformation; CM, capillary malformation; CNS, central nervous system; LM, lymphatic malformation; VM, venous malformation.

[a] These lesions belong to the *PIK3CA*-related overgrowth spectrum (PROS).

vascular anomalies, and some syndromes are included in this categorization.[4,5] Interestingly, there are some disorders (e.g., hereditary hemorrhagic telangiectasia), which may indeed be syndromes, yet "syndrome" is not in their nomenclature.

Syndromes may be heritable, in which case genomic mutations can be identified, as discussed in Chapter 10. Identification of a causative mutation in these cases enables the opportunity to screen family members and offer prenatal testing—amniocentesis/chorionic villus sampling in female patients and/or preimplantation genetic testing. Nonheritable syndromes may have somatic mutations identified in affected tissue. Genetic information may be necessary to establish eligibility for novel pharmacological therapeutic protocols. However, there is lack of clarity, even in the ISSVA classification, as to which diagnoses are truly syndromes. Nonetheless, awareness of the phenotypic expression of syndromic vascular anomalies remains an important aspect in the field.[2,6–9]

Table 3.3 lists many vascular anomaly syndromes, their clinical criteria, and associated genetic mutation(s), when known. Many postzygotic somatic mutations in vascular anomaly–related growth disorders are involved in the receptor tyrosine kinase and phosphatidylinositol 3-kinase (PI3K)/Akt/mTOR signaling pathways.[1,9–11] Tables 3.4 and

3.5 delineate *PIK3CA*-related overgrowth spectrum (PROS) disorders, which represent heterogeneous segmental overgrowth phenotypes, the majority of which have vascular anomalies and somatic *PIK3CA* activating mutations.[1,12]

The utility of characterizing the accurate phenotype and genotype translates into target effective therapies, as demonstrated by the study by Venot et al., whereby a *PIK3CA* inhibitor improved several clinical parameters in treated animals and patients.[13]

Table 3.4 *PIK3CA*-related overgrowth spectrum (PROS) disorders

- Fibroadipose hyperplasia or overgrowth (FAQ)
- Hemihyperplasia multiple lipomatosis (HHML)
- Congenital lipomatous overgrowth, vascular malformations, epidermal nevi, scoliosis/skeletal and spinal (CLOVES) syndrome
- Macrodactyly
- Fibroadipose infiltrating lipomatosis/facial infiltrative lipomatosis
- Megalencephaly-capillary malformation (MCAP or M-CM)
- Dysplastic megalencephaly (DMEG)
- Klippel–Trenaunay syndrome

Table 3.5 *PIK3CA*-related overgrowth spectrum (PROS) disorders—Diagnostic criteria

Required criteria:

Presence of somatic *PIK3CA* mutation (if mutation cannot be defined, categorized as presumptive PROS disorder)

Congenital or early childhood onset

Sporadic, without family history, mosaic distribution

One or more findings from category A or B

A. Spectrum (two or more features)

Overgrowth: Adipose, muscle, nerve, skeletal

Vascular malformations: Capillary, venous, arteriovenous malformation, lymphatic

Epidermal nevus

B. Isolated features

Large isolated lymphatic malformation

Isolated macrodactyly or overgrown splayed feet/hands, overgrown limbs

Truncal adipose overgrowth

Hemimegalencephaly (bilateral)/dysplastic megalencephaly/focal cortical dysplasia

Epidermal nevus

Seborrheic keratoses

Benign seborrheic keratoses

Source: From Keppler-Noreuil KM et al. *Am J Med Genet A.* 2015;167A(2):287–295.

REFERENCES

1. Keppler-Noreuil KM, Rios JJ, Parker VE et al. *PIK3CA*-related overgrowth spectrum (PROS): Diagnostic and testing eligibility criteria, differential diagnosis, and evaluation. *Am J Med Genet A.* 2015;167A(2):287–295.
2. Happle R. Lethal genes surviving by mosaicism: A possible explanation for sporadic birth defects involving the skin. *J Am Acad Dermatol.* 1987;16(4):899–906.
3. Jones GE, Mansour S. An approach to familial lymphoedema. *Clin Med (Lond).* 2017;17(6):552–557.
4. Wassef M, Blei F, Adams D et al. Vascular anomalies classification: Recommendations from the International Society for the Study of Vascular Anomalies. *Pediatrics.* 2015;136(1):e203–e214.
5. International Society for the Study of Vascular Anomalies (ISSVA). ISSVA classification for vascular anomalies, April 2014, last revision May 2018. http://www.issva.org/UserFiles/file/ISSVA-Classification-2018.pdf.
6. Frank SA. Somatic mosaicism and disease. *Curr Biol.* 2014;24(12):R577–R581.
7. Spinner NB, Conlin LK. Mosaicism and clinical genetics. *Am J Med Genet C Semin Med Genet.* 2014;166C(4):397–405.
8. Mitchell CB, Phillips WA. Mouse models for exploring the biological consequences and clinical significance of *PIK3CA* mutations. *Biomolecules.* 2019;9(4):158.
9. Zuniga-Castillo M, Teng CL, Teng JMC. Genetics of vascular malformation and therapeutic implications. *Curr Opin Pediatr.* 2019;31(4):498–508.
10. Kang HC, Baek ST, Song S, Gleeson JG. Clinical and genetic aspects of the segmental overgrowth spectrum due to somatic mutations in *PIK3CA*. *J Pediatr.* 2015;167(5):957–962.
11. Vahidnezhad H, Youssefian L, Uitto J. Molecular genetics of the PI3K-AKT-mTOR pathway in genodermatoses: Diagnostic implications and treatment opportunities. *J Invest Dermatol.* 2016;136(1):15–23.
12. Bezniakow N, Gos M, Obersztyn E. The RASopathies as an example of RAS/MAPK pathway disturbances—Clinical presentation and molecular pathogenesis of selected syndromes. *Dev Period Med.* 2014;18(3):285–296.
13. Venot Q, Blanc T, Rabia SH et al. Targeted therapy in patients with *PIK3CA*-related overgrowth syndrome. *Nature.* 2018;558(7711):540–546.

4

Consensus on contemporary classification

BYUNG-BOONG LEE AND LEONEL VILLAVICENCIO

GENERAL CONSIDERATION

Through the last half-century, advanced diagnostic technology and therapeutic modalities (e.g., embolo-/sclerotherapy) based on a rapidly expanding medical technology provided crucial information for gaining a better understanding of congenital vascular malformations (CVMs). They are inborn disorders involving the arterial, venous, lymphatic, and/or capillary system. Based on all new information, a contemporary concept and classification of the CVMs were established.[1-4]

Following the workshop held in Hamburg in 1988, two new classifications emerged to help precise evaluation, diagnosis, and therapy of CVMs. These replaced the old name-based eponyms/classifications.[4,5] The first classification was limited to the CVMs, later named the Hamburg classification;[6,7] the second classification was for vascular anomalies to accommodate both the CVMs and vascular tumors/hemangiomas, subsequently adopted by the International Society for the Study of Vascular Anomalies (ISSVA) as their official classification.[8,9]

The ISSVA classification provides a comprehensive picture of vascular malformations and vascular tumors together under one umbrella of "vascular anomalies,"[1-4,8,9] in addition to the flow-based classification of the CVMs. This new classification was a major contribution through clear differentiation between the vascular tumors/hemangiomas and the CVMs.

The Hamburg classification defined two distinctively different groups of the CVM lesions, initially based on the morphological as well as anatomical differences: one group of the lesions involving the main vessel trunks, named *truncular* lesion, and another group with no direct involvement of the vessel trunk remaining independently as a cluster of amorphous vascular structures, named *extra-truncular* lesions.[10,11]

The truncular lesion represents the outcome of defective development during the vascular trunk formation period along the *later* stage of embryogenesis. The extra-truncular lesion is the embryonic tissue remnant following the developmental arrest during the reticular/plexiform network stage while the primitive vascular structures are still in the "undifferentiated capillary network so that it would keep such unique condition of the growth."[12,13] This new term *extra-truncular*, previously called *angioma*, cleared decades-long confusion caused often by the misleading terms *angioma* versus *hemangioma*.

The Hamburg classification extended its original scope of the classification based on morphological concepts/differences of the CVMs further to accommodate a new embryological concept with the two stages of embryogenesis;[14,15] it interprets the critical difference between two morphologically as well as functionally different truncular and extra-truncular lesions based on different embryological characteristics depending on the embryological stages when the developmental arrests occurred.[16,17]

The extra-truncular lesion following developmental arrest in its "early" stage of embryogenesis continues to possess unique mesenchymal cell characteristics with the growth tendency when the condition is met with proper stimulation. High recurrence rates as the trademark of all CVMs following treatment are due to this unique embryological characteristic of the embryonic tissue remnants derived from an early stage of embryogenesis.[18,19]

The totally unpredictable behavior of the extra-truncular lesions is now correctly interpreted based on their unique embryonic characteristics, and over the last three decades this new embryological concept/interpretation has critically contributed to the management of "recurrence" risk with much better vision throughout the decades.[1-4]

While the Hamburg classification is based on morphological characteristics, the ISSVA classification adopted a new classification of the CVMs based on flow characteristics, fast-flow and slow-flow lesions,[8,9,20,21] and further subclassified the arteriovenous malformation (AVM) to AV fistula (AVF) and AV malformation to recognize two morphologically and functionally different groups of AVMs.[8,9]

However, the AVF and AVM are both the same AVMs, but they originate from two different stages of embryogenesis; both have the same (AV) fistulous condition, and the only difference between them is the morphological differences existing either with the nidus or without the nidus as the outcome of developmental arrests in two different stages of embryogenesis.

Due to the ISSVA classification of the AVM to AVF and AVM, many physicians remain confused, erroneously interpreting that there are two different AVMs; AVF as a fistulous lesion and AVM as a nonfistulous lesion. But all the AVM lesions are "fistulous" lesions by definition to allow for AV shunting either *directly* between the arterial and venous system as the outcome of defective development in the *later* stage of embryogenesis or *indirectly* through dysplastic capillary structure as the outcome of defects during the *earlier* reticular stage of the embryogenesis, known as "nidus."[2,3,22]

Hence, the "AVF" lesion of ISSVA classification is the same as the "truncular" AVM lesion of the Hamburg classification with *no* nidus (e.g., ductus Botalli, pulmonary AVM), while the "AVM" lesion of the ISSVA classification is also the same as the extra-truncular AVM lesion of the Hamburg classification with nidus.[4,22]

The ISSVA classification has been widely modified throughout the years, and the last versions adopted the new term *malformations* to designate lesions equivalent to the extra-truncular lesions of the Hamburg classification, and "malformations of major named vessels" to the lesions equivalent to the "truncular" one.[21,23]

Nevertheless, the ISSVA classification still holds most of the old name-based eponyms/classifications through its syndromic classification of the CVMs, despite strong advocation by many experts to abolish them to reduce unnecessary confusion and keep the original principles/concepts held through the Hamburg consensus workshop of 1988. Such "name-based" syndromes as part of the CVM classification remain, with substantial confusion regarding the clinical implementation of CVM management together with the complexity of the classification.[2,4,22]

SYNDROME-BASED CLASSIFICATION

Throughout the last century, name-based syndromes were inevitable outcomes/dividends of the descriptions of the vascular malformations based solely on clinical observations/findings, with insufficient knowledge; these syndromes were often named after the physicians credited for first reporting them.

Vascular malformation, however, presents not only with great variability and various combinations among many different types, often involving more than one type of CVM, but also with a variety of underlying diseases as well as systemic nonvascular abnormalities.[1–4]

Hence, with the lack of proper diagnostic tools early in the last century, many are confused, giving different names to similar if not the same conditions/diseases or giving the same name to different diseases. Therefore, correct understanding of the vascular malformation components in these name-based syndromes is necessary for the safe management of syndromic CVMs together with their secondary outcome involving the affected organs/systems (e.g., gastrointestinal [GI] bleeding).[24,25]

Exclusive use of these eponyms (e.g., Klippel–Trenaunay syndrome) alone would lead to incorrect identification of its vascular malformation components. Therefore, the eponyms should be used along with precise diagnostic information of each involved CVM lesion based on modern laboratory tests to help properly understand the syndrome in order to develop a rational management strategy.

Every syndrome, therefore, has to be described precisely by its vascular malformation components as well as nonvascular malformation components together with their active and passive clinical problems involved. And proper assessment is warranted for the secondary effects of the primary pathology to the various systems: GI system (e.g., GI bleeding, chylous ascites, malabsorption syndrome); cardiopulmonary system (e.g., pleural effusion, chylothorax); musculoskeletal system (e.g., long bone length discrepancy, joint involvement, scoliosis, pelvis tilt); and genitourinary system (e.g., lymph leak: chyluria, chylorrhagia).[1–4]

GENETIC PROSPECT OF CLASSIFICATION

Increased knowledge of the genetic mutations involved in vascular malformation pathogenesis has brought substantial improvements in the understanding of the relationship between vessel embryology and genetic mutations affecting vessel development. Although further studies are necessary for better understanding these genetic mechanisms, recent genetic theory explains such a tendency for growth with the gene mutations within the tissues based on newly identified causative genes.[1,3,5]

Recent data from genetic studies show the regulatory genes of vasculogenesis and angiogenesis (TIE-2/PDGFB) play an important role in the development of the extra-truncular type of venous malformations;[1,26] further, we can speculate that the genes involved in stages of angiogenesis will have an important role in the pathogenesis of "truncular" vascular malformations following the stage of mesenchymal cell maturation.

Currently available genetic data are not yet sufficient to draw a conclusive determination of the exact underlying genetic and molecular mechanisms responsible for differentiation between truncular and extra-truncular lesions. Although localized genetic defects seem to play a critical role in the pathophysiology of the CVMs,[27] the exact pathophysiological and genetic mechanism responsible for the development of both truncular and extra-truncular subtypes remains to be clarified.

However, the Hamburg classification based on their morphology with different anatomical and pathological characteristics as well as the process of vasculogenesis will remain the same regardless of the genetic mutation, although it may affect the process.[1,4]

Hence, there is an increasing consensus on the need for discussion of further subclassification of CVMs according

Table 4.1 Congenital vascular malformation (CVM) integrated classification system

Congenital vascular malformations					
Low flow			**High flow**		
Venous (VM)	Extra-truncular	Diffuse/infiltrating	Arterial (AM)	Extra-truncular	Diffuse/infiltrating
		Localized			Localized
	Truncular	Obstruction/narrowing		Truncular	Obstruction/narrowing
		Dilatation			Dilatation
Lymphatic (LM)	Extra-truncular	Diffuse/infiltrating	Arteriovenous (AVM)	Extra-truncular	Diffuse/infiltrating
		Localized			Localized
	Truncular	Obstruction/narrowing		Truncular	Obstruction/narrowing
		Dilatation			Dilatation
Capillary (CM)					
Combined					
Syndrome associated			Syndrome associated		

Source: Cited from Lee BB et al. Int Angiol. 2015;34(2):97–149.

to the stage of abnormal embryogenesis and shifting of the focus to the role of genetic defects in determining the characteristics of CVMs and their syndromes.[27]

INTEGRATED CLASSIFICATION SYSTEM: NEW CONSIDERATION

Two new classifications have successfully replaced the old classification of the CVMs with the name-/syndrome-based concept and have become the new guidelines for contemporary management of CVMs. Although there are substantial differences between the two classifications, both are mutually complementary, one with embryological criteria and the other with hemodynamic criteria for CVMs. Many clinicians use parts of both classification systems together.[1–4]

These advanced classification systems provide critical information on accurate diagnosis, treatment, and prognosis of CVMs.[28] The clinicians now can predict the clinical course and response to treatment of CVMs quite accurately by properly understanding the vascular embryology of CVMs based on pathophysiology depending in large part on the embryogenesis of the vasculature.

Recent advances in diagnostic imaging technologies and treatment modalities of CVMs helped form a better understanding of the pathophysiology as well as the embryology combined with genetics, only to confirm that the current classification is far from being perfect and mandates further modification as our knowledge of the CVMs continues to grow (e.g., hemodynamics and genetics).

In addition, the relatively new concept of the multidisciplinary team approach based on full integration of different medical specialists confirmed the urgent need for a *unified* classification system to fully integrate two different classification systems for the contemporary management of CVMs.

The integrated classification system (Table 4.1), proposed through the International Union of Phlebology (IUP) commissioned consensus for venous malformation 2013,[1] has a prospective value of the utilization as the basis for the diagnostic protocols and therapeutic algorithms for the CVMs. It would allow for a streamlined evaluation process as well as facilitated communications among caretakers using the same language and would deliver fully integrated multimodality treatment, open surgical and endovascular, with no further confusion on the treatment options.[1–4]

To facilitate a streamlined approach, we recommend upholding the terms *low flow* and *high flow* rather than using *slow flow* and *fast flow*, respectively, when flow patterns of CVMs are described. Multiple terms to describe identical hemodynamic characteristics in the same lesion with two mutually exclusive hemodynamic statuses only add to the risk of misinterpretation.

REFERENCES

1. Lee BB, Baumgartner I, Berlien P et al. Diagnosis and treatment of venous malformations consensus document of the International Union of Phlebology (IUP): Updated 2013. Int Angiol. 2015;34(2):97–149.
2. Lee BB, Baumgartner I, Berlien HP et al. Consensus document of the International Union of Angiology (IUA)-2013. Current concept on the management of arterio-venous management. Int Angiol. 2013;32(1): 9–36.
3. Lee BB, Antignani PL, Baraldini V et al. ISVI-IUA consensus document—Diagnostic guidelines on vascular anomalies: Vascular malformations and hemangiomas. Int Angiol. 2015;34(4):333–374.
4. Lee BB. New classification of congenital vascular malformations (CVMs). Rev Vasc Med. 2015;3(3):1–5.

5. Lee BB, Laredo J. Classification of congenital vascular malformations: The last challenge for congenital vascular malformations. *Phlebology*. 2012;27(6):267–269.

6. Belov S. Classification of congenital vascular defects. *Int Angiol*. 1990;9:141–146.

7. Belov St. Anatomopathological classification of congenital vascular defects. *Semin Vasc Surg*. 1993;6:219–224.

8. Enjolras O, Wassef M, Chapot R. Introduction: ISSVA classification. In: Enjolras O, Wassef M, Chapot R, eds. *Color Atlas of Vascular Tumors and Vascular Malformations*. New York, NY: Cambridge University Press; 2007:1–11.

9. Mulliken JB. Classification of vascular birthmarks. In: Mulliken JB, Young AE, eds. *Vascular Birthmarks: Hemangiomas and Malformations*. Philadelphia, PA: WB Saunders; 1988:24–37.

10. Lee BB, Laredo J. Venous malformation: Treatment needs a bird's eye view. *Phlebology*. 2013;28:62–63.

11. Lee BB. All congenital vascular malformations should belong to one of two types: "Truncular" or "extra-truncular", as different as apples and oranges! [Editorial]. *Phlebological Rev*. 2015;23(1):1–3.

12. Bastide G, Lefebvre D. Anatomy and organogenesis and vascular malformations. In: Belov St, Loose DA, Weber J, eds. *Vascular Malformations*. Reinbek, Germany: Einhorn-Presse Verlag GmbH; 1989:20–22.

13. Woollard RH. The development of the principal arterial stems in the forelimb of the pig. *Contrib Embryol*. 1922;14:139–154.

14. Lee BB, Laredo J, Lee TS, Huh S, Neville R. Terminology and classification of congenital vascular malformations. *Phlebology*. 2007;22(6):249–252.

15. Leu HJ. Pathoanatomy of congenital vascular malformations. In: Belov S, Loose DA, Weber J, eds. *Vascular Malformations*. vol 16. Reinbek, Germany: Einhorn-Presse Verlag; 1989:37–46.

16. Van Der Stricht J. Classification of vascular malformations. In: Belov St, Loose DA, Weber J, eds. *Vascular Malformations*. Reinbek, Germany: Einhorn-Presse Verlag GmbH; 1989:23.

17. Belov S. Classification, terminology, and nosology of congenital vascular defects. In: Belov S, Loose DA, Weber J, eds. *Vascular Malformations*. Reinbek, Germany: Einhorn-Presse; 1989:25–30.

18. Gloviczki P, Duncan AA, Kalra M et al. Vascular malformations: An update. *Perspect Vasc Surg Endovasc Ther*. 2009;21(2):133–148.

19. Rutherford RB. Classification of peripheral congenital vascular malformations. In: Ernst C, Stanley J, eds. *Current Therapy in Vascular Surgery*. 3rd ed. St. Louis, MO: Mosby; 1995:834–838.

20. Enjolras O, Riche MC, Merland JJ, Escandej P. Management of alarming hemangiomas in infancy: A review of 25 cases. *Pediatrics*. 1990;85:491–498.

21. Wassef M, Blei F, Adams D et al.; on behalf of the ISSVA Board and Scientific Committee. Vascular anomalies classification: Recommendations from the International Society for the Study of Vascular Anomalies. *Pediatrics*. 2015;136(1):e203–e214.

22. Lee BB, Lardeo J, Neville R. Arterio-venous malformation: How much do we know? *Phlebology*. 2009;24:193–200.

23. Dompmartin A, Vikkula M, Boon L. Venous malformations: Update on etiopathogenesis, diagnosis and management. *Phlebology*. 2010;25(5):224–235.

24. Garzon MC, Huang JT, Enjolras O, Frieden IJ. Vascular malformations: Associated syndromes. *J Am Acad Dermatol*. 2007;56(4):541–564.

25. Lee BB, Laredo J, Lee SJ, Huh SH, Joe JH, Neville R. Congenital vascular malformations: General diagnostic principles. *Phlebology*. 2007;22(6):253–257.

26. Uebelhoer M, Natynki M, Kangas J et al. Venous malformation-causative *TIE2* mutations mediate an *AKT*-dependent decrease in PDGFB. *Hum Mol Genet*. September 1, 2013 22(17):3438–3448.

27. Limaye N, Boon LM, Vikkula M. From germline towards somatic mutations in the pathophysiology of vascular anomalies. *Hum Mol Genet*. 2009;18(R1):R65–R74.

28. Villavicencio JL. Primum non nocere: Is it always true? The use of absolute ethanol in the management of congenital vascular malformations. *J Vasc Surg*. 2001;33(4):904–906.

Diagnosis

5

How extensive study should be included in initial assessment for congenital vascular malformations

BYUNG-BOONG LEE AND JAMES LAREDO

GENERAL CONSIDERATIONS

Congenital vascular malformations (CVM) represent a garden variety of vascular defects occurring during two different stages of embryogenesis, affecting the entire circulation system: artery, vein, lymphatics, and capillary vessels. Naturally, it presents as various forms of vascular disorder throughout the body, often noticeable upon birth in various extents and severity.[1-4]

Hence, the precise diagnosis of a CVM is a major challenge requiring substantial knowledge of its clinical, hemodynamic, and morphological features in addition to its embryology as well as pathophysiology.

But a thorough history taking and detailed physical examination should provide most of the critical information necessary to reach the suspicion for CVMs. Further confirmation of a clinical impression of CVMs can be achieved with basic laboratory tests. Such evaluation should start with a differential diagnosis to first rule out a similar vascular condition known as (infantile) hemangioma, especially when encountered during the neonatal period. Infantile hemangioma can be mostly diagnosed based on careful history alone through proper confirmation on its new appearance *after* the birth as a newly developed vascular tumor and if not, with further findings of its unique clinical progress with rapid growth. But occasionally, Duplex ultrasonography might be added to make its final confirmation.[1-4]

However, if this vascular lesion suggests a CVM, further careful physical examination should be conducted to identify the type of the CVM involved, and further assessment can proceed with a proper combination of various non- to less-invasive laboratory tests indicated to confirm the clinical diagnosis, as follows:

Basic tests:

- Duplex ultrasonography (arterial and venous)
- Standard magnetic resonance imaging (MRI) of T1 and T2 image with no contrast

- Standard computed tomography (CT)
- Soft tissue plain radiography
- Bone scanogram
- Radionuclide lymphoscintigraphy (LSG)

Optional tests:

- MR angiography/MR arteriography (MRA) and MR venography (MRV)
- CT angiography with contrast enhancement, and/or three-dimensional CT reconstruction
- Whole-body blood pool scintigraphy (WBBPS)
- Transarterial lung perfusion scintigraphy (TLPS)

The basic evaluation to confirm the nature of the CVMs can be carried on before the age of 2 if not 3 years, based on the noninvasive tests alone, mostly with the combination of duplex ultrasonography and standard MRI. Occasionally, MRI can be replaced with standard CT scan, especially for a lesion that is suspicious for arteriovenous malformation (AVM), but in general, MRI is preferred for baseline evaluation for CVMs across the board, and CT/CT angiography is added as an option for AVM lesions.[1-4]

But, always, regardless of age, the AVM should be ruled out first since most of them are potentially life- if not limb-threatening conditions throughout the life span. If there is any doubt of the risk of the AVM, further evaluation with various invasive tests (e.g., arteriography) should be included as part of the initial diagnostic procedure, even before reaching the age of 2 years with proper indication, although such invasive tests are generally saved/deferred until needed later to serve as a road map when treatment is indicated:

- Ascending, descending, and/or segmental venography/phlebography
- Standard and/or selective and superselective arteriography

- Percutaneous direct puncture angiography: arteriography, phlebography
- Varicography, lymphography

If the lesion should be confirmed as an AVM, such invasive tests should be repeated in proper intervals per indication to assess the progress (e.g., micro-shunting AVM lesions among Parkes Weber syndrome) as a due diagnostic procedure.

In addition, when the CVM lesions accompany the risk of angio-osteo-dystrophy (= hypertrophy or hypotrophy), also called *vascular bone syndrome*, to cause limb length discrepancy, full diagnostic assessment/procedures should be completed even before the age of 5 years so that timely management of the CVM lesion to minimize the length discrepancy can be carried on with no further delay.[1–4]

Otherwise, necessary evaluation to confirm the clinical diagnosis may be deferred until the lesion(s) is indicated for treatment, and a proper combination/section of various non- to less-invasive tests as listed is more than enough to make the diagnosis, except for the AVMs.

DUPLEX ULTRASONOGRAPHY

Congenital vascular malformation lesion: General

Duplex ultrasonography (DUS) is the most essential tool to initiate primary examination of the CVM.[1–6] Its unique function allows verification of the flow characteristics of the lesions as high flow (AVM), low flow (VM), or no flow (LM), in addition to obtaining the dimensions of the lesion. But it has a limited role in defining the extent of lesions located in locations other than the extremities, so MRI is often needed to aid in locating the lesion (e.g., deep intramuscular lesions) in such cases.

Venous malformation

Following basic evaluation of the venous system, clinically detected venous malformation (VM) lesions should be assessed separately for the surrounding soft tissue/structure/organ, especially in proximity to vital structures (e.g., airway); additional efforts should be made to look for hidden VM lesions elsewhere, as well as the phleboliths and/or intravascular thrombus.

Lymphatic malformation

Precise assessment of fluid movement within a cystic lesion is mandated for differential diagnosis with VM if not with mixed condition. Additional efforts should be given to assess the surrounding soft tissue/structure/organ, especially on the extent/proximity to the vital structures (e.g., airway, eyesight) in addition to looking for hidden lymphatic malformation (LM) lesions elsewhere (e.g., neck, axilla, buttock).

Arteriovenous malformation

Additional and detailed documentation on the feeding artery and draining veins of the AVM are warranted, together with the circulation status distal to the lesion, specifically looking for the subclinical status of distal arterial insufficiency/steal syndrome and distal venous hypertension/chronic venous insufficiency.

Capillary malformation

Thorough evaluation should include the hidden VM, LM, and/or AVM throughout the soft tissue beneath the capillary malformation (CM) lesion with documentation of even the negative findings.

STANDARD MAGNETIC RESONANCE IMAGING WITH NO CONTRAST

MRI is the procedure of choice for all CVM assessment, providing a better spatial resolution/definition with a wider field of view than ultrasound. All CVMs regardless of type should have standard MRI with no contrast as a routine part of the investigation together with DUS before a conclusive diagnosis is made.[7,8]

T2-weighted imaging is essential for all VM and LM diagnoses. The coronal view is mandatory for the assessment of periarticular VM with or without joint involvement.

However, certain conditions of VM and LM will be indicated for the MRI with the contrast, especially for the mixed condition of VM and LM.

STANDARD COMPUTED TOMOGRAPHY

Advanced forms of CT could provide more information on the CVMs than MRI,[9,10] especially when the test is combined with the contrast. Additional information on the skeletal system together with the soft tissue is more advantageous than the standard MRI, ideal for high-flow CVM, in particular with bone involvement.

CONVENTIONAL SOFT TISSUE PLAIN RADIOGRAPHY

This test remains essential to identify the phleboliths as a hallmark of VMs.[11,12] It is also useful to identify abnormal findings in the soft tissue other than the calcifications in the soft tissues and other malformation-related abnormalities along the skeletal system besides phleboliths.

BONE SCANOGRAM

A scanogram is a long bone radiograph used to provide an accurate measurement of the long bone length.[13,14] Any CVM condition combined with abnormal long bone growth with a leg/arm length discrepancy should have the baseline measurement with scanogram and repeat every 2 years until the bone growth is finished.

WHOLE-BODY BLOOD POOL SCINTIGRAPHY

WBBPS using Tc99 is able to detect abnormal blood pool throughout the body to confirm the presence of a vascular malformation.[15,16] Hence, it is essential for the general assessment of the VM and also the LM to be ruled out. It is also essential for follow-up assessment on each session/therapy as well as its natural course/recurrence.

TRANSARTERIAL LUNG PERFUSION SCINTIGRAPHY

TLPS is the most accurate way to assess the AV-shunting percentage of the AVM lesion located in the limb by quantifying the shunt volume;[17,18] it has a special value to detect and assess a micro-AV shunting lesion, frequently existing among Parkes Weber syndrome and often difficult to detect with conventional techniques.[19,20]

TLPS is, therefore, able to replace the substantial role of traditional arteriography as a follow-up assessment tool, providing quantitative measurement of the shunting status during therapy and treatment results on extremity AVMs.

RADIONUCLIDE LYMPHOSCINTIGRAPHY

The role of LSG for CVM evaluation is limited for the assessment of primary lymphedema, involved in the Klippel–Trenaunay Syndrome (KTS) as a truncular LM. But, the LSG is the essential test to evaluate lymphatic dysfunction, from clearance rate to general status of the lymph vessels/nodes, including dermal backflow. It is therefore a mandatory test for a hemolymphatic malformation (HLM), combined form of the VM and LM.[1–4,21,22]

COAGULOPATHY ASSESSMENT

Localized intravascular coagulopathy (LIC) associated with the VM lesion is the result of "consumptive" coagulopathy caused by blood stagnation within the VM lesion, resulting in thrombosis and subsequent phlebolith formation. The assessment of coagulation abnormalities is particularly indicated among the VM lesions with extensive involvement to a large surface area and deep tissue structures.[23,24]

HISTOPATHOLOGY

A biopsy should be considered whenever the differential diagnosis with malignant tumor is needed besides a noninvoluting vascular tumor (e.g., a noninvoluting congenital hemangioma [NICH]). Conclusive genetic tests can be added to make a further assessment on the inherited form of the VMs.[25,26]

REFERENCES

1. Lee BB, Baumgartner I, Berlien P et al. Diagnosis and treatment of venous malformations consensus document of the International Union of Phlebology (IUP): Updated 2013. *Int Angiol.* 2015;34(2): 97–149.

2. Lee BB, Baumgartner I, Berlien HP et al. Consensus document of the International Union of Angiology (IUA)-2013. Current concept on the management of arterio-venous management. *Int Angiol.* 2013;32(1): 9–36.

3. Lee BB, Antignani PL, Baraldini V et al. ISVI-IUA consensus document—Diagnostic guidelines on vascular anomalies: Vascular malformations and hemangiomas. *Int Angiol.* 2015;34(4):333–374.

4. Lee BB, Baumgartner I. Contemporary diagnosis of venous malformation. *J Vasc Diagn.* 2013;1:25–34.

5. Gold L, Nazarian LN, Johar AS, Rao VM. Characterization of maxillofacial soft tissue vascular anomalies by ultrasound and color Doppler imaging: An adjuvant to computed tomography and magnetic resonance imaging. *J Oral Maxillofac Surg.* 2003;61(1):19–31.

6. Lee BB, Mattassi R, Choe YH et al. Critical role of duplex ultrasonography for the advanced management of a venous malformation (VM). *Phlebology.* 2005;20:28–37.

7. Yonetsu K, Nakayama E, Miwa K et al. Magnetic resonance imaging of oral and maxillofacial angiomas. *Oral Surg Oral Med Oral Pathol.* 1993;76(6):783–789.

8. Lee BB, Choe YH, Ahn JM et al. The new role of MRI (magnetic resonance imaging) in the contemporary diagnosis of venous malformation: Can it replace angiography? *J Am Coll Surg.* 2004;198(4):549–558.

9. Rubin PA, Bilyk JR, Dunya IM, Weber AL. Spiral CT of an orbital venous malformation. *Am J Neuroradiol.* 1995;16:1255–1257.

10. Napoli A, Fleischmann D, Chan FP et al. Computed tomography angiography: State-of-the-art imaging using multidetector-row technology. *J Comput Assist Tomogr.* 2004;28(Suppl 1):S32–S45.

11. Scolozzi P, Laurent F, Lombardi T, Richter M. Intraoral venous malformation presenting with multiple phleboliths. *Oral Surg Oral Med Oral Pathol Oral Radiol Endod.* 2003;96(2):197–200.

12. Chava VR, Shankar AN, Vemanna NS, Cholleti SK. Multiple venous malformations with phleboliths: Radiological-pathological correlation. *J Clin Imaging Sci.* 2013;3(Suppl 1):13.

13. Mattassi R. Differential diagnosis in congenital vascular-bone syndromes. *Semin Vasc Surg.* 1993;6:233–244.

14. Mattassi R, Vaghi M. Vascular bone syndrome-angiosteodystrophy: Current concept. *Phlebology.* 2007;22:287–290.

15. Lee BB, Mattassi R, Kim BT, Kim DI, Ahn JM, Choi JY. Contemporary diagnosis and management of venous and AV shunting malformation by whole body blood pool scintigraphy (WBBPS). *Int Angiol.* 2004;23(4): 355–367.

16. Inoue Y, Wakita S, Ohtake T et al. Use of whole-body imaging using Tc-99m RBC in patients with soft-tissue vascular lesions. *Clin Nucl Med.* 1996;21(12): 958–959.

17. Partsch H, Lofferer O, Mostbeck A. Determination of the shunt volume in congenital angiodysplasias of the extremities. (An aid to the differential diagnosis between the Klippel–Trenaunay syndrome and the F.P. Weber syndrome) [author's transl]. *Wien Klin Wochenschr.* 1973;85(31):544–547.

18. Lee BB, Mattassi R, Kim BT, Park JM. Advanced management of arteriovenous shunting malformation (AVM) with transarterial lung perfusion scintigraphy (TLPS) for follow-up assessment. *Int Angiol.* 2005;24(2):173–184.

19. Gloviczki P, Driscoll DJ. Klippel–Trenaunay syndrome: Current management. *Phlebology.* 2007;22:291–298.

20. Ziyeh S, Spreer J, Rossler J et al. Parkes Weber or Klippel–Trenaunay syndrome? Non-invasive diagnosis with MR projection angiography. *Eur Radiol.* 2004;14(11):2025–2029.

21. Choi JY, Lee BB, Hwang JH et al. Risk assessment of dermatolymphangioadenitis by lymphoscintigraphy in patients with lower extremity lymphedema. *Kor J Nucl Med.* 1999;33(2):143–151.

22. Lee BB, Laredo J. Contemporary role of lymphoscintigraphy: We can no longer afford to ignore! *Phlebology.* 2011;26:177–178.

23. Hermans C, Dessomme B, Lambert C et al. Venous malformations and coagulopathy. *Ann Chir Plast Esthet.* 2006;51(4–5):388–393.

24. Mazoyer E, Enjolras O, Bisdorff A et al. Coagulation disorders in patients with venous malformation of limbs and trunk: A study in 118 patients. *Arch Dermatol.* 2008;144:861–867.

25. Leu HJ. Pathomorphology of vascular malformations: Analysis of 310 cases. *Int Angiol.* 1990;9:147–155.

26. Stein JA, Heidary N, Pulitzer M, Schaffer JV, North P. Noninvoluting congenital hemangioma. *Dermatol Online J.* 2013;14(5):7.

6

Should hemangiomas be included in initial differential diagnosis for congenital vascular malformations?

FRANCINE BLEI

The classification of vascular anomalies has been recognized as essential into two large classes of lesions, vascular tumors and vascular malformations, since the 1980s, based on Mulliken and Glowacki's observations.[1] This categorization was based on the premise that vascular tumors demonstrate endothelial proliferation, and vascular malformations represent developmental abnormalities of one or more vascular channels. We now recognize that vascular malformations may also exhibit proliferation; thus, the distinction based on vascular growth is less apparent.

The International Society for the Study of Vascular Anomalies (ISSVA) classification separates vascular malformations from vascular tumors, with hemangiomas in the latter group.[2] The ISSVA classification is updated regularly to incorporate new genetic information and insights in the etiopathology of vascular anomalies (https://www.issva.org/classification) (Table 6.1).

INFANTILE HEMANGIOMA

The most common type of hemangioma is the infantile hemangioma (hemangioma of infancy), which has a rather predictable life cycle of postnatal proliferation followed by gradual involution. Infantile hemangiomas have distinctive histological features and are glucose transporter-1 (GLUT-1) positive. Factors modulating *in utero* quiescence and the growth/improvement after birth are not fully understood, and hemangiomas may also exhibit late growth after involution.[3-6] Hemangiomas of infancy are typically sporadic; however, inheritance and an increased relative risk in siblings of affected proband have been recognized in some studies.[7,8]

CONGENITAL HEMANGIOMA

Congenital hemangiomas proliferate *in utero*, are present at birth, and rapidly improve, partially improve, or remain stable postnatally. Congenital hemangiomas may have a high flow component, may have transient hematologic abnormalities, may have ulcerations with bleeding, and are GLUT-1 negative.[9,10] Rarely, congenital hemangiomas exhibit postnatal growth.[9-12] Mutations in *GNAQ*, *GNA11*, and *GNNA14* have been identified in congenital hemangiomas.[13-15] Cheraghlou et al. reviewed the Ras-mitogen-activated protein kinase (Ras-MAPK) pathway. An updated review of clinical behavior and management of hemangiomas was recently published by the American Academy of Pediatrics.[16]

SYNDROMIC HEMANGIOMAS

The two major hemangioma syndromes are PHACE (posterior fossa, brain malformations; hemangioma, segmental; arterial anomalies of the head and/or neck, abnormalities of the blood vessels in the neck or head; cardiac abnormalities/aortic coarctation, abnormalities of the heart or the blood vessels that are attached to the heart; eye abnormalities) syndrome and LUMBAR (lower-body hemangioma and other cutaneous defects, urogenital anomalies, myelopathy, bone deformities, anorectal malformations, arterial anomalies, renal anomalies) syndrome, which are associated with large segmental hemangiomas and accompanying structural defects.[17,18] Genomic and somatic mutations have been characterized in many vascular malformation syndromes (e.g., CLOVES [congenital, lipomatous, overgrowth, vascular malformations, epidermal nevi, and spinal/skeletal

25

Table 6.1 International Society for the Study of Vascular Anomalies classification of vascular anomalies—Vascular tumors

Benign Vascular Tumors 1[a]

Infantile hemangioma/hemangioma of infancy	*see details*
Congenital hemangioma	*GNAQ/GNA11*
Rapidly involuting (RICH)[b]	
Noninvoluting (NICH)	
Partially involuting (PICH)	
Tufted angioma[b,c]	*GNA14*
Spindle-cell hemangioma	*IDH1/IDH2*
Epithelioid hemangioma	*FOS*
Pyogenic granuloma (also known as lobular capillary hemangioma)	*BRAF/RAS/GNA14*
Others	*see details*

Benign Vascular Tumors 2[d]

Others
   Hobnail hemangioma
   Microvenular hemangioma
   Anastomosing hemangioma
   Glomeruloid hemangioma
   Papillary hemangioma
   Intravascular papillary endothelial hyperplasia
   Cutaneous epithelioid angiomatous nodule
   Acquired elastotic hemangioma
   Littoral cell hemangioma of the spleen

Related Lesions
   Eccrine angiomatous hamartoma
   Reactive angioendotheliomatosis
   Bacillary angiomatosis

Locally Aggressive or Borderline Vascular Tumors[a]

Kaposiform hemangioendothelioma[b,c]	*GNA14*
Retiform hemangioendothelioma	
Papillary intralymphatic angioendothelioma (PILA), Dabska tumor	
Composite hemangioendothelioma	
Pseudomyogenic hemangioendothelioma	*FOSB*
Polymorphous hemangioendothelioma	
Hemangioendothelioma not otherwise specified	
Kaposi sarcoma	
Others	

Malignant Vascular Tumors

Angiosarcoma	(Postradiation) *MYC*
Epithelioid hemangioendothelioma	*CAMTA1/TFE3*
Others	

Source: The Classification for Vascular Anomalies by the International Society for the Study of Vascular Anomalies (ISSVA) is licensed under a Creative Commons Attribution 4.0 International License. http://www.issva.org/UserFiles/file/ISSVA-Classification-2018.pdf.

[a] Reactive proliferative vascular lesions are listed with benign tumors. Causal genes in italics.
[b] Some lesions may be associated with thrombocytopenia and/or consumptive coagulopathy, see details.
[c] Many experts believe that tufted angioma and kaposiform hemangioendothelioma are part of a spectrum rather than distinct entities.
[d] The tumoral nature of some of these lesions is not certain. Reactive proliferative vascular lesions are listed with benign tumors.

anomalies and/or scoliosis] syndrome, Proteus syndrome, hereditary hemorrhagic telangiectasia, venous malformations). To date, a causative gene has not been identified in PHACE or LUMBAR syndrome.[19] Perhaps there is a somatic mutation causing a field defect, with developmental timing or concentration of the mutation contributing to the gradation of abnormalities.

MESENCHYMAL STEM CELLS AND HEMANGIOMAS

Mesenchymal stem cells have been purported to be involved in the development of hemangiomas. The role of hypoxia angiogenesis and other factors, including hypoxia inducible factor (HIF1α), vascular endothelial growth factor (VEGF), *AKT* signaling, as well as the renin-angiotensin pathway have been implicated in hemangioma growth and are being studied as therapeutic targets[20–34] (Table 6.2).

DISTRIBUTION

Patterns of distribution exhibited by hemangiomas may provide insight to their development. Waner et al. observed the nonrandom distribution of hemangiomas (focal or segmental), with the former occurring in zones of mesenchymal or mesenchymal-ectodermal embryonic fusion.[35] Reimer et al. reviewed the anatomical distribution of hemangiomas in the extremities and attributed the observed patterns of distribution to areas of regional hypoxia related to embryonic arterial supply, which stimulates hemangioma stem cell proliferation.[36] The "biker glove" pattern of hemangiomas on distal extremities ascribed to by Weitz et al. suggests the developmental error occurs "*after the*

finger rays are formed, yet *before* the interweb spaces are completely developed and the distal digits have differentiated."[37] Additionally, Reimer and colleagues propose that multifocal (small disseminated) hemangiomas differ from traditional hemangiomas of infancy, in that "their number correlates inversely with their size," and they are associated with other issues.[38]

INVOLUTION

Regarding involution of hemangiomas, several studies have documented the transition from proliferation to involution and adipogenesis (mesenchymal stem cells within hemangiomas differentiated into adipocytes).[39] England et al. demonstrated that β-blockers, used to treat hemangiomas of infancy, interfered with this process *in vitro*, causing apoptosis.[40] Studies by Zhang et al. suggested that insulin-like growth factor 2 promotes the adipogenesis of hemangioma-derived stem cells.[41]

GENETIC FACTORS

Cheraghlou et al. reviewed genetic factors taking part in hemangioma and related diagnoses, highlighting the Ras-MAPK pathway (Figure 6.1).[42] In this respect, hemangiomas demonstrate an overlap in the signaling pathways associated with many vascular malformations, specifically the PI3K/AKT/mTOR pathway. The history, clinical presentation, radiological findings, and clinical course should be emphasized when diagnosing vascular lesions, as hemangiomas are clearly distinct from vascular malformations. At present, medical therapy for hemangiomas and vascular malformations differ; however, in the future, similar pathways may be exploited in therapeutic trials.

Table 6.2 Expression of VEGF, VEGFR2, Ki-67, Glut-1, p-AKT, and p-ERK in human hemangioma

| Target | Group | Cases | n | | | | Positive rate (%) | X^2 | P |
			−	+	++	+++			
VEGF	Proliferating phase HAs	30	6	7	12	5	80.0	11.712	.001
	Involuting phase HAs	25	13	9	3	0	48.0		
VEGFR 2	Proliferating phase HAs	30	8	6	10	6	73.3	8.628	.003
	Involuting phase HAs	25	15	6	3	1	40.0		
Ki-67	Proliferating phase HAs	30	7	12	6	5	76.7	5.559	.018
	Involuting phase HAs	25	14	6	4	1	44.0		
Glut-1	Proliferating phase HAs	30	5	8	8	9	83.3	19.921	<.001
	Involuting phase HAs	25	18	5	2	0	28.0		
p-AKT	Proliferating phase HAs	30	8	13	7	2	73.3	8.512	.004
	Involuting phase HAs	25	16	7	2	0	36.0		
p-ERK	Proliferating phase HAs	30	10	13	5	2	66.7	8.913	.003
	Involuting phase HAs	25	18	6	1	0	28.0		

Source: Ou JM et al. *Eur J Histochem.* 2014;58(1):2263. This work is licensed under a Creative Commons Attribution-Non-Commercial 4.0 International License.
Abbreviation: HAs, hemangiomas.

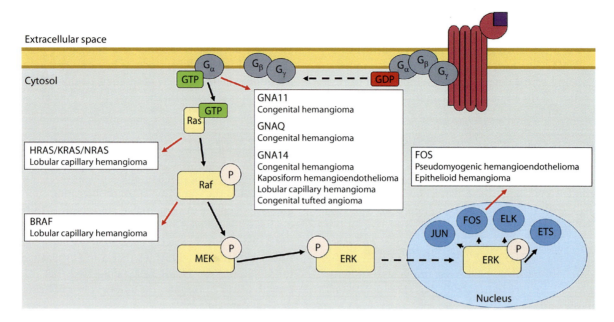

Figure 6.1 Positions of the Ras-MAPK pathway wherein mutations have been demonstrated to lead to childhood vascular tumors (red arrows). Unbroken arrows indicate activation, while broken arrows indicate migration. (From Cheraghlou S, Lim Y, Choate K. Genetic investigation of childhood vascular tumor biology reveals pathways for therapeutic intervention [version 1; peer review: 2 approved]. F1000Research. 2019(8[F1000 Faculty Rev]):590. https://doi.org/10.12688/f1000research.16160.1.)

REFERENCES

1. Mulliken JB, Glowacki J. Hemangiomas and vascular malformations in infants and children: A classification based on endothelial characteristics. *Plast Reconstr Surg.* 1982;69(3):412–422.
2. Wassef M, Blei F, Adams D et al. Vascular anomalies classification: Recommendations from the International Society for the Study of Vascular Anomalies. *Pediatrics.* 2015;136(1):e203–e214.
3. Mulliken JB, Enjolras O. Congenital hemangiomas and infantile hemangioma: Missing links. *J Am Acad Dermatol.* 2004;50(6):875–882.
4. Greenberger S, Bischoff J. Pathogenesis of infantile haemangioma. *Br J Dermatol.* 2013;169(1):12–19.
5. Leaute-Labreze C, Harper JI, Hoeger PH. Infantile haemangioma. *Lancet.* 2017;390(10089):85–94.
6. O'Brien KF, Shah SD, Pope E et al. Late growth of infantile hemangiomas in children >3 years of age: A retrospective study. *J Am Acad Dermatol.* 2019;80(2):493–499.
7. Grimmer JF, Williams MS, Pimentel R et al. Familial clustering of hemangiomas. *Arch Otolaryngol Head Neck Surg.* 2011;137(8):757–760.
8. Castren E, Salminen P, Vikkula M, Pitkaranta A, Klockars T. Inheritance patterns of infantile hemangioma. *Pediatrics.* 2016;138(5):e20161623.
9. Baselga E, Cordisco MR, Garzon M, Lee MT, Alomar A, Blei F. Rapidly involuting congenital haemangioma associated with transient thrombocytopenia and coagulopathy: A case series. *Br J Dermatol.* 2008;158(6):1363–1370.
10. Powell J, Blouin MM, David M, Dubois J. Bleeding in congenital hemangiomas: Crusting as a clinical predictive sign and usefulness of tranexamic acid. *Pediatr Dermatol.* 2012;29(2):182–185.
11. Cossio ML, Dubois J, McCuaig CC et al. Non-involuting congenital hemangioma (NICH) with postnatal atypical growth: A case series. *Pediatr Dermatol.* 2019;36:466–470.
12. Knopfel N, Walchli R, Luchsinger I, Theiler M, Weibel L, Schwieger-Briel A. Congenital hemangioma exhibiting postnatal growth. *Pediatr Dermatol.* 2019;36:548–549.
13. Funk T, Lim Y, Kulungowski AM et al. Symptomatic congenital hemangioma and congenital hemangiomatosis associated with a somatic activating mutation in *GNA11. JAMA Dermatol.* 2016;152(9):1015–1020.
14. Ayturk UM, Couto JA, Hann S et al. Somatic activating mutations in *GNAQ* and *GNA11* are associated with congenital hemangioma. *Am J Hum Genet.* 2016;98(4):789–795.
15. Lim YH, Bacchiocchi A, Qiu J et al. *GNA14* somatic mutation causes congenital and sporadic vascular tumors by MAPK activation. *Am J Hum Genet.* 2016;99(2):443–450.
16. Krowchuk DP, Frieden IJ, Mancini AJ et al. Clinical practice guideline for the management of infantile hemangiomas. *Pediatrics.* 2019;143(1):e20183475.
17. Garzon MC, Epstein LG, Heyer GL et al. PHACE syndrome: Consensus-derived diagnosis and care recommendations. *J Pediatr.* 2016;178:24–33.e2.
18. Iacobas I, Burrows PE, Frieden IJ et al. LUMBAR: Association between cutaneous infantile heman-

giomas of the lower body and regional congenital anomalies. *J Pediatr.* 2010;157(5):795–801.e1–7.

19. Siegel DH. PHACE syndrome: Infantile hemangiomas associated with multiple congenital anomalies: Clues to the cause. *Am J Med Genet C Semin Med Genet.* 2018;178(4):407–413.

20. Itinteang T, Brasch HD, Tan ST, Day DJ. Expression of components of the renin-angiotensin system in proliferating infantile haemangioma may account for the propranolol-induced accelerated involution. *J Plast Reconstr Aesthet Surg.* 2011;64(6):759–765.

21. Dornhoffer JR, Wei T, Zhang H, Miller E, MAC, Richter GT. The expression of renin-angiotensin-aldosterone axis components in infantile hemangioma tissue and the impact of propranolol treatment. *Pediatr Res.* 2017;82(1):155–163.

22. de Jong S, Itinteang T, Withers AH, Davis PF, Tan ST. Does hypoxia play a role in infantile hemangioma? *Arch Dermatol Res.* 2016;308(4):219–227.

23. Diaz-Gonzalez JA, Russell J, Rouzaut A, Gil-Bazo I, Montuenga L. Targeting hypoxia and angiogenesis through HIF-1α inhibition. *Cancer Biol Ther.* 2005;4(10): 1055–1062.

24. Drolet BA, Frieden IJ. Characteristics of infantile hemangiomas as clues to pathogenesis: Does hypoxia connect the dots? *Arch Dermatol.* 2010;146(11):1295–1299.

25. Herbert A, Ng H, Jessup W et al. Hypoxia regulates the production and activity of glucose transporter-1 and indoleamine 2,3-dioxygenase in monocyte-derived endothelial-like cells: Possible relevance to infantile haemangioma pathogenesis. *Br J Dermatol.* 2011;164(2):308–315.

26. Kleinman ME, Greives MR, Churgin SS et al. Hypoxia-induced mediators of stem/progenitor cell trafficking are increased in children with hemangioma. *Arterioscler Thromb Vasc Biol.* 2007;27(12):2664–2670.

27. Xia HF, Zhu JY, Wang JN et al. Association of ATF4 expression with tissue hypoxia and M2 macrophage infiltration in infantile hemangioma. *J Histochem Cytochem.* 2017;65(5):285–294.

28. Yamashita T, Jinnin M, Makino K et al. Serum cytokine profiles are altered in patients with progressive infantile hemangioma. *Biosci Trends.* 2018;12(4): 438–441.

29. Sulzberger L, Baillie R, Itinteang T et al. Serum levels of renin, angiotensin-converting enzyme and angiotensin II in patients treated by surgical excision, propranolol and captopril for problematic proliferating infantile haemangioma. *J Plast Reconstr Aesthet Surg.* 2016;69(3):381–386.

30. Oszajca K, Szemraj J, Wyrzykowski D, Chrzanowska B, Salamon A, Przewratil P. Single-nucleotide polymorphisms of VEGF-A and VEGFR-2 genes and risk of infantile hemangioma. *Int J Dermatol.* 2018;57(10): 1201–1207.

31. Ou JM, Yu ZY, Qiu MK et al. Knockdown of VEGFR2 inhibits proliferation and induces apoptosis in hemangioma-derived endothelial cells. *Eur J Histochem.* 2014;58(1):2263.

32. Ye X, Abou-Rayyah Y, Bischoff J et al. Altered ratios of pro- and anti-angiogenic VEGF-A variants and pericyte expression of DLL4 disrupt vascular maturation in infantile haemangioma. *J Pathol.* 2016;239(2):139–151.

33. Jinnin M, Medici D, Park L et al. Suppressed NFAT-dependent VEGFR1 expression and constitutive VEGFR2 signaling in infantile hemangioma. *Nat Med.* 2008;14(11):1236–1246.

34. Lu S, Chen L, Tang L. Upregulation of *AKT1* and downregulation of *AKT3* caused by dysregulation of microRNAs contributes to pathogenesis of hemangioma by promoting proliferation of endothelial cells. *J Cell Physiol.* 2019;234:21342–21351.

35. Waner M, North PE, Scherer KA, Frieden IJ, Waner A, Mihm MC Jr. The nonrandom distribution of facial hemangiomas. *Arch Dermatol.* 2003;139(7):869–875.

36. Reimer A, Fliesser M, Hoeger PH. Anatomical patterns of infantile hemangioma (IH) of the extremities (IHE). *J Am Acad Dermatol.* 2016;75(3):556–563.

37. Weitz NA, Bayer ML, Baselga E et al. The "biker-glove" pattern of segmental infantile hemangiomas on the hands and feet. *J Am Acad Dermatol.* 2014;71(3):542–547.

38. Reimer A, Hoeger PH. Lesion morphology in multifocal infantile hemangiomas. *Pediatr Dermatol.* 2016; 33(6):621–626.

39. Yu Y, Fuhr J, Boye E et al. Mesenchymal stem cells and adipogenesis in hemangioma involution. *Stem Cells.* 2006;24(6):1605–1612.

40. England RW, Hardy KL, Kitajewski AM et al. Propranolol promotes accelerated and dysregulated adipogenesis in hemangioma stem cells. *Ann Plast Surg.* 2014;73(Suppl 1):S119–S124.

41. Zhang K, Wang F, Huang J et al. Insulin-like growth factor 2 promotes the adipogenesis of hemangioma-derived stem cells. *Exp Ther Med.* 2019;17(3):1663–1669.

42. Cheraghlou S, Lim Y, Choate K. Genetic investigation of childhood vascular tumor biology reveals pathways for therapeutic intervention [version 1; peer review: 2 approved]. F1000Research. 2019;8[F1000 Faculty Rev]):590. https://doi.org/10.12688/f1000research.16160.1.

7

To what extent should genetic studies be incorporated for assessment of venous and arteriovenous malformations, and when?

SANDRO MICHELINI, STEFANO PAOLACCI, AND MATTEO BERTELLI

Venous malformations (VMs) have an estimated incidence of 1/5,000–10,000 and are the most frequent vascular malformations.[1] They usually affect skin and mucosa but can also involve the brain, bones, or muscle.[2] They are characterized by enlarged channels lined with endothelium surrounded by an irregular layer of smooth muscle cells.[3] These disorders can be divided into sporadic VMs, multiple cutaneous and mucosal VMs, glomuvenous malformations, blue rubber bleb nevi, cerebral cavernous malformations, and verrucous VMs.[4]

Arteriovenous malformations (AVMs) are rare malformations (prevalence and incidence are not known) characterized by abnormal connections between arteries and veins, bypassing high-resistance capillary beds. Isolated AVMs are usually sporadic and may be localized or regional.[4] With time, arterial to venous shunting causes tissue ischemia that may lead to pain, ulceration, bleeding, and destruction of adjacent tissues.[5] AVMs can also be found in association with other conditions such as in capillary malformation/AVM (CM/AVM) and in hereditary hemorrhagic telangiectasia (HHT).

Both VMs and AVMs may be diagnosed by clinical and histological examinations, and most of these malformations are sporadic; however, there may be cases of inherited VMs (glomuvenous malformations or multiple cutaneous VMs) or AVMs (CM/AVM or HHT-associated AVMs) (Table 7.1). Genetic testing, therefore, would be important to identify the molecular causes and establish recurrence risk in the families.[6] Genetic testing should also be used because drugs that target a specific protein or pathway may be specifically used for patients with known mutations in order to give better treatments. For instance, VMs are mostly caused by mutations in *TEK* or *PIK3CA* that are

members of the PI3K/AKT/mTOR pathway;[7,8] whereas, extracranial and cerebral AVMs are mainly caused by somatic activating mutations in *MAP2K1* and *KRAS*,[5,9] respectively, and both genes encode members of the RAS/MAPK pathway.

In 2015, Boscolo and coworkers began a clinical study to test rapamycin.[10] Rapamycin was chosen because of its inhibitor effects on the PI3K/AKT/mTOR pathway that is hyperactivated in VMs by mutations in *TEK* or *PIK3CA*. The study suggests that rapamycin can reduce VM signs and symptoms.[10] Rapamycin is currently being tested under the name of Sirolimus in a multicenter clinical trial on lymphatic-vascular malformations (NCT00975819).

There are many drugs (at least 23), used in cancer therapies, that target the RAS/MAPK pathway and that may be used in patients with AVMs. For instance, bevacizumab (commercial name: Avastin) is going to be tested in patients with brain AVMs (NCT02314377). Bevacizumab directly binds vascular endothelial growth factor (VEGF) to inhibit angiogenesis. VEGF, when it binds to its receptor, VEGFR, initiates angiogenesis through various pathways, such as the RAS/MAPK pathway.

In conclusion, patients with VMs and AVMs should always be subject to genetic testing for two main reasons:

1. To identify if the VMs and AVMs are caused by somatic or germline mutations. In case of germline mutations, genetic testing should be performed in other family members to assess the carrier status and establish recurrence risk.
2. To identify the mutated gene in order to choose the most appropriate drug that specifically targets the mutated protein or pathway.

Table 7.1 Summary of the molecular and genetic features, and possible pharmacological treatments of venous malformations (VMs) and arteriovenous malformations (AVMs)

Venous malformation (VM)/arteriovenous malformation (AVM)	Disease (OMIM ID)	Mutated genes (OMIM ID)	Mutation type	Inheritance	Percentage/number of reported cases[a]	Potential drugs (ClinicalTrial.gov ID)
VM	Sporadic VMs	TEK (600221), PIK3CA (171834)	S	S	50% (TEK), ~25% (PIK3CA)	Sirolimus (NCT00975819), Regorafenib (NCT02736305), ARQ 092 (NCT03317366), everolimus, MK2206, BEZ235, infliximab, taselisib, pictilisib, SF1126, bpV(phen), bpV(pic), VO-Ohpic, SF1670, crizotinib, ruxolitinib
	Multiple cutaneous and mucosal VMs (600195)	TEK	G, G+S, S	AD, PD, sp	90%	/
	Blue rubber bleb nevus syndrome (112200)	TEK	S	Sp	87%	
	Glomuvenous malformations (138000)	GLMN (601749)	G, G+S	AD, PD	~95%	
	Verrucous VM	MAP3K3 (602539)	S	Sp	3/6	CI-1040, PD-0325901, ARRY-438162, AZD6244, RDEA119, GSK1120212, TAK-733, GDC-0973, AZD8330, RO5126766, RO4987655, RO5068760, AS703026, trametinib, dabrafenib, selumetinib, MEK162, CEP-11981, regorafenib, ruxolitinib
	Cerebral cavernous malformations (116860)	KRIT1 (604214), CCM2 (607929), PDCD10 (609118)	G, G+S	AD, PD	65% (KRIT1), 20% (CCM2), 15% (PDCD10)	Propranolol (NCT03474614, NCT03523650), simvastatin (NCT01764451), H-1152, fasudil, Y-27632, sorafenib, NSC-23766, EHT1864
	Primary intraosseous vascular malformation (606893)	ELMO2 (606421)	G	AR	Five families	/
AVM	Capillary malformation-AVM (608354, 618196)	RASA1 (139150), EPHB4 (600011)	G, G+S	AD, PD	68% (RASA1), 16% (EPHB4)	Trametinib, selumetinib, MEK162, dabrafenib, CEP-11981, regorafenib, ruxolitinib, rapamycin, GDC0941, BEZ235

(Continued)

Table 7.1 (Continued) Summary of the molecular and genetic features, and possible pharmacological treatments of venous malformations (VMs) and arteriovenous malformations (AVMs)

Venous malformation (VM)/arteriovenous malformation (AVM) Disease (OMIM ID)	Mutated genes (OMIM ID)	Mutation type	Inheritance	Percentage/number of reported cases[a]	Potential drugs (ClinicalTrial.gov ID)
Hereditary hemorrhagic telangiectasia (HHT, 187300, 600376, 615506)	ENG (131195), ACVRL1 (601284), GDF2 (605120)	G, G+S	AD, PD	39%–59% (ENG), 25%–57% (ACVRL1), 2/38 (GDF2)	TRC105, dalantercept, PF-03446962, tamoxifen (NCT00375622), N-acetyl-cysteine, sorafenib, GW771806, thalidomide, bevacizumab, metformin, propranolol, soluble endoglin, raloxifene hydrochloride, bazedoxifene, tacrolimus, G6.31, infliximab, lenalidomide
Juvenile polyposis/HHT syndrome (175050)	SMAD4 (600993)	G	AD	2%	
Extracranial AVMs	MAP2K1 (176872)	S	Sp	16/25	CI-1040, PD-0325901, ARRY-438162, AZD6244, RDEA119, GSK1120212, TAK-733, GDC-0973, AZD8330, RO5126766, RO4987655, RO5068760, AS703026, trametinib, dabrafenib, selumetinib, MEK162, CEP-11981, U0126
Cerebral AVMs (108010)	KRAS (190070)	S	Sp	45/72	Trametinib, selumetinib, MEK162, dabrafenib, CEP-11981, regorafenib, ruxolitinib, doxycycline, minocycline, marimastat

Source: Adapted from Table I and Table III from Paolacci S et al. *Int Angiol.* 2019;38(2):157–170.

Abbreviations: AD, autosomal dominant; AR, autosomal recessive; G, germline; G+S, somatic second hit in addition to germline mutation; PD, paradominant; S, somatic; Sp, sporadic.

[a] Number of cases/percentage of patients with a mutation in the genes listed in the table.

REFERENCES

1. Brouillard P, Vikkula M. Genetic causes of vascular malformations. *Hum Mol Genet*. 2007;16(2):140–149.

2. Boon L, Mulliken J, Enjolras O et al. Glomuvenous malformation (glomangioma) and venous malformation. *Arch Dermatol*. 2004;140(8):971–976.

3. Vikkula M, Boon LM, Carraway KL et al. Vascular dysmorphogenesis caused by an activating mutation in the receptor tyrosine kinase TIE2. *Cell*. 1996;87(7):1181–1190.

4. Paolacci S, Zulian A, Bruson A et al. Vascular anomalies: Molecular bases, genetic testing and therapeutic approaches. *Int Angiol*. 2019;38(2):157–170.

5. Couto JA, Huang AY, Konczyk DJ et al. Somatic *MAP2K1* mutations are associated with extracranial arteriovenous malformation. *Am J Hum Genet*. 2017;100(3):546–554.

6. Mattassi R, Manara E, Colombo PG et al. Variant discovery in patients with Mendelian vascular anomalies by next-generation sequencing and their use in patient clinical management. *J Vasc Surg*. 2018;67(3): 922-932.

7. Limaye N, Wouters V, Uebelhoer M et al. Somatic mutations in angiopoietin receptor gene *TEK* cause solitary and multiple sporadic venous malformations. *Nat Genet*. 2009;41(1):118–124.

8. Limaye N, Kangas J, Mendola A et al. Somatic activating *PIK3CA* mutations cause venous malformation. *Am J Hum Genet*. 2015;97(6):914–921.

9. Nikolaev SI, Vetiska S, Bonilla X et al. Somatic activating *KRAS* mutations in arteriovenous malformations of the brain. *N Engl J Med*. 2018;378(3):250–261.

10. Boscolo E, Limaye N, Huang L et al. Rapamycin improves *TIE2* -mutated venous malformation in murine model and human subjects. *J Clin Invest*. 2015;125(9):1–14.

8

Indications for genetic testing in evaluation of lymphatic and hemolymphatic malformations

STANLEY G. ROCKSON

Lymphatic malformations (LMs) are localized lesions composed of dilated channels that are lined by lymphatic endothelial cells and that contain lymph. However, these vascular structures do not drain into the central lymphatic system.[1] LMs are congenital developmental anomalies. In recognition of the fact that these do not have familial distribution, it has been conjectured that LMs might result from somatic mutations that would be lethal if they appeared in the germline.[2] There is now substantial confirmation of this hypothesis.

LMs can be structurally either micro- or macrocystic or have a mixture of these attributes. They can be localized, but a diffuse distribution is observed in generalized lymphatic anomalies (GLAs, formerly known as lymphangiomatosis).[3] Combined malformations also exist, such as the condition formerly known as Klippel–Trenaunay syndrome.[3] In these capillary-lymphaticovenous malformations, overgrowth of the affected limb might also be present.

PIK3CA MUTATIONS

In recent years, it has become evident that most patients with LMs have mutations in *PIK3CA* (see Chapters 10 and 43).[4] In addition, Klippel–Trenaunay syndrome (KTS) has a number of phenotypic features that overlap with those observed in patients with activating mutations in the PI3K-AKT pathway.[5] Such mutations, frequently encountered in neoplastic disease, are also found in nonmalignant presentations.[6] There is ever-mounting evidence that, in several congenital malformation and overgrowth syndromes, including CLOVES syndrome (whose acronym underscores the frequent presence of vascular malformation), there is disordered vascular growth on a genetic basis.[6] The *PIK3CA*-related overgrowth spectrum (PROS),[7] which constitutes the differential diagnostic cluster for capillary-lymphaticovenous malformations (KTS), is presented in Table 8.1. Progressive overgrowth occurs throughout childhood, producing segmental overgrowth of mesodermal tissues. These conditions typically affect adipose

tissue, fibroblasts, muscle, and bone. However, the most common tissues affected are the vasculature (capillaries, veins, and lymphatics).[6] The phenotype of this spectrum ranges from isolated disease, such as macrodactyly, megalencephaly, or vascular malformations, to syndromes defined by tissue overgrowth, vascular malformations, and epidermal nevi.[7-9]

Most of the individuals with KTS, CLOVES syndrome, or isolated lymphatic malformations have somatic mosaic PiIK3CA mutations. Five recurrent mutations account for most cases; these can be inexpensively screened by droplet digital polymerase chain reaction (PCR).[10] Gene-focused next-generation sequencing (NGS) with single molecule molecular inversion probes has identified additional *PIK3CA* mutations. NGS technology has revolutionized the ability to analyze mutational presentations.[10]

Testing eligibility criteria for somatic *PIK3CA* mutations have been established:[4] these include combined vascular lesions, including the large lymphatic malformations. This is a nontrivial consideration,[9] inasmuch as these diagnostic maneuvers entail tissue biopsy.

NON-*PIK3CA* MUTATIONS

In addition to the consideration of somatic *PIK3CA* mutation, there are KTS-like disorders, with overgrowth and cutaneous vascular lesions, caused by mutations in genes other than *PIK3CA*.[5] These would potentially include capillary malformations (*GNAQ* mutation),[11] as well as segmental overgrowth, lipomatosis, arteriovenous malformation, and epidermal nevus (SOLAMEN) syndrome (*PTEN* mutation).[12] Parkes Weber syndrome, originally described as the Klippel–Trenaunay–Weber syndrome (also known as Parkes Weber syndrome) is recognized to depend on *RASA1* mutations.[13] Furthermore, mutations in the RAS/MAPK/MEK signaling pathway have also been identified in patients with complex vascular anomalies.[14] Mutations that dysregulate the RAS pathway, including those in *EPHB4, KRAS, HRAS, NRAS, BRAF, RAF1, PTPN11,*

Table 8.1 *PIK3CA*-related overgrowth spectrum (PROS)

- Klippel–Trenaunay syndrome (capillary lymphaticovenous malformation)
- CLOVES (congenital lipomatous overgrowth, vascular malformations, epidermal nevi, scoliosis/skeletal and spinal) syndrome
- Megaencephaly-capillary malformation (M-CAP; M-CM)
- Hemihyperplasia multiple lipomatosis (HHML)
- Fibroadipose hyperplasia or overgrowth (FAO)
- Macrodactyly
- Fibroadipose infiltrating lipomatosis/facial infiltrative lipomatosis
- Dysplastic megalencephaly (DMEG)

Table 8.2 Identified causal somatic mutations in lymphatic malformations and related disorders

• *PIK3CA*	• *BRAF*
• RAS/MAPK/MEK signaling pathway	• *RAF1*
• *EPHB4*	• *PTPN11*
• *KRAS*	• *SOS1*
• *HRAS*	• *GNAQ*
• *NRAS*	• *PTEN*

and *SOS1*, have been recognized in vascular anomalies. These mutations have been found in kaposiform lymphangiomatosis (KLA), central conducting lymphatic anomalies (CCLAs) and other lymphedema syndromes.[15–17]

GENETIC TESTING

Identification of causal somatic mutations (Table 8.2) opens the door to effective pharmacotherapeutic interventions (see Chapter 72). Accordingly, genetic testing, including involved tissue biopsy, should be strongly considered by the clinician who evaluates these patients with lymphatic malformations, KTS, and other complex vascular anomaly presentations.

REFERENCES

1. Boon L, Vikkula M. Vascular anomalies. In: Wolff K, Goldsmith L, Katz L, Gilchrest B, Paller A, Leffell D, eds. *Fitzpatrick's Dermatology in General Medicine.* New York, NY: McGraw-Hill Professional Publishing; 2008:1651–1666.
2. Brouillard P, Boon L, Vikkula M. Genetics of lymphatic anomalies. *J Clin Invest.* 2014;124:898–904.
3. Hammer J, Seront E, Duez S et al. Sirolimus is efficacious in treatment for extensive and/or complex slow-flow vascular malformations: A monocentric prospective phase II study. *Orphanet J Rare Dis.* 2018;13:191.
4. Luks VL, Kamitaki N, Vivero MP et al. Lymphatic and other vascular malformative/overgrowth disorders are caused by somatic mutations in *PIK3CA*. *J Pediatr.* 2015;166:1048-54.e1–5.
5. Vahidnezhad H, Youssefian L, Uitto J. Klippel–Trenaunay syndrome belongs to the *PIK3CA*-related overgrowth spectrum (PROS). *Exp Dermatol.* 2016;25:17–19.
6. Mitchell CB, Phillips WA. Mouse models for exploring the biological consequences and clinical significance of PIK3CA mutations. *Biomolecules.* 2019;9(4):158.
7. Nathan N, Keppler-Noreuil KM, Biesecker LG, Moss J, Darling TN. Mosaic disorders of the PI3 K/PTEN/AKT/TSC/mTORC1 signaling pathway. *Dermatol Clin.* 2017;35:51–60.
8. Keppler-Noreuil KM, Sapp JC, Lindhurst MJ et al. Clinical delineation and natural history of the *PIK3CA*-related overgrowth spectrum. *Am J Med Genet A.* 2014;164A:1713–1733.
9. Keppler-Noreuil KM, Rios JJ, Parker VE et al. *PIK3CA*-related overgrowth spectrum (PROS): Diagnostic and testing eligibility criteria, differential diagnosis, and evaluation. *Am J Med Genet A.* 2015;167A:287–295.
10. Giardina T, Robinson C, Grieu-Iacopetta F et al. Implementation of next generation sequencing technology for somatic mutation detection in routine laboratory practice. *Pathology.* 2018;50:389–401.
11. Nakashima M, Miyajima M, Sugano H et al. The somatic GNAQ mutation c.548G>A (p.R183Q) is consistently found in Sturge–Weber syndrome. *J Hum Genet.* 2014;59:691–693.
12. Caux F, Plauchu H, Chibon F et al. Segmental overgrowth, lipomatosis, arteriovenous malformation and epidermal nevus (SOLAMEN) syndrome is related to mosaic PTEN nullizygosity. *Eur J Hum Genet.* 2007;15:767–773.
13. Eerola I, Boon LM, Mulliken JB et al. Capillary malformation-arteriovenous malformation, a new clinical and genetic disorder caused by RASA1 mutations. *Am J Hum Genet.* 2003;73:1240–1249.
14. Adams DM, Ricci KW. Vascular anomalies: Diagnosis of complicated anomalies and new medical treatment options. *Hematol Oncol Clin North Am.* 2019;33:455–470.
15. Barclay SF, Inman KW, Luks VL et al. A somatic activating *NRAS* variant associated with kaposiform lymphangiomatosis. *Genet Med.* 2019;21:1517–1524.
16. Manevitz-Mendelson E, Leichner GS, Barel O et al. Somatic *NRAS* mutation in patient with generalized lymphatic anomaly. *Angiogenesis.* 2018;21:287–298.
17. Taghinia AH, Upton J, Trenor C 3rd et al. Lymphaticovenous bypass of the thoracic duct for the treatment of chylous leak in central conducting lymphatic anomalies. *J Pediatr Surg.* 2019;54:562–568.

Management

9

Importance of interdisciplinary team approach for evaluation and management of vascular malformations

MEGHA M. TOLLEFSON, PETER GLOVICZKI, AND DAVID J. DRISCOLL

In order that the sick may have the benefit of advancing knowledge, union of forces is necessary

William J. Mayo MD, 1910

Vascular malformations are difficult to diagnose and challenging to treat. Patients may present with a multitude of signs and symptoms, diagnosis requires expertise and experience, and treatment can be so diverse that more than one specialist involved in the care of vascular malformations is frequently needed. In this chapter, we briefly discuss advantages of a multidisciplinary approach and provide a template used at our institution to set up an interdisciplinary vascular malformation clinic. The term *interdisciplinary clinic* is used throughout this document, emphasizing the necessity of consultation and collaboration between all health-care providers, for the best interest of the patient.

ADVANTAGES OF INTERDISCIPLINARY COLLABORATION

Patients with vascular malformations may just have a small, asymptomatic, and superficial lesion, or they may present with a limb- or life-threatening complex vascular malformation, affecting the skin, bones, and soft tissues and leading to bleeding or infectious or thrombotic complications (Figure 9.1). While a thorough history taking and physical examination by an experienced physician frequently defines the nature of the disorder, important decisions in these patients, who are often children, have to be made about the need for ultrasound evaluation, genetic testing, or more sophisticated imaging using magnetic resonance angiography (MRA), computed tomographic angiography (CTA) or

catheter-directed contrast angiography to establish a definitive diagnosis. Up to 80% of patients with a vascular malformation have incorrect or incomplete diagnosis before presentation at an interdisciplinary clinic.[1,2] Accurate diagnosis is critical to avoid complications, predict prognosis, and guide appropriate and effective therapy.

Management may include observation, physical therapy, compression, local skin care, drug treatment, pain management, or endovascular, surgical, or hybrid therapy. All patients with anything more than small superficial skin lesions require interdisciplinary care. The heterogeneity of vascular malformations when it comes to location and extent of involvement, types of vessels affected, and potential complications requires individualized management. When patients are counseled at an interdisciplinary clinic, a thorough assessment of the risks and benefits of each management option are discussed in real time. This leads to improved patient satisfaction and clinical outcomes, while limiting rates of complications.[3,4] The advantages of "one-stop shopping" in an interdisciplinary vascular malformation clinic at a tertiary care center have been voiced by many authors,[1–7] and they cannot be overemphasized. Cost saving for the patient is obvious, and a recent cost analysis of the multidisciplinary vascular anomaly clinic of the George Washington University, Washington, DC, revealed a net positive margin.[8] In addition to cost-effective care, vascular malformation clinics have educational and research values, and they bring together multiple professionals in a stimulating and learning environment that reinforces the benefits of teamwork and decreases the need for asking for "special favors" from different practitioners (Figure 9.2).

Because patients who visit vascular malformation clinics may have vascular tumors, a pathology that is not discussed

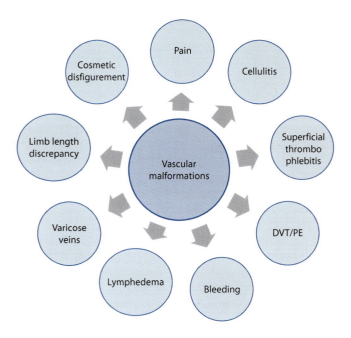

Figure 9.1 Different clinical presentations of vascular malformations. (DVT, deep vein thrombosis; PE, pulmonary embolism.)

here and is distinctly different from malformations, most interdisciplinary clinics function as vascular anomaly clinics, and thus evaluate and treat patients with a wide spectrum of benign and malignant vascular tumors, as well.[1,2,7]

COMPONENTS AND FUNCTION OF INTERDISCIPLINARY VASCULAR MALFORMATION CLINIC

While a dedicated team consisting of physicians, healthcare professionals, and an appointment coordinator is

needed to establish a functioning center, access to sophisticated diagnosis and therapy within the institution is also required to provide comprehensive and frequently complex care. Decisions on laboratory testing and diagnostic imaging studies should be made with much care and planning, frequently with consultation with a pediatrician, dermatologist, and vascular specialist or surgeon. Since most patients are infants, children, or adolescents, a pediatrician who is expert in vascular malformations is an ideal person to run a clinic. Depending on local expertise, several other specialists who are experts in management of vascular malformations may either serve as director or participate as members of the physicians' team (Table 9.1). At our institution, the clinic was organized by a pediatric dermatologist, with long-term experience in the evaluation and treatment of vascular malformations, and our physician members include a pediatric cardiologist; diagnostic and interventional radiologists; pathologists; a vascular medicine specialist; a geneticist; plastic, general, and vascular surgeons; ENT specialists; orthopedic and pediatric orthopedic surgeons; and a pediatric neurosurgeon. Immediate access to other specialists, listed in Table 9.1, is also available.

The actual sequence of care at the clinic starts with evaluation of all medical records of new patients, referred from another institution or by a primary care physician or a pediatrician. Self-referral is also accepted. Up to 12 new patients with complex malformations are set up for interdisciplinary consultations during the same day (or spread over 2 days if necessary) each month and listed for our vascular malformation conference, held at noon on Tuesday of the selected week. During the consultation time, all consultants when possible see the patient together in real time (Figure 9.3). Imaging studies, performed on Monday, if needed, are available for review prior to the consultations and presentation at the Tuesday conference, where they are reviewed by

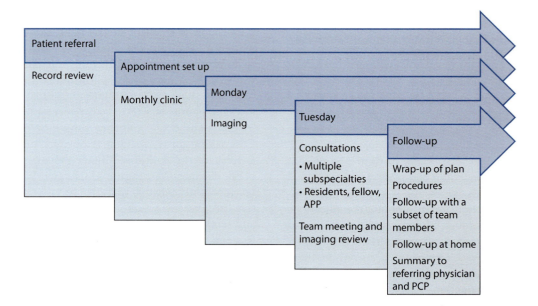

Figure 9.2 The benefits of an interdisciplinary vascular malformation clinic. (APP, allied patient provider; PCP, primary care provider.)

Table 9.1 List of specialties and clinics that may be involved in interdisciplinary care of vascular malformations

- Diagnostic radiology
- Interventional vascular radiology
- Vascular and endovascular surgery
- Interventional cardiology
- Dermatology
- Pediatric surgery
- Pediatrics
- Cardiology
- Vascular medicine
- Orthopedic surgery
- Plastic surgery
- ENT
- Genetics
- Physical medicine
- Urology
- Gastroenterology
- Hematology
- Oncology
- General surgery
- Lymphedema clinic
- Thrombophilia clinic
- Pain clinic
- Pathology

the entire team. The plan is then discussed as a group and communicated with the patient.

EPILOGUE

The landscape of vascular malformation evaluation, diagnosis, and treatment is rapidly changing. In recent years, the importance of genomics involvement as well as those with expertise in the medical treatment of vascular anomalies has become increasingly evident. Thus, multispecialty clinics that take care of these complex patients must be open to the contributions of others who may be directly or indirectly involved, and the format of the clinic itself may need to be fluid. It is additionally important that colleagues involved in taking care of these patients are up to date with the latest terminology and treatment literature. Thus, those who are interested, motivated, and able to learn from colleagues are often strong and valuable additions to interdisciplinary vascular malformations clinics. Vascular malformations are specifically suited for management at interdisciplinary clinics. As we noted in a previous editorial,[5] the team approach, so fit for management of vascular malformations, is not new to medicine, it has been time tested and has proven to be extremely effective. As William Mayo

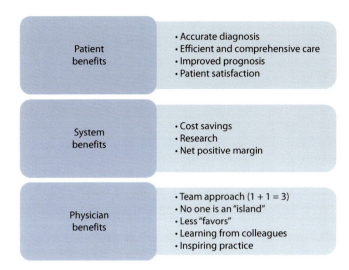

Figure 9.3 Weekly schedule of the interdisciplinary vascular malformation clinic.

said more than 100 years ago, "In order that the sick may have the benefit of advancing knowledge, union of forces is necessary."

REFERENCES

1. Mattila KA, Kervinen K, Kalajoki-Helmio T et al. An interdisciplinary specialist team leads to improved diagnostics and treatment for paediatric patients with vascular anomalies. *Acta Paediatr.* 2015;104:1109–1116.
2. Mathes EF, Haggstrom AN, Dowd C, Hoffman WY, Frieden IJ. Clinical characteristics and management of vascular anomalies: Findings of a multidisciplinary vascular anomalies clinic. *Arch Dermatol.* 2004;140: 979–983.
3. Ranieri M, Wohlgemuth W, Muller-Wille R et al. Vascular malformations of upper and lower extremity— From radiological interventional therapy to surgical soft tissue reconstruction—An interdisciplinary treatment. *Clin Hemorheol Microcirc.* 2017;67:355–372.
4. Lidsky ME, Markovic JN, Miller MJ Jr, Shortell CK. Analysis of the treatment of congenital vascular malformations using a multidisciplinary approach. *J Vasc Surg.* 2012;56:1355–1362; discussion 62.
5. Gloviczki P. Union of forces. *Phlebology.* 2010;25: 217–218.
6. Lee BB, Baumgartner I, Berlien P et al. Diagnosis and treatment of venous malformations. Consensus document of the International Union of Phlebology (IUP): Updated 2013. *Int Angiol.* 2015;34:97–149.
7. Mamlouk MD, Lee PW. Developing a multidisciplinary vascular anomalies clinic and reviewing the radiologist's clinic role. *Curr Probl Diagn Radiol.* 2018;47:378–381.
8. Straughan AJ, Mudd PA, Silva AL, Callicott SS, Krakovsky G, Bauman NM. Cost analysis of a multidisciplinary vascular anomaly clinic. *Ann Otol Rhinol Laryngol.* 2019;128:401–405.

10

How will genetics influence management of vascular malformations?

FRANCINE BLEI

Capillary, venous, arterial, and lymphatic vessel dysmorphogenesis may cause vascular malformations, affecting one or multiple vascular groups. In addition to abnormally formed vasculature, skeletal, cutaneous, or parenchymal abnormalities can arise. Vascular malformations may be familial or sporadic. Nonfamilial vascular malformations can be sporadic or caused by postzygotic (somatic) mutations. Somatic genetic mutations are generally identified in the affected tissue. Tissue expression of the affected mutation is often low, and genetic diagnosis is based on biopsy samples of involved areas. However, newer technologies will likely enable detection of somatic mutations by studying cell-free DNA in peripheral blood.[1,2]

Disorders such as many vascular malformations are described as a "segmental manifestation of lethal genes surviving by mosaicism" by Happel.[3] That is to say that the disorders would not survive as autosomal mutations and can only persist in the mosaic condition, mixed with normal cells. Happel states that "the underlying mutation, when present in all cells of the embryo, acts as a lethal factor, resulting in early intrauterine death," and terms these disorders "Lethal Autosomal Mutations Surviving as Segmental Mosaics, Confirmed at the Molecular Level."[3,4] Several vascular anomalies are in this category (Sturge–Weber syndrome, CLOVES syndrome, Klippel–Trenaunay syndrome, Maffucci syndrome, Proteus syndrome, arteriovenous malformations, and others).[5–10] Familial vascular anomalies also exist: hereditary hemorrhagic telangiectasia, *RASA1* or *EPHB4* mutation-related capillary malformation-arteriovenous malformation (AVM), *PTEN* hamartoma syndrome, cerebral cavernous malformations, mucocutaneous venous malformations, glomuvenous malformations, many lymphedema syndromes, and others.[11–13] These mutations are summarized in Table 10.1.

PIK3CA MUTATIONS

The phosphatidylinositol 3-kinase (PI3K) pathway is one of the major signaling pathways implicated in the development of vascular anomalies (*PIK3CA*-related overgrowth syndromes [PROS]) (Figure 10.1).[14,15] Interestingly, this pathway and mutations therein are often associated with human malignancies; however, malignancy is not a predominant presentation or occurrence in patients with vascular anomalies (Figure 10.2).[16,17] Hotspot mutations in the *PIK3CA* gene include E542K and E545K as well as H1047R, as depicted in Figure 10.3.[15] *PIK3CA* mutations in vascular anomalies are generally postzygotic somatic mutations, expressed in a mosaic fashion in the affected tissue.[18] Arbiser et al. identified an activation mammalian target of rapamycin (mTOR) in cutaneous vascular malformations *in vivo*.[19] Use of the mTOR inhibitor sirolimus in patients with lymphangioleiomyomatosis was promising and led to trials using this medication in patients with complex vascular malformations.[20,21] Although the results are variable, this therapy has been especially promising for patients with malformations having a strong lymphatic component.

OTHER SOMATIC MUTATIONS

Somatic *GNAQ* mutations have been identified in capillary malformations (including Sturge–Weber syndrome), congenital hemangiomas, and other diagnoses. Venous malformations have been associated with mutations in the *TIE2* gene. More recently, MAP2K mutations have been identified in mainly arterial malformations (RASopathies), expanding therapeutic options to medications targeting.[8,22]

Table 10.1 Genetic mutations in vascular anomalies

Syndrome	Mutation	Transmission	OMIM	Gene	Reference
Capillary malformation ("port-wine stain"), nonsyndromic capillary malformation	GNAQ	Somatic	163000	9q21.2	Couto et al.[28]
Sturge–Weber syndrome	GNAQ	Somatic	185300	9q21.2	Shirley et al.[29]
Congenital hemangioma	GNAQ, GNA11				
Diffuse capillary malformation with overgrowth (DCMO)	GNA11	Somatic		19p13.3	Couto et al.[30]
CM with bone and/or soft tissue hyperplasia	GNA11				
Phakomatosis pigmentovascularis and extensive dermal melanocytosis	GNA11 and GNAQ	Somatic		9q21.2, 19p13.3	Thomas et al.[31]
Pyogenic granuloma	BRAF, RAS, GNA14				
Tufted angioma (TA)	GNA14				Lim et al.[32]
Kaposiform hemangioendothelioma (KHE)	GNA14				Lim et al.[32]
Epithelioid hemangioendothelioma (EHE)	CAMTA1-WWTR1, FOS, TFE3	Somatic		t(1;3)(p36.3;q25)	Errani et al., Shibuya et al., Flucke et al.[33-35]
Pseudomyogenic hemangioendothelioma	FOSB				Walther et al.[36]
Postradiation angiosarcoma	MYC				
Arteriovenous fistula	MAP2K1	Somatic			Al-Olabi et al.[8], Nikolaev et al.[55], Hong et al.[56], Walther et al.[36]
Arteriovenous malformation Capillary malformation	RASA1	AD	608354	5q14.3	Revencu et al., Amyere et al.[11,37]
	RASA1 and MEF2C			5q14.3 microdeletion	Carr et al., Park et al.[38,39]
Arteriovenous malformation Capillary malformation	EPHB4	AD			Amyere et al.[11]
Parkes Weber syndrome	RASA1	AD	608355	5q14.3	Revencu et al.[40]
Hereditary hemorrhagic telangiectasia[a]					McDonald et al.[12]
HHT1	ENG	AD	187300	9q34.11	
HHT2	ACVRL1	AD	600376	12q13.13	
HHT3		AD	601101	5q31.3-q32	
Juvenile polyposis syndrome	SMAD4	AD	175050	18q21.2	
HHT-like	GDF2/BMP9	AD	615506	10q11.22	

(Continued)

Table 10.1 (*Continued*) Genetic mutations in vascular anomalies

Syndrome	Mutation	Transmission	OMIM	Gene	Reference
Arteriovenous malformation (extracranial)	MAP2K1	Somatic		15q22.31	Couto et al.[22]
Cerebral cavernous malformations	KRIT1 (CCM1), Malcavernin (CCM2), CCM3 (PDCD10)	AD	116860	7q21.2	
Venous malformation (VM)					
Common VM	PIK3CA	Somatic		3q26.32	Castillo et al.[41]
Common VM	TIE2/TEK	Somatic			
Familial mucocutaneous	TIE2/TEK	AD	600195	9p21.2	Soblet et al.[42]
BRBNS (blue rubber bleb nevus syndrome)	TIE2/TEK	Somatic	12200	9p21.2	Couto et al.[43]
Verrucous venous malformation	MAP3K3	Somatic			Brouillard et al.[44,45]
Glomuvenous malformation	Glomulin	AD	138000	1p22.1	Lindhurst et al.[6]
Proteus syndrome	AKT1	Somatic	176920	14q32.33	Amyere et al.[46]
Maffucci syndrome, spindle cell "hemangioma"	IDH1, IDH2	Somatic	614569	2q34,15q26.1	Kurek et al., Pilarski et al., Nathan et al.[7,47,48]
PTEN hamartoma syndrome	PTEN				
PTEN (type) hamartoma of soft tissue/"angiomatosis" of soft tissue		AD	158350	10q23.31	
Bannayan-Riley-Ruvalcaba syndrome		AD	153480	10q23.31	
SOLAMEN syndrome (segmental overgrowth, lipomatosis, arteriovenous malformation, and epidermal nevus)		AD + second hit somatic			Caux et al.[49]
CLOVES (congenital, lipomatous, overgrowth, vascular malformations, epidermal nevi, and spinal/skeletal anomalies and/or scoliosis)	PIK3CA	Somatic	612918	3q26.32	Kurek et al.[50]
Klippel–Trenaunay	PIK3CA	Somatic	149000	3q26.32	Luks et al.[51]
CLAPO syndrome	PIK3CA	Somatic			Rodriguez-Laguna et al.[57]
Fibro-adipose vascular anomaly	PIK3CA	Somatic			
Lymphatic malformation	PI3 K, PIK3CA	Somatic			
Megalencephaly-capillary malformation-polymicrogyria syndrome (MCAP)	PIK3CA	Somatic	602501	3q26.32	Mirzaa et al.[52]
MICCAP (microcephaly-capillary malformation)	STAMBP	AR	614261	2p13.1	McDonell et al.[53]
Familial intraosseous vascular malformation (vascular malformation osseous [VMOS])	ELMO2	AR	606893	20q13.12	Cetinkaya et al.[54]

[a] http://www.arup.utah.edu/database/HHT/index.php

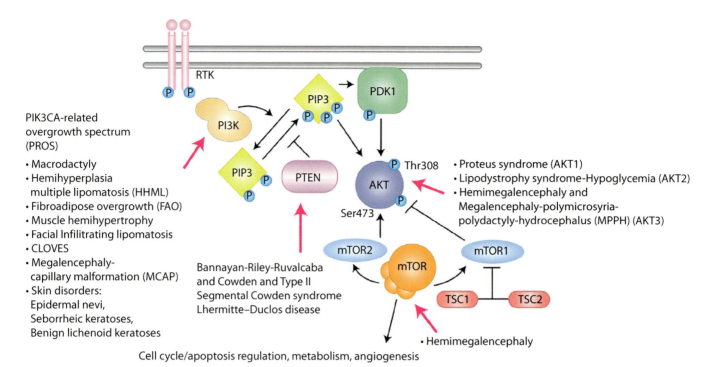

Figure 10.1 PI3K-AKT signaling pathway and associated clinical overgrowth disorders. (From Keppler-Noreuil et al. *Am J Med Genet A.* 2015;167A[2]:287–295.)

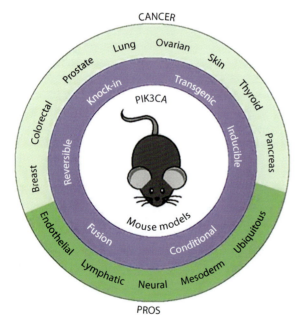

Figure 10.2 Graphical abstract: *PIK3CA*—the gene encoding the p110α catalytic subunit of PI3K—is one of the most commonly mutated human oncogenes. (From Mitchell et al. *Biomolecules.* 2019;9[4]:158.)

GENETICS

Genetics will greatly influence the management of patients with vascular malformations. New therapies target the implicated signaling pathways (Figure 10.4). In addition to antiangiogenic agents, inhibitors of vascular endothelial growth factor (VEGF) or proteins along the PI3K/AKT/mTor or RAS/BRAF/MAPK/ERK pathways are emerging as therapeutic options. Thus far, inhibitors of mTor, *AKT1*, and *PIK3CA* (sirolimus, miransertib [ARQ 092], and BYL719) show promise for patients with complex vascular malformations. Eligibility for clinical trials investigating these treatments requires genotype documentation.[8,21,23–26]

Genetics is also important for the option of prenatal genetic diagnosis for familial vascular malformations with a known mutation in a proband (e.g., *RASA1*, HHT mutations, and others).[27] Preimplantation *in vitro* genetic testing of embryos is also an option for interested families.

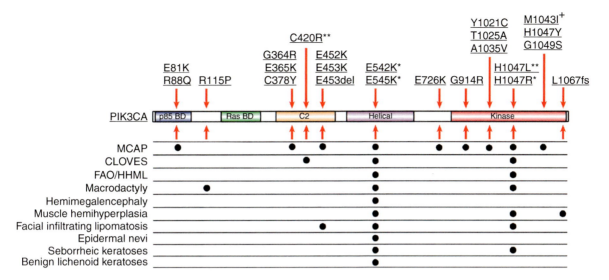

Figure 10.3 *PIK3CA*-related overgrowth spectrum (PROS). *PIK3CA*-predicted protein mutations and associated clinical overgrowth disorders to date. Oncogenic potency: *hot spot mutations, **strong mutations, and +intermediate. (Adopted from Gymnopoulos et al., 2007; from Keppler-Noreuil et al. *Am J Med Genet A.* 2015;167A[2]:287–295.)

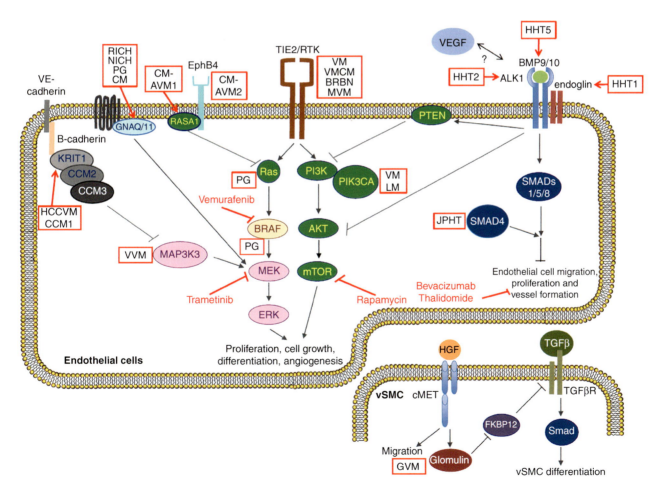

Figure 10.4 Mutations and signaling pathways involved in vascular diseases and vascular tumors and hypothetical treatment options. (From Queisser et al. *Otolaryngol Clin North Am.* 2018;51[1]:41–53. Copyright permission granted.)

REFERENCES

1. Giardina T, Robinson C, Grieu-Iacopetta F et al. Implementation of next generation sequencing technology for somatic mutation detection in routine laboratory practice. *Pathology*. 2018;50(4): 389–401.

2. Breveglieri G, D'Aversa E, Finotti A, Borgatti M. Non-invasive prenatal testing using fetal DNA. *Mol Diagn Ther*. 2019;23(2):291–299.

3. Happle R. Lethal genes surviving by mosaicism: A possible explanation for sporadic birth defects involving the skin. *J Am Acad Dermatol*. 1987;16(4): 899–906.

4. Happle R. The categories of cutaneous mosaicism: A proposed classification. *Am J Med Genet A*. 2016; 170A(2):452–459.

5. Boon LM, Mulliken JB, Vikkula M. RASA1: Variable phenotype with capillary and arteriovenous malformations. *Curr Opin Genet Dev*. 2005;15(3):265–269.

6. Lindhurst MJ, Sapp JC, Teer JK et al. A mosaic activating mutation in AKT1 associated with the Proteus syndrome. *N Engl J Med*. 2011;365(7): 611–619.

7. Nathan N, Keppler-Noreuil KM, Biesecker LG, Moss J, Darling TN. Mosaic disorders of the PI3K/ PTEN/AKT/TSC/mTORC1 signaling pathway. *Dermatol Clin*. 2017;35(1):51–60.

8. Al-Olabi L, Polubothu S, Dowsett K et al. Mosaic RAS/MAPK variants cause sporadic vascular malformations which respond to targeted therapy. *J Clin Invest*. 2018;128(4):1496–1508.

9. Soblet J, Limaye N, Uebelhoer M, Boon LM, Vikkula M. Variable somatic TIE2 mutations in half of sporadic venous malformations. *Mol Syndromol*. 2013;4(4):179–183.

10. Gordo G, Rodriguez-Laguna L, Agra N et al. Constitutional mosaicism in RASA1-related capillary malformation-arteriovenous malformation. *Clin Genet*. 2019;95:516–519.

11. Revencu N, Boon LM, Mendola A et al. RASA1 mutations and associated phenotypes in 68 families with capillary malformation-arteriovenous malformation. *Hum Mutat*. 2013;34(12):1632–1641.

12. McDonald J, Wooderchak-Donahue W, VanSant Webb C, Whitehead K, Stevenson DA, Bayrak-Toydemir P. Hereditary hemorrhagic telangiectasia: Genetics and molecular diagnostics in a new era. *Front Genet*. 2015;6:1.

13. Queisser A, Boon LM, Vikkula M. Etiology and genetics of congenital vascular lesions. *Otolaryngol Clin North Am*. 2018;51(1):41–53.

14. Keppler-Noreuil KM, Sapp JC, Lindhurst MJ et al. Clinical delineation and natural history of the PIK3CA-related overgrowth spectrum. *Am J Med Genet A*. 2014;164A(7):1713–1733.

15. Keppler-Noreuil KM, Rios JJ, Parker VE et al. PIK3CA-related overgrowth spectrum (PROS): Diagnostic and testing eligibility criteria, differential diagnosis, and evaluation. *Am J Med Genet A*. 2015;167A(2):287–295.

16. Mitchell CB, Phillips WA. Mouse models for exploring the biological consequences and clinical significance of PIK3CA mutations. *Biomolecules*. 2019; 9(4):158.

17. Blatt J, Finger M, Price V, Crary SE, Pandya A, Adams DM. Cancer risk in Klippel–Trenaunay syndrome. *Lymphat Res Biol*. 2019. https://doi.org/10.1089/lrb.2018.0049.

18. Erickson RP. Somatic gene mutation and human disease other than cancer: An update. *Mutat Res*. 2010;705(2):96–106.

19. Shirazi F, Cohen C, Fried L, Arbiser JL. Mammalian target of rapamycin (mTOR) is activated in cutaneous vascular malformations in vivo. *Lymphat Res Biol*. 2007;5(4):233–236.

20. Adams DM, Trenor CC 3rd, Hammill AM et al. Efficacy and safety of Sirolimus in the treatment of complicated vascular anomalies. *Pediatrics*. 2016;137(2):e20153257.

21. Hammer J, Seront E, Duez S et al. Sirolimus is efficacious in treatment for extensive and/or complex slow-flow vascular malformations: A monocentric prospective phase II study. *Orphanet J Rare Dis*. 2018;13(1):191.

22. Couto JA, Huang AY, Konczyk DJ et al. Somatic MAP2K1 mutations are associated with extracranial arteriovenous malformation. *Am J Hum Genet*. 2017;100(3):546–554.

23. Lindhurst MJ, Yourick MR, Yu Y, Savage RE, Ferrari D, Biesecker LG. Repression of AKT signaling by ARQ 092 in cells and tissues from patients with Proteus syndrome. *Sci Rep*. 2015;5:17162.

24. Ranieri C, Di Tommaso S, Loconte DC et al. *In vitro* efficacy of ARQ 092, an allosteric AKT inhibitor, on primary fibroblast cells derived from patients with PIK3CA-related overgrowth spectrum (PROS). *Neurogenetics*. 2018;19(2):77–91.

25. Venot Q, Blanc T, Rabia SH et al. Targeted therapy in patients with PIK3CA-related overgrowth syndrome. *Nature*. 2018;558(7711):540–546.

26. Keppler-Noreuil KM, Sapp JC, Lindhurst MJ et al. Pharmacodynamic study of miransertib in individuals with Proteus syndrome. *Am J Hum Genet*. 2019;104(3):484–491.

27. Palmyre A, Eyries M, Senat MV et al. Prenatal molecular diagnosis in RASA1-related disease. *Prenat Diagn*. 2017;37(12):1261–1264.

28. Couto JA, Huang L, Vivero MP et al. Endothelial cells from capillary malformations are enriched for somatic GNAQ mutations. *Plast Reconstr Surg*. 2016; 137(1):77e–82e.

29. Shirley MD, Tang H, Gallione CJ et al. Sturge–Weber syndrome and port-wine stains caused by somatic mutation in GNAQ. *N Engl J Med.* 2013;368(21):1971–1979.

30. Couto JA, Ayturk UM, Konczyk DJ et al. A somatic GNA11 mutation is associated with extremity capillary malformation and overgrowth. *Angiogenesis.* 2017;20(3):303–306.

31. Thomas AC, Zeng Z, Riviere JB et al. Mosaic activating mutations in GNA11 and GNAQ are associated with phakomatosis pigmentovascularis and extensive dermal melanocytosis. *J Invest Dermatol.* 2016;136(4):770–778.

32. Lim YH, Bacchiocchi A, Qiu J et al. GNA14 somatic mutation causes congenital and sporadic vascular tumors by MAPK activation. *Am J Hum Genet.* 2016;99(2):443–450.

33. Errani C, Zhang L, Sung YS et al. A novel WWTR1-CAMTA1 gene fusion is a consistent abnormality in epithelioid hemangioendothelioma of different anatomic sites. *Genes Chromosomes Cancer.* 2011;50(8):644–653.

34. Shibuya R, Matsuyama A, Shiba E, Harada H, Yabuki K, Hisaoka M. CAMTA1 is a useful immunohistochemical marker for diagnosing epithelioid haemangioendothelioma. *Histopathology.* 2015;67(6):827–835.

35. Flucke U, Vogels RJ, de Saint Aubain Somerhausen N et al. Epithelioid hemangioendothelioma: Clinicopathologic, immunohistochemical, and molecular genetic analysis of 39 cases. *Diagn Pathol.* 2014;9:131.

36. Walther C, Tayebwa J, Lilljebjorn H et al. A novel SERPINE1-FOSB fusion gene results in transcriptional up-regulation of FOSB in pseudomyogenic haemangioendothelioma. *J Pathol.* 2014;232(5):534–540.

37. Amyere M et al. Germline loss-of-function mutations in EPHB4 cause a second form of capillary malformation-arteriovenous malformation (CM-AVM2) deregulating RAS-MAPK signaling. *Circulation.* 2017;136(11):1037–1048.

38. Park SM, Kim JM, Kim GW et al. 5q14.3 Microdeletions: A contiguous gene syndrome with capillary malformation-arteriovenous malformation syndrome and neurologic findings. *Pediatr Dermatol.* 2017;34(2):156–159.

39. Carr CW, Zimmerman HH, Martin CL, Vikkula M, Byrd AC, Abdul-Rahman OA. 5q14.3 neurocutaneous syndrome: A novel continguous gene syndrome caused by simultaneous deletion of RASA1 and MEF2C. *Am J Med Genet A.* 2011;155A(7):1640–1645.

40. Revencu N, Boon LM, Mulliken JB et al. Parkes Weber syndrome, vein of Galen aneurysmal malformation, and other fast-flow vascular anomalies are caused by RASA1 mutations. *Hum Mutat.* 2008;29(7):959–965.

41. Castillo SD, Tzouanacou E, Zaw-Thin M et al. Somatic activating mutations in Pik3ca cause sporadic venous malformations in mice and humans. *Sci Transl Med.* 2016;8(332):332ra43.

42. Soblet J, Kangas J, Natynki M et al. Blue rubber bleb nevus (BRBN) syndrome is caused by somatic TEK (TIE2) mutations. *J Invest Dermatol.* 2017;137(1):207–216.

43. Couto JA, Vivero MP, Kozakewich HP et al. A somatic MAP3K3 mutation is associated with verrucous venous malformation. *Am J Hum Genet.* 2015;96(3):480–486.

44. Brouillard P, Boon LM, Mulliken JB et al. Mutations in a novel factor, glomulin, are responsible for glomuvenous malformations ("glomangiomas"). *Am J Hum Genet.* 2002;70(4):866–874.

45. Brouillard P, Boon LM, Revencu N et al. Genotypes and phenotypes of 162 families with a glomulin mutation. *Mol Syndromol.* 2013;4(4):157–164.

46. Amyere M, Dompmartin A, Wouters V et al. Common somatic alterations identified in Maffucci syndrome by molecular karyotyping. *Mol Syndromol.* 2014;5(6):259–267.

47. Kurek KC, Howard E, Tennant LB et al. PTEN hamartoma of soft tissue: A distinctive lesion in PTEN syndromes. *Am J Surg Pathol.* 2012;36(5):671–687.

48. Pilarski R, Burt R, Kohlman W, Pho L, Shannon KM, Swisher E. Cowden syndrome and the PTEN hamartoma tumor syndrome: Systematic review and revised diagnostic criteria. *J Natl Cancer Inst.* 2013;105(21):1607–1616.

49. Caux F, Plauchu H, Chibon F et al. Segmental overgrowth, lipomatosis, arteriovenous malformation and epidermal nevus (SOLAMEN) syndrome is related to mosaic PTEN nullizygosity. *Eur J Hum Genet.* 2007;15(7):767–773.

50. Kurek KC, Luks VL, Ayturk UM et al. Somatic mosaic activating mutations in PIK3CA cause CLOVES syndrome. *Am J Hum Genet.* 2012;90(6):1108–1115.

51. Luks VL, Kamitaki N, Vivero MP et al. Lymphatic and other vascular malformative/overgrowth disorders are caused by somatic mutations in PIK3CA. *J Pediatr.* 2015;166(4):1048–1054.e1–5.

52. Mirzaa GM, Riviere JB, Dobyns WB. Megalencephaly syndromes and activating mutations in the PI3K-AKT pathway: MPPH and MCAP. *Am J Med Genet C Semin Med Genet.* 2013;163C(2):122–130.

53. McDonell LM, Mirzaa GM, Alcantara D et al. Mutations in STAMBP, encoding a deubiquitinating enzyme, cause microcephaly-capillary malformation syndrome. *Nat Genet.* 2013;45(5):556–562.

54. Cetinkaya A, Xiong JR, Vargel I et al. Loss-of-function mutations in ELMO2 cause intraosseous vascular malformation by impeding RAC1 signaling. *Am J Hum Genet.* 2016;99(2):299–317.

55. Nikolaev SI et al. Somatic activating KRAS mutations in arteriovenous malformations of the brain. *N Engl J Med.* 2018;378(3):250–261.

56. Hong T et al. High prevalence of KRAS/BRAF somatic mutations in brain and spinal cord arteriovenous malformations. *Brain.* 2019;142(1):23–34.

57. Rodriguez-Laguna L et al. CLAPO syndrome: Identification of somatic activating PIK3CA mutations and delineation of the natural history and phenotype. *Genet Med.* 2018;20(8):882–889.

PART **2**

Arteriovenous Malformations (AVMs)

Definition and Classification

11

Confusion with arteriovenous fistula versus arteriovenous malformation of ISSVA classification

DIRK A. LOOSE

Developmental disorders develop in different stages during embryonic development. If a disorder occurs in the development from hemangioblast to angioblast, a vasculogenous defect develops and thus an extra-truncular vascular malformation. There are *inter alia*, diffuse short-circuit connections of arteries and veins: extra-truncular arteriovenous (AV) malformations.

If the developmental disorder occurs at a later stage of maturity of the embryo, then the angioblast is disturbed in the differentiation of the vascular structures and an angiogenic defect arises: a truncular defect of differentiated vessels (e.g., veins and arteries, which may well have communications).

It must, therefore, be made clear in the International Society for the Study of Vascular Anomalies (ISSVA) classification that there are *single* malformed vascular structures in contrast to the combined ones, and that there are AV malformations as an entity, which, of course, have numerous AV fistulas. This eliminates the rubric for a single AV fistula.

> The beginning of wisdom lies in calling things by their correct name
>
> Konfuzius, 551 v.Chr.-479 v.Chr.

It is essential to state that in the embryonal development, there are ripening stages depending on the age of the embryo. If there are developmental defects, it is mandatory to know at which ripening stage the defect started (Figure 11.1).[1]

If the developmental defect, the inborn embryonic error,[2] starts in an early ripening stage, and if the affected cell material, the hemangioblasts, will be more differentiated, then this cell type is called *angioblast*. From this cell population, vascular structures start to develop,[3] which is called *vasculogenesis*. We call the resulting developmental malformation an *extra-truncular vascular malformation*.[4]

This disturbed developmental process can affect all vascular structures, which are going to differentiate into arteries, veins, and lymph vessels—the formation of the endothelial vascular plexus.[5] That is why all possible developmental vascular malformations exist, isolated or in every imaginable combination. There are also numerous microvascular or larger-caliber connections of veins and arteries, called *multiple AV fistulas* (Figure 11.2).[6]

Such extra-truncular AV malformations represent completely different challenges. They are active lesions, and they have a high tendency to progress, to worsen, and to re-expand after treatment.

If the developmental defect starts in a late stage of the developing embryo, and the affected structures are differentiated vessels with maturation of the vessel wall, named *angiogenesis* (Figure 11.1),[2] we call the resulting developmental malformation a *truncular* vascular malformation. This disturbed developmental process can affect only arteries (resulting in aneurysms, coarctations, arterial stenosis, arterial ectasias) or only veins (stenosis or obstruction) or it can even affect arteries and veins in the form of *single arteriovenous connections* (Figures 11.3 and 11.4):

1. *Extra-truncular multiple arteriovenous malformations* (AVMs) (Figure 11.2): Complex combined regional syndromes, early embryonal defects, and developmental malformations. We call them *vasculogenic*.
2. *Truncular arterial malformations* (AMs): Aneurysms, arterial coarctation, arterial ectasias, arterial stenosis, and single AV communications (Figures 11.3 and 11.4), late embryonal defects, and developmental malformations. We call them *angiogenic*.

Truncular AMs develop in the late phase of embryonic development, and they have a much better prognosis in terms of recurrence than the extra-truncular AVMs.

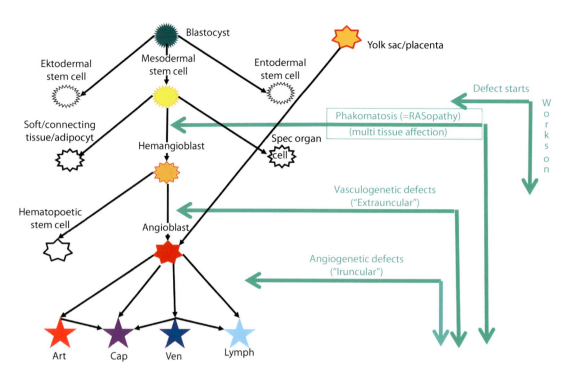

Figure 11.1 Algorithm showing the different steps of development of the angiogenesis according to P. Berlien.

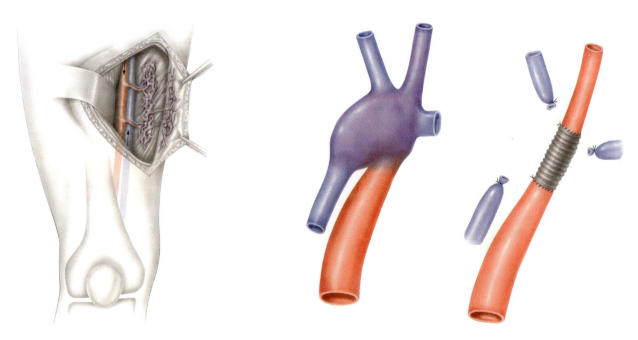

Figure 11.2 Extra-truncular arteriovenous malformation.

Figure 11.3 Truncular arteriovenous communication of major named vessels.

These truncular AMs occur as aneurysms, coarctations, and stenosis or ectasias or single AV communications. The surgical repair applies regular techniques of reconstructive vascular surgery, such as tangential resection of an aneurysm, resection of the aneurysm, and replacement by autologous interposition graft or an autologous venous patch angioplasty or an alloplastic bypass graft to treat an arterial or aortic stenosis or coarctation.

Congenital AV communications of major named vessels (ISSVA [Figure 11.5]) are also treated by standard vascular surgery techniques (e.g., interruption of the venous connection and reconstruction of the arterial defect by an alloplastic interposition graft [Figure 11.3]). AV communications of larger peripheral vessels can be treated by interventional catheter techniques as well as by open vascular surgery: ligation and interruption of each AV communication (Figure 11.6).

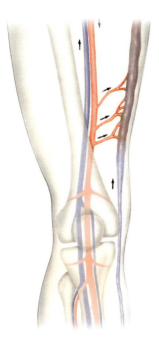

Figure 11.4 Single arteriovenous communications.

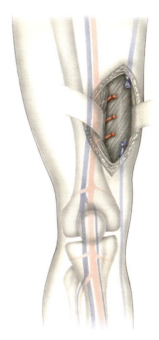

Figure 11.6 Ligation and interruption of each of the arteriovenous communications.

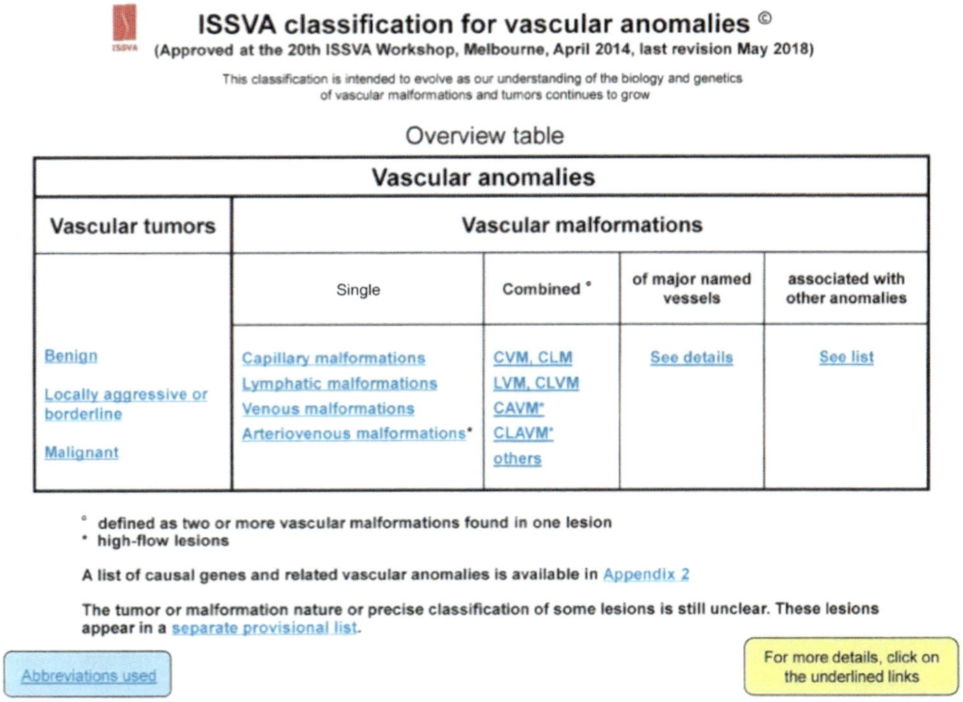

ISSVA classification for vascular anomalies ©
(Approved at the 20th ISSVA Workshop, Melbourne, April 2014, last revision May 2018)

This classification is intended to evolve as our understanding of the biology and genetics
of vascular malformations and tumors continues to grow

Overview table

Vascular anomalies				
Vascular tumors	**Vascular malformations**			
	Single	Combined °	of major named vessels	associated with other anomalies
Benign	Capillary malformations	CVM, CLM	See details	See list
Locally aggressive or borderline	Lymphatic malformations	LVM, CLVM		
	Venous malformations	CAVM*		
Malignant	Arteriovenous malformations*	CLAVM*		
		others		

° defined as two or more vascular malformations found in one lesion
* high-flow lesions

A list of causal genes and related vascular anomalies is available in Appendix 2

The tumor or malformation nature or precise classification of some lesions is still unclear. These lesions appear in a separate provisional list.

Abbreviations used

For more details, click on the underlined links

Figure 11.5 Corrected ISSVA classification for vascular anomalies.

That is why in the vascular anomalies overview presented in Figure 11.5, the term *vascular malformations* is given as "simple." This is a mistake, because it should be called "single."

The term *AV fistula* is misleading, and it should be deleted in the ISSVA classification (Figure 11.5).[7]

REFERENCES

1. Berlien P, Urban P, Poetke M et al. Classification of vascular malformations. *Phlebologie.* 2016;45(5):295–303.
2. Chun CZ, Sood R, Ramchandran R. Vasculogenesis and angiogenesis. In: North PE, Sander T, eds. *Vascular*

Tumors and Developmental Malformations. New York, NY: Springer Science and Business Media; 2016:77–99.

3. Wilting J, Männer J. Vascular embryology. In: Mattassi R, Loose DA, Vaghi M, eds. *Hemangiomas and Vascular Malformations.* 2nd ed. Milano, Italy: Springer; 2015:3–19.

4. Loose DA, Mattassi RE. Hamburg classification of vascular malformations. In: Kim YW, Lee BB, Yakes WF, Do YS, eds. *Congenital Vascular Malformation—Comprehensive Review on Current Management.* Heidelberg, Germany: Springer; 2017:51–54.

5. Mattassi R, Loose DA. Classification of vascular malformations. In: Mattassi R, Loose DA, Vaghi M, eds. *Hemangiomas and Vascular Malformations.* 2nd ed. Milano, Italy; 2015:181–186.

6. Loose DA, Surgical treatment for high-flow CVM. In: Kim YW, Lee BB, Yakes WF, Do YS, eds. *Congenital Vascular Malformation—Comprehensive Review on Current Management.* Heidelberg, Germany: Springer; 2017:275–282.

7. Wassef M, Blei F, Adams D et al. ISSVA Board and Scientific Committee: Vascular anomalies classification: Recommendations from the International Society for the Study of Vascular Anomalies. *Pediatrics.* 2015;136(1):203–214.

12

Nidus or no nidus: Is it a crucial issue for diagnostic assessment of arteriovenous malformations?

FURUZAN NUMAN

Arteriovenous malformations (AVMs) are one of various congenital vascular malformations (CVMs) seen at many sites in the body and result from birth defects involving the vessels of both arterial and venous origins. Direct communications between them or via a meshwork of abnormal vessels is termed a *nidus*. AVMs are characterized by the shunting of high-velocity low-resistance blood flow from the arterial vasculature into the venous system via the fistulous vascular network.[1-4]

The pathogenesis of AVM is still largely unknown, and no specific marker proteins have been identified for AVM.

The differentiating angioblasts aggregate into a primitive vascular plexus (vasculogenesis), which subsequently undergoes growth, migration, and sprouting (angiogenesis), resulting in the development of a functional circulatory system.

As angiogenesis progresses, vessels become surrounded by layers of mesenchyme-derived pericytes in smaller vessels and vascular smooth muscle cells (vSMCs) in larger vessels. They produce signals that are essential for the generation and stabilization of mature blood vessels.

Proper assembly of the vessel wall depends on reciprocal communication between endothelial cells and vSMCs. Endothelial cells cannot complete mature vessel formation independently. Endothelial cells differentiate from mesodermally derived angioblasts in response to signals provided by surrounding tissues and the extracellular matrix.

The initial stage of vascular development consists of the formation of a primitive vascular tube made of a single layer of endothelial cells. Vascular development consists of an early stage of vasculogenesis and a later stage of vascular maturation.

Expression of specific markers in endothelial cells determines their differentiation, either into an artery or into a vein in the early stage of vascular development.[4,5] The Dll4-Hey2-EphrinB2 pathway determines endothelial fate as an artery, and the *COUP-TFII* pathway signals endothelial cells to become veins.[6,7]

Blood vessel maturation is the later stage of vascular development. The reciprocal interactions between endothelial cells and vSMCs are essential for vessel maturation. This interaction strengthens vSMCs around the vascular tube and stabilizes the blood vessel. TGF-β and PDGF-β are two major genes involved in this maturation process.

Endoglin is a TGF-β coreceptor that is necessary for angiogenesis. Endoglin null embryos exhibit a loss of arteriovenous identity and defective vSMC recruitment. Examination of endoglin null embryos revealed ectopic arterial expression of the venous-specific marker COUP-TFII when endoglin reexpression in endothelial cells restored normal COUP-TFII expression. These findings suggest that endoglin plays distinct and cell-autonomous roles in vSMC recruitment and arteriovenous specification via COUP-TFII in angiogenesis.

As an example, polymorphism (mutations) in TGF-β coreceptors endoglin and activin receptor-like kinase 1 plays a critical role in the development of hereditary hemorrhagic telangiectasia (HHT) disease. These mutations commonly lead to loss of function in the genes associated with TGF-β signaling as shown in laboratory studies.

The possibility of combinatorial changes at genetic and epigenetic levels in vascular development leads to the abnormal phenotype of AVM. Studies suggest that the development of AVM requires stimuli to endothelial cells in blood vessels.[8,9] It could be at either the transcriptional level or the metabolite level in the cytoplasm of endothelial cells. Altered transcription may happen according to changes at epigenetic makeup or at gene level.

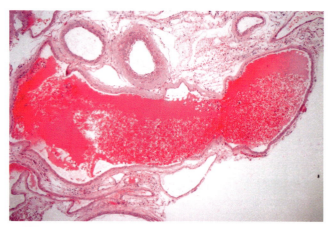

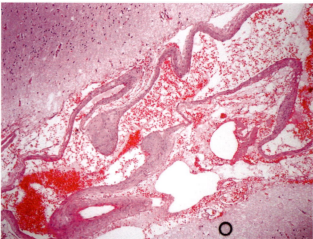

Figure 12.1 Arteriovenous malformation. The close juxtaposition of artery and vein and an associated small vessel component (H&EX40-100). (Courtesy of Prof. Nil Counoglu, MD, Istanbul University School of Medicine, Department of Pathology, Istanbul, Turkey.)

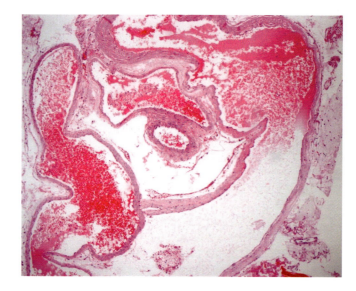

Figure 12.2 Venous component in arteriovenous malformation (H&EX100). (Courtesy of Prof. Nil Counoglu, MD, Istanbul University School of Medicine, Department of Pathology, Istanbul, Turkey.)

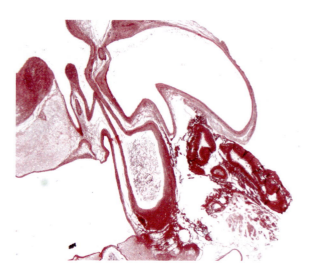

Figure 12.3 Elastic stain illustrated in arteriovenous malformation (EVGX40). (Courtesy of Prof. Nil Counoglu, MD, Istanbul University School of Medicine, Department of Pathology, Istanbul, Turkey.)

A series of changes in the metabolites in the endothelial cells, such as the DNA methylation and histone modifications in the genes, may also trigger AVM development.

Histological analysis showed that AVM nidus is a collection of aberrant vascular structures depicted as hypertrophic veins, with increased thickness of the media layer, arterial-like structures with reduced tunica media layer, and small arteriole and venules (Figures 12.1 and 12.2). In AVM nidus, EVG staining revealed the presence of large arteries and dysplastic veins with a discontinuous internal elastic lamina layer (Figure 12.3).

The α-SMA staining demonstrated aberrancy in the smooth muscle layer of AVM-associated blood vessels. As a conclusion, a nidus formation is the most important part of an AVM. Understanding its whole complex pathway of development will help us to find the best way to treat AVM now and may help to prevent development of AVM in the future by restoring defected genes and perigenetic factors.

REFERENCES

1. Lee BB, Laredo J, Deaton DH, Neville RF. Arteriovenous malformations: Evaluation and treatment. In: Gloviczki P, ed. *Handbook of Venous Disorders: Guidelines of the American Venous Forum.* 3rd ed. London, UK: A Hodder Arnold; 2009:649–662.
2. Lee BB, Do YS, Yakes W, Kim DI, Mattassi R, Hyun WS. Management of arterial-venous shunting malformations (AVM) by surgery and embolosclerotherapy. A multidisciplinary approach. *J Vasc Surg.* 2004;39:590–600.

3. Simon MC. Vascular morphogenesis and the formation of vascular networks. *Dev Cell*. 2004;6:479–482.

4. Conway EM, Collen D, Carmeliet P. Molecular mechanisms of blood vessel growth. *Cardiovasc Res*. 2001;49:507–521.

5. Shin D, Garcia-Cardena G, Hayashi S et al. Expression of ephrinB2 identifies a stable genetic difference between arterial and venous vascular smooth muscle as well as endothelial cells, and marks subsets of microvessels at sites of adult neovascularization. *Dev Biol*. 2001;230:139–150.

6. Davis RB, Curtis CD, Griffin CT. BRG1 promotes COUP-TFII expression and venous specification during embryonic vascular development. *Development*. 2013;140:1272–1281.

7. Mancini ML, Terzic A, Conley BA, Oxburgh LH, Nicola T, Calvin PH. Vary, endoglin plays distinct roles in vascular smooth muscle cell recruitment and regulation of arteriovenous identity during angiogenesis. *Dev Dyn*. 2009;238(10):2479–2493.

8. Thomas JM, Surendran S, Abraham M et al. Gene expression analysis of nidus of cerebral arteriovenous malformations reveals vascular structures with deficient differentiation and maturation. *PLOS ONE*. 2018;13(6):e0198617.

9. Thomas JM, Surendran S, Abraham M, Rajavelu A, Kartha CC. Genetic and epigenetic mechanisms in the development of arteriovenous malformations in the brain. *Clin Epigenetics*. 2016;8:78.

13

New classification of arteriovenous malformations based on angiographic findings: What are the advantages?

YOUNG SOO DO AND KWANG BO PARK

Angiography is the gold standard of confirmative diagnosis as well as therapeutic tools in the management of arteriovenous malformation (AVM). Typically, arteriography in AVM shows the feeding artery, nidus, and early draining veins. Angiographic findings of AVM are totally different in every patient, and the malformed vasculature is very complex to determine the detailed vascular connection at a glance. Therefore, types and patterns of different AVMs have been required to be classified systematically to correlate with the treatment response. Simplified angiographic classification of intracranial AVM proposed by Houdart et al. in 1993 is considered to be an adequate model for application in peripheral AVM.[1] In this simplified classification system, AVM was divided into three different types, and the number and size of the feeding artery and vein as well as the vascular connection between the feeding artery and vein were the main considerations for the angiographic description and classification. Based on this concept, Cho et al. and Ko et al. proposed modified angiographic classification for the AVMs in the torso and extremity in 2006 and 2019.[2,3]

Figure 13.1 illustrates the vascular anatomical connection between feeding artery and draining veins. A type I AVM is defined as an arteriovenous fistula that consists of not more than three different feeding arteries that shunt to a single draining vein: a single direct arteriovenous fistula. A type II AVM refers to arteriolovenous fistulae that consist of multiple arterioles shunting to the draining vein. According to the morphology of the draining vein, type II is subclassified into types IIa, IIb, and IIc.[3] Type IIa AVM indicates multiple arterioles shunt to the focal segment of the single draining vein. Type IIb AVM indicates multiple arterioles shunt to the venous sac with multiple draining veins. Type IIc AVM indicates multiple arterioles shunt along the long segment of the draining vein. Type III AVMs have multiple shunts between the arterioles and venules. In this type, if

the fistula unit of the nidus is observed as a blush or fine striation on angiography, it is categorized as type IIIa with a nondilated fistula; when the fistula unit of the nidus is observed as a complex vascular network, it is classified as type IIIb with a dilated fistula.

According to the angiographic classification of AVMs, treatment strategy should be different. Figure 13.2 presents a typical treatment approach and embolotherapy according to the angiographic types of AVM. The main target of type I AVM is the direct fistula between the artery and draining vein. The fistula is embolized with coils, or plugs, by the intraarterial approach. Generally, our treatment strategy for type II AVM is as follows: first, reduce the blood flow velocity in the venous segment of AVM with coils, and second, perform ethanol embolotherapy of the residual shunts, because the shunts are located at the venous wall of the draining vein. For type IIa AVM, the focal venous segment of the draining vein of the AVM is approached by direct puncture or transvenous approach, and the focal venous segment is embolized by packing with coils or core-removed guidewire. Because coil packing is not enough to occlude the shunts, additional injection of high concentration ethanol (80%–100%) is required through an intraarterial superselective microcatheter, percutaneous puncture needle, or transvenous catheter. For type IIb AVM, direct puncture of the venous sac would be the most effective approach. The procedure, which consists of coil packing of the venous sac followed by ethanol injection, is similar to that of type IIa AVM. In type IIc AVM, direct puncture or the transvenous approach to the draining vein and coil embolization and additional ethanol injection between the insertions of multiple coils along the long segment of the draining vein are effective. Type IIIa is treated by intraarterial catheterization of the feeding arteries and injection of diluted ethanol (50%–60%), because micro-fistulae are too small to puncture directly. Type IIIb is treated

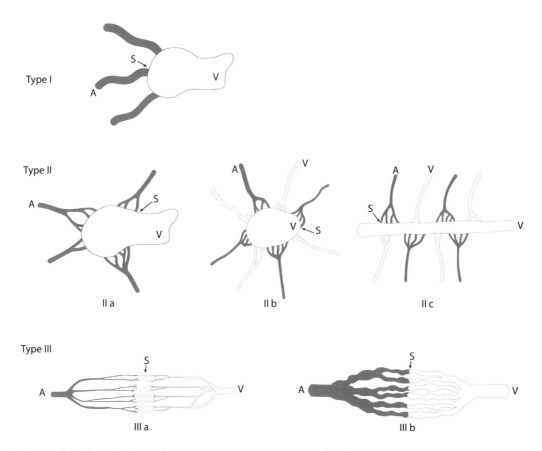

Figure 13.1 Angiographic classification of AVMs. Type I: arteriovenous fistulae with not more than three feeding arteries and a single draining vein. Type IIa: multiple arterioles shunt to the focal segment of the single draining vein. Type IIb: multiple arterioles shunt to the venous sac with multiple draining veins. Type IIc: multiple arterioles shunt along the long segment of the draining vein. Type IIIa: multiple arterioles shunt to the multiple draining veins through the multiple fine fistulae. Type IIIb: multiple arterioles shunt to the multiple draining veins through the multiple enlarged fistulae. (A, artery; S, shunt; V, vein.)

through either intraarterial or direct puncture approaches. A high concentration of ethanol (80%–100%) is injected through the intraarterial catheter or direct puncture needle. When the fistula is large, coil insertion is required to reduce the amount of ethanol.

In our experience, the treatment of peripheral AVMs in 306 patients resulted in an overall cure rate of 39% and a clinical success rate (cured + markedly improved) of 60%. Among them, type I AVM was rare (less than 2%), but cure rate after embolization of the fistula was 100%. The proportion of type II was 27%, and cure rate was up to 80%;[4] the cure rate of type IIa (95%) was significantly better than that of type IIc (65%; $p = 0.015$).[3] The proportions of type IIIa and IIIb were 5% and 40%, respectively. Types IIIa and IIIb showed less therapeutic response to embolotherapy. The cure rates of type IIIa and IIIb were 19% and 30%, respectively, and the clinical success rates of type IIIa and IIIb were 50% and 56%, respectively. Although the modified angiographic classification system defined a category for each type of AVM, not all the AVMs fall into these four specific types completely. Twenty seven percent of AVMs are classified as complex AVMs; that means more than two different types of

AVM are combined.[4] In terms of angiographic classification, those with type I and type II AVMs showed the best clinical results with ethanol embolotherapy with or without coils, and those with type IIIb also showed an acceptably good response rate. However, either alone or in combination with other types, type IIIa showed the poorest response rate.[4] One study showed that lesion extent is also related to treatment response.[5] Even with type IIIb AVM, localized lesion can show good results with repetitive treatment. However, a satisfactory result is difficult with extensive AVMs involving the whole extremity. The overall complication rate of ethanol embolotherapy was 23%, with 20% minor and 3% major complications. Skin necrosis and bullae formation were the most common minor complications.[4]

In conclusion, by using a different treatment strategy according to the types of AVMs, a high cure rate can be achieved with acceptable major and minor complications. This new classification and treatment strategy for peripheral AVMs may provide therapeutic teams with a standardized understanding of the characteristics of AVMs in the body and extremities, which is useful for planning the optimal therapeutic approach.

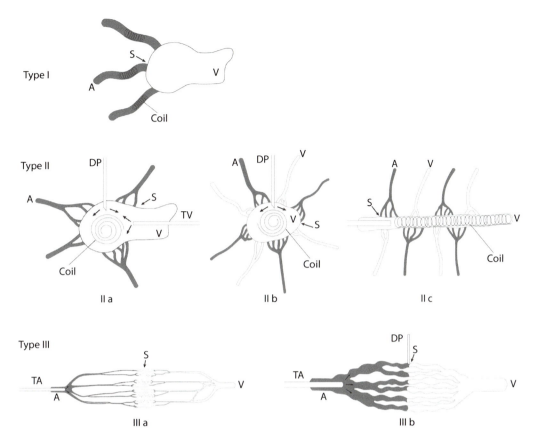

Figure 13.2 Strategy for embolotherapy according to each type of AVM. Type I: arteriovenous fistula is embolized with coils. Type IIa: focal venous sac is embolized with coils or core-removed guidewires through direct puncture or the transvenous catheter approach. Type IIb: venous sac is embolized with coils or core-removed guidewires through the direct puncture approach. Type IIc: long segment of the draining vein is occluded with coils or core-removed guidewires by the transvenous approach or direct puncture. Type IIIa: diluted ethanol (50%–60%) is injected through the transarterial catheter. Type IIIb: high concentration of ethanol (80%–100%) is injected through the transarterial catheter or direct puncture needle. When the fistula is large, coil insertion is required to reduce the amount of ethanol. (A, artery; DP, direct puncture; S, shunt; V, vein.)

REFERENCES

1. Houdart E, Gobin YP, Casasco A et al. A proposed angiographic classification of intracranial arteriovenous fistulae and malformations. *Neuroradiology.* 1993;35:381–385.
2. Cho SK, Do YS, Shin SW et al. Arteriovenous malformations of the body and extremities: Analysis of therapeutic outcomes and approaches according to a modified angiographic classification. *J Endovasc Ther.* 2006;13:527–538.
3. Ko SE, Do YS, Park KB et al. Sub-classification and treatment results of ethanol embolotherapy of type II arteriovenous malformations of the extremity and body. *J Vasc Interv Radiol.* 2019;30(9):1443–1451.
4. Park KB, Do YS, Kim DI et al. Endovascular treatment results and risk factors for complications of body and extremity arteriovenous malformations. *J Vasc Surg.* 2019;69:1207–1218.
5. Park KB, Do YS, Kim DI et al. Predictive factors for response of peripheral arteriovenous malformations to embolization therapy: Analysis of clinical data and imaging findings. *J Vasc Interv Radiol.* 2012;23: 1478–1486.

Diagnosis

14

Arteriographic assessment: Is it still the gold standard for diagnosis of arteriovenous malformations?

HENDRIK VON TENGG-KOBLIGK, SABRINA FREY, DOMINIK OBRIST, AND IRIS BAUMGARTNER

INTRODUCTION

Clinicians expect that diagnostic noninvasive imaging will differentiate between high-flow or low-flow congenital vascular malformations (CVMs) and will define its three-dimensional (3D) anatomy. If vascular structures are involved and the hemodynamic characteristics are unknown, a combination of functional and structural imaging methods should be applied.[1] Primary imaging aims at distinguishing between no- and low-flow or high-flow lesions, and it should also define the extent of the lesion to establish if it is uni- or multifocal.[2] Noninvasive imaging has emerged as an eminent initial diagnostic step,[3] and it helps the multidisciplinary team in treatment decisions and to support long-term management strategies.[2]

"The Holy Grail" of noninvasive, high-flow imaging of arterio-venous malformation (AVM) remains the detection of the nidus (arterio-venous transition) and the characterization of the angioarchitecture to classify AVM subtypes.[4] All being extremely relevant for therapy planning and outcome prediction. Since relevant hemodynamic aspects within the nidus change in the range of milliseconds, switching from the arterial to the venous system, high temporal and high spatial resolutions are key to allow proper visualization and quantification of vascular characteristics.

IMAGING METHODS

A multidisciplinary team needs to embrace more or less four different imaging methods that can be used for initial exploration, focused diagnostic workup, intervention, and follow-up. Each step has specific requirements.

Ultrasound-based techniques

Typically, ultrasound (US)-based techniques are applied first, because of excellent availability, high safety profile, and low cost. US is straightforward and allows hemodynamic evaluation using color and pulsed Doppler mode.[1] Continuous-wave (CW) Doppler can quickly determine the type of blood flow (*high flow* versus *low flow* or *no flow*) and is best suited during the initial diagnostic procedure. Venous malformation (VM) and lymphatic malformation (LM) will present with low flow or no flow, whereas AVMs will present with pulsatile high-flow characteristics.

Duplex ultrasound (DUS) remains the first choice for initial clinical evaluation and follow-up among the various noninvasive modalities. However, US has the disadvantages of a limited field of view, restricted penetration, and operator dependency. Power Doppler can be used to have a more sensitive detection of blood flow.

Digital subtraction arteriography

Dynamic two-dimensional (2D) catheter-based intra-arterial digital subtraction angiography (DSA) is still the gold standard for final diagnostic imaging to confirm or optimize the description of the nidus localization within the predefined AVM due to its high temporal resolution of up to 30 images/second (approximately 30 ms) at a spatial resolution of ca. 1 mm^3.[5,6] Recent technological improvements enabling four-dimensional (4D) DSA with improved spatial resolution to approximately 0.01 mm^3 (while maintaining the same temporal resolution) offer an unmet combination of both high spatial and temporal resolution. This and the ability to select the essential feeding vessel make catheter- and X-ray-based imaging still the method of choice. Nevertheless, its existing disadvantages, like ionizing radiation exposure to patient and interventional team, invasiveness, costs, and a pure intraluminal contrast are limiting its usage outside the interventional procedures, especially in young patients. The DSA technique is being used during selective and super-selective arteriography, percutaneous direct puncture arteriography, and percutaneous direct puncture phlebography.[4]

Computed tomography angiography

Technically, contrast-enhanced computed tomography angiography (ceCTA) can be applied as a 4D (3D + time) acquisition capturing the hemodynamics of a focused vascular bed (up to approximately 16 cm in z-scan direction). Maximum spatial resolution is around 0.4 mm^3 with a temporal resolution of approximately 50–80 ms, depending on the available CT scanner. Ionizing radiation, however, restricts the usage of this technology beyond rare individual decisions. Limited soft tissue contrast remains a limiting factor for ceCTA.

CT angiography can be very useful to evaluate AVM of bone.[1] CTA with 3D reconstructions can be useful to visualize diagnostic arteriography during evaluation and road-mapping of AVMs, reserving arteriography for when requirements for treatment are established.[6]

Structural and functional magnetic resonance imaging

Magnetic resonance imaging (MRI) allows detection and characterization of CVM and its surrounding soft tissue with great tissue contrast,[7] being the best technique to determine the extent of the lesions and their relationship to adjacent structures.[1,8] However, the main disadvantage is its low availability (in some countries), the need for sedation in pediatric patients, and time of acquisition.

If the malformation is predefined to be high flow, the protocol has to provide information on the hemodynamics besides detailed 3D structural information on the soft tissue components in and around a lesion. The 3D contrast-enhanced (CE) MR angiography is applied as a dynamic/multiphasic acquisition known (e.g., as TRICKS or TWIST).[9] Time-resolved (4D) MR angiography allows acquisition of one 3D dataset every 1–3 seconds at approximately 1 mm^3. This high temporal resolution enables improved separation of arterial inflow from venous drainage and detection

of early venous shunting, which acquires information about the contrast material arrival time. A test bolus is not needed. Dynamic intraluminal gadolinium enhancement allows identification of the feeding arteries and draining veins. Conventional CE MR angiography allows acquisition of one 3D dataset every 15–20 seconds at a higher spatial resolution around 0.8 mm^3, ideally in isotropy. Using a field strength of 3 T offers some advantages, especially for extensive AVMs.

On the horizon

Computer-augmented imaging offers new possibilities for better identification and characterization of CVM. To this end, computational models of blood flow in vascular networks are combined with established imaging methods to provide enhanced imaging data with information on flow rate, pulsatility, and pressure.

In the context of peripheral AVMs, it has been demonstrated that the computational analysis of DSA data can be used to support the identification of the AVM nidus and to characterize the angioarchitecture.[10,11] Figure 14.1 shows examples of computer-augmented DSA images where contrast agent (CA) transport and dispersion characteristics have been used to highlight different structures within the lesioned vascular tree.

Further computational analysis of these images can yield additional quantitative information on the AVM angioarchitecture.[1] Frey et al. have shown that histograms of time-of-arrival histograms from DSA exhibit characteristic structures that can be directly associated with different AVM types (Figure 14.2).

Computational analysis of DSA data can also be used to identify CVMs of the microcirculation, which are not directly visible on the images due to resolution limitations.[12] To this end, the microvascular angioarchitecture is inferred from the relationship between the arterial input (CA bolus) and the venous output (dispersed CA bolus). Figure 14.3 shows a comparison between classical high-flow AVMs and microvascular AVMs based only on clinical DSA data and synthetically generated angiograms.

Translation of these computer-augmented imaging techniques to clinical routine requires near real-time turnaround times for the underlying computational models. This can be enabled by employing dedicated computational hardware such as graphical processing units (GPUs), which can be integrated into existing imaging systems.

CONCLUSION

Proper characterization of high-flow and arteriovenous transitional zone (nidus) in AVM is still a challenge for noninvasive imaging methods. Today, we are still very confident in using the established catheter-based DSA to confirm or adjust the gained imaging impressions of preinterventional diagnostic workup. New and improved imaging and image processing methods are on the horizon to further reduce or eradicate diagnostic surprises in the interventional suite.

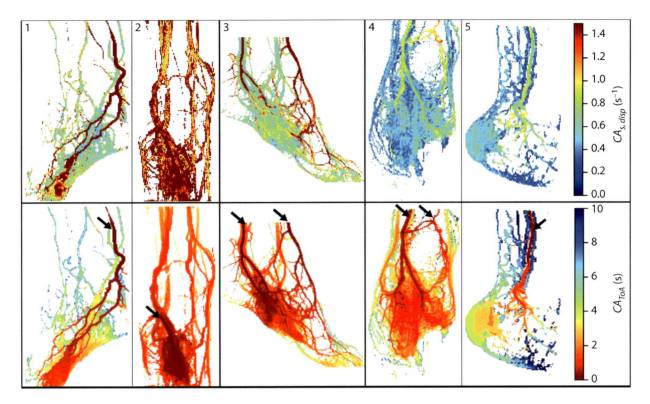

Figure 14.1 Examples of computer-augmented DSA for different AVMs of the foot: (1) and (2) type IIIb; (3) same patient as in (2) at an intermediate treatment stage; (4) same patient as in (2) and (3) at a later treatment stage with emerging type IV AVM; (5) type IV. $CA_{s,disp}$ quantifies the dispersion of the CA bolus as it passes through the AVM, CA_{ToA} indicates the time of arrival of the CA bolus. (Modified from Frey S. In: *Biomedical Engineering*. Bern, Switzerland: University of Bern; 2018.)

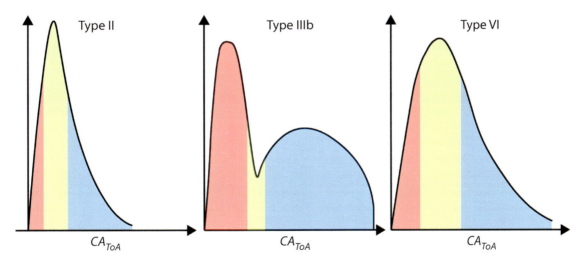

Figure 14.2 Comparison of characteristic shapes of histograms of CA time of arrival (CA_{ToA}) for different AVM types, as they can be obtained from computer-augmented DSA images shown in Figure 14.1. (Modified from Frey S. In: *Biomedical Engineering*. Bern, Switzerland: University of Bern; 2018.)

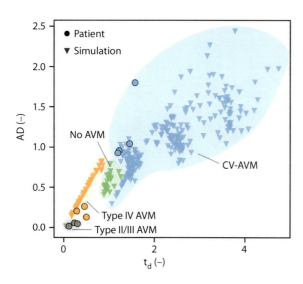

Figure 14.3 Classification of peripheral AVMs of type II/III/IV and hyperdynamic, capillary-venulous malformation (CV-AVM) based on the computational analysis of DSA data. (Patient: clinical data; simulation: synthetically generated data; AD: absolute dispersion; t_d, total delay.) (From Frey S et al. *PLOS ONE*. 2018;13:e0203368.)

REFERENCES

1. Madani H, Farrant J, Chhaya N et al. Peripheral limb vascular malformations: An update of appropriate imaging and treatment options of a challenging condition. *Br J Radiol*. 2015;88:20140406.
2. Lee BB, Baumgartner I, Berlien HP et al. Consensus Document of the International Union of Angiology (IUA)-2013. Current concept on the management of arterio-venous management. *Int J Angiol*. 2013; 32:9–36.
3. Dunham GM, Ingraham CR, Maki JH, Vaidya SS. Finding the nidus: Detection and workup of non-central nervous system arteriovenous malformations. *Radiographics*. 2016;36:891–903.
4. ISSVA Classification of Vascular Anomalies ©2018, International Society for the Study of Vascular Anomalies.The International Society for the Study of Vascular Anomalies (ISSVA)-2018 Classification. Available at issva.org/classification Accessed September 12, 2019.
5. Sandoval-Garcia C, Royalty K, Yang P et al. 4D DSA a new technique for arteriovenous malformation evaluation: A feasibility study. *J Neurointervent Surg*. 2016;8:300–304.
6. Khurana A, Hangge PT, Albadawi H et al. The use of transarterial approaches in peripheral arteriovenous malformations (AVMs). *J Clin Med*. 2018;7:1–2.
7. Dobson MJ, Hartley RW, Ashleigh R, Watson Y, Hawnaur JM. MR angiography and MR imaging of symptomatic vascular malformations. *Clin Radiol*. 1997;52:595–602.
8. Flors L, Leiva-Salinas C, Maged IM et al. MR imaging of soft-tissue vascular malformations: Diagnosis, classification, and therapy follow-up. *Radiographics*. 2011;31:1321–1340; discussion 1340–1341.
9. Lidsky ME, Spritzer CE, Shortell CK. The role of dynamic contrast-enhanced magnetic resonance imaging in the diagnosis and management of patients with vascular malformations. *J Vasc Surg*. 2012;56:757–764.e751.
10. Frey S, Haine A, Kammer R, von Tengg-Kobligk H, Obrist D, Baumgartner I. Hemodynamic characterization of peripheral arterio-venous malformations. *Ann Biomed Eng*. 2017;45:1449–1461.
11. Frey S. Hemodynamics in peripheral arterio-venous malformations. In: *Biomedical Engineering*. Dissertation/thesis. Bern, Switzerland: University of Bern; 2018.
12. Frey S, Cantieni T, Vuillemin N et al. Angioarchitecture and hemodynamics of microvascular arterio-venous malformations. *PLOS ONE*. 2018;13:e0203368.

15

Ultrasonographic assessment: New role for arteriovenous malformations. How far can it be implied?

ERICA MENEGATTI AND SERGIO GIANESINI

ULTRASOUND ASSESSMENT OF ARTERIOVENOUS MALFORMATION MORPHOLOGY AND HEMODYNAMIC CHARACTERISTICS

Arteriovenous malformations (AVMs) consist of a collection of abnormal vessels, in which the arterial circulation shunts directly into the venous circulation.[1] They are characterized by the presence of feeding arteries, draining veins, and a "nidus" composed of multiple dysplastic vascular channels that connect the arteries and veins, with the absence of a normal capillary bed. Despite the presence of a cluster of channels, there are no significant solid identifiable masses. The AVMs can be present in a dormant stage during birth but can also show rapid growth over a relatively short period of time during childhood or adulthood, as they increase in size proportionally with the growth of the patient. AVMs can be single, multiple, or part of a genetic disorder, and they are classified among high-flow malformations constituting about 10% of the whole malformations field.

The resulting hemodynamic changes, such as increased blood flow velocities and decreased hemodynamic resistance, can be detected by a conventional ultrasonography (US) method.[1,2]

ULTRASOUND EVALUATION OF AVMS

Doppler US is widely used together with other imaging modalities (magnetic resonance imaging [MRI], computed tomography [CT], radiographs) in the diagnosis, treatment, and follow-up of AVMs.[2,3] US is a noninvasive and cost-effective tool for examining vascular lesions, especially in the initial stages.[4]

Anomalies can be assessed by color and spectral Doppler describing the flow and velocity characteristics.[5] Some additional benefits of US are its lack of ionizing radiation and its ubiquity in clinical settings. Also, it does not require a great deal of cooperation on behalf of the patient, which is an important aspect in young patients.[6]

The use of a color code aims to confirm the vascular nature of the lesion, assessing flow characteristics and also identifying both feeding and draining vascular patterns. Moreover, spectral waveforms of feeding arteries can indicate low peripheral resistance, and dilated draining veins can show pulsatile flow, suggesting the presence of direct arteriovenous communications without an intervening capillary bed. The nidus is characterized by a "mosaic" pattern with a mixture of red and blue colors in the anechoic structure, as well as a buzzing sound at the Doppler acoustic signal.

Several hemodynamic parameters can be considered in US as helpful in the characterization of AVMs, which include peak systolic velocity, end-diastolic velocity, mean flow velocity, resistance index (RI), pulsatility index, and flow rate.[7]

In the color mode, the pathological vessels appear as different shades of multicolor patterns, corresponding to the different directions of the blood flow in the vessels of the AVMs. Additionally, because of the elevated systolic and diastolic blood flow velocities, the aliasing phenomenon (the change of red and blue color intensity) could be observed.

Doppler spectrum analysis of the AVMs can be detected by placing the sample volume in the pathological "color cloud" signal. It is characterized by increased peak velocities, systolic and diastolic, resulting in a decreased pulsatility and

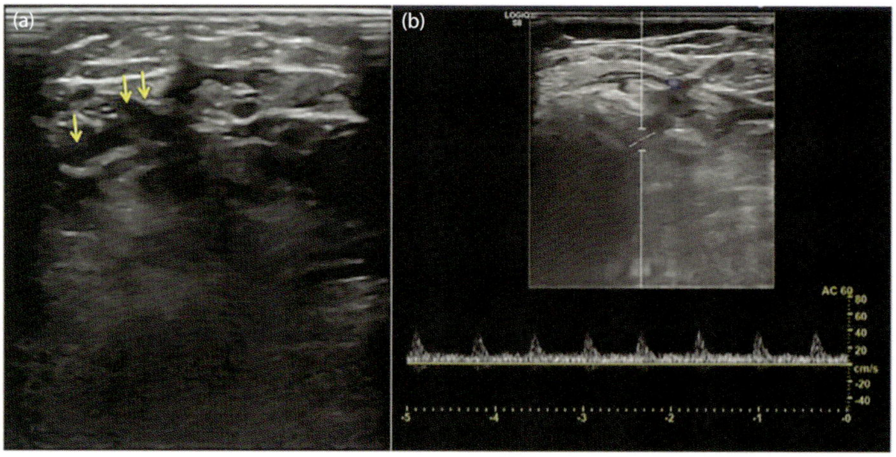

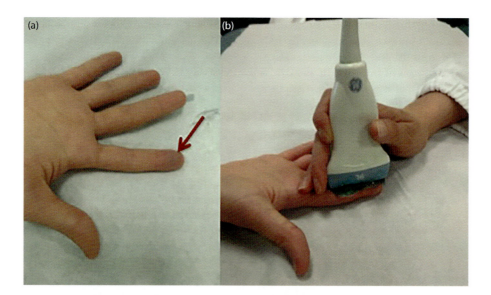

Figure 15.1 Ultrasonography of a vascular malformation in a pediatric patient who presented with a palpable right leg mass extending approximately 4 cm distally from the right lateral tibial condyle. (a) B-mode enhances multiple channels between superficial and deep muscular fascia, with feeding vessels large enough to be seen on grayscale (yellow arrow). (b) Doppler spectral waveform confirms the simultaneous presence of arterial and venous signals.

resistance index. The feeding arteries to the AVMs nidus could be identified with use of the same hemodynamic criteria.[3]

US is operator dependent; therefore, the US evaluation of AVMs can be challenging, with underestimation of the complexity and size of lesions.[2] Other typical limitations of US that may be encountered are related to the discrimination of the nearby structures, including nerves and bones.[6]

High-flow lesions can present mixed echogenicity with feeding vessels large enough to be seen on the grayscale, and color Doppler and spectral analysis can be used to confirm high-systolic flow. The arterialization of veins will also produce pulsatile venous flow and spectral broadening due to localized arterial and venous hypertrophy[8] (Figure 15.1).

DOPPLER EQUIPMENT, PATIENT POSITIONING, TIPS AND TRICKS FOR BEST IMAGE ACQUISITION

As regarding the Doppler equipment, a 5–7 MHz linear or phased array can be useful, especially in obese patients, for the investigation of deep intramuscular or periosteal malformations.

For those more superficial lesions with smaller surface area (hands, fingers, or feet) a higher-frequency microlinear array, up to 17 MHz, should be used for better resolution.[2]

Patient positioning is an important part of the examination, aimed to enhance the best visualization of the area of interest. Since the area of interest is frequently small, superficial, and with uneven surfaces, it is recommended

Figure 15.2 (a) The red arrow points at a lesion on a distal phalange of the right index finger. (b) It is important that the operator applies as little pressure as possible on a lesion while acquiring and maintaining a proper apposition of the probe to allow preservation of the anatomical shape of a lesion as much as possible. The operator can achieve this by applying a sufficient amount of the gel and by placing the little finger of the probe-holding hand between the probe and the examined area.

to use a generous amount of gel. To avoid pressure on both vessels and tissues, thus distorting the velocimetric and morphological data, the little finger of the operator might be used as an interface between the transducer and tissues (Figure 15.2).

HIGH-RESOLUTION B-MODE US

Exploration of parenchyma and soft tissue begins with a grayscale setting to delineate the margins of the malformation.[9] The use of brightness mode (B-mode) is aimed to characterize the extension of a lesion and to describe its echo-texture such as hypo-, iso-, or hyperechogeneities.[10,11] Additional comments should be done thoroughly on the homogeneity or nodularity and focal spots, such as calcifications or fluid collections.[9]

The AVMs present at B-mode US display variable characteristics; the most common location is the subcutaneous tissue, and due to the mechanical effect of AVM, the surrounding tissues may present as thickened or hyperechoic.[7]

COLOR DOPPLER US AND SPECTRAL WAVE ANALYSIS

After an accurate B-mode evaluation, the lesions must be qualified according to their vascularization pattern, using color Doppler and spectral wave analysis. The technical parameters such as pulse repetition frequency (PRF), Doppler-gain, and wall-filter have to be adjusted according to the flow irregularities typical of AVMs.

The lesion must be assessed including the type of vessels and the flow characteristics describing venous blood stasis or arterial blood flow accelerations, measuring also the flow velocities.[7,11]

The pathognomonic finding of AVM is arteriovenous shunt, presenting a spectrum of high peak systolic velocities and rather high diastolic flow velocities resulting in a low RI (<0.5). Especially with the existence of multiple shunts, a rather high flow volume can be detected in the main draining vein.

Making a differential diagnosis between AVM and malignant soft tissue formations can sometimes be difficult, particularly when in the presence of considerable vascularization. Moreover, evidence surrounding weak echoic tissue representing edema might be suspicious for a malignant process; the differential must be excluded by biopsy.[7]

POWER DOPPLER ANALYSIS

Power Doppler US (PDUS) is a technique that uses the amplitude of the Doppler signal to detect moving matter. PDUS is independent of flow velocity and direction, so there is no possibility of signal aliasing. It is also angle independent, allowing detection of smaller velocities than color Doppler, facilitating examinations in certain technically challenging clinical setting. PDUS has higher sensitivity than color Doppler, which makes a trade-off with flash artifacts. It is particularly useful in clinical practice when examining superficial structures, like thyroid, testis, renal grafts, and subcutaneous lesions; moreover, it may be used to look for tumor vessels and to evaluate tiny vessels such as in AVMs.[12] A PDUS device with at least a 10 MHz linear transducer can be used for joint assessment of superficial soft-tissue lesions including also AVMs.

B-FLOW ANALYSIS

B-Flow imaging is a non-Doppler technology for blood flow visualization that displays the blood flow echoes in grayscale imaging, with different gray intensities according

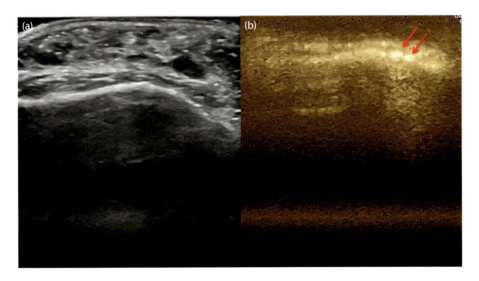

Figure 15.3 (a) Vascular malformation of the zygomatic region in B-mode and power Doppler mode demonstrates no significant color enhancement. (b) B-flow modalities highlight flow signal (hyperintense signal indicated by red arrows), leading to better flow characterization even in case of very weak flow signal.

to the reflector speed and dynamics. It was introduced on high-frequency transducers at the end of the last decade.[13]

B-flow technology is not plagued by some of the troublesome pitfalls often encountered during color and power Doppler flow imaging and appears promising in addition to Doppler evaluation with the following imaging advantages:

- Direct hemodynamic visualization
- No vessel wall overlap
- Less operator dependency or scanning angle
- Higher frame rate and spatial resolution than color Doppler

During the evaluation of hemodialysis shunts, the major advantage of this technique is its ability to avoid color artifacts such as aliasing and overwriting, and it provides superior evaluation compared with low- and high-PRF color and power Doppler sonography[14] (Figure 15.3). Some experiences exploring hepatic B-flow imaging indicate that this currently underused technology has the potential to substantially improve noninvasive blood flow evaluation. This application can contribute to better visualization of the true lumen size of a vessel, which is useful to depict vascular anatomy and bypasses some of the pitfalls of US.[15]

REFERENCES

1. Lee BB, Baumgartner I, Berlien HP et al. International Union of Angiology. Consensus Document of the International Union of Angiology (IUA)-2013. Current concept on the management of arterio-venous management. *Int Angiol.* 2013;32(1):9–36.
2. Madani H, Farrant J, Chhaya N et al. Peripheral limb vascular malformations: An update of appropriate imaging and treatment options of a challenging condition. *Br J Radiol.* 2015;88(1047):20140406.
3. Bartels E. Evaluation of arteriovenous malformations (AVMs) with transcranial color-coded duplex sonography: Does the location of an AVM influence its sonographic detection? *J Ultrasound Med.* 2005;24(11):1511–1517.
4. Lee BB, Baumgartner I, Berlien P et al. Diagnosis and treatment of venous malformations. Consensus document of the International Union of Phlebology (IUP): Updated 2013. *Int Angiol.* 2015;(34):97–149.
5. Fu B, Zhao J-Z, Yu L-B. The application of ultrasound in the management of cerebral arteriovenous malformation. *Neurosci Bull.* 2008;24(6):387.
6. Behravesh S, Yakes W, Gupta N et al. Venous malformations: Clinical diagnosis and treatment. *Cardiovasc Diagn Ther.* 2016;6(6):557–569.
7. Gruber H, Peer S. Ultrasound diagnosis of soft tissue vascular malformations and tumours. *Curr Med Imaging Rev.* 2009;5:55–61.
8. Legiehn GM, Heran MKS. A step-by-step practical approach to imaging diagnosis and interventional radiologic therapy in vascular malformations. *Semin Intervent Radiol.* 2010;27(2):209–231.
9. Dubois J, Soulez G, Oliva VL, Berthiaume MJ, Lapierre C, Therasse E. Soft-tissue venous malformations in adult patients: Imaging and therapeutic issues. *Radiographics.* 2001;21(6):1519–1531.
10. Trop I, Dubois J, Guibaud L et al. Soft-tissue venous malformations in pediatric and young adult patients: Diagnosis with Doppler US. *Radiology.* 1999;212: 841–845.
11. Paltiel HJ, Burrows PE, Kozakewich HP, Zurakowski D, Mulliken JB. Soft-tissue vascular anomalies: Utility of US for diagnosis. *Radiology.* 2000;214:747–754.
12. Toprak H, Kiliç E, Serter A, Kocakoç E, Ozgocmen S. Ultrasound and Doppler US in evaluation of superficial soft-tissue lesion. *J Clin Imaging Sci.* 2014;4:12–13.
13. Wachsberg RH. B-flow, a non-Doppler technology for flow mapping: Early experience in the abdomen. *Ultrasound Q.* 2003;19(3):114–122.
14. Yucel C, Oktar SO, Erten Y, Bursali A, Ozdemir H. B-flow sonographic evaluation of hemodialysis fistulas: A comparison with low- and high-pulse repetition frequency color and power Doppler sonography. *J Ultrasound Med.* 2005;24:1503–1508.
15. Morgan TA, Jha P, Poder L, Weinstein S. Advanced ultrasound applications in the assessment of renal transplants: Contrast-enhanced ultrasound, elastography, and B-flow. *Abdom Radiol (NY).* 2018;43(10): 2604–2614.

16

Magnetic resonance angiography and/or computed tomography angiography: New gold standard for arteriovenous malformations?

MASSIMO VAGHI

The diagnostic evaluation is aimed at confirming the presence of a vascular malformation, its precise localization, its morphology, and the extension of the malformation to plan a possible intervention. Vascular malformations may be considered a chronic pathology with the need for multiple interventions and multiple diagnostic assessments.

The diagnostic workup should minimize the risks of the diagnostic procedures and the exposition to ionizing radiations. Imaging in medicine is based on the use of physical energies (magnetic resonance, X-rays, ultrasound) and the postprocessing of the acquired images with the aid of a computer. Today we have two imaging studies that allow for the scanning of wide areas of the body: computed tomography (CT) and magnetic resonance imaging (MRI). The study of blood vessels with CT is possible only with the aid of contrast medium, and the examination is named CT angiography (CTA). In the 1990s, the slip ring was developed for helical scanning. Here, the X-rays tube/detector array is continuously rotated around the patient as the table is incrementally advanced, resulting in a continuous spiral scanning mechanism through the entire patient. Thus, CT scanning became much more rapid and efficient, and the introduction of multiple detector rows allowed further improvement in spatial resolution and quicker scanning times, as fewer slices were required to image a defined field of view. And finally, with advancements in computer technology, large image datasets could be quickly processed and manipulated in real time, thus providing a more complete understanding of the vascular anatomy than traditional invasive angiography, as the arterial wall itself may be visualized and the anatomy may be seen from any orientation.

The study of a blood vessel using magnetic resonance is named *MR angiography* (MRA), and it is possible with or without the injection of paramagnetic contrast.

The diagnostic possibilities are amplified by the continuous evolution of the imaging systems. The diagnostic capability of a tool is related to the integration of the resolution capabilities: temporal resolution, spatial resolution, and contrast resolution (Figure 16.1). Although the temporary and spatial resolution of MRA is not as high as that of CTA and angiography, MRA has the advantage of avoiding exposure to ionizing radiation, which may be important in patients who have chronic illness and need various

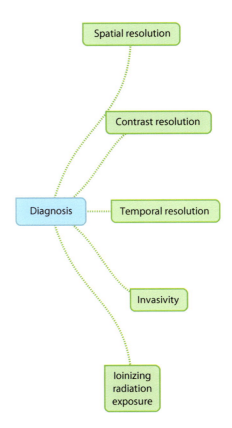

Figure 16.1 Properties of diagnostic capability of diagnostic tools.

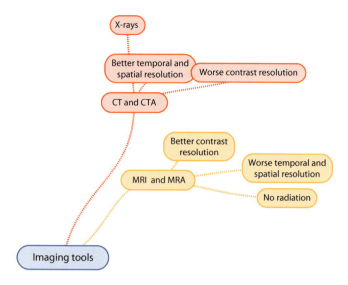

Figure 16.2 Characteristics of computed tomographic angiography and magnetic resonance angiography.

treatment and imaging controls, especially in those being treated since pediatric age.

The principal advantage of CTA is represented by the capillary diffusion of the diagnostic equipment on the territory and the velocity of the examination. In CTA and MRA, it is possible to use image reconstructions in order to plan the vascular access and the therapy (Figure 16.2). CTA is feasible only when using contrast media (Figure 16.3). In MRA, there are two methods in acquiring images: contrast-enhanced and non-contrast-enhanced methods. The non-contrast-enhanced methods are based on the motion of blood (phase-contrast MRA, time-of-flight [TOF] MRA) or the magnetic properties of blood (steady-state free precession MRA)

to differentiate signals from blood and stationary tissues, whereas contrast-enhanced methods require the intravenous injection of a contrast material to differentiate signals from blood and stationary tissues. MRI provides high-contrast images of soft tissues and some hemodynamic characteristics. We can perform MRI and MRA in a unique examination to have a complete picture of the morphology and the extension and limits of the malformation, together with the morphology of the vessels and the flow characteristics (Figure 16.4). This diagnostic tool is most valuable in children when compared to all age groups. It is clear that CT angiographic and conventional digital angiography cause considerable radiation exposure that is under the threshold for deterministic effects, but there is an increased risk for malignancy. We can estimate an increased sensitivity to radiation in children by a factor of three to five relative to adults.[1] This has more impact because of the frequent necessity of multiple diagnostic procedures to control the effects of the therapeutic interventions and the therapeutic approaches.

The goal of imaging studies in vascular malformations is to classify the malformations according to the involved vessels, to specify their anatomy with respect to feeding and draining vessels, and to evaluate their effect on other neighboring tissues.

Contrast-enhanced MRA (CE-MRA), just like digital subtraction angiography (DSA) and CTA, provides reliable enhancement of the arterial lumen during the arterial phase of the gadolinium bolus injection. Although MR imaging is slower than DSA or CTA, advances in magnet technology, gradient performance, pulse sequence design, parallel imaging, and MR contrast agents continue to improve CE-MRA image quality such that it rivals DSA in accuracy for diagnosing vascular anomalies and diseases.[2]

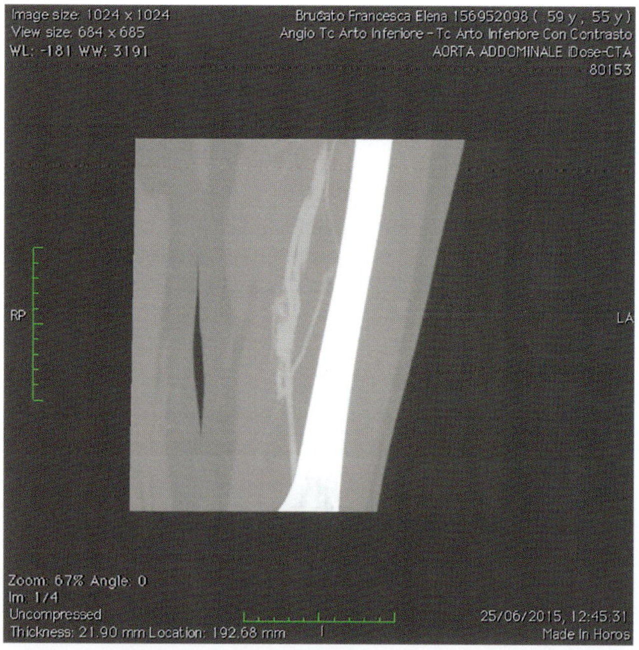

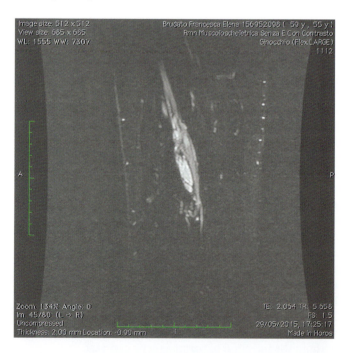

Figure 16.3 Computed tomographic angiography of arteriovenous malformation in the thigh.

Figure 16.4 Magnetic resonance angiography of the same (as in Figure 16.3) arteriovenous malformation in the thigh.

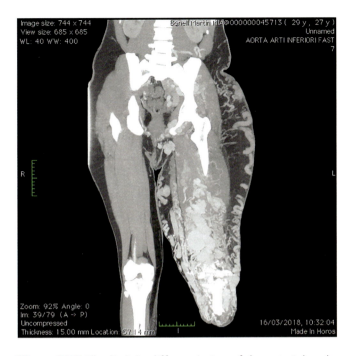

Figure 16.5 The limit in differentiation of the arterial and venous vessels is represented by the shunt volume. High shunt volume causes the acquisition at equilibrium both in computed tomography angiography and magnetic resonance angiography.

Unlike conventional MRA techniques that rely on blood flow or intrinsic blood relaxation properties to distinguish vasculature from background tissue, CE-MRA uses a magnetic contrast agent to shorten the T1 relaxation time of blood so that the intraluminal signal is brighter than that of surrounding tissues[1,2] on T1-weighted images. Blood can then be directly imaged using fast, three-dimensional, spoiled gradient echo or steady-state free precession pulse sequences. The short echo time of these three-dimensional gradient echo sequences minimizes blood motion (e.g., flow artifacts that are problematic on noncontrast techniques). Gradient echo processing is preferred over steady-state free precession, especially for large, field-of-view (FOV) applications to eliminate banding and susceptibility artifacts of steady-state free precession. The most useful sequences are time resolved; in these sequences, the injection of a test bolus of gadolinium is not necessary, but we can acquire imagines simultaneously and then select the desired set (arterial, venous, or both).[3] The diagnostic capability is similar to DSA imaging, which should be implemented only in case of discrepancy between the clinical picture, MRI images, duplex scanning evaluation, and MRA.[4,5]

Until now, we focused on the toxicity of ionic contrast media used for CT enhancement. But we are also aware that there is a toxicity related to gadolinium in patients suffering from renal failure, which causes systemic renal fibrosis, a progressive disabling illness.[6]

Both CT and MRA give a static vision of the malformation that may assume different morphological patterns during selective arteriography (Figure 16.5). MRA reveals fewer artifacts than CTA in visualizing vessels treated with Onyx, and this is a great advantage in the follow-up of these patients.[7]

High field strength imaging (up to 7 Tesla) is the new border for MRA imaging with the hype of a better spatial resolution with techniques not using contrast media or needing lower doses of contrast media in CE-MRA.

We can conclude that MRA provides a good diagnostic quality for diagnosis, subsequent treatment planning, and follow-up of arteriovenous malformations with the advantages of being noninvasive and not exposing patients to ionizing radiation. It now represents the gold standard in the diagnosis of vascular malformations.

REFERENCES

1. Hall EJ. Lessons we have learned from our children: Cancer risks from diagnostic radiology. *Pediatr Radiol*. 2002;32:700–706.
2. Zhang HL, Zhang W, Juluru K, Prince MR. Body magnetic resonance angiography. *Semin Roentgenol*. 2009;44:84–98.
3. Higgins LJ, Koshy J, Mitchell SE et al. Time-resolved contrast-enhanced MRA (TWIST) with gadofosveset trisodium in the classification of soft-tissue vascular anomalies in the head and neck in children following updated 2014 ISSVA classification: First report on systematic evaluation of MRI and TWIST in a cohort of 47children. *Clin Radiol*. 2016;71:32–39.
4. Hammer S, Uller W, Manger F, Fellner C, Zeman F, Wohlgemuth WA. Time-resolved magnetic resonance angiography (MRA) at 3.0 Tesla for evaluation of hemodynamic characteristics of vascular malformations: Description of distinct subgroups. *Eur Radiol*. 2017;27:296–305.
5. Riederer SJ, Haider CR, Borisch EA, Weavers PT, Young PM. Recent advances in 3D time-resolved contrast-enhanced MR angiography. *J Magn Reson Imaging*. 2015;42(1):3–22.
6. Juluru K, Vogel-Claussen J, Macura KJ, Kamel IR, Steever A, Bluemke DA. MR imaging in patients at risk for developing nephrogenic systemic fibrosis: Protocols, practices, and imaging techniques to maximize patient safety. *Radiographics*. 2009;29:9–22.
7. Saatci I, Saruhan Cekirge H, Ciceri EFM, Mawad ME, Gulsun Pamuk A, Aytekin Besim. CT and MR imaging findings and their implications in the follow-up of patients with intracranial aneurysms treated with endosaccular occlusion with onyx. *Am J Neuroradiol*. 2003;24:567–578.

17

Transarterial lung perfusion scintigraphy (TLPS): New role for follow-up assessment?

RAUL MATTASSI

Transarterial lung perfusion scintigraphy (TLPS) for study of arteriovenous malformations (AVMs) is based on the injection of TC-99m labeled macroaggregated albumin (MAA) in the artery proximal to the shunt/lesion. If there is no AVM lesion(s), albumin will be trapped in the peripheral capillary; if a shunt exists, the radiotracer will pass the shunt, enter the venous system, and be trapped in the lung with local increase in radioactivity, which can be quantified using a gamma camera.

Technically, the first injection is performed into a vein, in order to get a baseline activity in the lung; then the second injection is done in the proximal artery, and the increase of radioactivity in the lung, if any, detected by the labeled albumin is recoded with the gamma camera. The result is presented as an activity curve in the lung with two increases: the first after the endovenous injection and a second increase after the intra-arterial injection. The second curve depends on the size of the shunt and can be quantified by a simple relation of the activity between the two increases. That allows for numerical evaluation of the shunt as a percentage[1,2] (Figure 17.1).

The test can only be done to assess a limb lesion, because proximal arterial injection other than in the femoral or brachial artery is not technically easy in other parts of the body using the percutaneous technique. An alternative is the injection of the radiotracer by catheter, but then the method becomes invasive and is not practical. A limitation to this diagnostic test is that it cannot be performed in regional or general anesthesia as both induce vasodilatation and cause a significant degree of arteriovenous (AV) shunting in normal extremities.[3]

The technique is not new; it was described many years ago but was poorly understood and has not been used for the detection of congenital vascular malformations (CVMs) until more recently.[2,3] At the beginning of this century, it was rediscovered by a few groups.[4-6] In addition to diagnostic use of TLPS for AVMs, the technique has been used as a postprocedure (surgical resection or embolization for the AVM) appraisal method, in order to confirm effective removal of the defect/lesion or to determine if some fistulous areas should have remained.[5,6]

TLPS is also well recognized for follow-up assessment of the natural course of the progress and evaluation of treated AVM lesions. Patients with Parkes Weber syndrome, who often present with various extents of *microshunting* AVM lesions as one of the vascular malformation components, are ideal candidates for this unique test to replace an invasive arteriography to provide periodic follow-up on progress and to choose the right time for further intervention.

The ability to quantify the AV shunting and to compare its data with former tests results is helpful in assessing the evolution of an AVM, as the AVM lesion has a tendency to recur following the intervention, often in an unpredictable form (Figure 17.2).

A study performed on 21 cases of AVM tested with TLPS before and after treatment demonstrated the efficacy of the method. Angiography and duplex scan performed in these cases confirmed the data obtained by TLPS.[7]

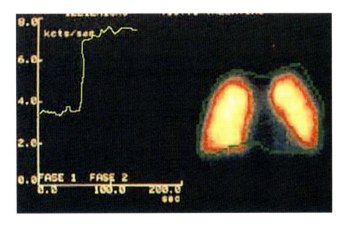

Figure 17.1 Transarterial lung perfusion scintigraphy in a case of arteriovenous malformation of a lower limb. Shunt is 94.5%. On the right, the activity of tracer in lungs.

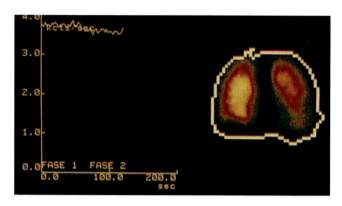

Figure 17.2 TLPS in a case of limited AVM after complete surgical removal of the defect. The curve demonstrates no shunt (no increase after the intra-arterial injection). (AVM, arteriovenous malformation; TLPS, transarterial lung perfusion scintigraphy.)

However, even if it is a simple, effective, and less invasive procedure and with the advantage to quantify the shunt, it is rarely used, even today. Only a few groups have adopted this unique method to assess AVM lesions, as a diagnostic or as a follow-up routine procedure. As nuclear medicine tests are rarely used in angiology as hemodynamic studies, physicians are unaware of the proper clinical implementation of this useful diagnostic method. Much more common and familiar to doctors are duplex ultrasonography and/or computed tomography/magnetic resonance angiography.

However, TLPS as an additional method for AVM diagnosis and follow-up provides unique advantages, like the quantification of AV shunting percentage and simplicity of the test to deliver clear-cut, reproducible outcomes.[8]

REFERENCES

1. Choi JY. Radionuclide scintigraphy for congenital vascular malformations. In: Kim YW, Lee B-B, Yakes WF, Do Y-S, eds. *Congenital Vascular Malformations.* Heidelberg, Germany: Springer; 2017:165–172.
2. Rutherford RB. Noninvasive testing in the diagnosis and assessment of arteriovenous fistula. In: Berenstein EF, ed. *Noninvasive Diagnostic Techniques in Vascular Disease.* St. Louis, MO: Mosby; 1982:430–432.
3. Rutherford RB, Anderson BO. Diagnosis of congenital vascular malformations of the extremities: New perspectives. *Int Angiol.* 1990;9(3):162–167.
4. Dentici R, Mattassi R, Vaghi M. Diagnostica per immagini in medicina nucleare (Nuclear medcine diagnostcs). In: Mattassi R, Belov St, Loose DA, Vaghi M. *Malformazione Vascolare Ed Emangiomi.* Milan, Italy: Springer; 2003:32–39.
5. Lee BB, Mattassi R, Kim YW, Kim BT, Park JM, Choi JY. Advanced management of arteriovenous shunting malformations with transarterial lung perfusion scintigraphy for follow-up assessment. *Int Angiol.* 2005;24(2):173–184.
6. Vaišnytė B, Vajauskas D, Palionis D et al. Diagnostic methods, treatment modalities, and follow-up of extracranial arteriovenous malformations. *Medicina (Kaunas).* 2012;48(8):388–398.
7. Chung JW, Choi JY, Kim YW et al. Diagnosis and post therapeutic evaluation of arteriovenous malformations in extremities using transarterial lung perfusion scintigraphy. *Nucl Med Mol Imaging.* 2006;40:316–321.
8. Dentici R, Mattassi R. Nuclear medicine diagnostics. In: Mattassi R, Loose DA, Vaghi M, eds. *Hemangiomas and Vascular Malformations: An Atlas of Diagnosis and Treatment.* Milan, Italy: Springer; 2015:223–236.

Management: 1

18

Do all the arterio-venous malformations mandate the therapy? Is there any contraindication for the therapy?

BYUNG-BOONG LEE AND JAMES LAREDO

An arteriovenous malformation (AVM) is one of many different types of congenital vascular malformations (CVMs). It is much different from the rest of the CVMs in its clinical behavior due to its unique anatomic defect involving vessels of both arterial and venous origin, resulting in direct communications to allow shunting of arterial blood to the venous system, mostly via a meshwork of abnormal vessels termed a *nidus*.[1-4]

Such arteriovenous (AV) shunting is mostly of high-velocity, low-resistance flow from the arterial vasculature into the venous system through the primitive anatomical structure of the reticular network in a variety of fistulous conditions. It is the outcome of defective development during embryogenesis with a lack of a normal capillary system in between.

This unique condition of "high-flow" AV shunting through micro- or macrofistulous communications between the arterial and venous systems causes a complicated anatomical, pathophysiological, and hemodynamic status with vastly different clinical presentations from other CVMs.[1-4]

Therefore, AVM lesions are hemodynamically much more complicated than all other CVMs with broad hemodynamic impacts throughout the entire cardiovascular system, causing cardiac failure, arterial insufficiency (e.g., ulceration, gangrene), venous insufficiency, and/or lymphatic overload/hypertension depending on lesion location. Such hemodynamic complexity involving the arterial, venous, and lymphatic systems with altered cardiovascular hemodynamics, centrally, peripherally, and locally, makes the lesion a potentially limb- if not life-threatening condition.[5,6]

AVM lesions also cause various degrees of mechanical impact to the surrounding tissues and organs, by direct expansion/compression and/or infiltration with much higher morbidity and recurrence following treatment, by their unique embryological characteristics.[7,8]

An "extra-truncular" lesion as an embryonal tissue remnant from an "early stage" of embryogenesis[9,10] retains the mesenchymal cell characteristics with the potential to proliferate/grow when the condition is met with enough stimulation.[1-4] Various stimulations by extrinsic (e.g., trauma, surgery) as well as intrinsic (e.g., menarche, pregnancy) origins can precipitate the recurrence and/or progression of the extra-truncular lesion accordingly, causing its clinical behavior to be totally unpredictable.[11,12]

Improper treatment based on a poor understanding of the unique nature of the extra-truncular lesion, ignoring such critical embryological characteristics, stimulates/provokes the AVM lesion in a dormant state to become activated to a proliferative state; for example, the ligation of the feeding arteries rather than the precise control of the nidus of the lesion itself only leads to an erratic response by the lesion with massive explosive growth with uncontrollable complications.

The old strategy of shutting off the feeding artery alone allows the nidus to be left intact and subsequently stimulates the surviving primitive lesion to take a more aggressive neovascular response, making the condition worse.[1,3]

Also, AVMs infrequently coexist with other CVMs like venous malformation, lymphatic malformation, and/or capillary malformation, although the vast majority of AVMs exist as extra-truncular lesions in independent conditions. Such mixed conditions (e.g., Parkes Weber syndrome) make their proper diagnosis and management more difficult, with often disappointing treatment results (e.g., microshunting AVM).[2,3,13,14]

AVMs, therefore, remain the most challenging and dangerous as potential limb- or life-threatening CVM lesions despite their relative rarity in the range of 10%–20% of all CVMs. Clinicians should remain alert to the fact that an AVM is not only different from other CVMs in etiology, anatomy, and pathophysiology, but it also takes entirely different clinical courses with different long-term prognoses and warrants a fundamentally different management strategy.[15,16]

An "infiltrating" AVM lesion in particular is far more complicated, carrying a higher risk of recurrence and/or fast deterioration/progression with more destructive potential due to this embryologic characteristic, so that an accurate diagnosis and precise assessment of the nature, extent, and severity of this unique condition are warranted to avoid such high risks of complication and morbidity.[17,18]

Even though AVM is classified as one of the CVMs together with other "relatively benign" -natured CVMs affecting only one of the circulation systems, the AVM is entirely different from the rest of the CVM group. It has a wide range of clinical presentations, with unpredictable clinical courses and erratic responses to treatment, with a high risk of recurrence and morbidity.[2,3]

Therefore, AVM should be ruled out first whenever CVMs are encountered, and if there is any chance that an AVM is detected based on the clinical evaluation, the lesion should be pursued as an AVM until proven otherwise, because almost all AVM lesions will eventually progress to the point of anatomical, physiological, and hemodynamic deterioration to become limb-if not life-threatening with this virulent nature.

The AVM is "the most dangerous" primitive CVM with a high risk of recurrence. As it can cause serious consequences, ideally an early aggressive approach is favored for all AVM lesions with either macro- or micro-AV shunting whenever feasible.[1–4]

Currently available treatments for AVMs in general carry significant risks of complication and morbidity in various degrees. Complete eradication of the AVM "nidus" is often difficult, if not impossible, using a conventional surgical approach treatment alone, and it has a high likelihood of recurrence.[19,20]

Therefore, careful planning to minimize the risks of complication and morbidity is critical for a successful outcome of treatment. Aggressive management should be limited to when the treatment benefit outweighs the associated risks of complication and morbidity (e.g., ethanol sclerotherapy), even though early aggressive control of the nidus of the AVM lesion is generally warranted for the majority of patients in order to reduce the consequence of its hemodynamic impact by delaying treatment.[1,3]

AVMs are more serious than any other CVMs with a more dismal long-term outcome due to their nature/progress, so all AVMs should take priority over all other CVMs for treatment. But the presence of an AVM does not always mandate treatment, and a calculated "controlled" aggressive approach should remain within the acceptable boundary of the "palliative" concept only.

The temptation to intervene on an AVM radically must be waived with the realistic long-term goal of the treatment plan, unless the treatment is indicated for a life- or limb-threatening condition (e.g., hemorrhage, high cardiac output failure). Otherwise, an accurate assessment of the risk-to-benefit ratio prior to initiating treatment is essential for success along with clearly defined treatment goals and realistic expectations.

The decision for treatment as well as selection of the treatment modalities should be made by a multidisciplinary team approach based on the proper indications and should proceed only when the benefit exceeds the associated morbidity of the proposed treatment to achieve effective control of AVM lesions. Such a fully integrated specialty team will be able to deliver maximum coordination among the various CVM-related specialists, providing the full spectrum of advanced diagnosis and treatment of AVMs.[3,5,21]

REFERENCES

1. Lee BB, Baumgartner I, Berlien HP et al. Consensus document of the International Union of Angiology (IUA)-2013. Current concept on the management of arterio-venous management. *Int Angiol.* 2013;32(1): 9–36.
2. Lee BB, Antignani PL, Baraldini V et al. ISVI-IUA consensus document—Diagnostic guidelines on vascular anomalies: Vascular malformations and hemangiomas. *Int Angiol.* 2015;34(4):333–374.
3. Lee BB, Lardeo J, Neville R. Arterio-venous malformation: How much do we know? *Phlebology.* 2009;24:193–200.
4. Lee BB, Antignani PL. Not all the vascular malformations are AV malformation! Editorial. *Acta Phlebol.* 2014;15:1–2.
5. Lee BB, Do YS, Yakes W et al. Management of arterial-venous shunting malformations (AVM) by surgery and embolosclerotherapy. A multidisciplinary approach. *J Vasc Surg.* 2004;39(3):590–600.
6. Lee BB. Statues of new approaches to the treatment of congenital vascular malformations (CVMs)—Single center experiences (Editorial Review). *Eur J Vasc Endovasc Surg.* 2005;30(2):184–197.
7. Loose DA. Combined treatment of congenital vascular defects: Indications and tactics. *Semin Vasc Surg.* 1993;6(4):260–265.
8. Lee BB, Laredo J, Lee SJ, Huh SH, Joe JH, Neville R. Congenital vascular malformations: General diagnostic principles. *Phlebology.* 2007;22(6):253–257.
9. Belov S. Classification of congenital vascular defects. *Int Angiol.* 1990;9:141–146.
10. Lee BB. All congenital vascular malformations should belong to one of two types: "Truncular" or "extra-truncular", as different as apples and oranges! Editorial. *Phlebological Rev.* 2015;23(1):1–3.
11. Bastide G, Lefebvre D. Anatomy and organogenesis and vascular malformations. In: Belov St, Loose DA, Weber J, eds. *Vascular Malformations.* Reinbek, Germany: Einhorn-Presse Verlag GmbH; 1989: 20–22.
12. Woolard HH. The development of the principal arterial stems in the forelimb of the pig. *Contrib Embryol.* 1922;14:139–154.

13. Lee BB. Critical issues on the management of congenital vascular malformation. *Ann Vasc Surg.* 2004;18(3): 380–392.

14. Lee BB, Mattassi R, Kim BT, Park JM. Advanced management of arteriovenous shunting malformation with Transarterial Lung Perfusion Scintigraphy (TLPS) for follow up assessment. *Int Angiol.* 2005;24(2): 173–184.

15. Kim JY, Kim DI, Do YS, Kim YW, Lee BB. Surgical treatment for congenital arteriovenous malformation: 10 years' experience. *Eur J Vasc Endovasc Surg.* 2006;32(1):101–106.

16. Park KB, Do YS, Lee BB et al. Predictive factors for response of peripheral arteriovenous malformations to embolization therapy: Analysis of clinical data and imaging findings. *J Vasc Interv Radiol.* 2012;23: 1478–1486.

17. Koskinen EVS, Tala P, Siltanen P. The effect of massive arteriovenous fistula on hemodynamics and bone growth. *Clin Orthop.* 1967;50:305.

18. Sumner D. Hemodynamics and pathophysiology of arteriovenous fistulas. In: Rutherford RB, ed. *Vascular Surgery.* 5th ed. Philadelphia, PA: WB Saunders; 2000:1400–1425.

19. Vollmar JF, Stalker CG. The surgical treatment of congenital arterio-venous fistulas in the extremities. *J Cardiovasc Surg.* 1976;17:340.

20. Loose DA, Weber J. Indications and tactics for a combined treatment of congenital vascular malformations. In: P. Balas, ed. *Progress in Angiology.* Torino, Italy: Minerva Medica; 1992:373–378.

21. Lee BB, Bergan JJ. Advanced management of congenital vascular malformations: A multidisciplinary approach. *Cardiovasc Surg.* 2002;10(6):523–533.

19

How much is too much for arteriovenous malformation management?

YOUNG-WOOK KIM

Arteriovenous malformation (AVM) is a type of congenital vascular malformation (CVM) that causes direct communication between arteries and veins. These lesions are defined by the shunting of blood with high-flow velocity from the arterial vasculature into the venous system in a variety of forms of fistulous conditions, and they are characterized by a progressive, unpredictable clinical course.[1]

An AVM is usually composed of feeding arteries (feeders), nidus (a complex, primary network of arteriovenous connections), and draining veins.

Nidus is an angiographic term describing a bundle or cluster of small-sized arteriovenous connections seen on arteriographic images rather than an anatomical or histological term.[2–4]

Despite the vast knowledge we have accumulated on vascular embryology, the pathogenesis of AVMs is still unclear. Our current understanding of the pathogenesis of AVMs usually is attributed to defects in the development of the vascular system in fetal life.

The initial stage of vascular development consists of the formation of a primitive vascular tube made of a single layer of endothelial cells. Predetermined genetic factors expressed in the endothelial cells decide whether the fate of the endothelial tube will be to develop into the arterial or venous system. The later stage of vascular development includes blood vessel maturation by an interaction between endothelial cells and smooth muscle cells. This interaction is essential for vessel maturation and recruits more smooth muscle cells around the vascular tube, thus stabilizing the primitive blood vessel.[5–7]

Vascular malformations could occur when there is a defect in either an early or late phase of vascular development. Previous studies on AVM suggest that multiple pathways rather than a single pathway are involved in AVM pathogenesis. In animal studies, various signaling molecules were reported to be involved in the early and later stages of vascular development.[8,9]

Unlike other types of vascular malformation, AVMs show more progressive clinical features. Clinically, AVMs

are present at birth in 40% of cases[10] and present with various symptoms or signs in later life, which can range from an asymptomatic birthmark to life-threatening organ failure.

Schöbinger et al.[11] classified an AVM lesion into four stages (Table 19.1). An AVM lesion is usually asymptomatic and dormant during early life. In this stage, it seems to give no or little harm to the patient. Characteristically, it grows with the patient's growth. In some patients, an AVM lesion shows an episodic accelerated growth that may be related to trauma (e.g., blunt trauma or surgical intervention to the AVM lesion), hormonal changes (e.g., puberty, pregnancy, use of contraceptive pill, or female hormone replacement therapy), infection, or local ischemia (e.g., surgical ligation or endovascular embolization of the feeding artery of the AVM lesion).

In the later stages of an AVM, the clinical features are a mixture of a progressed AVM lesion and secondary changes of the connecting blood vessels or surrounding musculoskeletal tissues, which were caused by continuous abnormal

Table 19.1 Schöbinger's clinical grading system of arteriovenous malformation (AVM)

Stage	Clinical feature
Stage I: Quiescence	Usually no discoloration; pink or blue skin spot and warm; arteriovenous shunting on Doppler examination
Stage II: Expansion	Stage I plus engorgement, pulsation, thrill, bruit, tortuous and tense veins
Stage III: Destruction	Stage II plus dystrophic skin change, ulceration, bleeding, pain, necrosis; osteolytic lesions may occur
Stage IV: Decompensation	Stage III plus high-output congestive heart failure and left ventricular hypertrophy

(a)

(b)

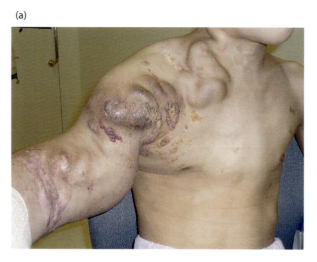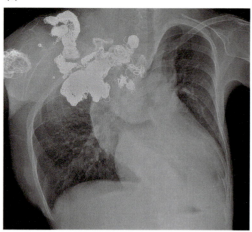

Figure 19.1 (a) An 18-year-old male patient with AVMs around the neck base and right shoulder who presented with symptoms and signs of congestive heart failure; (b) chest computed tomography of the patient shows cardiomegaly with multiple coils in the AVM lesions, which were percutaneously inserted through multiple sessions of endovascular treatment.

arteriovenous shunting. At the last stage of an AVM, it can cause remote organ complications such as congestive heart failure (Figure 19.1).

In practice, treatment of AVMs is usually considered when clinical symptoms or signs develop. Clinical manifestation depends on the location and size of AVMs. Patients with quiescent AVM lesions in Schöbinger stage I or asymptomatic lesions in stage II are typically managed conservatively with initial diagnostic workup and subsequent periodic follow-up evaluation. Definitive treatment for AVMs is generally reserved for symptomatic AVMs in stage III and IV lesions in practice.[12]

The goal of AVM treatment is complete obliteration or removal of the AVM nidus, without significant complications or recurrence. Unlike low-flow-type vascular malformations such as venous malformation (VM), it is not easy to achieve these goals in AVMs. It is difficult to remove an AVM surgically due to the risk of intraoperative bleeding and damages to the surrounding tissue (e.g., nerve or muscle). Furthermore, surgical treatment of AVM lesions carries a high rate of recurrence. It has been reported that 98% of AVMs will enlarge or recur within 5 years following surgical resection and embolic therapy.[13,14]

A localized small AVM lesion in the same anatomical plane with a single feeder and well-defined borders can be a good candidate for surgical excision. Surgical removal is usually recommended after prior embolization of the AVMs with endovascular means. Endovascular therapy has become the first-line treatment for most patients with advanced AVM lesions. Endovascular procedures used for AVM treatment are different from those used in VM treatment due to there being more complicated vascular anatomy and high blood flow through AVMs.

As previously described, an AVM lesion is composed of arterial feeders, nidus, and draining veins, although they are not always clearly visible on the angiographic images. The target of the current endovascular treatment of AVM

is the nidus of the AVMs. Various endovascular techniques have been used depending on the angiographic type, anatomic location, and catheter accessibility of the AVM lesion.

A recent report[15] from a specialized CVM center cited a decreased complication rate and higher clinical success rate after endovascular treatment of extremity or torso AVMs compared to those performed in the last decade. They reported an 18.5% rate of minor complications and a 2.4% rate of major complications after endovascular treatment of the AVMs in the last 10 years. According to the authors, the reasons for the improved treatment results included use of an angiographic types-based treatment strategy; diverse access routes to the AVM lesion including transarterial, transvenous, and/or direct puncture to the AVMs nidus; and use of variable concentrations of the ethanol rather than a fixed high concentration compared to treatment performed in the last decade.

When we assess treatment options, we usually consider the risks and benefits of the treatment. If the risk of treatment is greater than the benefit, the treatment is "too much." However, it is difficult to predict the risk of complication before AVM treatment. In the treatment of AVM, patient age, anatomical location, surrounding anatomical structures, angiographic features, degree of arteriovenous shunting, and catheter accessibility to the AVMs are related to the risks and results of the AVM treatment.

The age of the patient at the diagnosis of AVM is an important prognostic factor. Compared with adult patients, patients experiencing AVM exacerbation early in life will have a worse prognosis, will require a significantly higher number of interventions for treatment, and will have higher morbidity and sequelae.[1]

In addition, the vascular approach is more challenging in pediatric AVM patients due to small-sized vessels, greater radiation hazards, and a relatively narrow safety margin in the use of sclerosing or embolic agents and anesthesia. Depending on the anatomical location of the AVM, expected complications may differ. Figure 19.2 shows AVMs at various

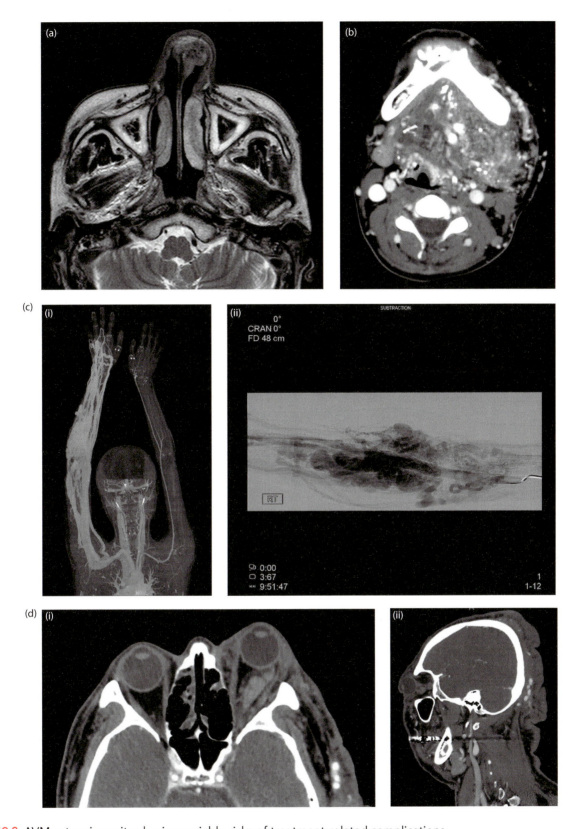

Figure 19.2 AVMs at various sites having variable risks of treatment-related complications.

locations, each of which carries the potential risk of specific complications after treatment. An AVM at the nose tip (a) carries the risk of nasal cartilage damage and nasal deformity through the sclerotherapy of the AVM. AVMs in the oral cavity (b) carry the risk of upper airway obstruction after endovascular treatment of AVMs. For this reason, we have to consider a prolonged endotracheal intubation or tracheotomy after endovascular treatment of the AVM.

AVMs at the upper extremity (c) carry higher risk of nerve palsy than in treatment of lower extremity (LE) AVMs after ethanol sclerotherapy. This may be because there are more nerves in a narrow compartment in the upper extremity (UE) compared to the LE. And nerve palsy in the UE is clinically more remarkable than that in the LE. Utmost caution must be exercised in endovascular treatment of UE AVMs to avoid permanent nerve palsy. Most nerve palsy is transient. However, it can be permanent in patients who undergo repeated treatment.

A patient with orbital AVMs (d) presented with pulsatile exophthalmos that carries the risk of optic nerve damage and blindness after endovascular treatment of the intraorbital, retrobulbar AVM.

Regarding catheter accessibility to the AVM nidus, it differs according to the angiographic type of AVM. Our group suggested three types of AVMs based on the presence of visible nidus and number and size of the feeders and draining veins on angiographic images. Endovascular treatment of AVMs was recommended according to the angiographic type.[15,16]

To overcome the difficulties in the transarterial approach, transvenous, percutaneous direct puncture to the AVM nidus or combined techniques have been used in the treatment of AVMs.

For the treatment of AVMs with a large amount of arteriovenous shunt, arterial compression with a proximal tourniquet or temporary occluding balloons in the draining veins can be used during the endovascular procedure to slow down the blood flow and prolong the retention time of the sclerosing agent in the AVM lesions.

In determining the optimal timing of treatment for patients with asymptomatic, dormant AVMs, the dilemma can be whether to treat or defer the treatment to the time when complications or symptoms occurred. One study on the natural course of AVMs described that almost all AVMs eventually progressed, with nearly half becoming Schöbinger stage 3. They recommended the early treatment of AVM regardless of stage.[17] Early treatment of AVM lesions has the theoretical merit of possible eradication of AVM but carries the risk of AVM aggravation by an improper treatment. Delayed treatment of AVM is usually performed after development of symptoms or signs of AVM. Most AVM treatment belongs in this category. Although we cannot completely eradicate whole AVMs at this time, we can control complications of the AVM and occlude prominent AVM nidus with endovascular means in current practice. For example, a very small facial AVM lesion entices doctors to intervene either surgically or with laser ablation with the intent of complete cure of the AVM lesion.

However, the cosmetic results of plastic surgery on a small forehead skin AVM are not always satisfactory. AVMs that are difficult to delineate by imaging are not good candidates for surgical resection, because the surgical margin is too elusive to have an effective surgical outcome.[18]

And the surgical management of AVMs is commonly complicated by wound dehiscence and early postoperative recurrence. Poor oxygen tension and the aberrant local environment of the AVMs are thought to contribute to poor wound healing and the recurrence of AVMs. Furthermore, bleeding from residual AVMs of the mucosa (nasal or oral) may be particularly difficult to control.

Recently, the use of Onyx has enabled the partial or complete control of AVMs in anatomically challenging areas. Onyx can be used in preoperative embolization before targeted resection of AVMs. This can reduce intraoperative bleeding and assists in demonstrating margins for resection. However, the use of Onyx is not free of complications such as infections, bleeding, skin discoloration, or skin necrosis.[19]

Attempts have been made to use angiogenesis inhibitors in the treatment of AVMs. Of the various angiogenesis inhibitors, it was demonstrated that the anti-vascular endothelial growth factor (VEGF) monoclonal antibody (bevacizumab, Avastin) can prevent the formation of AVMs and cease the progression of AVM development in an animal model of hereditary hemorrhagic telangiectasia 2 (HHT-2).[20,21] There have been anecdotal clinical reports that a VEGF inhibitor (bevacizumab, Avastin) reduced epistaxis, telangiectasias, and iron-deficiency anemia in patients with HHT. However, bevacizumab is still in the middle of clinical trial only for patients with brain AVMs who are not candidates for other proven treatment modalities. Its efficacy in the treatment of peripheral AVMs should be determined in the future. The use of doxycycline (MMP-9 inhibitor),[22] thalidomide, and interferon-α[23] has also been attempted to prevent AVM formation and arrest the progression of AVM development.

So far, there has been no prospective study comparing treatment results for patients with asymptomatic dormant AVM between an initial observative treatment and late endovascular or multimodal treatment if required versus primary curative treatment before symptoms appear. As such, it is difficult at this point to say how much is too much in the treatment of dormant AVMs. However, most dormant AVM lesions are treated with initial observative treatment in current practice.

To answer the question of how much treatment is too much for patients with symptomatic AVMs, in the author's opinion, it is "too much" when significant complications or permanent sequelae develop or AVMs progress in their symptoms or appearance after the treatment.

In the treatment of AVMs, what we have to always keep in mind is that an improper treatment such as incomplete resection, ligation, or embolization of the feeding arteries may aggravate the AVMs and make further treatment more difficult. Before the treatment of AVMs, we have to consider patient age, the risks of radiation, and the risks and benefits of the treatment based on the anatomical location, clinical stage, and angiographic features of the AVM lesions.

REFERENCES

1. Lee BB, Baumgartner I, Berlien HP et al. Consensus document of the International Union of Angiology (IUA)-2013 current concepts on the management of arteriovenous malformations. *Int Angiol.* 2013;32:9–36.

2. John L, Doppman JL. The nidus concept of spinal cord arteriovenous malformations. A surgical recommendation based upon angiographic observations. *Br J Radiol*. 1971;44:758–763.

3. Valavanis A, Schubiger O, Wichmann W. Classification of brain arteriovenous malformation nidus by magnetic resonance imaging. *Acta Radiol Suppl*. 1986; 369:86–89.

4. Geibprasert S, Pongpech S, Jiarakongmun P, Shroff MM, Armstrong DC, Krings T. Radiologic assessment of brain arteriovenous malformations: What clinicians need to know. *RadioGraphics*. 2010;30:483–501.

5. Darland DC, D'Amore PA. Blood vessel maturation: Vascular development comes of age. *J Clin Invest*. 1999;103:157–158.

6. Bergers G, Song S. The role of pericytes in blood-vessel formation and maintenance. *Neuro Oncol*. 2005;7:452–464.

7. Wu J, Bohanan CS, Neumann JC, Lingrel JB. KLF2 transcription factor modulates blood vessel maturation through smooth muscle cell migration. *J Biol Chem*. 2008;283:3942–3950.

8. Berg JN, Gallione CJ, Stenzel TT et al. The activin receptor-like kinase 1 gene: Genomic structure and mutations in hereditary hemorrhagic telangiectasia type 2. *Am J Hum Genet*. 1997;61:60–67.

9. Lamouille S, Mallet C, Feige JJ, Bailly S. Activin receptor-like kinase 1 is implicated in the maturation phase of angiogenesis. *Blood*. 2002;100:4495–4501.

10. Frieden I, Enjolras O, Esterly N. Vascular birthmarks and other abnormalities of blood vessels and lymphatics. In: Schacner LA, Hanson RC, eds. *Pediatric Dermatology*. 3rd ed. St Louis, MO: Mosby; 2003:833–862.

11. Schöbinger MP, Hansen M, Pribaz JJ, Mulliken JB. Arteriovenous malformations of the head and neck: Natural history and management. *Plast Reconstr Surg*. 1998;102:643–654.

12. Mulligan PR, Prayapati HJS, Martin LG, Patel TH. Vascular anomalies: Classification, imaging characteristics and implications for interventional radiology treatment approaches. *Br J Radiol*. 2014;87:20130392.

13. Greene AK, Orbach DB. Management of arteriovenous malformations. *Clin Plast Surg*. 2011;38;95–106.

14. Liu AS, Mulliken JB, Zurakowski D, Fishman SJ, Greene AK. Extracranial arteriovenous malformations: Natural progression and recurrence after treatment. *Plast Reconstr Surg*. 2010;125:1185–1194.

15. Park KB, Do YS, Kim DI et al. Endovascular treatment results and risk factors for complications of body and extremity arteriovenous malformations. *J Vasc Surg*. 2019;69:1207–1218.

16. Cho SK, Do YS, Shin SW et al. Arteriovenous malformations of the body and extremities: Analysis of therapeutic outcomes and approaches according to modified angiographic classification. *J Endovasc Ther*. 2006;13:527–538.

17. Liu AS, Mulliken JB, Zurakowski D et al. Extracranial arteriovenous malformations: Natural progression and recurrence after treatment. *Plast Reconstr Surg*. 2010;125:1185–1194.

18. Uller W, Ahmad I, Alomari AI, Richter GT. Arteriovenous malformations. *Semin Pediatr Surg*. 2014; 23:203–207.

19. McMillan K, Dunphy L, Nishikawa H, Monaghan A. Experiences in managing arteriovenous malformations of the head and neck. *Br J Oral Maxillofacial Surg*. 2016;54:643–647.

20. Han C, Choe S-W, Kin Y-H et al. VEGF neutralization can prevent and normalize arteriovenous malformations in an animal model for hereditary hemorrhagic telangiectasia 2. *Angiogenesis*. 2014;17:823–830.

21. Williams BJ, Park DM, Sheehan JP. Bevacizumab used for the treatment of severe, refractory perilesional edema due to an arteriovenous malformation treated with stereotactic radiosurgery. *J Neurosurg*. 2012;116:972–977.

22. Lee CZ, Xue Z, Zhu Y, Yang G-Y, Young WL. Matrix metalloproteinase-9 inhibition attenuates vascular endothelial growth factor-induced intracerebral hemorrhage. *Stroke*. 2007;38:2563–2568.

23. Adam Z, Pour L, Krejci M, Pourova E, Synek O, Zahradova L. Successful treatment of angiomatosis with thalidomide and interferon-α. A description of five cases and overview of treatment of angiomatosis and proliferating hemangiomas. *Vnitr Lek*. 2010;56:810–823.

20

Ethanol sclerotherapy: Is it gold standard for arteriovenous malformation management?

IRIS BAUMGARTNER, MIHAI CONSTANTINESCU, JOCHEN KARL RÖSSLER, AND HENDRIK VON TENGG-KOBLIGK

Arteriovenous malformation (AVM) is defined as high-flow, low-resistance communication of the arterial and venous system without an intervening normal capillary system. An ill-planned and improper treatment strategy (incomplete resection, surgical ligation/skeletonization, and/or proximal coil embolization of the feeding arteries) will result in lesion recurrence and enlargement by neovascular stimulation and needs to be abandoned (Figure 20.1).[1–3] Endovascular therapy is the preferred therapeutic solution for the vast majority of patients. Precise delivery of the embolic agent to ablate the AVM nidus is required for successful therapy. To perform nidus embolization, supraselective intra-arterial microcatheter, direct percutaneous nidus puncture, transvenous retrograde access, or a combination utilizing any of the three routes of delivery may be required (Figure 20.2).[2,4]

Although there is not a single gold standard embolic agent, absolute ethanol (96%–98% dehydrated ethyl alcohol) with or without coiling is by far the most commonly used endovascular ablative technique to treat AVM with curative intention.[5–9] The curative potential of ethanol is explained by its protein denaturing properties inducing permanent vessel wall damage. With the destruction of endothelial cells, the phenomena of neovascular stimulation due to secretion of angiogenic factors is noticeably absent, and a permanent occlusion of the AVM is the result.[10]

Despite unique features of ethanol, other embolic agents have been used for endovascular treatment of AVM.[11–15] Polyvinyl alcohol (PVA) particles, microspheres, Gelfoam, and collagen powders, alone or in combination with other agents, are documented, all being palliative with high recurrence rates. Moreover, particles are often either too large, and occlude the vessels proximal to the nidus, or too small, and travel through the AV shunt causing nontarget embolization. The use of polymerizing agents such as nBCA glue (n-butyl-2-cyanoacrylate, Histoacryl) or EVOH (ethylene vinyl alcohol, Onyx) are suitable for embolization. However, due to their viscosity and precipitation, embolization and filling of the nidus often remain incomplete. Moreover, the advantage of less toxicity as compared to absolute ethanol is counterbalanced by more frequent recurrences as dissolution of these agents can occur, allowing neovascular stimulation and growth of massive networks of small arteries.[16–18] Coils are designed to mechanically occlude larger vessels. When used as a transarterial embolic occlusive device to treat an AVM, they will imitate a proximal arterial ligation, rather worsening the situation by neovascular stimulation. In contrast to the transarterial approach, coiling can be extremely effective in those AVMs where multiple arteries connect to a single enlarged or aneurysmal draining vein if direct percutaneous puncture of the nidus using 18 G needles or a retrograde transvenous catheterization of the nidus comes to the application. Particularly, direct percutaneous puncture of the nidus has demonstrated extraordinary precision and safety with the positioning of puncture needles at almost any site within the body. By injecting contrast through a proximally positioned arterial catheter or by ultrasound guidance, the needle can be guided directly into the nidus. Pulsatile flow followed by selective arteriography through the needle verifies the correct position. Densely packed coils (eventually combined with J-guided wires to reduce the number of coils needed to pack large volumes) can completely block flow, thereby even being curative by itself. In AVMs that have an aneurysmal dilatation along the draining vein, with multiple outflow veins arising from it, coil embolization can be used in combination with ethanol to secure definitive closure.[17] Once flow has been slowed in the outflow veins by the placement of the coils, the injection of absolute ethanol can then reflux into the many vein fistulae in the wall of this aneurysmal vein to allow permanent occlusion. This "retrograde vein occlusion" technique in the curative treatment of high-flow vascular malformations was first described by Yakes et al. in 1990 and later confirmed by Jackson et al. in 1996 and Cho et al. in 2008.[3,19–21]

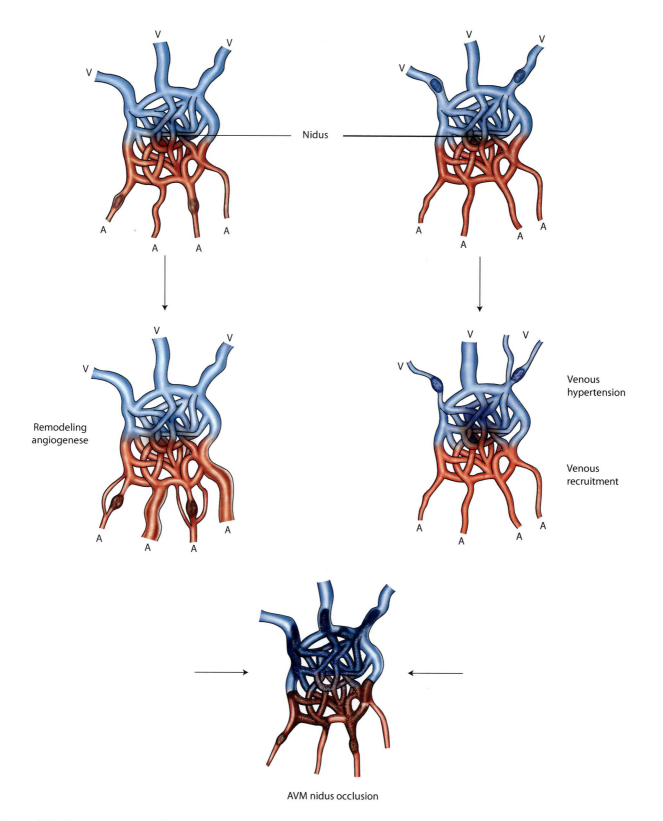

Figure 20.1 Arteriovenous malformation (AVM) with multiple arterial feeder and draining veins. Incomplete embolization of a dominant arterial feeder leads to remodeling angiogenesis and enlargement of innumerable smaller-sized feeders. Incomplete embolization of the venous drainage will induce profound venous hypertension. Complete filling of the nidus will occlude the AVM and prevents development of collaterals. (A, artery; V, vein.) (Adjusted from Doppman JL, Pevsner P. *Am J Roentgenol.* 1983;140:773–778.)

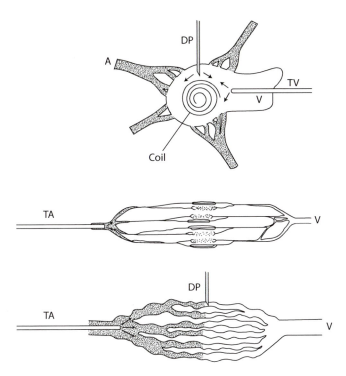

Figure 20.2 Adjusted supra-selective access for ethanol and/or coil embolization of the nidus according to the angioarchitecture of an arteriovenous malformation. (A, artery; DP, direct puncture; TA, transarterial; TV, transvenous; V, vein.) (With kind permission from Springer Science+Business Media: *Congenital Vascular Malformations. A Comprehensive Review of Current Management*, New arteriographic classification of AVM based on the Yakes classification system, 2017, 62–69, Yakes WF, Vogelzang RL, Ivancev K, Yakes A. In: Kim Y-W, Lee B-B, Yakes WF, Do Y-S, eds. Berlin, Germany: Springer Verlag.)

Direct arteriovenous fistulous connections without interposition of a multi-channeled nidus are typically seen in pulmonary and renal AVMs (Yakes type I). In these AVMs, interruption of blood flow using coils, plugs, or other mechanical devices alone is curative per se.[22,23] The most difficult variant of AVM to be treated is the micro-fistulous, infiltrative type (Yakes type IV). Multiple arteries/arterioles form innumerable microfistulae that diffusely infiltrate the affected tissue. Interspersed within these innumerable microfistulae are capillary beds that maintain the viability of the affected tissue. It is recommended to use a diluted 50/50% mixture of ethanol with nonionic contrast. Mixing nonionic contrast with absolute ethanol changes the viscosity. Being more viscous allows for preferential flow to the microfistulous parts of the AVM, whereas nutritive capillaries are conditionally protected due to their higher resistance.[2] As ethanol is rather an unforgiving embolic agent, the experience of the operator is of particular importance, and ill-considered application is to be avoided. Close to neural structures, in intracranial or spinal lesions, ethanol is contraindicated. If injection at the level of the nidus is not possible, ethanol is not useful.

Absolute ethanol is associated with systemic and local complications related to the tissue being embolized and the size of the AVM. Precise delivery to minimize complications but a sufficient amount of ethanol to achieve long-term cure is required. Multisession therapy is preferred, and every effort has to be made to minimize risks of ethanol embolosclerotherapy during each session. Pulmonary hypertension is a potentially fatal complication associated with ethanol embolization and occurs when a significant dose of ethanol is allowed to reach the lungs. The etiology of pulmonary hypertension is felt to be related to either pulmonary arterial spasm or extensive microthromboembolization. A total dose of ethanol during an embolization procedure should be less than 1 mL/kg as the maximum volume that can be safely given during a procedure. Limiting ethanol bolus injections to 0.14 mL ethanol/kg ideal body weight every 10 minutes usually obviates the need for a pulmonary artery catheter.[24–26] Adhering to these principles, the risk of ethanol flowing to the pulmonary circulation, thus causing pulmonary vascular spasm with subsequent acute right heart failure, is negligible. Accurate and meticulous embolization requires precise injection solely in the AVM nidus vasculature that is nonnutritive and without capillaries. Proximal injection of ethanol into a feeding artery causes severe tissue necrosis by destroying nutritive capillary beds. Avoidance of ethanol embolization of nutritive capillary beds, and a combined use of coils in Yakes type I, IIIa, and IIIb AVMs, limit complications.[2] The most frequently encountered complications are skin blistering or necrosis and transient nerve palsy in about 10%–30% of treatment sessions. Hemoglobinuria is described, but clinically relevant hemoglobinuria is rarely seen. In a recently published long-term evaluation of several hundred patients with AVMs, the rates of minor (18.5%–20.1%) and major (2.4%–3.15%) complications were described to be relatively constant over the 20-year assessment period. To decrease postembolization swelling in the endovascularly treated area and to prevent nerve injuries due to edema, routine use of IV dexamethasone before the procedure, as well as nonsteroidal anti-inflammatory drugs and steroid medical therapy for 5 days after the procedure, are recommended.

REFERENCES

1. Lee BB, Baumgartner I, Berlien HP et al. Consensus document of the International Union of Angiology (IUA)-2013 current concepts on the management of arterio-venous malformations. *Int Angiol.* 2013;32(1): 9–36.
2. Yakes WF, Vogelzang RL, Ivancev K, Yakes A. New arteriographic classification of AVM based on the Yakes classification system. In: Kim Y-W, Lee B-B, Yakes WF, Do Y-S, eds. *Congenital Vascular Malformations. A Comprehensive Review of Current Management.* Berlin, Germany: Springer Verlag; 2017: 62–69.

3. Doppman JL, Pevsner P. Embolisation of arteriovenous malformations by direct percutaneous puncture. *Am J Roentgenol.* 1983;140:773–778.

4. Yakes WF, Pevsner P, Reed M, Donohue HJ, Ghaed N. Serial embolizations of an extremity AVM with alcohol via direct puncture. *Am J Roentgenol.* 1986;146:1038–1044.

5. Yakes WF, Luethke JM, Merland JJ et al. Ethanol embolization of arteriovenous fistulas: A primary form of therapy. *J Vasc Intervent Radiol.* 1990;1:89–96.

6. Yakes WF. Endovascular management of high-flow AVMs. *Semin Intervent Radiol.* 2004;21:49–58.

7. Do YS, Park KB, Park HS, Cho SK, Shin SW, Moon JW. Ethanol embolization of arteriovenous malformations: Interim results. *Radiology.* 2005;235:674–682.

8. Vogelzang RL, Atassi R, Vouche M, Resnick S, Salem R. Ethanol embolotherapy of vascular malformations: Clinical outcomes at a single center. *J Vasc Interv Radiol.* 2014;25:206–213.

9. Yakes W, Huguenot M, Yakes A, Continenza A, Kammer R, Baumgartner I. Percutaneous embolization of arterio-venous malformations at the plantar aspect of the foot. *J Vasc Surg.* 2016;64:1478–1482.

10. Ellman BA, Parkhill BJ, Marcus PB. Renal ablation with absolute ethanol: Mechanism of action. *Invest Radiol.* 1984;19:416–423.

11. Zanetti PH. Cyanoacrylate/iophenylate mixtures: Modification and in vitro evaluation as embolic agents. *J Int Radiol.* 1987;2:65–68.

12. Widlus DM, Murray RR, White RI Jr et al. Congenital arteriovenous malformations: Tailored embolotherapy. *Radiology.* 1988;169:511–516.

13. Jacobowitz GR, Rosen RJ, Rockman CB et al. Transcatheter embolization of complex pelvic vascular malformations: Results and long-term follow-up. *J Vasc Surg.* 2001;33:51–55.

14. Numan F, Omeroglu A, Kara B, Cantademir M, Adalet- li I, Kantarci F. Embolization of peripheral vascular malformations with ethylene vinyl alcohol copolymer (Onyx). *J Vasc Interv Radiol.* 2004;15:939–946.

15. Giurazza F, Corvino F, Cangiano G et al. Transarterial embolization of peripheral high flow malformation with ethylene vinyl alcohol copolymer (Onyx®): Single-center 10-year experience. *Radiol Med.* 2019;124(2):154–162.

16. Rao VRK, Mandalan KR, Gupta AK, Kumar S, Joseph S. Dissolution of isobutyl 2-cyanoacrylate on long term follow-up. *Am J Neuroradiol.* 1989;10:135–141.

17. Germano IM, Davis RL, Wilson CB, Hiershima GB. Histopathological follow up study of 66 cerebral arteriovenous malformations after therapeutic embolization with polyvinyl alcohol. *J Neurosurg.* 1992;76:607–614.

18. Davidson GS, Terbrugge KG. Histologic long-term follow-up after embolization with polyvinyl alcohol particles. *Am J Neuroradiol.* 1995;16(4 Suppl): 843–846.

19. Jackson JE, Mansfield AO, Allison DJ. Treatment of high-flow vascular malformations aided by flow occlusion techniques. *Cardiovasc Intervent Radiol.* 1996;19:323–328.

20. Cho SK, Do YS, Kim DI et al. Peripheral arteriovenous malformations with dominant outflow vein: Results of ethanol embolization. *Korean J Radiol.* 2008;9:258–267.

21. Lee SY, Do YS, Kim CW, Park KB, Kim YH, Cho YJ. Efficacy and safety of transvenous embolization of type II renal arteriovenous malformations with coils. *J Vasc Interv Radiol.* 2019;30(6):807–812.

22. Meek ME, Meek JC, Beheshti MV. Management of pulmonary arteriovenous malformations. *Semin Intervent Radiol.* 2011;28(1):24–31.

23. Lacombe P, Lacout A, Marcy PY et al. Diagnosis and treatment of pulmonary arteriovenous malformations in hereditary hemorrhagic telangiectasia: An overview. *Diagn Interv Imaging.* 2013;94(9):835–848.

24. Shin BS, Do YS, Lee BB, Kim DI, Chung IS, Cho HS. Multistage ethanol sclerotherapy of soft-tissue arterio-venous malformations: Effect on pulmonary arterial pressure. *Radiology.* 2005;235:1072–1077.

25. Ko JS, Kim JA, Do YS, Kwon MA, Choi SJ, Gwak MS. Prediction of the effect of injected ethanol on pulmonary arterial pressure during sclerotherapy of arterio-venous malformations: Relationship with dose of ethanol. *J Vasc Interv Radiol.* 2009;20:39–45.

26. Shin BS, Do YS, Cho HS, Hahm TS, Kim CS. Effects of repeat bolus ethanol injections on cardiopulmonary hemodynamic changes during embolotherapy of arterio-venous malformations of the extremities. *J Vasc Interv Radiol.* 2010;21:81–89.

N-butyl cyanoacrylate versus Onyx embolotherapy

FURUZAN NUMAN

The first prospective study was performed by Loh and Duckwiler as Onyx Trial Investigators. These authors came to the conclusion that Onyx is equivalent to N-butyl cyanoacrylate (NBCA) in safety and efficacy as a preoperative embolic agent by reducing brain arteriovenous malformation (AVM) volume by at least 50%.[1]

Among different available embolic agents, liquid agents seem most appropriate for AVMs because of their ability to form a cast penetrating the nidus and occluding the different feeders. Both of them have the same indications for embolization of lesions; vascular pathologies such as AVMs, aneurysms, pseudoaneurysms (PAs), arteriovenous fistulas (AVFs) of head and neck and the peripheral, and also type I and II endoleaks, portal veins, bleeding, and tumors.[3-5]

N-BUTYL CYANOACRYLATE

Cyanoacrylate glues are liquid alkyl-2-cyanoacrylate monomers that, on contact with ionic mediums (e.g., water, blood), form flexible polymers with strong adhesive bonds to soft tissues. These liquid monomers in isolation are nonviscous, radiolucent, and rapidly polymerize. Consequently, they are combined as a two-component embolic agent with either tantalum powder or ethiodized oil (Lipiodol; Andre Guerbet, Aulnay-sous-Bois, France). The added agent prolongs polymerization time, opacifies the liquid agent, and allows for its visualization under fluoroscopy. The NBCA mixture ratio is also guided by the polymerization times described by Pollak and White, who suggested that the estimated *in vivo* polymerization time for NBCA to iodize oil mixtures between 1:1 and 1:4 was 1–4 seconds, with a linear relationship between time and mixture ratio.[2,6,9]

N-butyl-2-cyanoacrylate (n-BCA) liquid embolic system (Trufill, Cordis Neurovascular) is approved by the U.S. Food and Drug Administration (FDA) for embolization of cerebral arteriovenous malformations (AVMs).[8] There are also other off-label liquid embolic agents such as Glubran2 (GEM, Viareggio, Italy) and Histoacryl (B/Braun, Tuttlingen, Germany).

For embolization, a coaxial combination of 4 F macro- and microcatheter is recommended. Flushing microcatheter with nonheparinized 5% dextrose (D5) prior to injection is mandatory to prevent polymerization of the mixture in contact with residual blood or saline in the catheter tip. This maneuver also helps to slow the glue polymerization and allows for deeper penetration and distal embolization. Once the injection is complete, the microcatheter is aspirated and withdrawn rapidly.[9]

If the coaxial macrocatheter and microcatheter are blocked with refluxed or high concentrated glue, the whole coaxial system should be withdrawn.[7] If the microcatheter is blocked due to the user not following the steps, the microcatheter should be withdrawn from the macrocatheder. Any attempt to clear the lumen of either of the catheters may cause nontarget embolization as an unwanted complication. Even if used by skilled hands, there may be unwanted complications, such as nontarget embolization, delayed polymerization, and catheter tip entrapment within the polymerized glue.

Nontarget embolization is the most clinically significant complication with the potential to precipitate end-organ ischemia and bacterial sepsis.[9]

Size, shape, and location of fragments need to be identified if fragmentation and embolization are detected. Relocating the embolus back to the target site, positioning the embolus in a suitable vascular side, or retracting the glue embolus through a catheter are the troubleshooting options.

Venous outflow blockage by migrated polymerized embolic agent through the nidus is wanted at peripheral AVMs, opposite of brain AVMs, which causes an increased risk of hemorrhage.[10]

ONYX

Onyx is an ethylene vinyl alcohol copolymer (EVOH: Onyx; ev3-Covidien, Irvine, California) dissolved in dimethyl sulfoxide (DMSO). It is a nonadhesive and radiolucent liquid embolic agent that has been used since the early 1990s.[11,12]

Onyx-based closure of the lumen of the targeted vessel is obtained by means of precipitation, initiated after diffusion of DMSO in the presence of water. The process is enhanced peripherally to the main flux of the injected mixture. These properties facilitate angiographic monitoring of embolization at any stage. Fluoroscopic visualization of the injected Onyx mass is possible through the addition of tantalum filings.[15]

There are three different FDA-approved Onyx types with different viscosities: Onyx 18, 34, and 34L. Onyx 34L has a reduced tantalum amount in comparison to Onyx 34, which causes no artifacts on computed tomography (Figure 21.1a and b) and good visibility during the injection.

We published that it is safe to use Onyx in pediatric patients. Onyx is not indicated for use with premature infants (<1500 g) or individuals with significant liver function impairment.[14]

Onyx embolization is done mostly via a transarterial approach. The other techniques are a direct percutaneous puncture, a transvenous approach, an external compression (bandage), and balloon protection.

We prefer a coaxial system using 4 Fr. Berenstein as a macrocatheter with any of the DMSO-compatible microcatheters (Echelon-14 or Echelon-10, ev3, Irvine, California) to perform super-selective catheterization. The Berenstein macrocatheter's short arm and appropriate angulation help to anchor the feeding artery ostium distally. This creates a safe distance to protect the parent artery from untarget end-organ embolization. The microcatheter has to be placed as close as possible to the nidus.[12,13]

According to flow velocity within the AVM (AFVs), which can vary from low to high, it is necessary to decide the concentration and viscosity of the copolymer. There is no quantitative calculation parameter. The test with the contrast agent is not efficient. Onyx 18 should be preferred in cases with tiny feeding arteries for distal penetration. Onyx 34/34L is recommended in high-flow lesions. The vials of Onyx are shaken for 20 minutes using a shaker (Vortex-Genie,

Scientific Industries, Bohemia, New York) to make the tantalum powder homogenous within the suspension.

Steps to the procedure are flushing the microcatheter with saline solution and filling the "dead space" with an adequate volume of DMSO, followed by injecting Onyx slowly, using a 1 mL syringe.

DMSO's chemical irritation causes pain. General anesthesia helps to comfort the patient while following the procedural steps.

A cast of Onyx guide to applying further injections on roadmap imaging. The injections continue until the feeding arteries, the nidus, and the drainage vein or veins are completely occluded. Changing the magnification during the injection will also help to observe if the Onyx is migrated through the unattended minuscule fistula to a normal artery because of altered hemodynamic stress.

For low flow and big AVMs with tiny niduses and feeding arteries not suitable to reach with a microcatheter, we prefer to use the "modified Onyx technique." In this technique, we further dilute Onyx 18 in a 1 mL syringe (60% Onyx, 40% DMSO) in order to embolize as many niduses as quickly as possible. After finishing embolization within the first feeding artery, we flush the microcatheter via DMSO and move on to embolization in other feeding arteries with the same microcatheter.

Clearing up the lumen with DMSO has benefits such as pushing and diluting Onyx more distally and having an angiogram without changing the place of the microcatheter (Figures 21.2a,b and 21.3a,b).

With this technique, we lower the cost and procedure time, decreasing the radiation dose given to the patient, which makes using Onyx more efficient against NBCA. Onyx has several advantages, such as the microcatheter tip is not glued within the vessel and it is easier to handle during surgery because of the lower inflammatory reaction, which makes surgical dissection easier without surrounding tissue reaction.

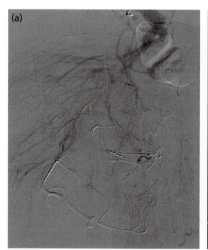
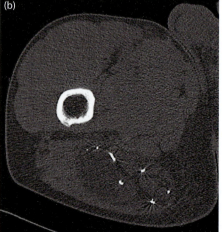

Figure 21.1 **(a)** Right buttocks arteriovenous malformation (AVM) treated using Onyx 34L. Digital subtraction angiography showed the cast of Onyx 34L during the embolization. **(b)** Postprocedural computed tomography showed significantly reduced AVM (demonstrated by reduced tantalum amount).

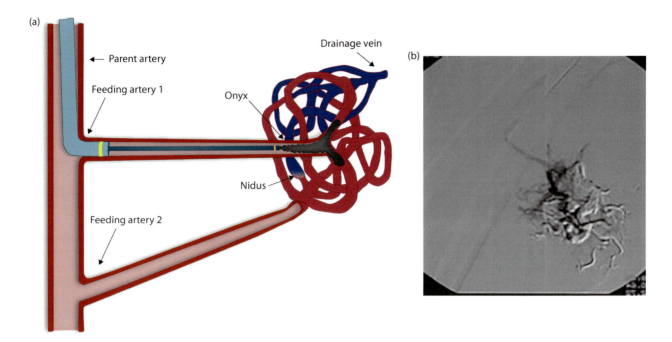

Figure 21.2 (a) Distal nidus was accessed first by coaxial catheter system and was successfully occluded by Onyx. **(b)** Digital subtraction angiography of the left forearm arteriovenous malformation (AVM) involving soft tissue (note AVM nidus).

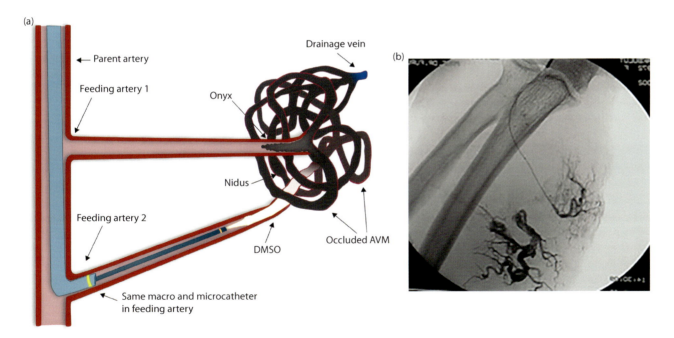

Figure 21.3 (a) The second nidus was embolized with the same coaxial catheter system. Catheter was flushed with dimethyl sulfoxide to clear Onyx from the microcatheter. **(b)** Digital subtraction angiography demonstrates successful embolization of the second nidus.

The elimination of DMSO from the body via respiration and sweat causes a garlic-like smell that may last for a few days.

Discoloration of the dark skin, bullous formation, and nerve palsy are mostly seen at superficial AVMs because of untargeted embolization through minuscule fistulas. Discoloration faded spontaneously by leaving a faint mark on the skin (Figure 21.4).

Large fistulas may be a source of the pulmonary embolism, which is the reason why fluoroscopic observation during the injection is mandatory (Figure 21.5).

In conclusion, transcatheter embolization with Onyx is a promising treatment option for peripheral AVMs. Onyx seems to provide controlled embolization due to slow polymerization, which enables deep penetration in the

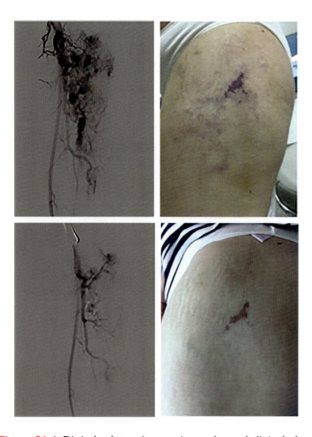

Figure 21.4 Digital subtraction angiography and clinical photographs of the skin during Onyx embolization (before) and during a follow-up (after) of the left thigh arteriovenous malformation (AVM) treatment (note AVM feeding arteries from the left profunda femoral artery branches). Discoloration of the skin faded over time, and a small faint mark remained.

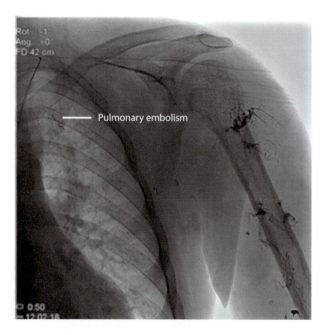

Figure 21.5 During the Onyx embolization of the left shoulder AVM, fistula caused nonfatal pulmonary embolism that was detected during the procedural fluoroscopy. (AVM, arteriovenous malformation; DSA, digital subtraction angiography.)

nidus with less risk of catheter gluing due to its nonadhesive nature. It has been proven that off-label, these products are safe and effective to use for the embolization of vascular pathologies.

REFERENCES

1. Loh Y, Duckwiler GR, Onyx Trial Investigators. A prospective, multicenter, randomized trial of the Onyx liquid embolic system and N-butyl cyanoacrylate embolization of cerebral arteriovenous malformations. *J Neurosurg.* 2010;113(4):733–741.
2. Pollak JS, White RI Jr. The use of cyanoacrylate adhesives in peripheral embolization. *J Vasc Interv Radiol.* 2001;12:907–913.
3. Numan F, Cakirer S, Işlak C et al. Posttraumatic high-flow priapism treated by N-butyl-cyanoacrylate embolization. *Cardiovasc Interven Radiol.* 1996;19(4):278–280.
4. Kish JW, Katz MD, Marx MV, Harrell DS, Hanks SE. N-butyl cyanoacrylate embolization for control of acute arterial hemorrhage. *J Vasc Interv Radiol.* 2004;15:689–695.
5. Lee B-B, Do YS, Yakes W et al. Management of arteriovenous malformations: A multidisciplinary approach. *J Vasc Surg.* 2004;39:590–600.
6. Mattamal GJ. US FDA perspective on the regulations of medical-grade polymers: Cyanoacrylate polymer medical device-tissue adhesives. *Expert Rev Med Devices.* 2008;5(1):41–49.
7. Takeuchi Y, Morishita H, Sato Y et al. Committee of Practice Guidelines of the Japanese Society of Interventional Radiology. Guidelines for the use of NBCA in vascular embolization devised by the Committee of Practice Guidelines of the Japanese Society of Interventional Radiology (CGJSIR). *Jpn J Radiol.* 2014;32(8):500–517.
8. Loffroy R. Glubran2, histoacryl or trufill: Which cyanoacrylate glue for endovascular use? *Diagn Interv Imag.* 2016;97:119.
9. Hill H, Chick JFB, Hage A, Srinivasa RN. N-butyl cyanoacrylate embolotherapy: Techniques, complications, and management. *Diagn Interv Radiol.* 2018; 24(2):98–103.
10. Yata S, Ohuchi Y, Adachi A et al. Is glue embolization safe and effective for gastrointestinal bleeding? *Gastrointest Intervent.* 2018;7(3):158–161.
11. Terada T, Nakamura Y, Nakai K et al. Embolization of arteriovenous malformations with peripheral aneurysms using ethylene vinyl alcohol copolymer. Report of three cases. *J Neurosurg.* 1991;75: 655–660.
12. Numan F, Omeroglu A, Kara B, Cantaşdemir M, Adaletli I, Kantarci F. Embolization of peripheral vascular malformations with ethylene vinyl alcohol copolymer (Onyx). *J Vasc Interv Radiol.* 2004;15(9): 939–946.

13. Bratby MJ, Lehmann ED, Bottomley J et al. Endovascular embolization of visceral artery aneurysms with ethylene-vinyl alcohol (Onyx): A case series. *Cardiovasc Intervent Radiol.* 2006;29:1125–1128.

14. Cantasdemir M, Gulsen F, Solak S, Gulsen GY, Kantarci F, Numan F. The use of Onyx for embolization of peripheral vascular malformations in pediatric patients. *Pediatr Surg Int.* 2012;28(5):477–487.

15. Szajner M, Roman T, Markowicz J, Szczerbo-Trojanowska M. Onyx® in endovascular treatment of cerebral arteriovenous malformations—A review. *Pol J Radiol.* 2013;78(3):35–41.

Management: 2

22

Surgical therapy combined with embolo-/sclerotherapy: Multidisciplinary approach

PAUL MARJI, JAMES LAREDO, AND BYUNG-BOONG LEE

INTRODUCTION

The arteriovenous malformation (AVM) is considered the most virulent of all congenital vascular malformations (CVMs), causing not only profound local effects that threaten surrounding tissues and organs but also alterations that affect the entire cardiovascular system leading to functional impairment.[1,2] The extra-truncular AVM lesions, with the "nidus" that constitutes them, comprise most AVM cases, with truncular AVM lesions, the true fistulous lesions, encompassing a smaller subset.[3]

TREATMENT GUIDELINES

The approach to treatment of all extra-truncular AVM lesions should be elimination of the nidus. Incomplete excision, limited ligation, or proximal embolic occlusion of feeding vessels is unsatisfactory management, as this often leads to nidus proliferation and recurrence. A poorly planned management strategy will lead to stimulation of the extra-truncular AVM lesion, transforming it from a dormant to a proliferative state, resulting in a growth phase that complicates treatment.

The approach to managing truncular AVM lesions is relatively uncomplicated, requiring elimination of the AV shunt via excision, embolization, or covered stent, with virtually no risk of recurrent progression if initial treatment is executed successfully.

Ultimately, an aggressive but controlled approach to treatment should be implemented that encompasses an integrated, multidisciplinary effort with calculated selection of treatment modalities to improve outcomes, reducing morbidity, mortality, and recurrence.[3–6] Subsequent to assessing the indications and urgency of treatment, the full spectrum of available endovascular treatments in conjunction with traditional surgical resection should be appraised.[3,4]

ENDOVASCULAR TREATMENT

Endovascular embolo-/sclerotherapy is the sole modality of choice for *surgically inaccessible* extra-truncular lesions, those with prohibitive surgical risks (diffuse, infiltrating type), as well as for extensive lesions that extend beyond the deep fascia with involvement of muscle, tendon, or bone. This treatment modality is a vital adjunct to treating lesions also amenable to resection. In the adjuvant setting, its precise delivery via a combination of transarterial, transvenous, and direct puncture approaches reduces nidus size preoperatively, minimizing the morbidity of a complex resection. Additionally, it may also be used postoperatively. Multiple, limited administrations should be implemented to avoid collateral damage and potential systemic complications, utilizing the minimally effective volume of embolization/sclerotherapy agents during each session to minimize morbidity.[7–12] Selection of the most appropriate agent is often determined by lesion location, morphology, and overall clinical scenario.

Embolization improves the effectiveness of other therapies by altering the hemodynamics of the lesion. Coils, polyvinyl alcohol particles, microspheres, Gelfoam, and collagen powders may focally occlude large feeding vessels leading to their thrombosis, but they do not penetrate the lesion nidus and may even result in nontarget embolization. In addition, a sustained endothelial injury does not occur with coiling, which may lead to future recanalization and eventual recurrence. However, primary sequential treatment with coils is effective for successful obliteration of truncular-type lesions, and in combination with absolute ethanol for definitive treatment of arteriographic type II AVM lesions, with coils placed in a single draining vein.

Liquid agents, which include either sclerosants or polymerizing agents, possess the intrinsic property to penetrate the nidus. N-butyl cyanoacrylate (nBCA) exothermically polymerizes on contact with blood, causing a mechanical effect and inducing an acute inflammatory response. It is typically administered via direct puncture into the AVM nidus. Chronically, it stimulates an antigenic inflammatory response, promoting its long-term efficacy. Additionally, the cast-like nature of the polymerized glue plays a role in the long-term obliteration of the vasculature. Embolization of a lesion with nBCA glue facilitates surgical dissection and helps minimize intraoperative blood loss. When used as single therapy, it is typically deemed more of a palliative measure[13-16] and is only curative in very small and therefore typically resectable AVMs.[3]

Onyx, another preoperative or palliative embolic liquid adhesive, has the advantage of a slower, more controlled, and precise administration, with less risk of propagation compared to nBCA. Onyx is renowned for its effectiveness in reaching a large portion of the nidus via macroshunting and has a much lower risk of pulmonary embolism relative to other particulate embolization agents.[3]

Absolute ethanol therapy, a robust sclerosant with curative capacity, denudes the endothelial lining of the vessel wall and causes intimal fracturing, leading to thrombosis and cessation of angiogenic chemotaxis.[17-21] Multiple sessions at low dosages are typically implemented to limit cardiopulmonary toxicity and ischemic complications, as this modality carries the highest risk of potentially fatal consequences. The maximal dose of ethanol should not exceed 1 mg/kg of body weight per treatment session, and it may be diluted when used to treat superficial AVMs with a high risk of cutaneous necrosis, as well as those in close vicinity to nerves.[3]

Endovascularly placed covered stents are effective in the treatment of direct communicating truncular AVMs, much in the way as they are useful in controlling "aquired" AV fistulas of the subclavian, iliac, or femoral arteries. However, their use in extra-truncular lesions is limited, as the "nidus" is left intact, and recurrence ultimately results. Therefore, stents are reserved as a last resort and life-saving option in such AVMs.

SURGICAL TREATMENT

Surgical excision of extra-truncular AVMs remains the "gold standard" to *surgically accessible* and amenable lesions and is the ideal treatment modality for establishing a "cure"; however, it harbors the prospective morbidity associated with a radical resection. Preoperative embolo-/scelerotherapy improves the safety and effectiveness of surgery and is now an integral component in the management of surgically accessible lesions, improving outcomes. This modern strategy mitigates the potentially indiscriminate and invasive nature of traditional surgical therapy and takes advantage of the inherent advantages of both approaches.

There exist four categories of extracranial AVM, each with varying characteristics related to a specified approach, excisional intervention, and reconstruction: head and neck, visceral, upper limb, and lower limb. In general, an *en bloc* resection is advised, including surrounding soft tissues,

unless adequate preoperative embolo-/sclerotherapy has been conducted with a respectable outcome.[3] Additionally, silicone-based balloon tissue expansion is beneficial in preparation for reconstruction of not only the face and neck but also the upper and lower extremities. Reconstruction entails restoration of vascular flow, boney fixation, and repair of any specialized tissue including nerve, tendon, and muscle, followed by definitive soft tissue coverage either by local tissue rearrangement or autologous tissue transfer.[3]

REFERENCES

1. Lee BB. Statues of new approaches to the treatment of congenital vascular malformations (CVMs): Single center experiences. *Eur J Vasc Endovasc Surg.* 2005; 30:184–197.
2. Lee BB, Kim DI, Huh S et al. New experiences with absolute ethanol sclerotherapy in the management of a complex form of congenital venous malformation. *J Vasc Surg.* 2001;33:764–772.
3. Lee BB, Baumgartner I, Berlien HP et al. Consensus document of the International Union of Angiology (IUA)-2013. Current concept on the management of arterio-venous management. *Int Angiol.* 2013;32(1): 9–36.
4. Lee BB, Laredo J, Neville R. Arterio-venous malformation: How much do we know? *Phlebology.* 2009; 24:193–200.
5. Lee BB, Do YS, Yakes W et al. Management of arterial-venous shunting malformations (AVM) by surgery and embolosclerotherapy. A multidisciplinary approach. *J Vasc Surg.* 2004;39:590–600.
6. Lee BB. Advanced management of congenital vascular malformation (CVM). *Int Angiol.* 2002;21:209–213.
7. Gloviczki P, Duncan AA, Kalra M et al. Vascular malformations: An update. *Perspect Vasc Surg Endovasc Ther.* 2009;21(2):133–148.
8. Lee BB, Laredo J, Kim YW, Neville R. Congenital vascular malformations: General treatment principles. *Phlebology.* 2007;22(6):258–263.
9. Cho SK, Do YS, Kim DI, Kim YW, Shin SW, Park KB. Peripheral arteriovenous malformations with a dominant outflow vein: Results of ethanol embolization. *Korean J Radiol.* 2008;9:258–267.
10. Burrows P. Endovascular treatment of vascular malformations of the female pelvis. *Semin Intervent Radiol.* 2008;25:347–360.
11. Fan XD, Su LX, Zheng JW, Zheng LZ, Zhang ZY. Ethanol embolization of arteriovenous malformations of the mandible. *Am J Neuroradiol.* 2009;30:1178.
12. Numan F, Omeroglu A, Kara B, Cantaşdemir M, Adaletli I, Kantarci F. Embolization of peripheral vascular malformations with ethylene vinyl alcohol copolymer (Onyx). *J Vasc Interv Radiol.* 2004;15:939–946.
13. Velat GJ, Reavey-Cantwell JF, Sistrom C, Smullen D, Fautheree GL, Whiting J. Comparison of N-butyl cyanoacrylate and Onyx for the embolization of intracranial arteriovenous malformations: Analysis

of fluoroscopy and procedure times. *Neurosurgery.* 2008;63(Suppl 1):ONS7378; discussion ONS78–80.

14. Han MH, Seong SO, Kim HD, Chang KH, Yeon KM, Han MC. Craniofacial arteriovenous malformation: Preoperative embolization with direct puncture and injection of n-butyl cyanoacrylate. *Radiology.* 1999;211:661–666.

15. Natarajan SK, Born D, Ghodke B, Britz GW, Sekhar LN. Histopathological changes in brain arteriovenous malformations after embolization using Onyx or N-butyl cyanoacrylate. Laboratory investigation. *J Neurosurg.* 2009;111:105–113.

16. Loh Y, Duckwiler GR, Onyx Trial Investigators. A prospective, multicenter, randomized trial of the Onyx liquid embolic system and N-butyl cyanoacrylate embolization of cerebral arteriovenous malformations. Clinical article. *J Neurosurg.* 2010;113:733–741.

17. Yakes WF, Pevsner P, Reed M, Donohue HJ, Ghaed N. Serial embolizations of an extremity AVM with alcohol via direct puncture. *Am J Roentgenol.* 1986;146:1038–1044.

18. Yakes WF, Haas DK, Parker SH, Gibson MD, Hopper KD, Mulligan JS. Symptomatic vascular malformations: Ethanol embolotherapy. *Radiology.* 1989;170:1059–1066.

19. Yakes WF, Takebayashi S, Hosaka M, Ishizuka E. AVMs of the kidney: Ablation with alcohol. *Am J Roentgenol.* 1988;150:587–590.

20. Vinson AM, Rohrer DG, Willcox CW, Sigfred SV, Wheeler JR, Jacobs JS. Absolute ethanol embolization for peripheral AVM: Report of 2 cures. *South Med J.* 1988;1:1052–1055.

21. Do YS, Park KB, Park HS, Cho SK, Shin SW, Moon JW. Ethanol embolization of arteriovenous malformations: Interim results. *Radiology.* 2005;235:674–682.

23

Indications for amputation in patients with arterio-venous malformations

YOUNG-WOOK KIM

Limb amputation is usually the last option in the treatment of common vascular diseases affecting the extremity. This operation can be adopted for the purpose of achieving better functional or symptomatic results by removing the diseased part of the body, rather than repairing the vascular lesions, and preserving the affected limb.

In vascular surgery, most limb amputations are performed for patients with irreversible ischemia due to arterial occlusive disease, severe diabetic foot infection, or mangled trauma of the limb.

Although better functional results are reported after limb amputation than before because of improvements of the prostheses, limb amputation results in psychosocial problems in addition to the physical disability due to limb loss.

Limb amputation in patients with arteriovenous malformation (AVM) is different from that in patients with arterial occlusive disease. As described in other chapters in this book, AVM is characterized by high-flow vascular malformation and often presents with remarkable hemodynamic abnormality and more progressive clinical features than other types of vascular malformation (e.g., venous or lymphatic malformations). AVMs show episodic fast growth or lesion progression by a provoking event such as hormonal, traumatic, or ischemic stimulation. Improper surgical or endovascular treatment of AVMs can produce traumatic or ischemic stimuli to the AVM lesions. Due to these characteristics, it is more difficult to manage AVMs than other types of vascular malformations.

Most AVM patients present with pulsatile vascular mass, bleeding, toe or finger ischemic pain due to arterial shunting, extremity deformity including limb length discrepancy, or even symptoms or signs of congestive heart failure.

For patients with AVMs affecting the limb presenting with severe pain or complications that cannot be corrected with current surgical or endovascular treatment, limb amputation may be considered as a practical solution. However, limb amputation may not completely remove the AVM lesions; furthermore, it carries a higher rate of recurrence. Unlike amputation for patients with peripheral artery occlusive disease (PAOD), it is usually difficult to determine an optimal level of amputation in AVM patients due to extensive and infiltrative involvement of subcutaneous tissue, muscle, or even long bone in the extremity.

In the past, extensive surgical removal of AVMS, such as hip disarticulation or hemipelvectomy[1] under cardiopulmonary bypass[2] or deep hypothermic circulatory arrest,[3,4] has been reported for the purpose of complete removal of the AVM lesions. In current practice, such extensive surgery is rarely performed. When surgical removal of AVMs is required, a strategy of preoperative endovascular embolization and later surgical removal of AVM is more often used instead of extensive surgery. When residual or recurrent AVMs developed after limb amputation, staged endovascular therapy can be performed.

In some patients with AVM, the affected limb may be nonfunctioning or deformed due to associated limb hypertrophy, limb length discrepancy (LLD), and/or joint contracture.

Table 23.1 shows type and distribution of the extracranial congenital vascular malformation (CVM) registered in a database at Samsung Medical Center (SMC) in Seoul, Korea, during the period from 1994 to 2018. Of 2,854 patients with extracranial CVMs, 596 (21%) patients were AVMs. Of 596 AVM patients, 333 (56%) patients had AVMs affecting the extremity: 184 (55%) lower extremity (LE) and 149 (45%) upper extremity (UE) AVMs (Table 23.1).

Among patients with extremity AVMs, limb, finger, or toe amputation was required in 6.6% (UE AVMs, 11%; LE AVMs, 3%). When major amputation is defined as LE amputation above the ankle or UE amputation at or above the wrist, major amputation was performed in 3.9% (UE, 5%; LE, 3%) of patients with extremity AVMs. The most common indications for major limb amputation were severe intractable foot or hand pain combined with frequent episodes of large amounts of external bleeding, a nonfunctioning limb with deformity, or multiple fractures (Table 23.2).

Table 23.1 Type and distribution of extracranial congenital vascular malformations (CVMs) (1994–2018 at SMC, Seoul, Korea)

CVM (N = 2,854 patients)		Number (%)
Type	Venous predominant malformation	1,579 (55)
	Arteriovenous malformation	596 (21)
	Lymphatic malformation	541 (19)
	Miscellaneous (e.g., capillary malformation, etc.)	239 (5)
Distribution	Head (extracranial) and neck	777 (27)
	Extremity	1,759 (62)
	Upper extremity	472 (27)
	Lower extremity	1,287 (73)
	Trunk	279 (10)
	Thorax	192 (69)
	Abdomen and pelvis	87 (3)
	Multifocal	39 (1)

When we reviewed the clinical features of the patients who underwent major limb amputation, all patients had severe foot or hand pain of ischemic nature with various other clinical symptoms or signs (Table 23.3).

In patients who are undergoing limb amputation, preoperative assessment of surgical risk is necessary including cardiac and renal risk assessment. Due to continuous arteriovenous shunting, reopening of an atrial septal defect (ASD) or ventricular septal defect (VSD), and right heart failure should be suspected in all AVM patients.

We should be prepared for unexpected hemodynamic changes during the amputation surgery due to large amounts of bleeding or stopping the large amount of arteriovenous shunting.

Table 23.2 Distribution of arteriovenous malformations (AVMs) and frequency of amputation due to AVMs (1994–2018; at SMC, Seoul, Korea)

AVM (N = 596 patients)	Number of patients (%)
Distribution of AVMs	
Head and neck	179 (30)
Extremity	333 (56)
Upper extremity	149 (45)
Lower extremity	184 (55)
Trunk	81 (13.5)
Multifocal	3 (0.5)
Amputation required among extremity AVMs	22/333 (6.6)
Upper extremity	16/149 (11)
Lower extremity	6/184 (3)
Major limb amputation[a]	13/333 (3.9)
Upper extremity	7/149 (5)
Lower extremity	6/184 (3)
Indications for Major Amputation	
Severe pain	13 (100)
Frequent external arterial bleeding	5 (38)
Uncorrectable limb deformity	6 (46)
Multiple bone fractures	1 (7.7)
Combined	13 (100)
Iatrogenic distal ischemia[b]	1 (7.7)

[a] Major limb amputation denotes lower limb amputation above ankle or upper limb amputation at or above wrist.
[b] Upper extremity major amputation performed in a 25-year-old female patient due to skin necrosis and repeated arterial bleeding from the skin lesion after three sessions of endovascular embolo-/sclerotherapy of the forearm AVMs with coils and a high concentration of ethanol.

Table 23.3 Clinical features of the patients who required major limb amputation and their outcomes (at SMC, Seoul, Korea)

	Upper extremity (n = 7)	Lower extremity (n = 6)
Clinical Features		
Severe pain	7 (100%)	6 (100%)
Multiple skin ulcers	5 (71%)	5 (83%)
Frequent arterial bleedings	3 (43%)	2 (33%)
Nonfunctioning hand or foot	2 (29%)	3 (50%)
Limb length discrepancy	3 (43%)	1 (17%)
Knee and hip joint contracture	NA	1 (17%)
Multiple bone fractures	1 (14%)	0
Outcomes of Amputations		
Residual AVM	0	1 (17%)
Walkable with prosthesis	NA	100%
Required redo embolic or sclerotherapy	0	1 (17%)

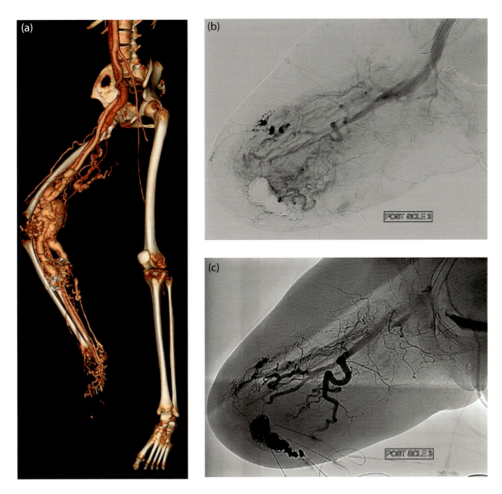

Figure 23.1 A 16-year-old female with right leg arteriovenous malformations (AVMs). **(a)** Preoperative computed tomography angiogram (three-dimensional reconstruction) reveals an AVM lesion affecting the right leg with right knee contracture. **(b)** Postoperative angiogram shows prior coil embolization and residual AVMs at the posterior thigh with a feeding artery (a branch of the deep femoral artery). **(c)** Repeated coil embolization and ethanol sclerotherapy was performed to treat the residual AVMs close to the amputation stump.

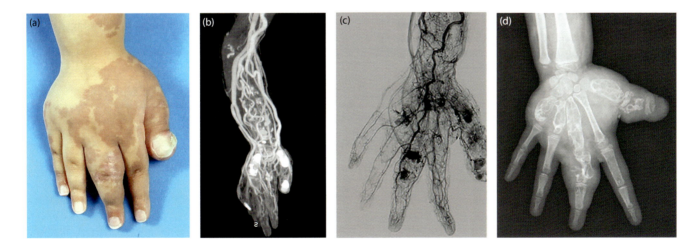

Figure 23.2 Arteriovenous malformations (AVMs) in the right hand and forearm. **(a)** Clinical findings of the right hand show hand and finger hypertrophy and capillary malformations ("port-wine stains") at the hand dorsum. **(b)** Computed tomography angiogram shows AVMs in the right forearm and hand. **(c)** Angiogram demonstrates that AVM involved multiple sites of carpal and metacarpal bones. **(d)** X-ray reveals fracture-dislocation of the first and third metacarpophalangeal joints and severe osteolytic changes of the metacarpal bones in the AVM-affected hand.

Figure 23.1 shows a three-dimensional formatted computed tomography (CT) angiogram in a 16-year-old girl with AVMs around the popliteal area, thigh, and calf. She presented to us with a severe painful ulcer at the right forefoot and the right knee contracture. After six sessions of endovascular coiling and ethanol sclerotherapy, we decided to perform an above-the-knee amputation due to intractable severe foot pain, nonhealing foot ulcer, and contracted, nonfunctioning right leg.

Figure 23.2 shows photogram and imaging studies of a girl having AVMs in the right hand and forearm. Initially, the patient presented to us with a brown skin spot at the right-hand dorsum and mild hypertrophy of the right hand. Clinical symptoms and signs of AVMs progressed over time. We performed 23 sessions of ethanol sclerotherapy to treat AVMs of the forearm and hand. At her age of 12 years, we decided to perform an amputation at the wrist level due to uncontrollable hand pain and nonfunctioning, and deformation of the hand due to multiple pathological fractures of carpal and metacarpal bones.

In summary, major limb amputation was uncommon (3.9%) in patients with extremity AVMs. The most common indication for the limb amputations was severe uncontrollable pain that was often combined with other complications of the AVMs such as frequent episodes of external bleeding and a nonfunctioning or deformed affected limb.

After limb amputation, postoperative surveillance is required to find residual or recurrent AVMs. We observed that an AVM lesion close to the amputation stump may be aggravated by wearing a prosthesis. It is recommended that the residual or recurrent AVM close to the limb amputation stump be treated with sclerotherapy rather than coil embolization because embolic material can give discomfort to the patients while walking with a prosthetic leg.

REFERENCES

1. Lee YO, Hong SW. Treatment of large arteriovenous malformation in right lower limb. *Korean J Thorac Cardiovasc Surg.* 2014;47:66–70.
2. Ismail MS, Sharaf I, Thambidorai CR et al. Cardiopulmonary bypass in surgery for complex-combined vascular malformation of the lower limb: Case report. *Pediatr Surg Int.* 2005;21:392–395.
3. McCready RA, Fehrenbacher JW, Divelbiss JL, Bryant A, Savader S. Surgical resection of a large recurrent pelvic arteriovenous malformation using deep hypothermic circulatory arrest. *J Vasc Surg.* 2004;39:1348–1350.
4. Schwentker EP, Bahnson HT. Total circulatory arrest for treatment of advanced arteriovenous fistulae. *Ann Surg.* 1972;175:70–74.

24

How much pharmacological therapy can be incorporated into arteriovenous malformation management?

JOCHEN KARL RÖSSLER AND IRIS BAUMGARTNER

Pharmacological therapy for arteriovenous malformations (AVMs) remains experimental. There have been quite a lot of efforts to identify a drug or molecules with selective activity for AVM. However, identification of an effective drug is still pending.

Historically, angiogenic inhibitors have been administered in single patients with AVMs, such as marimastat, doxycycline, or bevacizumab (Avastin).[1] This list can be enlarged adding vascular endothelial growth factor (VEGF) receptor tyrosine kinase inhibitors such as sorafenib and other molecules that stop formation of blood vessels such as thalidomide. Nevertheless, confirmation of these drugs by any clinical trial to be effective in AVM is still lacking, and they have not been included in any guideline or standard of care for AVM patients.

For treatment of AVMs of the gastrointestinal tract, the effect of octreotide (OCT), a synthetic analogue of somatostatin, has been studied. The mechanism of action of this drug is inhibition of angiogenesis. Some authors reported on regression of AVM volume and discontinuation of bleedings.[2,3]

Infantile hemangioma therapy entered a new era in 2008 with the discovery of propranolol as an effective drug for complicated cases,[4] and this approach has recently been applied for AVM. Single case reports on the positive effect of the vasoconstrictive and antiangiogenic effect can be found.[5] However, these data have to be confirmed in a larger patient cohort.

Rapamycin (Sirolimus) has been reported as effective in the treatment of lymphatic and venous malformations.[6] Later, the molecular mechanism became obvious when somatic mutations in PI3KCA were discovered in venous and lymphatic malformations.[7,8] In a retrospective study on 41 vascular anomalies, the overall response rate was 80.4% with rapamycin. However, four aggressive AVMs did not show any response.[9] An explanation for this failure could be the lack of these mutations in AVM.

Finally, the most promising discovery is the description of somatic mutations in *MAP2K1* in extracranial AVM.[10] These mutations lead to increased MEK1 activity. MEK1 inhibitors are available for several malignant tumors, and this could therefore be a potential drug for patients with AVM.

REFERENCES

1. Lee BB, Baumgartner I, Berlien HP et al. Consensus document of the International Union of Angiology (IUA)-2013. Current concept on the management of arterio-venous management. *Int Angiol.* 2013;32(1): 9–36.
2. Danesi R, Del Tacca M. The effects of the somatostatin analog octreotide on angiogenesis *in vitro*. *Metabolism*. 1996;45(8 Suppl 1):49–50.
3. Bon C, Aparicio T, Vincent M et al. Long-acting somatostatin analogues decrease blood transfusion requirements in patients with refractory gastrointestinal bleeding associated with angiodysplasia. *Aliment Pharmacol Ther.* 2012;36(6):587–593.
4. Leaute-Labreze C, Hoeger P, Mazereeuw-Hautier J et al. A randomized, controlled trial of oral propranolol in infantile hemangioma. *N Engl J Med.* 2015;372(8):735–746.
5. Lu J, Anvari R, Wang J et al. Propranolol as a potentially novel treatment of arteriovenous malformations. *JAAD Case Rep.* 2018;4(4):355–358.
6. Adams DM, Trenor CC 3rd, Hammill AM et al. Efficacy and safety of sirolimus in the treatment of complicated vascular anomalies. *Pediatrics.* 2016;137(2):e20153257.

7. Blesinger H, Kaulfuss S, Aung T et al. *PIK3CA* mutations are specifically localized to lymphatic endothelial cells of lymphatic malformations. *PLOS ONE.* 2018;13(7):e0200343.

8. Limaye N, Kangas J, Mendola A et al. Somatic activating *PIK3CA* mutations cause venous malformation. *Am J Hum Genet.* 2015;97(6):914–921.

9. Triana P, Dore M, Cerezo VN et al. Sirolimus in the treatment of vascular anomalies. *Eur J Pediatr Surg.* 2017;27(1):86–90.

10. Couto JA, Huang AY, Konczyk DJ et al. Somatic *MAP2K1* mutations are associated with extracranial arteriovenous malformation. *Am J Hum Genet.* 2017;100(3):546–554.

25

Secondary changes in arteriovenous malformations: Arteries, veins, tissues, bones, when do they have to be treated?

DIRK A. LOOSE

In the treatment of AVMs the main interest has to be the occlusion of the arterial feeders. This is a task that can be fulfilled by different techniques. The main option is the interventional catheter embolotherapy.[1] Even if the main feeders are controlled, however, during the existence of the AVM over years, different secondary damages of the involved tissues will arise. These have great importance concerning recurrences or complaints.[2] The secondary changes affect the following:

1. Arterial system
2. Venous system
3. Bones
4. Skin

Of course, each of the different manifestations of the damage has its special indication for treatment. An important point is that they have to be treated as early as possible but at least when they become symptomatic.

AVMs can result in arterial aneurysm that can be treated interventionally or by reconstructive vascular surgery.[2]

AVMs produce a high pressure in the venous system. This can lead to venous aneurysms (Figures 25.1 and 25.2) or to numerous venectasias (Figures 25.3 and 25.4), which can cause considerable congestion problems. Venous aneurysms can be treated by resection and reconstruction. The secondary venectasias are best treated by meticulous extirpation by surgery. Here a sclerotherapy is not indicated.

The bone system is influenced by AVMs by an increased length growth of a limb (see Chapter 41, Figure 41.5). Early treatment of the AVMs can normalize the length discrepancy so that a temporary epiphysiodesis can be avoided.

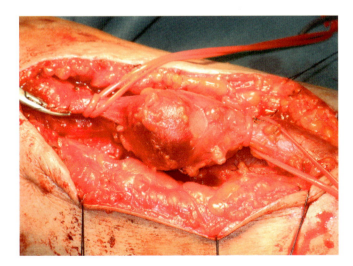

Figure 25.1 Venous aneurysm secondary to the elevated pressure in arteriovenous malformation.

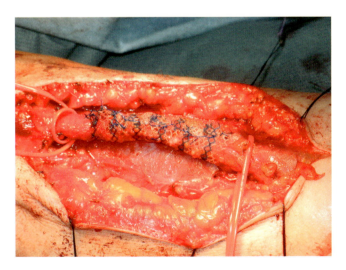

Figure 25.2 Postoperative findings after tangential resection of a venous aneurysm and reinforcement with a plastic mesh.

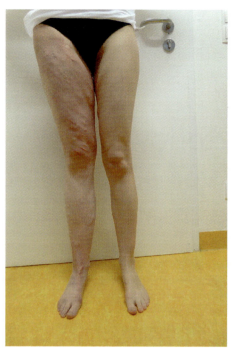
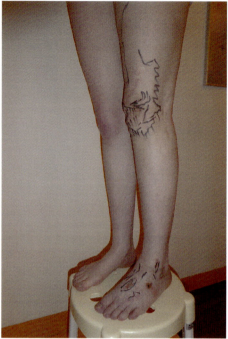

Figure 25.3 Clinical findings of two patients who presented with venectasias of the lower extremities secondary to the elevated pressure in the arteriovenous malformation.

Skin damage is caused by AVM ischemia in the area of the skin and subcutaneous tissue. The cause of ischemia, namely, the arteriovenous fistulas, has to be eliminated.[3] Subsequently, the skin defect can be healed with conservative measures (Figure 25.5).

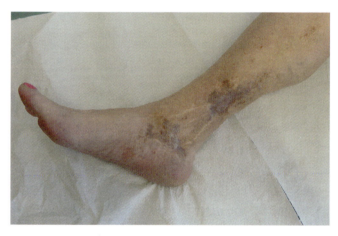

Figure 25.5 Clinical findings show healed ischemic ulcers, on the medial perimalleolar region of the right lower extremity, after embolization of arteriovenous malformation.

REFERENCES

1. Clemens RK, Meier TO, Pfammatter T, Giovanoli P, Amann-Vesti BR. Arteriovenöse Mißbildungen, Therapie ist selten kurativ, sondern zielt auf Symptom- und Grössenkontrolle. *Cardiovasc.* 2016;15(2):23–26.
2. Kleinschmidt F, Loose DA, Steinmeyer C, Müller E. Problems in the therapy of central ectasias and elongations in long-lasting arteriovenous fistulas. *Chirurg.* 1976;47(9):496–501.
3. Kotteck H, Clemens RK, Valentin H, Meier TO, Amann-Vesti BR. Importance of non-vascular tissue on vascular malformations. *VASA.* 2015;44(Suppl 89):48.a

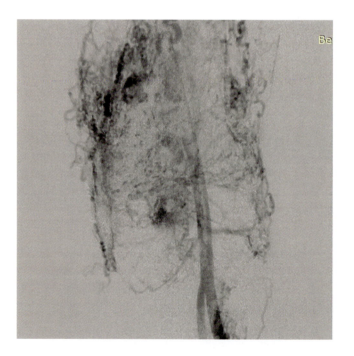

Figure 25.4 Venous phase of arteriography after multiple embolizations of arteriovenous malformation (AVM) demonstrates extensive venectasias secondary to elevated pressure in the AVM.

Venous Malformations

Definition and Classification

26

Capillary and cavernous hemangioma and venous malformations

BYUNG-BOONG LEE AND JAMES LAREDO

The term *cavernous/capillary* hemangioma was freely used throughout the last century for "venous malformation" (VM) *by mistake* and still causes substantial confusion together with many of the name-based eponyms of the old classification for the congenital vascular malformations (CVMs).[1-4]

The term *cavernous/capillary* hemangioma is the most frequently abused/misused terminology for the VM, especially during the era of "angiodysplasia," by misunderstanding the nature of the VM, which is different from that of a genuine "hemangioma."[5-8]

A genuine "hemangioma" is not a vascular malformation but represents a vascular tumor, although vascular malformation and hemangioma are classified together to one group of vascular anomalies. The vascular tumor is represented by "infantile/neonatal" hemangioma together with "congenital" hemangioma. They are fundamentally different from vascular malformation, not only in their anatomical, histological, and pathophysiological findings, but also in their clinical courses.[9-12]

A hemangioma originates from endothelial cells like all other vascular tumors. It is usually not present at birth but generally appears during the early neonatal period as a rapidly growing tumor in 3–5:1 of the female-to-male ratio. It progresses with a distinctive growth cycle characterized by early rapid growth through the proliferation phase, soon followed by slow regression through the involutional phase. In other words, hemangiomas undergo "self-limited" growth as newly developed lesions in the postnatal period, with subsequent involution in the majority before reaching the age of 5–10 years[11] (Figure 26.1).

The VM is generally noticeable at birth in an equal gender distribution as an inborn error so that it always presents at birth (even though initially it may not be apparent) like other CVMs; therefore, it never goes away like a hemangioma but continues to grow commensurably at a rate that is proportional to the growth rate of the body, as the outcome of a birth defect involved with the venous system during embryogenesis (vasculogenesis/angiogenesis)[13-16] (Figure 26.2).

When the defective development occurs through the "early" stage of embryogenesis, these embryonic tissue remnants possess a unique mesenteric characteristic: they have "self-perpetuating" growth throughout the rest of the life cycle. Like all other "extra-truncular" types of CVM, this extra-truncular VM lesion also proliferates when challenged by various growth stimuli, both internally (e.g., female hormones, menarche, pregnancy) and externally (e.g., trauma, injury, surgery, etc.).[17-20]

Hence, the (extra-truncular) VM lesion will never involute/regress but will remain throughout life. It will persist as an amorphous vascular structure/tuft so that it was previously called an "angioma." It was later properly renamed with a new embryological term, *extra-truncular*, by the Hamburg classification[13-16] to define its unique embryological/mesenchymal cell characteristics with high risks for growth/progress as well as "recurrence" as the major clinical issue.

Therefore, the use of the term *hemangioma* should be limited to the vascular tumor represented by a genuine "hemangioma." The erroneously used term of *capillary* or *cavernous* hemangioma for the VMs should be terminated to avoid confusion between (a genuine) hemangioma and vascular malformation and to prevent an incorrect diagnosis.[6,7]

The terms *hemangioma*, which remains the most abused term among various names for the VM and has become a constant source of confusion, and *cavernous/capillary* hemangioma should be discarded once and for all.

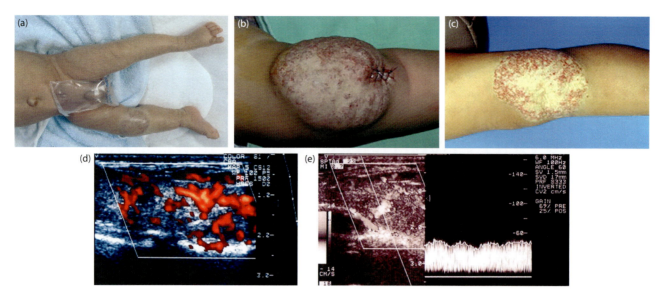

Figure 26.1 Infantile hemangioma—Clinical course. Hemangioma appears abruptly in the early neonatal period as a rapid growing *de novo* tumor as shown in **(a)**. It takes a distinctive growth cycle starting with a proliferation phase of early rapid growth as shown in **(b)**. But it soon transitions into an involutional phase to take slow regression as shown in **(c)** and in most cases, it disappears before a patient reaches the age of 5 years. The nature of hemangioma can be further confirmed by unique ultrasonographic findings as shown in **(d)** and **(e)**.

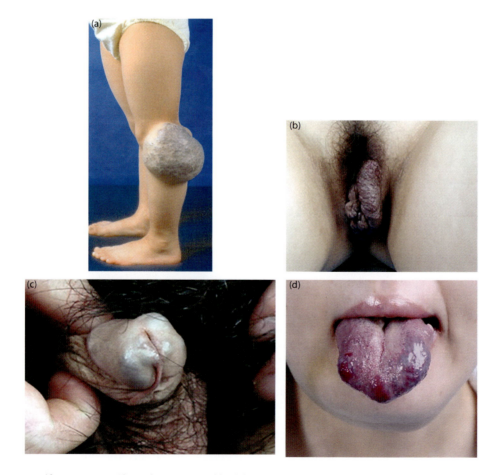

Figure 26.2 Venous malformation—Clinical course. Unlike hemangiomas, venous malformation (VM) can be apparent at birth as an "inborn" vascular defect affecting the venous system throughout the body as shown in **(a)** through **(d)**. As the outcome of a birth defect developed from the "early" stage of the embryogenesis, VMs do not spontaneously regress, instead they continue to grow at a rate that is proportional to the growth rate of the body throughout the life, like all other congenital VMs belonging to the "extra-truncular" type carrying mesenchymal cell characteristics.

REFERENCES

1. Lee BB, Baumgartner I, Berlien P et al. Diagnosis and treatment of venous malformations consensus document of the International Union of Phlebology (IUP): Updated 2013. *Int Angiol.* 2015;34(2):97–149.
2. Lee BB, Antignani PL, Baraldini V et al. ISVI-IUA consensus document—Diagnostic guidelines on vascular anomalies: Vascular malformations and hemangiomas. *Int Angiol.* 2015;34(4):333–374.
3. Lee BB. New classification of congenital vascular malformations (CVMs). *Rev Vasc Med.* 2015;3(3):1–5.
4. Lee BB, Laredo J. Classification of congenital vascular malformations: The last challenge for congenital vascular malformations. *Phlebology.* 2012;27(6):267–269.
5. Lee BB, Bergan J, Gloviczki P et al. Diagnosis and treatment of venous malformations—Consensus document of the International Union of Phlebology (IUP)-2009. *Int Angiol.* 2009;28(6):434–451.
6. Lee BB, Laredo J. Hemangioma and venous/vascular malformation are different as an apple and orange! [Editorial]. *Acta Phlebol.* 2012;13:1–3.
7. Lee BB, Laredo J, Lee TS, Huh S, Neville R. Terminology and classification of congenital vascular malformations. *Phlebology.* 2007;22(6):249–252.
8. Lee BB, Laredo J. Venous malformation: Treatment needs a bird's eye view. *Phlebology.* 2013;28:62–63.
9. Mulliken JB. Treatment of hemangiomas. In: Mulliken JB, Young AE, eds. *Vascular Birthmarks, Hemangiomas and Malformations.* Philadelphia, PA: WB Saunders; 1988:88–90.
10. Mulliken JB, Young AE, eds. *Vascular Birthmarks: Hemangiomas and Malformations.* Philadelphia, PA: WB Saunders; 1988.
11. Mulliken JB, Glowacki J. Hemangiomas and vascular malformations in infants and children: A classification based on endothelial characteristics. *Plast Reconstr Surg.* 1982;69:412–422.
12. Mulliken JB, Zetter BR, Folkman J. *In vivo* characteristics of endothelium from hemangiomas and vascular malformations. *Surgery.* 1982;92:348–353.
13. Belov S. Classification, terminology, and nosology of congenital vascular defects. In: Belov S, Loose DA, Weber J, eds. *Vascular Malformations.* Reinbek, Germany: Einhorn-Presse; 1989:25–30.
14. Belov St. Classification of congenital vascular defects. *Int Angiol.* 1990;9:141–146.
15. Rutherford RB. Editorial introduction. *Sem Vasc Surg.* 1993;6:197–198.
16. Belov St. Anatomopathological classification of congenital vascular defects. *Sem Vasc Surg.* 1993;6:219–224.
17. Bastide G, Lefebvre D. Anatomy and organogenesis and vascular malformations. In: Belov St, Loose DA, Weber J, eds. *Vascular Malformations.* Reinbek, Germany: Einhorn-Presse Verlag GmbH; 1989:20–22.
18. Woolard HH. The development of the principal arterial stems in the forelimb of the pig. *Contrib Embryol.* 1922;14:139–154.
19. Leu HJ. Zur Morphologie der arteriovenösen Anastomosen bei kongenitalen Angiodysplasien. *Morphol Med.* 1982;2:99–107.
20. Van Der Stricht J. Classification of vascular malformations. In: Belov St, Loose DA, Weber J, eds. *Vascular Malformations.* Reinbek, Germany: Einhorn-Presse Verlag GmbH; 1989:23.

27

Angiographic classification of venous malformations based on venous drainage status: What are the advantages?

KWANG BO PARK AND YOUNG SOO DO

Venous malformations (VMs) make up the largest population of the congenital vascular anomalies and are responsible for more than 50% of patient referrals to vascular anomaly centers.[1,2] VMs are composed of abnormal veins that show variable luminal diameter and wall thickness, and they usually lack venous valves.[1] Certain VMs consist of fine, small-diameter dysplastic veins, but a large proportion of VMs consist of markedly ectatic and serpentine venous channels. Dysplastic veins are connected with each other in an irregular and disorganized pattern, and VMs have normal venous connections with superficial or deep venous systems.

Although with full-shot arteriography for arteriovenous malformation (AVM) it is easy to get an overall image for the vascular malformation, a VM is hard to be imaged in a single-injection phlebography done through a transvenous approach. Also, the routine ascending or descending phlebography cannot show the whole VM in a single image because the venous flow is exiting the VM frequently. Therefore, direct puncture phlebography is useful to understand the dysplastic venous connection of the VM in detail, but even with direct puncture phlebography, the whole VM cannot be filled with contrast media because the venous drainage of the VM component that is apart from the needle insertion point passes through the different venous connections. Furthermore, direct puncture venography is an invasive procedure so that the exact phlebographic classification can be obtained with simultaneous sclerotherapy in many cases. Direct puncture phlebographic findings in VM are very complex in most patients; however, careful analysis of direct puncture phlebography provides detailed information for the patterns of normal venous connection and the appearances of dysplastic vein. Phlebographic evaluation sometimes requires manual compression or dispersion of

contrast media to the rest of the nonopacified VM component and nonopacified normal venous connection. Unless adequate phlebographic evaluation is done, VM cannot be characterized thoroughly. Former biological and clinical classification systems like the Hamburg classification or the International Society for the Study of Vascular Anomalies (ISSVA) classification did not reflect venous anatomical and hemodynamic factors.[3]

Phlebographic classification for the VM has few data. In 1991, Dubois et al. suggested classification for the VM according to the type of venous drainage, as type I was an excluded, well-circumscribed VM without visible draining veins; type II was venous lakes drained into a normal venous system; and type III was VM having ectatic abnormal draining veins.[4] In 2001, Dubois et al. described direct phlebographic findings in three simplified categories: cavitary, spongy, and dysmorphic veins.[5] However, this simple description is insufficient for stratifying the complex malformed venous structures in torso and extremity VMs. In 2003, Puig proposed a modified phlebographic classification system.[6] Puig also considered the pattern of venous drainage and normal venous connection as a clue to stratify four different types of VMs. Figure 27.1 shows the typical phlebographic appearance of four types of VMs. Type I VM was defined as an isolated malformation without peripheral venous drainage (Figure 27.1a). Type II was a VM that drains into normal veins (Figure 27.1b). Type III was a VM that drains into dysplastic veins (Figure 27.1c). Type IV was a VM that represents a venous dysplasia (Figure 27.1d). Incidences of each type of VMs were reported as 30% for type I, 37% for type II, 21% for type III, and 12% for type IV.[6] However, these incidences can vary from center to center because the data were derived from a small population (43 patients) phlebographic study. The

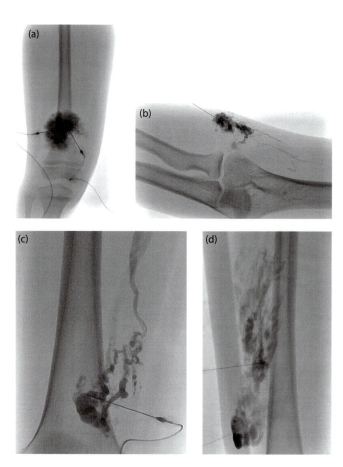

Figure 27.1 Phlebographic classification of venous malformations (VMs). **(a)** Type I isolated VM without peripheral venous drainage. **(b)** Type II VM in the right elbow that drains into normal superficial veins (arrows). **(c)** Type III VM that drains into dysplastic veins (arrows). **(d)** Type IV VM with diffuse venous dysplasia. Complex, irregular, and ectatic veins are extensively affecting the left thigh.

importance of the Puig classification was that it emphasized venous anatomical factors including normal venous communication with dysplastic veins. Understanding the vascular anatomy of VM and the hemodynamic connection between dysplastic veins and the normal venous channel is helpful to establish the treatment scheme. The Puig classification (reference) is well correlated with percutaneous sclerotherapy results. Types I and II show good therapeutic response to sclerotherapy because the sclerosing agent can be confined within the VM for a sufficient time, and sclerosant washout into the normal venous system can be minimized. Type I and II VMs showed higher cure rates with lower numbers of treatment sessions.[4] However, sclerosing agent is hard to stay enough in type III and IV VMs that lead to less therapeutic response. Furthermore, type III and IV VMs have risks for embolic material spillage into the normal venous system that gives rise to systemic complications. Therefore, the rate of exclusion from sclerotherapy is higher (up to half of patients) in type III and IV VMs.[6] This phlebographic classification system can be applied to simple VMs on ISSVA classification 2014,[3,7] not for the combined types. Combined VMs are often more complex in phlebographic findings, and some of the lesions are difficult to get direct puncture venography because the dysplastic veins are too small. Current phlebographic classification lacks consideration of lesion extent, location, and multiplicity. In a simple manner, phlebographically localized VMs are easy to treat, and the therapeutic response is better because the lesion extent is restricted, and the sclerosing effect can be maximized. However, diffuse VMs are less likely to show good therapeutic response because the lesion extent is too broad. Diffuse VMs require too many treatment sessions to achieve satisfactory results or are even impossible to treat with either sclerotherapy or surgery. The number of treatment sessions and the invasiveness of treatment are also related to the quality of life of the individual patient. There is a limitation that the phlebographic classification considers only the dysplastic vein, but some VMs have a large proportion of solid or fibrous connective tissue stroma as a component of the lesion. The ratio of vascular component and solid component also affects the result of sclerotherapy.[8] It is difficult to get direct puncture phlebography with certain types of VM because of the abundant stroma with relative paucity of the dysplastic venous channel. Therefore, further research, discussion, and agreement would be required to make an improved, reliable, and outcome-related phlebographic classification system for VMs.

APPENDIX-ACKNOWLEDGMENTS

Reprinted by permission from Kim YW, Lee BB, Yakes WF, Do YS. 2017. *Congenital Vascular Malformations*. Springer Nature, Springer, Berlin: Germany.

REFERENCES

1. Legiehn GM, Heran MKS. Venous malformations: Classification, development, diagnosis, and interventional radiologic management. *Radiol Clin North Am.* 2008;46:545–597.
2. Vikkula M, Boon LM, Mulliken JB. Molecular basis of vascular anomalies. *Trends Cardiovasc Med.* 1998; 8:218–292.
3. Lee BB, Baumgartner I, Berlien P et al. Diagnosis and treatment of venous malformations consensus document of the International Union of Phlebology (IUP): Updated 2013. *Int Angiol.* 2013;32:1–53.
4. Dubois JM, Sebag GH, Prost YD, Teillac D, Chretien B, Brunelle FO. Soft-tissue venous malformations in children: Percutaneous sclerotherapy with Ethibloc. *Radiology.* 1991;180:195–198.
5. Dubois JM, Soulez G, Oliva VL, Berthiaume MJ, Lapierre C, Therasse E. Soft-tissue venous malformations in adult patients: Imaging and therapeutic issues. *Radiographics.* 2001;21:1519–1531.

6. Puig S, Aref H, Chigot V, Bonin B, Brunelle F. Classification of venous malformations in children and implications for sclerotherapy. *Pediatr Radiol.* 2003; 33:99–103.

7. Wassef M, Blei F, Adams D et al. Vascular anomalies classification: Recommendations from the International Society for the Study of Vascular Anomalies. *Pediatrics.* 2015;136(1):e203–e214.

8. Park HS, Do YS, Park KB et al. Clinical outcome and predictors of treatment response in foam sodium tetradecyl sulfate sclerotherapy of venous malformations. *Eur Radiol.* 2016;26(5):1301–1310.

Diagnosis

28

Ultrasonographic assessment: Mandatory test to lead the assessment of the venous malformations?

PIER LUIGI ANTIGNANI

Venous malformation (VM) is the most common type of congenital vascular malformation (CVM).[1,2] VMs can cause significant morbidity, pain, and discomfort to patients as they can lead to serious local and systemic complications. Although present at birth, they are not always clinically evident until later in life and tend to grow in concert with the child and without spontaneous regression.[3]

In the last decade, there has been an increase in knowledge of different aspects of vascular anomalies, including histopathology, etiology, and their treatment. Due to its low incidence and heterogenous presentation of clinical and imaging findings, misdiagnosis is common; therefore, correct classification and terminology are paramount for proper clinical management.[4]

VMs are composed of ectatic venous channels found usually in the head, neck, limbs, and trunk and are thought to be sporadic in most cases, though familial inheritance patterns exist.[5]

Accurate diagnosis has been a limiting factor in VM management.[6,7] An increased emphasis has been placed on creating comprehensive classification systems for diagnostic and therapeutic purposes of this chronic condition.

Duplex scanning (DS) and magnetic resonance imaging (MRI) are key imaging methods used to characterize and diagnose VMs.[7,8]

Although imaging is not critical for the clinical diagnosis of cutaneous VMs, it is necessary to detect and evaluate deeper lesions. X-rays can image calcified phleboliths and the degree of dystrophic calcification in VMs, which can be useful in suggesting the presence of VMs, as it has been shown that over one-third of VMs have bony changes.[9]

CT does not have significant use in discerning VMs, unless there is intraosseous involvement, and it may be superior to MRI of bone.[10]

The imaging evaluation predominantly involves DS and MRI. Magnetic resonance angiography (MRA)/magnetic resonance venography (MRV) is useful in mapping the venous system and has supplanted the diagnostic role of conventional angiography in many cases.[7,11]

The duplex scanning test is a safe, reliable, noninvasive imaging technique and should be used as the first modality when investigating the presence of a vascular malformation, especially for superficial lesions or those in the extremities.[5] Other benefits are its ubiquity in clinical settings, low cost, and lack of ionizing radiation, which is an important aspect in young patients.[12,13] Conversely, depth and spatial resolution are low, resulting in a narrow field of vision. Limitations in discerning the involvement of nearby structures including nerves and bone are inherent with the use of DS.[14]

DS is widely used for initial screening and can help in planning for further imaging assessment.[7,16] DS should be able to evaluate vascularity if it includes grayscale, color Doppler, and spectral Doppler tracings.[7] VMs typically composed of small chambers on ultrasound (US) and phleboliths are detected as a mass with acoustic shadowing and are typical of venous malformations.

Another advantage of DS is that it can evaluate the response to treatment by detecting changes in size and flow characteristics.[7] However, the limited field of view for large lesions and operator-dependent examination are major limitations as a primary diagnostic modality.[7]

DS is used as the first-line modality to diagnose venous malformations, and they appear as slow flow with multiple chambers. Doppler sonography helps the physicians to distinguish high-flow from slow-flow VM and to differentiate lymphatic from venous malformations.[7,12,16]

DS is the first diagnostic test for all patients with VMs involving the limbs, to assess the deep and superficial veins; to identify any aberrant vein, obstruction, dilation, or valvular incompetence; and to define the feeding or draining veins of the VM.

Priority should be given to identification of the nature of an anomaly, and if a vascular malformation is detected, to ascertain the type of malformation. To this end, B-mode ultrasonography is particularly useful in being able to discern tumors/hemangiomas from vascular malformations.

B-mode ultrasonography reveals the mass, borders, and size of a lesion. Soft tissue solid mass indicates a tumor, while vascular channels with minimal soft tissue point to a VM. The presence of heterogenous and hypo- or anechoic vascular spaces typically represents compressible subcutaneous or intramuscular vascular spaces that are the hallmarks of VMs on B-mode or high-resolution grayscale US.[5,7,12] The range in appearance includes purely solid to multicystic, localized, and well defined to infiltrative, or cavitary (most common) to dysplastic lesions.[6,7]

B-mode ultrasonography shows the location and the depth of the lesion in the tissue (subcutaneous, intramuscular, intermuscular, periarticular, intra-articular, etc.), the compressibility of vascular channels, and the presence/absence of thrombus within the channels; the evidence of previous treatments (hyperechoic walls/segments), sclerothrombus, and surgical scarring should be identified and commented on.[6,7,12]

The presence of other vessels in the vicinity and their contribution to the lesion and normal anatomy should be identified and excluded. It is mandatory to also study the arterial vessels, and comparison with the contralateral side should be performed to make sure the vessel is part of the normal anatomy.

The B-mode is elicited to discover disorders of the main vessels like hypoplasia, aplasia, and diffuse dilation or aneurysmal dilatation.[6,7] In the presence of dilated vessels or the presence of cysts, the compression of these structures with the probe will reveal if these are thrombosed (incompressible tubes) or, in case of dilated spaces, there are lymph cysts (not compressible).

The B-mode evaluation allows visualization of the dynamic of involved muscles and the presence of major nervous trunks around the malformation. It is also possible to highlight the presence of accessory vessels, as marginal vein, persistent after birth.[6,7,15,16]

Extra-truncular malformations usually infiltrate neighboring tissues. They are prone to developing thrombosis. Thrombosed vessels should be described by the flow pattern, which may be spontaneous, present after augmentation, or absent.

The presence of soft tissues calcifications called *phlebolith* is typical of venous malformations and is the result of multiple episodes of thrombosis.

Doppler mode, conversely, is better used to discern hemodynamics, identifying high- or low-flow lesions.[7] Flow has been demonstrated in the majority of lesions, with monophasic and biphasic flow.

Spectral, color, and power Doppler examinations should confirm the flow characteristics (low flow versus high flow);

assessment of flow direction under different postural and respiratory conditions should be included in the evaluation.

In case of VMs involving the lower limbs, a separate venous incompetence study needs to be done to map the incompetent pathways. This is especially relevant when investigating complex malformations such as Klippel–Trenaunay syndrome.[6,7]

Tubular, tortuous, anechoic formations are sometimes observed in the surrounding subcutaneous fat, muscles, tendons, and other tissues. The presence of acoustically shadowing phleboliths postapplication of compression is a strong diagnostic clue for venous lesions.[6,7] Valsalva or manual compression can be required at times to induce visible flow.[7]

Finally, comments should be made regarding whether the lesion is unilateral or bilateral and if the underlying tissue shows hypertrophy or atrophy.

DS findings should be corroborated by MRI, and in the case of deep intramuscular lesions, MRI should be the first-choice imaging modality to ensure that the lesion is accurately localized.[10,11]

In conclusion, a dedicated vascular laboratory with expertise in the diagnosis of vascular anomalies should be performing these studies. Sonographers should be trained specifically in this field and should appreciate the complexity and the range of conditions they may encounter. This training allows for increased accuracy in the testing and a better-quality laboratory. The limits of the investigation are related to a limited spatial resolution and a limited investigation field. The temporal resolution is very high and allows real-time examinations and precise hemodynamic evaluation.

It is important to highlight that the procedure is operator dependent, and the results of the investigation are related not only to the technical skills of the operator but more to the operator's knowledge of the pathology. There is some agreement for the necessity to standardize the examination and to perform it according to different depths.[7]

The first step in the diagnosis of a vascular malformation is to recognize its presence. The differential diagnosis is represented by hemangiomas and malignant tumors.

The second step is to characterize the malformation according to the hemodynamic parameters (slow flow/high flow) and the vessels involved. It is mandatory to define the malformation according to the embryological development into truncular or extra-truncular malformations. In truncular malformation, hemodynamic impairment is predominant; in extra-truncular malformations, organ involvement is predominant.

The third step is the guide for therapy (percutaneous, endovascular, surgical). Hemodynamic evaluation of all the vessels of the anatomical area involved by the malformation is crucial to plan a therapeutic intervention. Finally, the DS allows for confirmation of the results of treatment and for follow-up of patients.

REFERENCES

1. Richter GT, Friedman AB. Hemangiomas and vascular malformations: Current theory and management. *Int J Pediatr.* 2012;2012:645678.
2. Cox JA, Bartlett E, Lee EI. Vascular malformations: A review. *Semin Plast Surg.* 2014;28:58–63.
3. Legiehn GM, Heran MK. Venous malformations: Classification, development, diagnosis, and interventional radiologic management. *Radiol Clin North Am.* 2008;46:545–597, vi.
4. Lee BB, Baumgartner I, Berlien HP et al. Consensus document of the International Union of Angiology (IUA)-2013. Current concept on the management of arterio-venous management. *Int Angiol.* 2013;32:9–36.
5. Eivazi B, Fasunla AJ, Hundt W et al. Low flow vascular malformations of the head and neck: A study on brightness mode, color coded duplex and spectral Doppler sonography. *Eur Arch Otorhinolaryngol.* 2011;268:1505–1511.
6. Lee BB, Baumgartner I, Berlien P et al. Diagnosis and treatment of venous malformations. Consensus document of the International Union of Phlebology (IUP): Updated 2013. *Int Angiol.* 2015;34:97–149.
7. Lee BB, Antignani PL, Baraldini V et al. ISVI-IUA consensus document diagnostic guidelines of vascular anomalies: Vascular malformations and hemangiomas. *Int Angiol.* 2015;34(4):333–374.
8. Samadi K, Salazar GM. Role of imaging in the diagnosis of vascular malformations (VM). *Cardiovasc Diagn Ther.* 2019;9(Suppl 1):S143–S151.
9. Dubois J, Kulungowski AM. Vascular anomalies: What a radiologist needs to know. *Pediatr Radiol.* 2010;40:895–905.
10. Flors L, Leiva-Salinas C, Maged IM et al. MR imaging of soft-tissue vascular malformations: Diagnosis, classification, and therapy follow up. *RadioGraphics.* 2011;31:1321–1340.
11. Lidsky ME, Spritzer CE, Shortell CK. The role of dynamic contrast-enhanced magnetic resonance imaging in the diagnosis and management of patients with vascular malformations. *J Vasc Surg.* 2012;56:757–764.e1.
12. McCafferty I. Management of low-flow vascular malformations: Clinical presentation, classification, patient selection, imaging and treatment. *Cardiovasc Intervent Radiol.* 2015;38:1082–1104.
13. Lee BB. Venous malformation and haemangioma: Differential diagnosis, diagnosis, natural history and consequences. *Phlebology.* 2013;28:176–187.
14. Mendonca DA, McCafferty I, Nishikawa H et al. Venous malformations of the limbs: The Birmingham experience, comparisons and classification in children. *J Plast Reconstr Aesthet Surg.* 2010;63:383–389.
15. Hassanein AH, Mulliken J, Fishman S et al. Venous malformations: Risk of progression during childhood and adolescence. *Ann Plast Surg.* 2012;68:198–201.
16. Behravesh S, Yakes W, Gupta N et al. Venous malformations: Clinical diagnosis and treatment. *Cardiovasc Diagn Ther.* 2016;6(6):557–569.

29

Conventional and dynamic contrast enhanced magnetic resonance imaging (dceMRI) and/or magnetic resonance venography: Diagnostic modalities with different objectives? Can they replace phlebography?

JOVAN N. MARKOVIC AND CYNTHIA K. SHORTELL

One of the most important steps in the diagnostic evaluation of venous malformations (VMs) is to exclude the arterial component with a high degree of accuracy. Failure to identify the presence of arterial flow can lead to serious adverse events and a catastrophic outcome of the treatment. To this end, multiple diagnostic modalities are used to evaluate VMs: ultrasonography (US), computed tomography (CT) scans, phlebography, and magnetic resonance imaging (MRI) were utilized either alone or combined, to identify the lesion and its hemodynamic characteristics, as well as its morphology and relationship to surrounding anatomic structures.[1,2]

Ultrasonography is widely available, relatively inexpensive when compared to the previously mentioned diagnostic modalities, and is useful to confirm the initial diagnosis based on clinical presentation. US is fast, easy, and demonstrates the flow velocity and vascularization. However, its major limitation is that it is inadequate to determine the true extent of the lesion and to precisely delineate surrounding anatomical structures. Therefore, US is frequently followed by another diagnostic modality that can provide the details that are inaccessible by US. CT (and contrast-enhanced CT scans) can identify the location of the malformation, osteo-involvement, vessel ectasia, and aneurysm formation. However the true extent of the VM into soft tissue is often underestimated as only contrast-enhanced vessels opacity. Phlebography clearly demonstrates hemodynamic characteristics of a lesion, and it has been used to distinguish low-flow from high-flow lesions with a high degree of accuracy. Its major limitation is that it does not provide information about the extent of the malformation with regard to the surrounding tissue involvement and the relationship to normal anatomy, all of which are very important for definitive treatment selection and preoperative planning in VMs where treatment is indicated.

Specific to MRI, the parenchymal components of VMs appear bright on T2-weighted images, and when T1 and T2 (or short T1 inversion recovery [STIR]) images are acquired, the extent of tissue involvement is shown.[3] VMs characteristically have an increased intraluminal signal on T2-weighted images. There is likely an intraluminal signal on the T1-weighted images as well. VMs enhance with contrast and typically do not contain flow voids.[4] A low signal in such malformations is concerning for thrombosis, although a very focal area of the abnormal signal could also be derived from a phlebolith. It is very important to mention that arterial flow characteristically contains flow voids on T1- and T2-weighted sequences.[5] These characteristics are used to distinguish them from VMs. Other MRI radiographic characteristics indicative of arterial components are dilated feeding arteries and draining veins with a paucity of venous lakes. In addition to providing information used to exclude the arterial component, MRI delineates the extent of the malformation throughout the involved tissues, and importantly, it shows the relation between the malformation and normal vascular and nonvascular structures as well as providing good soft tissue definition. However, there are certain factors that may affect MRI findings that are important to mention. For example, a blood vessel that courses within the MRI imaging plane may give false-negative results by suggesting a VM despite arterial blood flow within the malformation.[6] Therefore, in more complex cases, distinguishing between low-flow and high-flow malformation based on conventional MRI can be difficult, and was traditionally done by catheter-based angiography. To avoid this, magnetic resonance venography or dynamic contrast-enhanced MRI (dceMRI) can be used. The techniques used by dceMRI, TRICKS (time-resolved imaging of contrast kinetics), and TREAT (time-resolved echo-shared angiographic technique), are required to more accurately assess flow within the lesion even in the most complex cases.[7] The previously mentioned techniques have the advantage of being able to delineate dominant or multiple feeding vessels in malformations, which can potentially facilitate intervention. At our medical center, we employ the following technique: 1.5 T and 3 T scanners are used to initially acquire noncontrast multiplanar T1-weighted spin echo and T2-weighted fast spin echo or fast STIR images. Following this, gadolinium-based contrast (5–20 mL) is intravenously administered using a power injector. Next, dynamic sequencing images are obtained from the arterial to venous phases utilizing either TRICKS, TREAT, or time-resolved angiography with stochastic trajectories. We use temporal resolution ranging from 3 to 8 seconds. To complete the imaging acquisition, postcontrast T1-weighted spin echo images are acquired after the contrast run.

To evaluate the accuracy of dceMRI, Rijswijk et al. reviewed in a prospective study conventional MRI and dceMRI by blinding two independent observers as they reviewed conventional MRI and dceMRI imaging studies from 27 patients with clinically suspected arteriovenous malformations.[8] Selective and superselective angiography, with digital subtraction techniques, was performed in all 27 patients, and the results of venography were integrated with the angiographic findings. Data from this study showed an increase in the specificity of MRI from 24%–33% to 95% with the addition of dynamic contrast-enhanced sequences and sensitivity of 83%.[8]

More recently, at our institution we evaluated a large number of malformations in 122 patients (92 lesions [85.3%] were low flow).[6] All patients underwent dceMRI. Additional imaging studies performed selectively included diagnostic catheter-based arteriography, US and CT scan in 13 (10.7%), 17 (13.9%), and 8 (6.6%) cases, respectively.[6] Data from our study demonstrated that dceMRI accurately characterized lesion flow in 89.3% (109/122) of cases. In 10.7% (13/122) of the patients, hemodynamic characteristics were indeterminate based on dceMRI. These patients underwent diagnostic angiography. Overall, our data showed that dceMRI sensitivity and specificity for high-flow lesions were 78.6% and 85.2%, respectively. For low-flow lesions, dceMRI sensitivity and specificity were 85.2% and 78.6%, respectively.[6]

Traditionally, catheter-based phlebography has been used for assessing vascular malformations in complex cases. However, such procedures are not entirely benign and carry risk to the patient. Complications observed with endovascular procedures occur in 1.5%–9% of patients and include groin hematoma, pseudoaneurysm, arteriovenous fistula, acute arterial occlusion or thrombosis, embolic events, and infection.[9] Although some of these complications can be managed conservatively, approximately 11% of groin hematomas and 61% of pseudoaneurysms will require treatment.[9] Subjecting patients with VMs to these (even small) risks adds to the morbidity of the vascular lesions from which they are already suffering. Catheter-based phlebography is limited in its ability to delineate a lesion relative to its adjacent structures. This is a critical limitation, as vascular malformations can infiltrate muscle, circumscribe nerves, or infiltrate neighboring vital tissues. Since not all types of vascular malformation require catheter-based interventions for treatment, the ability to distinguish between high-flow and low-flow lesions noninvasively in order to avoid catheter-related morbidity for low-flow lesions is advantageous.

In summary, imaging modalities utilized in the management of VMs, including US, CT, and MRI, provide variable degrees of diagnostic accuracy and frequently insufficient information for preprocedural planning, leaving a significant number of patients who required evaluation with a catheter-based angiography.[10] The relatively recently introduced technique of dceMRI has been validated as being clinically applicable to definitively distinguish high-flow from low-flow lesions with high accuracy, leaving a relatively small number of inconclusive cases that require confirmatory angiogram. In addition to flow characteristics, dceMRI yields more information regarding the extent of the malformation, the soft tissue involvement, and the relationship to normal anatomy, all of which become important in treatment planning.[10] By using dceMRI, a significant number of patients can be spared the expense, risk, and inconvenience of a catheter-based diagnostic study, as well as delayed or erroneous diagnosis.

REFERENCES

1. Lee BB, Mattassi R, Loose D, Yakes W, Tasnadi G, Kim HH. Consensus on controversial issues in contemporary diagnosis and management of congenital vascular malformation—Seoul communication. *Int J Angiol.* 2004;13:182–192.
2. Rutherford RB. Congenital vascular malformations: Diagnostic evaluation. *Semin Vasc Surg.* 1993;6:225–232.
3. Konez O, Burrows PE. Magnetic resonance of vascular anomalies. *Magn Reson Imaging Clin N Am.* 2002;10:363–388. vii.
4. Breugem CC, Maas M, Reekers JA, van der Horst CM. Use of magnetic resonance imaging for the evaluation of vascular malformations of the lower extremity. *Plast Reconstr Surg.* 2001;108:870–877.
5. Lidsky ME, Markovic JN, Miller MJ Jr, Shortell CK. Analysis of the treatment of congenital vascular malformations using a multidisciplinary approach. *J Vasc Surg.* 2012;56:1355–1362.

6. Lidsky M, Spritzer C, Shortell C. The role of dynamic contrast-enhanced magnetic resonance imaging in the diagnosis and management of patients with vascular malformations. *J Vasc Surg.* 2012;56: 757–764.

7. Prince MR. Contrast-enhanced MR angiography: Theory and optimization. *Magn Reson Imaging Clin N Am.* 1998;6:257–267.

8. van Rijswijk CS, van der Linden E, van der Woude HJ, van Baalen JM, Bloem JL. Value of dynamic contrast-enhanced MR imaging in diagnosing and classifying peripheral vascular malformations. *Am J Roentgenol.* 2002;178:1181–1187.

9. Lumsden A. Complications of endovascular procedures. In: Rutherford R, ed. *Rutherford's Vascular Surgery.* 6th ed. Philadelphia, PA: Elsevier Saunders; 2005:809–820.

10. Burrows PE. Endovascular treatment of slow-flow vascular malformations. *Tech Vasc Interv Radiol.* 2013;16(1):12–21.

30

Computed tomography (CT) and CT venography: How are these diagnostic modalities different from magnetic resonance imaging (MRI) for evaluation of venous malformations?

JOVAN N. MARKOVIC AND CYNTHIA K. SHORTELL

With the relatively recent advancements in the management of venous malformations, it may be possible to avoid unnecessary invasive catheter-based procedures during the diagnostic evaluation and treatment for the majority of patients with venous malformations (VMs).[1] The introduction of magnetic resonance imaging (MRI) has led to significant advances in the noninvasive diagnosis of venous malformations.[2] The high temporospatial resolution of MRI allows for improved visualization of the extent of VM and its relationship with surrounding anatomical structures.[3–6] Malformations and soft tissue delineation are greatly enhanced when compared to computed tomography (CT). Nonionizing radiation exposure is also avoided, and three-dimensional reconstruction is superior to CT scans.

MRI and dynamic contrast-enhanced MRI (dceMRI) findings used to evaluate VMs are described in Chapter 29. Briefly, VMs are usually hypointense on T1-weighted images and markedly hyperintense on T2-weighted MRI images. VMs are best captured using short T1 inversion recovery (STIR) sequences and T2-W imaging with fat suppression. Images should be acquired in at least two orthogonal planes. On nonenhanced CT, VMs appear as hypoattenuating or heterogeneous lesions that predominately depend on the degree of fatty infiltration. Phleboliths are visible on CT scans as rounded to oval hyperdense masses. The most significant benefit of CT scan is the characterization of dystrophic calcifications within the lesion and involvement of adjacent bony structures. After contrast administration, gradual peripheral enhancement is noted.[7] Therefore, the benefit of CT in the evaluation of VMs is limited to better defining intraosseous involvement and may be superior to MR imaging of bone. However, the relationship of these vascular lesions to muscle groups, fascial planes, tendons, and neurovascular structures can be more accurately defined with MRI.

Van Rijswijk et al. showed that conventional MRI had 100% sensitivity and 24%–33% specificity in differentiating venous from nonvenous malformations in the study that included 27 patients with peripheral venous malformations.[8] Authors of this study also demonstrated that by adding dceMRI, specificity significantly increases. In this particular study, specificity increased to 95% by adding dceMRI.[8]

In a large series of patients, Lee et al. evaluated 294 MRI findings in 196 patients with clinically suspected VMs.[9] Data from this study showed sensitivity and positive predictive values of 98.9% and 98.9%, respectively. Respective rates for specificity and negative predictive value were equal, 90% and 90%. Authors of this study also demonstrated that MRI was an excellent imaging modality in the assessment of treatment outcomes.[9] The reduction in size of the malformation is noted on MRI as treated segments have an elevated heterogeneity, diminished STIR and T2 signal intensity, and decreased contrast enhancement. These characteristics allow for planning a future procedure for the untreated segments. Although superior to CT and CT venography, conventional MRI has its limitations as it does not provide clear differentiation between high-flow and low-flow lesions in complex cases. To this end, MRI specificity can be increased by adding dceMRI.[10] At our institution, we evaluated dceMRI in 122 patients ranging in age from 1 day to 70 years with congenital VMs. Data from our study showed that we were able to successfully distinguish between high-flow and low-flow

VMs using dceMRI alone in 83.8% of patients, minimizing the need for unnecessary invasive catheter-based procedures.[10] When dceMRI is not definitive in assessing hemodynamic status, arteriography can be performed not only to confirm the diagnosis but also to provide an opportunity to intervene. This diagnostic algorithm avoids unnecessary imaging and significantly reduces the need for catheter-based venography in most patients.

REFERENCES

1. Lidsky ME, Spritzer CE, Shortell CK. The role of dynamic contrast-enhanced magnetic resonance imaging in the diagnosis and management of patients with vascular malformations. *J Vasc Surg.* 2012;56(3):757–764.
2. Burrows PE, Laor T, Paltiel H, Robertson RL. Diagnostic imaging in the evaluation of vascular birthmarks. *Dermatol Clin.* 1998;16:455–488.
3. Legiehn GM, Heran MK. Venous malformations: classification, development, diagnosis, and interventional radiologic management. *Radiol Clin North Am.* 2008;46:545–597; vi.
4. Moukaddam H, Pollak J, Haims AH. MRI characteristics and classification of peripheral vascular malformations and tumors. *Skeletal Radiol.* 2009;38:535–547.
5. Lee BB. New approaches to the treatment of congenital vascular malformations (CVMs)—A single centre experience. *Eur J Vasc Endovasc Surg.* 2005; 30:184–197.
6. Lee BB, Baumgartner I, Berlien HP et al. Consensus document of the International Union of Angiology (IUA)-2013. Current concept on the management of arterio-venous management. *Int Angiol.* 2013;32:9–36.
7. Dubois J, Soulez G, Oliva VL, Berthiaume MJ, Lapierre C, Therasse E. Soft-tissue venous malformations in adult patients: Imaging and therapeutic issues. *RadioGraphics.* 2001;21(6):1519–1531.
8. van Rijswijk CS, van der Linden E, van der Woude HJ et al. Value of dynamic contrast-enhanced MR imaging in diagnosing and classifying peripheral vascular malformations. *Am J Roentgenol.* 2002;178:1181–1187.
9. Lee BB, Choe YH, Ahn JM et al. The new role of magnetic resonance imaging in the contemporary diagnosis of venous malformation: Can it replace angiography? *J Am Coll Surg.* 2004;198(4):549–558.
10. Lidsky ME, Markovic JN, Miller MJ Jr, Shortell CK. Analysis of the treatment of congenital vascular malformations using a multidisciplinary approach. *J Vasc Surg.* 2012;56:1355–1362.

31

Whole-body blood pool scintigraphy (WBBPS): Special role for management of venous malformations?

RAUL MATTASSI

Whole-body blood pool scintigraphy (WBBPS) is a nuclear medicine technique based on erythrocyte labeling with a radionuclide, most frequently Technetium-99 m (TC 99), which makes it possible to visualize the distribution of the labeled red cells in the body. The technique is commonly used for the functional study of organs—the heart, liver or kidney, and others, by focusing a γ-camera on the examined organ. A total-body study allows for the visualization of abnormal blood pooling in vascularized areas, a sign of a vascular malformation.[1,2]

The exam has been shown to be effective for recognizing the location and extension of extra-truncular venous malformations (VMs), as the tracer "accumulates" in pathological areas, providing a clear view of the extent of the dysplasia. Some studies demonstrate that the detection of VMs by this exam is over 96%[3] (Figures 31.1 and 31.2). The study can also be focused on specific areas to investigate (Figure 31.3). Truncular VMs can also be visualized, such as aplasia, hypoplasia, or aneurysm of the main veins. Three-dimensional images are also possible and can improve the accuracy of the diagnosis.

The study can be extended by a new scan on the following day, due to the remaining activity of the radiolabeled erythrocytes, in order to visualize lymphovenous anomalies that are not visible immediately because of the slow recirculation time and mixture among the two pathological districts (venous and lymphatic).[4]

Another unique value of WBBPS is that the negative findings of abnormal blood pool on WBBPS indirectly rule *out* the VM lesions and confirm the (extra-truncular) lymphatic malformation (LM) as an ultimate differential diagnosis, which is frequently overlooked even by T2-weighted magnetic resonance imaging (MRI) with contrast.[4,5]

The main liability/disadvantage of the procedure is, however, the low resolution of the images, as this technique is not

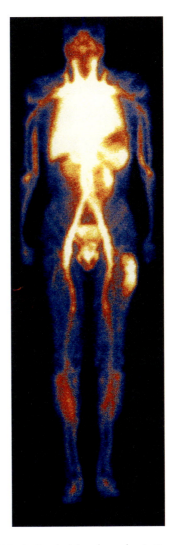

Figure 31.1 Whole-body blood pool scintigraphy demonstrates the area of venous malformation on the lateral side of the left thigh.

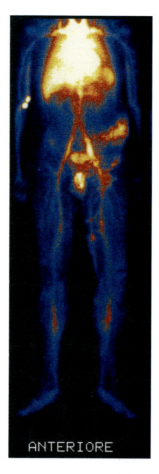

Figure 31.2 Whole-body blood pool scintigraphy demonstrates a venous malformation on the abdominal wall.

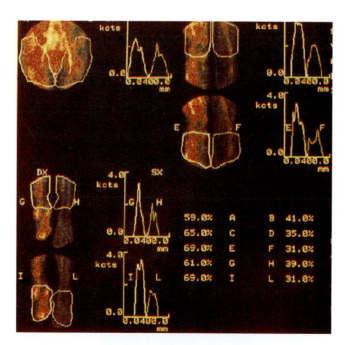

Figure 31.3 Whole-body blood pool scintigraphy in a case of diffuse venous malformation of the lower limb. Comparison right/left of radiotracer activity in specific areas of the lower limb. Notice the quantity curves.

able to detect and appraise small VM lesions. Radiation exposure of the patient is low, as the half-life of TC 99 is only 6 hours.

Nevertheless, WBBPS has been conveniently used for very efficient postoperative as well as post-embolosclerotherapy assessment of the treatment results; it can visualize the extent of the vascular occlusion of an extra-truncular VM after percutaneous alcohol sclerotherapy, for example[6] (Figures 31.4 through 31.6).

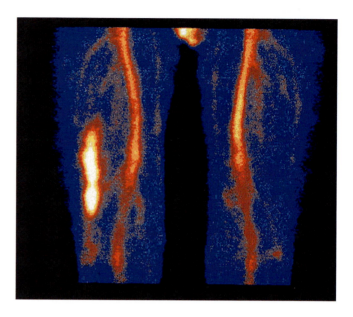

Figure 31.4 Whole-body blood pool scintigraphy of the lower limbs. Area of venous malformation on the lateral side of the right thigh.

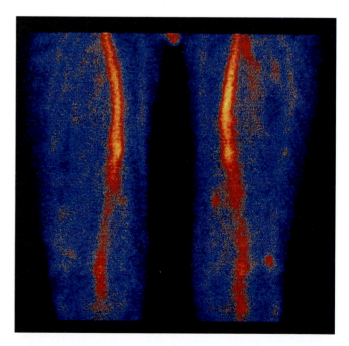

Figure 31.5 Whole-body blood pool scintigraphy after four alcohol sclerotherapy treatments. No sign of malformation.

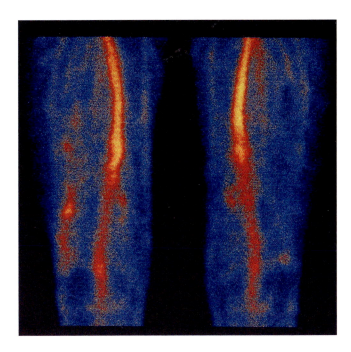

Figure 31.6 Follow-up after 1 year. Small area of recurrence.

WBBPS is a safe, less-invasive, and useful diagnostic and post-treatment follow-up tool for the management of VM.[1,2,4] However, this method has been used only rarely, mainly due to a limited knowledge of the procedure. Other diagnostic methods, like Duplex ultrasonography and computed tomography (CT)/magnetic resonance imaging (MRI) are preferred, are better known, and are much more frequently used in angiology. However, WBBPS remains an effective diagnostic tool, including the follow-up assessment of the natural untreated lesions, and should be considered as an effective alternative test to duplex scanning and MRI in VM management.

REFERENCES

1. Lee BB, Mattassi R, Kim BT et al. Contemporary diagnosis and management of venous and arteriovenous shunting malformation by whole body blood pool scintigraphy. *Int Angiol.* 2004;23(4):355–367.
2. Kim YH, Choi JY, Kim YW et al. Characterization of congenital vascular malformation in the extremities using whole body blood pool scintigraphy and lymphoscintigraphy. *Lymphology.* 2009;42(2):77–84.
3. Kim YH, Choi JY, Kim YW et al. Diagnosis and whole body screening using blood pool scintigraphy for evaluating congenital vascular malformations. *Ann Vasc Surg.* 2014;28:673–678.
4. Dentici R, Mattassi R. Nuclear medicine diagnostics. In: Mattassi R, Loose DA, Vaghi M, eds. *Hemangiomas and Vascular Malformations: An Atlas of Diagnosis and Treatment.* Rome, Italy: Springer Verlag; 2015:223–236.
5. Lee Y, Choi JY, Kim YH et al. Characterization of congenital lymphatic and blood vascular malformations in the head and neck using blood pool scintigraphy and SPECT. *Lymphology.* 2010;43(4):149–157.
6. Yun WS, Kim YW, Lee KB et al. Predictors of response to percutaneous ethanol sclerotherapy (PES) in patients with venous malformations: Analysis of patient self-assessment and imaging. *J Vasc Surg.* 2009;50(3):581–589, 589.e1.

Management: 1

32

Do all venous malformations require treatment?

KUROSH PARSI AND MINA KANG

INTRODUCTION

Venous malformations (VMs) are low-flow congenital vascular malformations involving the venous branch of the vascular system.[1] The vessels are dysplastic and may be very thin walled. The valves may be completely missing, small, and hypoplastic.

Truncular VMs involve mature vessels and are present as agenesis, hypoplasia, duplication, or aneurysms of named veins. Examples include the lateral marginal vein, duplicated femoral veins, and venous aneurysms. Extra-truncular VMs may present as lesions such as those seen in blue rubber bleb (BRB) syndrome or glomuvenous malformations (GVMs) (Figure 32.1). They may also present as diffuse and infiltrative venous spaces involving or completely replacing other tissues (Figure 32.2).

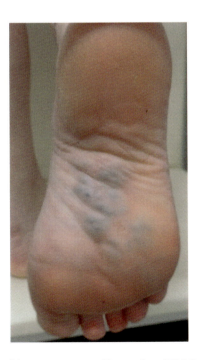

Figure 32.1 Glomuvenous malformation (GVM) on the sole of the right foot.

Typical sites of involvement are skin, subcutaneous layer, muscle, bone, and organs. Some patients present with a combination of truncular and extra-truncular anomalies (Figure 32.3).

VMs can be found in isolation or combined with other vascular malformations (capillary, lymphatic, and/or arteriovenous) and soft tissue or bony anomalies. A common syndromic presentation is Klippel–Trenaunay syndrome (KTS). These patients present with an extensive and diffuse VM involving most frequently one limb, in addition to soft tissue and bony hypertrophy. Extensive lymphatic and capillary malformations may coexist.

INVESTIGATIONS

Key diagnostic modalities used to assess VMs are discussed in the following sections.[2]

Duplex ultrasound

All patients with VMs, truncular as well as extra-truncular, should undergo a comprehensive duplex ultrasound (DUS) assessment that would include the following:

- B-mode and Doppler flow assessment of VMs. This should include careful B-mode assessment of the morphology, architecture, and wall thickness. Calcified thrombi, phleboliths, would present as echogenic lesions with a strong shadow artifact.
- Assessment of deep and superficial vein patency, valvular incompetence and reflux, thrombosis, and/or aneurysmal vein segments. Special diagnostic consideration includes assessment for aplasia and hypoplasia of deep and superficial veins.

Magnetic resonance imaging

Magnetic resonance imaging (MRI) in combination with venography (MRV) should be performed in all patients

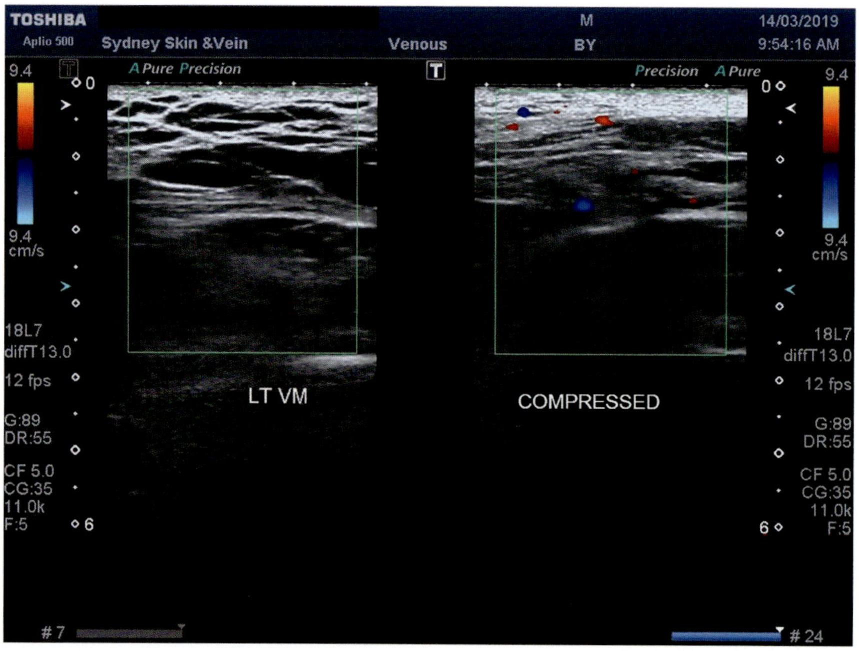

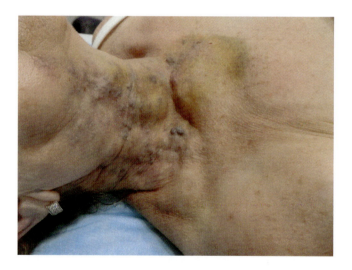

Figure 32.2 Extensive venous malformation (VM) infiltrating the entire depth of subcutaneous tissue as visualized on duplex ultrasound. Note the compressibility of the lesion in the subcutaneous layer due to the VM.

Figure 32.3 Combined truncular and extra-truncular venous malformation involving the jugular venous system.

with extensive VMs to determine the extent of the condition, involvement of other structures, and to guide intervention.

D-dimer, coagulation, and thrombophilia screening

Coagulation disorders are frequently found in patients with VM and especially in patients with KTS. These patients will often have elevated levels of D-dimer secondary to ongoing thrombus formation within the malformation and subsequent fibrinolysis. The major concern with this coagulopathy is the risk of silent pulmonary embolism (PE),[3] which can be potentially lethal. The process of thrombus formation and subsequent lysis within the VM is termed *localized intravascular coagulopathy* (LIC). At our institution, we perform thrombophilia screening for every patient who is at high risk for venous thromboembolism (VTE) or before the treatment of high-risk lesions, such as VMs located in the neck where a malformation drains into major neck veins or a VM that affects the eyelid, due to the risk of orbital vein or cavernous sinus thrombosis. For more details about coagulation disorders associated with VMs and KTS, please see Chapter 83.

Tissue biopsy

Tissue biopsy may be required to exclude other vascular anomalies such as vascular tumors or to differentiate similar conditions such as BRB and GVM.

TREATMENT

Not all VMs mandate therapy, as they may be asymptomatic. Indications for treatment include pain, swelling, recurrent thrombophlebitis, bleeding, and complications secondary to chronic venous hypertension such as ulceration. Lesions may interfere with function requiring palliative treatment. VMs can also result in significant cosmetic disfigurement necessitating treatment.

Treatment options range from conservative measures such as compression therapy for symptomatic management, interventional procedures using image-guided sclerotherapy, embolization, and endovenous laser ablation (EVLA). We prefer the use of EVLA and n-BCA glue for larger lesions and lesions with thicker walls and foam sclerosants for small-to-medium-sized veins and for diffuse lesions. Surgical excision is not a feasible option in most VMs due to the diffuse nature and high likelihood of recurrence. Most procedures can be safely performed using ultrasound guidance. Concurrent fluoroscopy may be required for deeper lesions.

Sirolimus (rapamycin) has emerged in recent years as a medical treatment option for complex vascular anomalies, in particular, hemangiomas refractory to or unfeasible for conventional or interventional therapy. Sirolimus is an inhibitor of mTOR, a serine/threonine kinase in the PI3K/AKT pathway. This pathway is responsible for the regulation of cellular motility, angiogenesis, as well as vascular cell growth.[4] It is worth emphasizing that since VMs are not proliferative tumors, treatment with sirolimus is palliative and goal oriented rather than curative, especially for extensive and diffuse lesions in terms of complete lesion eradication or disappearance (like in treatment of vascular tumors). Data from a relatively recent review by Seront et al. showed that rapamycin demonstrated significant ability to interrupt lesions' growth.[4] This study also showed (based on analysis of data from several other clinical trials) that rapamycin may be considered as a "gold standard" for treatment of recalcitrant VMs on a molecular level.[4] Data from studies that used MRI to evaluate efficacy of rapamycin treatment with regard to reduction of VM size, demonstrated substantial size reduction of the lesions treated with rapamycin.[5,6] The role of sirolimus in the management of VMs is in reducing vessel ectasia and secondary inflammation that can clinically result in pain, inflammation, and thrombophlebitis.[6] Recent clinical studies have demonstrated the efficacy of sirolimus in improving quality-of-life parameters such as severe pain, bleeds, oozing, and infection rates in patients with venous malformations.[4,5,7–9] Although VM treatment with sirolimus seems promising, further studies are needed for more accurate assessment of sirolimus safety and efficacy in VM management.

Ethanol sclerotherapy is associated with a higher risk of complications including cutaneous necrosis and systemic adverse effects. Ethanol sclerotherapy for VMs should be used only where no better options are suitable (e.g., recurrence). Most patients with dermal, subdermal, subcutaneous, and intramuscular VMs, however, can be managed with various therapeutic modalities: EVLA, foam sclerotherapy, and/or n-butyl cyanoacrylate (n-BCA) glue, either alone or in combination, depending on the extent of the lesions with reasonable outcomes (e.g., surgical excision of the localized lesion combined with preoperative n-BCA embolization).

A significant number of VMs require multiple and/or multimodal treatment sessions. In cases where multiple treatment sessions are required, the treatment should be properly planned with a minimum interval of 14–21 days apart. Longer time gaps between the treatment sessions may lead to recanalization and subsequent lack of treatment progress.

Routine intervention should only be performed in patients older than two and a half years of age to reduce the risk of paradoxical embolism via a patent foramen ovale (PFO).

Risks can be classified as procedure related, lesion related, and patient related. An example of a high-risk procedure is ethanol sclerotherapy requiring high volumes of ethanol. Neck VMs involving the jugular, subclavian, or superior vena cava pose a high risk of thrombosis and embolization. Patient-related contraindications include hypersensitivity to the sclerosing or embolic agents, acute VTE, ischemic neurological or myocardial events following previous intervention, acute systemic illness or infection, and chronic limb-threatening ischemia when treating leg lesions. Relative contraindications include pregnancy, postpartum, breastfeeding, high risk of VTE, and neurological adverse events.

CONCLUSION

In conclusion, most VMs can be safely treated using modern modalities of EVLA, foam sclerosants, and n-BCA under ultrasound guidance. Adequate training, familiarity with the treatment modalities, careful patient selection, and optimal image guidance are essential elements to achieve the best outcomes.

REFERENCES

1. Lee BB, Baumgartner I, Berlien P et al. Diagnosis and treatment of venous malformations. Consensus document of the International Union of Phlebology (IUP): Updated 2013. *Int Angiol.* 2015;34:97–149.
2. Lee BB, Antignani PL, Baraldini V et al. ISVI-IUA consensus document diagnostic guidelines of vascular anomalies: Vascular malformations and hemangiomas. *Int Angiol.* 2015;34:333–374.
3. Douma RA, Oduber CE, Gerdes VE et al. Chronic pulmonary embolism in Klippel–Trenaunay syndrome. *J Am Acad Dermatol.* 2012;66:71–77.
4. Seront ME, Van Damme MA, Boon ML et al. Rapamycin and treatment of venous malformations. *Curr Opin Hematol.* 2019;26(3):185–192.
5. Hammer J, Seront E, Duez S et al. Sirolimus is efficacious in treatment for extensive and/or complex slow-flow vascular malformations: A monocentric prospective phase II study. *Orphanet J Rare Dis.* 2018;13:191.
6. Boscolo E, Limaye N, Huang L et al. Rapamycin improves TIE2-mutated venous malformation in murine model and human subjects. *J Clin Invest.* 2015;125:3491–3504.
7. Adams DM, Trenor CC III, Hammill AM et al. Efficacy and safety of sirolimus in the treatment of complicated vascular anomalies. *Pediatrics.* 2016;137:e20153257.
8. Salloum R, Fox CE, Alvarez-Allende CR et al. Response of blue rubber bleb nevus syndrome to sirolimus treatment. *Pediatr Blood Cancer.* 2016;63:1911–1914.
9. Yesil S, Tanyildiz HG, Bozkurt C et al. Single-center experience with sirolimus therapy for vascular malformations. *Pediatr Hematol Oncol.* 2016;33:219–225.

33

How much is too much for venous malformation management?

PIER LUIGI ANTIGNANI

Low-flow lesions such as venous malformations (VMs) are some of the most common types of vascular malformations, with an overall prevalence of up to 1% in the general population.[1,2] The extremities encompass approximately 40% of the sites involved. Other locations include the head and neck (40% of cases) and the trunk (20%).[1,2]

Venous malformations are the result of errors in endothelial cell morphogenesis, causing disorganized angiogenesis and intimal smooth muscle proliferation. This results in the formation of dilated networks of venous lakes that are hemodynamically nonfunctional.[3] Depending on location, they may go unnoticed for years prior to presentation and range from asymptomatic superficial varicosities to large deforming craniofacial lesions.

They usually present at childhood or early adulthood with functional or cosmetic symptoms related to their size and location, including pain, reduced joint mobility, and skeletal deformity.[3–6] On examination, they are soft and compressible masses with blue discolorations of the skin. They characteristically decompress with elevation and local compression and enlarge on Valsalva maneuver. Palpable phleboliths and thrombi may also be present. They can cross tissue planes and invade adjacent tissues, including fat, muscle, tendon, and even bone. Joint swelling can be caused by venous engorgement, localized thrombosis/thrombophlebitis, mass effect, or local hemorrhage. Any connection to the deeper limb venous system can also precipitate the risk of deep vein thrombosis.[3–5]

Recurrent or chronic pain and swelling are often the presenting symptomatology.[7] Thrombus formation within a VM may initiate an inflammatory response along with swelling, which may cause pain and mass effect on adjacent structures such as nerves.

The slow-flow hemodynamics and abnormal venous architecture of VMs often trigger thrombosis. Recurrent induction of the coagulation cascade depletes coagulation factors and increases fibrinolysis. Continual thrombus turnover within VM may lead to localized intravascular coagulopathy (LIC), characterized by decreased plasma fibrinogen, factor V, factor VIII, factor XIII, and increased D-dimer.[9]

Localized intravascular coagulopathy increases the risk of intralesional thrombosis and peri-interventional risk for severe hemorrhage, as it may progress to disseminated intravascular coagulation.[9]

Clinically, an elevated D-dimer may be a useful marker of LIC if the patient is otherwise free of confounding comorbidities such as pulmonary embolism, malignancy, or inflammatory diseases.[8,9]

D-dimer elevations have been reported in 33%–42% of patients and are most common in large, multifocal VMs with palpable phleboliths or in patients with Klippel–Trenaunay syndrome.[9] In patients with large VMs, it is critical to obtain a coagulation profile, platelet count, fibrinogen, and D-dimer levels in the preprocedural setting.

The initial diagnosis may often be achieved on physical examination alone, with ultrasonography and magnetic resonance imaging (MRI) used to reveal the extent of interaction with surrounding structures as well as for procedural planning.

Occasionally, other investigations such as blood testing are required. Rarely, patients are referred for genetic counseling. VMs can sometimes be detected on antenatal scanning in a baby before birth.

Differentiation of VMs from lymphatic malformations may be challenging even in experienced hands, as the pathognomonic signs (e.g., noncompressible, cysts with thick septa, and liquid levels) are not always present or may be complicated by intracystic bleeding.[8]

Doppler sonography is useful to confirm the VM that exhibits slow monophasic flow.

In approximately 16% of cases, however, no flow is detectable, and this may be a sign of thrombosis, ongoing LIC, or flow that is simply too slow to detect.[7,8] Detection of a number of high-flow vessels may indicate an alternative diagnosis, such as an arteriovenous malformation or hemangioma.

MRI is the gold standard in the diagnosis of VMs. In large studies, MRI demonstrated 98.9% sensitivity and 90% specificity for the diagnosis of VMs.[10–14] MRI with spin-echo T1- and T2-weighted sequences is preferred over MR angiography, as the flow-sensitive images do not aid in the diagnosis or assessment of the VM.[13]

There are several treatment options to consider for patients with VMs. Some patients require no specific treatment as they may have no problems related to the VM.

Treatment modalities include systemic targeted drugs, open surgery, sclerotherapy, cryoablation, and laser photocoagulation.

Given the diversity in presentation, symptomatology, location, and extent of VMs, risks with therapy, and various treatment options, an individualized treatment plan should be devised using a multidisciplinary approach.[8]

The size and extent of the lesion determine the prescribed therapy, with small well-localized VMs often treated successfully in a single session with a single modality (e.g., resection, sclerotherapy). In contrast, large extensive VMs that involve surrounding structures are rarely curable and may require multiple treatment modalities. In any case, it is vital to discuss goals of care with the patient.

The primary goal in complex cases should be the alleviation of symptoms rather than eradication of the lesion. In some instances, however, cosmesis may have a dramatic impact on the patient's quality of life and should be considered when making treatment decisions.

Treatment is very much based on the impact of the lesions on the patients' quality of life, weighed against the risk of complications. In most cases, conservative treatment is recommended, but when a patient suffers clinical complications, treatment needs to be considered. Lee outlined absolute and relative indications for therapy.[8]

The goals of VM medical management are pain control, the prevention of venous ectasia and its associated localized intravascular coagulopathy, and treatment of secondary symptoms (e.g., anemia caused by bleeding).[13] When possible, compression therapy should be utilized to aid in the treatment of swelling and thrombophlebitis. Appropriate selection of a compression method may be difficult. Common types include bandages, garments, and pneumatic compression devices. The compression helps to reduce swelling and pain in many patients with extensive VMs. Compression garments can also improve blood clotting abnormalities that can be seen sometimes in VMs.[13]

In patients whose pain is associated with VM thrombosis, low-dose aspirin may provide relief though the efficacy is poorly described.[14] If pain is associated with localized intravascular coagulopathy, low-molecular-weight heparin may be administered for 2 weeks. However, if the pain persists, it should be reevaluated to rule out other possible causes; if the investigation continues to support the LIC as the most possible cause, we would continue treatment for 2 months and check the outcome of clinical as well as laboratory responses.[8–10] This may also prevent progression to disseminated intravascular coagulation (DIC) in severe cases.[13]

Recently, mTOR inhibitors have shown promising results in the management of vascular anomalies that respond poorly to other treatments. More recently, an increasing amount of data, including a single-center prospective phase II study, demonstrate that sirolimus is effective in treatment for extensive and/or complex low-flow vascular malformations.[15] Further studies are required to determine safety, efficacy, and optimal dosing.[8]

Image-guided percutaneous and interventional treatments of vascular malformations are now widely accepted as first-line therapy when combined with a multidisciplinary approach to treatment.

Many VMs can be treated by injection sclerotherapy alone or in combination with surgery. A few VMs may be suitable for surgical excision alone. As VMs can involve skin, mucous membranes (such as the lining of the inside of the mouth), tissues beneath the skin, muscles, joints, and bones, surgery may be difficult, and injection sclerotherapy may be a preferred option. As VMs can surround nerves and vital structures, surgery may not be an option.

The results of treatment vary depending on the type of vascular malformation being treated, but with the exception of capillary-based lesions, all types of vascular malformations can be considered.[16,17] To be effective, the treatments need to be repeated, usually at frequent intervals. Sometimes, surgical excision of the VM may be possible either without or following injection sclerotherapy. For patients with frequent, disabling pain who have significant abnormalities of blood clotting seen on blood testing, blood thinner medication given by injection may be prescribed.

Often surgical excision is part of a staged, multimodal treatment plan that is tailored to correct the specific cosmetic deformity, dysfunction, or pain.[8,17] There are instances where surgical excision alone is appropriate and preferred over sclerotherapy, such as when the VM is small (2–4 cm), accessible, and does not involve vital structures. In these cases, wide local excision results in cure rates near 100%.

Also, there are specific locations where partial or complete surgical excision is appropriate, including submandibular VMs or VMs of the temporalis muscle, as sclerotherapy in these locations may possibly lead to nerve injury.

Surgical excision of large, invasive VMs may be challenging even with multimodal therapy due to poorly defined tissue planes and proximity to important structures. In these cases, preoperative sclerotherapy may reduce intraoperative blood loss and improve visualization of vital structures. For example, preoperative sclerotherapy of facial VMs is associated with less operative time per lesion volume and less operative blood loss.[17] Alternately, lesions may be embolized with n-butyl cyanoacrylate glue prior to partial and/or complete resection of the VM.[8]

Long-term durability of this technique in large cohorts, however, remains poorly described.

Sclerotherapy is performed by percutaneously injecting a sclerosant directly into the lesion and is the treatment modality of choice for most VMs with the goal either being curative as a stand-alone procedure or preoperative with the intent to create a more well-defined, thrombosed mass that is easier to surgically excise.[8,18]

In general, the effectiveness of sclerotherapy is related to the potency of the agent used. There are many different sclerosants, including alcohols, detergents, and antitumor agents. Although pure ethanol is considered to be the most effective sclerosant with the lowest recurrence rates, complication rates are comparatively higher.[18]

Detergents are milder sclerosants with more favorable complication rates, though the rate of VM recanalization and recurrence is greater.

Antitumor agents also have utility, though there is a lack of large randomized control trials comparing these against well-studied agents.[14]

Sclerosants may also be used in combination with embolic agents or occlusion devices. Choice of sclerotherapy agent should be based on depth of the VM from the skin surface as well as the ability to adequately control the venous drainage to limit complications and inadvertent venous thrombosis. More potent sclerosants such as alcohol should be reserved for deeper VMs, as lesions near the skin surface are at risk for injury with extravasation.[8]

Standards for patient selection, technical considerations, and long-term efficacy are, however, still poorly described.

Cryoablation may be performed under ultrasound guidance with general anesthesia. Endovenous diode laser treatment of VMs has been reported in several small retrospective studies with promising results.[19]

Additionally, reasonable success has also been reported using percutaneous interstitial laser photocoagulation using Nd:YAG lasers. Laser therapy may benefit a select subset of patients; however, there is a lack of clinical trials comparing laser methods to sclerotherapy.[8]

In conclusion, given the diversity in presentation, symptomatology, location, and extent of VMs, an individualized treatment plan should be devised using a multidisciplinary approach. Treatment options available include medications, surgery, sclerotherapy, cryoablation, and laser photocoagulation.

REFERENCES

1. Clemens RK, Pfammatter T, Meier TO et al. Vascular malformations revisited. *VASA*. 2015;44:5–22.
2. Dompmartin A, Vikkula M, Boon LM. Venous malformation: Update on aetiopathogenesis, diagnosis and management. *Phlebology*. 2010;25(5):224–235.
3. Ernemann U, Kramer U, Miller S et al. Current concepts in the classification, diagnosis and treatment of vascular anomalies. *Eur J Radiol*. 2010;75:2–11.
4. Behravesh S, Yakes W, Gupta N et al. Venous malformations: Clinical diagnosis and treatment. *Cardiovasc Diagn Ther*. 2016;6:557–569.
5. Ali S, Mitchell SE. Outcomes of venous malformation sclerotherapy: A review of study methodology and long-term results. *Semin Intervent Radiol*. 2017;34(3):288–293.
6. Dasgupta R, Patel M. Venous malformations. *Semin Pediatr Surg*. 2014;23(1):24–30.
7. Foley LS, Ann M. Vascular anomalies in pediatrics. *Adv Pediatr*. 2015;62:227–255.
8. Lee BB, Antignani PL, Baraldini V et al. ISVI-IUA consensus document diagnostic guidelines of vascular anomalies: Vascular malformations and hemangiomas. *Int Angiol*. 2015;34(4):333–374.
9. Lee BB, Baumgartner I, Berlien P et al. Diagnosis and treatment of venous malformations. Consensus document of the International Union of Phlebology (IUP): Updated 2013. *Int Angiol*. 2015;34: 97–149.
10. Dompmartin A, Vikkula M, Boon LM. Venous malformation: Update on aetiopathogenesis, diagnosis and management. *Phlebology*. 2010;25(5):224–235.
11. Lowe LH, Marchant TC, Rivard DC, Scherbel AJ. Vascular malformations: Classification and terminology the radiologist needs to know. *Semin Roentgenol*. 2012;47:106–117.
12. Flors L, Leiva-Salinas C, Maged IM et al. MR imaging of soft-tissue vascular malformations: Diagnosis, classification, and therapy follow-up. *RadioGraphics*. 2011;31:1321–1340.
13. Madani H, Farrant J, Chhaya N et al. Peripheral limb vascular malformations: An update of appropriate imaging and treatment options of a challenging condition. *Br J Radiol*. 2015;88:20140406.
14. McCafferty IJ, Jones RG. Imaging and management of vascular malformations. *Clin Radiol*. 2011;66:1208–1218.
15. Hammer J, Seront E, Duez S et al. Sirolimus is efficacious in treatment for extensive and/or complex slow-flow vascular malformations: A monocentric prospective phase II study. *Orphanet J Rare Dis*. 2018;13(1):191.
16. Dabus G, Benenati JF. Interventional treatment options for vascular malformations. Approaches, techniques, and sclerosing and embolic agents that can be used in low- and high-flow vascular malformations. *Endovasc Today*. 2013;50–64.
17. Legiehn GM, Heran MK. A step-by-step practical approach to imaging diagnosis and interventional radiologic therapy in vascular malformations. *Semin Intervent Radiol*. 2010;27:209–231.
18. Qiu Y, Chen H, Lin X et al. Outcomes and complications of sclerotherapy for venous malformations. *Vasc Endovascular Surg*. 2013;65:34–39.
19. Cornelis FH, Labrèze C, Pinsolle V et al. Percutaneous image-guided cryoablation as second-line therapy of soft-tissue venous vascular malformations of extremities: A prospective study of safety and 6-month efficacy. *Cardiovasc Intervent Radiol*. 2017;8:354–359.

34

What is the first option for venous malformation management?

SARAH BERNHARD, ALEKSANDRA TULEJA, JOCHEN KARL RÖSSLER, AND IRIS BAUMGARTNER

As the natural history of congenital venous malformations (VMs) is generally benign, the first option for management should be conservative, as discussed in previous chapters. The conservative approach should comprise symptomatic therapy with compression garments for extensive VM of the extremities, anticoagulation in prophylactic dosage for patients with evidence of localized intravascular coagulation (LIC), and adequate pain management by specialized consultations in the absence of other therapeutic options. Anticoagulation should be initiated, especially during painful episodes caused by thrombosis due to LIC as well as before and after invasive procedures or in case of severe illness in patients with elevated D-dimers. In the case of chronic LIC with lowered fibrinogen levels, long-term treatment with prophylactic doses of anticoagulants is recommended. Anticoagulation can be initiated using the low-molecular-weight heparin (LMWH) at a dose of 100 anti-factor Xa units/kg/day[1] or by prescription of direct oral anticoagulants (rivaroxaban 10 mg, once daily[2,3]; dabigatran 75–110 mg, twice a day[4]) as documented in small case series.

If more aggressive treatment is indicated due to the following symptoms limiting the patient's quality of life, the exact treatment strategy should always be determined by an interdisciplinary board of vascular specialists, plastic surgeons, hematologists, oncologists, and other supporting disciplines depending on the region, extent of lesion, age of the patient, and feasibility of intervention[5]:

- Signs and symptoms of chronic venous insufficiency (CVI)
- Recurrent painful episodes due to localized thrombosis
- Bleeding
- Life-threatening location with involvement of vital organs or obstruction of their venous outflow
- Locations with high risk of complications such as hemarthrosis or thromboembolism in truncular VM
- Vascular bone syndrome or destructive angiodysplastic arthritis

- Thromboembolisms
- Consumptive localized intravascular coagulopathy
- Persistent lymphatic leakage in hemolymphatic malformation (VM and LM)

Treatment should always aim for complete occlusion or resection of VM, while taking into consideration risks and benefits of the different therapeutic options in terms of functional and cosmetic outcomes.

If conservative management fails, endovascular embolo-sclerotherapy is the first-line treatment of symptomatic extra-truncular VM. The role of surgery has been decreasing since Wayne Yakes et al. described the first case series of successful VM treatment with undiluted ethanol in 1984.[6] Although ethanol provides an effective method with long-lasting effect, it has threatening local and systemic side effects such as skin necrosis, pain and blistering, peripheral nerve injury, muscle contracture, deep vein thrombosis, pulmonary embolus, and cardiopulmonary collapse.[7-9] Complications with ethanol led to the introduction of other liquid sclerosants in the treatment of VM. In terms of functional outcome, endovascular sclerosing treatment strategies remain the most important therapeutic tool.[10] Standards for assessment of these lesions are under development.[11,12]

ENDOVASCULAR EMBOLO-SCLEROTHERAPY

Highly concentrated ethanol (60%–96%) injected directly into the VM provides local protein denaturation, which due to vascular wall destruction, leads to thrombosis, inflammation, and fibrosis. The destruction is in consequence irreversible, guaranteeing long-lasting effect.[13] Several monocentric studies analyzed treatment efficacy of ethanol embolo-sclerotherapy, starting from case series[14] to large retrospective group analysis[15,16] and prospective studies.[17]

Some authors describe use of an ethylcellulose (gelified ethanol) to prolong contact time with vasculature, permitting a reduction in the total amount of ethanol.[18,19]

Randomized controlled trials (RCTs) with appropriate blinding are missing. Only one prospective randomized trial directly compared ethanol with another sclerosant (bleomycin).[20] The use of ethanol was connected to better effectiveness (improvement of symptoms in 71/73 versus 41/63 cases) but at the same time a higher rate of complications (14/73 versus 5/63 concerning skin necrosis). Systematic reviews aiming to compare ethanol and other sclerosants remain inconclusive due to major differences in outcome definitions and variation in inclusion criteria.[21]

Summarizing the available literature from the last 10 years, ethanol is an effective substance to reduce the volume of VMs and patients' symptoms. All studies showed at least mild to good improvement of one of those two endpoints. A repetitive session of phlebography followed by direct percutaneous injection of ethanol under general anesthesia seem to be preferable. As previously mentioned, local complications include skin lesions (from blisters to necrosis), transient or persistent nerve injury, edema, and other signs of inflammation. Extravasation can result in muscle contraction or atrophy. Intentionally caused local thrombosis by injection of 96% ethanol can progress to the deep venous system and result in pulmonary embolism.[22] It is recommended not to exceed the maximal dose of 0.5–1 mL/kg body weight of ethanol. The risk of local and systemic complications is triggered not only by the amount of ethanol injected but also by localization and depth of the VM as well as drainage characteristics of the lesion in question (Figure 34.1).

Other sclerosing agents that have been developed and studied for the treatment of varicose veins are used for the treatment of VMs based on retrospective analysis and small case series.[23–25] Sclerosants include detergents, such as Ethibloc (an emulsion of zein, ethanol, oleum papaveris, propylene glycol, and a contrast medium) and Aethoxysklerol (lauromacrogol, ethanol 96% sodium hydrogen phosphate, and potassium hydrogen phosphate), microfoams such as polidocanol, sodium tetradecyl sulfate (STS), and chemotherapeutics such as bleomycin. As previously mentioned, the latter has been evaluated in a prospective randomized trial in comparison to undiluted ethanol.[20] One other prospective randomized trial compared the efficacy of ultrasound-guided foam sclerotherapy with 1% polidocanol to ultrasound-guided liquid sclerotherapy with 10% ethanolamine oleate in the treatment of symptomatic VMs.[26] A total of 89 patients were treated with either polidocanol or ethanolamine oleate with a significantly higher rate of total occlusion after 6 months of follow-up in the polidocanol group.

Complication rates ranged from 0%–6% compared to 8%–28% for embolo-sclerotherapy with undiluted ethanol,[27] but severe adverse events have also been reported related to all sclerosants mentioned.[28–31] Their superiority in terms of effectiveness compared with ethanol, especially regarding long-term outcomes, has yet to be demonstrated.[7,32,33]

OTHER ENDOVASCULAR THERAPIES

Embolization using coils, glue, or particles is not ideal for the treatment of VMs, as lesions are usually low flow, with high volume, and of large diameter. Consecutively, there is

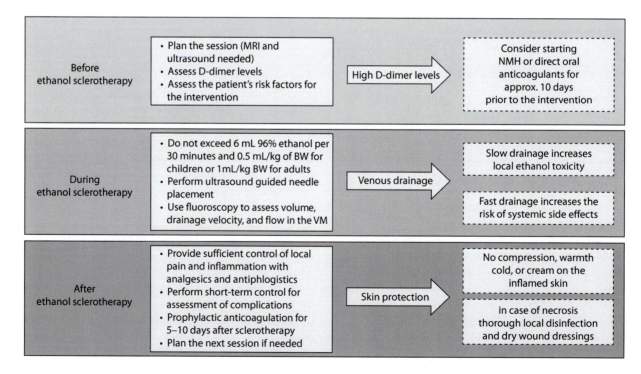

Figure 34.1 Recommendation on safety measures before, after, and during ethanol sclerotherapy.

an unproportionate risk of washing out coils or particles with embolization of VMs.[34]

Transdermal therapy with neodymium:yttrium-aluminum-garnet (Nd:YAG) lasers is especially useful for cosmetic improvement of associated intradermal capillary components[35,36] and can be applied in glomuvenous malformations.[37,38]

Endovascular laser sclerosation is an interesting option in the treatment of tubular components of venous malformations but especially for the occlusion of the marginal vein and residual embryonic veins if surgical resection is not feasible due to prior interventions.[39–41]

In the treatment of stenosing truncular VM, reconstruction of the hypo- or dysplastic deep venous system to restore venous outflow can be necessary, and endovenous stenting has shown to be effective in other contexts of venous stenosis.[42,43] If endovascular therapy fails, surgical reconstruction by bypass grafting is the treatment of choice.

SURGICAL TREATMENT

The success of surgical treatment depends on size, location, and type of the venous malformation. Small (less than 2–4 cm), well-bordered, superficial lesions are appropriate for a primary surgical approach.[44] Glomuvenous malformation (GVM) due to its characteristics is primarily dedicated for surgical treatment.[45]

Surgery plays an important role in the multimodal approach, with excision of scarred tissue or reconstruction of skin and tissue after primary embolo-sclerotherapy. Combined therapy with glue embolization followed directly by excision in the same session shows good results in well-selected patients based on single-center experiences.[46,47] Surgery of VM, in comparison to embolo-sclerotherapy, has a higher risk of major blood loss during the procedure and extensive resection causing deformation, which can be worse in functional outcomes than the symptomatic VM itself. But complete excision has an almost 100% success rate and limits the need for repetitive embolo-sclerotherapy.

Surgeons are a crucial part of the interdisciplinary consultation for VM patients to identify the lesions suitable for primary resection and to plan an eventual tailored multimodal approach.[48]

TARGETED MEDICAL THERAPY

In the absence of endovascular or surgical treatment options, because of location or extension of VM, but in the presence of symptoms severely affecting the patient's quality of life, treatment with the mammalian target of rapamycin (mTOR) inhibitor sirolimus (rapamycin) could be an option.[49]

The last decade brought a large number of published monocentric case series.[50–53] The best available evidence presents a prospective phase II study on 19 patients with refractory-to-standard-care slow-flow vascular malformations, which showed a complication rate of less than 10%,

and effectiveness was observed in 16 patients with maximum follow-up of 48 months on ongoing therapy.[54] A prospective multicentric phase III trial (VASE, NCT02638389; European Union Drug Regulation Authorities Clinical Trials [EudraCT] Number: 2015–001703-32) is conducted in Europe to evaluate the efficacy of sirolimus in pediatric and adult patients with VMs that are refractory to standard treatment.

The results are promising, but as long as blinded placebo-controlled trials are missing, we can only confirm the safety of the drug.

In summary, the best option is to avoid interventional treatment whenever possible. If symptoms are limiting the patient's quality of life or threatening life, organs, or limbs, endovascular embolo-sclerotherapy is recommended as first-line treatment of VMs. Various sclerosing agents are well described in terms of efficacy and safety, but large, randomized trials are missing.[21,55]

Undiluted ethanol represents the most aggressive and consequently likely most effective long-term approach. If handled cautiously, complications can be limited. Figure 34.1 shows suggestions for a practical and safe approach to ethanol embolo-sclerotherapy.

Less aggressive sclerosants should be used in high-risk regions such as head, neck, or superficial cutaneous involvement, perhaps combined with diluted ethanol and embolo-sclerotherapy using undiluted ethanol of deeper parts of the lesion and/or surgical treatment for improvement of cosmetic and functional outcomes.

For truncular lesions and marginal veins, endovascular laser therapy and surgical resection remain the treatment of choice. A targeted medical therapy with sirolimus can be discussed in case of interventional therapy failure or the absence of interventional therapeutic options.

REFERENCES

1. Dompmartin A, Acher A, Thibon P et al. Association of localized intravascular coagulopathy with venous malformations. *Arch Dermatol.* 2008;144(7):873–877.
2. Mack JM, Richter GT, Crary SE. Effectiveness and safety of treatment with direct oral anticoagulant rivaroxaban in patients with slow-flow vascular malformations: A case series. *Lymphat Res Biol.* 2018;16(3):278–281.
3. Vandenbriele C, Vanassche T, Peetermans M, Verhamme P, Peerlinck K. Rivaroxaban for the treatment of consumptive coagulopathy associated with a vascular malformation. *J Thromb Thrombolysis.* 2014;38(1):121–123.
4. Binet Q, Lambert C, Hermans C. Dabigatran etexilate in the treatment of localized intravascular coagulopathy associated with venous malformations. *Thromb Res.* 2018;168:114–120.
5. Dompmartin A, Vikkula M, Boon LM. Venous malformation: Update on aetiopathogenesis, diagnosis and management. *Phlebology.* 2010;25(5):224–235.

6. Yakes WF, Haas DK, Parker SH et al. Symptomatic vascular malformations: Ethanol embolotherapy. *Radiology.* 1989;170(3 Pt 2):1059–1066.

7. Burrows PE, Mason KP. Percutaneous treatment of low flow vascular malformations. *J Vasc Interv Radiol.* 2004;15(5):431–445.

8. Hammer FD, Boon LM, Mathurin P, Vanwijck RR. Ethanol sclerotherapy of venous malformations: Evaluation of systemic ethanol contamination. *J Vasc Interv Radiol.* 2001;12(5):595–600.

9. Mason KP, Michna E, Zurakowski D, Koka BV, Burrows PE. Serum ethanol levels in children and adults after ethanol embolization or sclerotherapy for vascular anomalies. *Radiology.* 2000;217(1):127–132.

10. Behravesh S, Yakes W, Gupta N et al. Venous malformations: Clinical diagnosis and treatment. *Cardiovasc Diagn Ther.* 2016;6(6):557–569.

11. Horbach SER, van der Horst CMAM, Blei F et al. OVAMA Consensus Group. Development of an international core outcome set for peripheral vascular malformations: The OVAMA project. *Br J Dermatol.* 2018;178(2):473–481.

12. Lokhorst MM, Horbach SER, van der Horst CMAM, Spuls PI; OVAMA Steering Group. Finalizing the international core domain set for peripheral vascular malformations: The OVAMA project. *Br J Dermatol.* 2019 Apr 25. doi: 10.1111/bjd.18043.

13. Dasgupta R, Patel M. Venous malformations. *Semin Pediatr Surg.* 2014;23(4):198–202.

14. Wang D, Su L, Han Y et al. Direct intralesional ethanol sclerotherapy of extensive venous malformations with oropharyngeal involvement after a temporary tracheotomy in the head and neck: Initial results. *Head Neck.* 2017;39(2):288–296.

15. Ali S, Weiss CR, Sinha A, Eng J, Mitchell SE. The treatment of venous malformations with percutaneous sclerotherapy at a single academic medical center. *Phlebology.* 2016;31(9):603–609.

16. Steiner F, FitzJohn T, Tan ST. Ethanol sclerotherapy for venous malformation. *ANZ J Surg.* 2016;86(10):790–795.

17. Orlando JL, Caldas JGMP, Campos HG do A, Nishinari K, Wolosker N. Ethanol sclerotherapy of superficial venous malformation: A new procedure. *Dermatology.* 2010;220(4):376–380.

18. Dompmartin A, Blaizot X, Théron J et al. Radio-opaque ethylcellulose-ethanol is a safe and efficient sclerosing agent for venous malformations. *Eur Radiol.* 2011;21(12):2647–2656.

19. Teusch VI, Wohlgemuth WA, Hammer S et al. Ethanol-gel sclerotherapy of venous malformations: Effectiveness and safety. *Am J Roentgenol.* 2017;209(6):1390–1395.

20. Zhang J, Li H-B, Zhou S-Y et al. Comparison between absolute ethanol and bleomycin for the treatment of venous malformation in children. *Exp Ther Med.* 2013;6(2):305–309.

21. van der Vleuten CJM, Kater A, Wijnen MHWA, Schultze Kool LJ, Rovers MM. Effectiveness of sclerotherapy, surgery, and laser therapy in patients with venous malformations: A systematic review. *Cardiovasc Intervent Radiol.* 2014;37(4):977–989.

22. Greene AK, Alomari AI. Management of venous malformations. *Clin Plast Surg.* 2011;38(1):83–93.

23. Duffy DM. Sclerosants: A comparative review. *Dermatol Surg.* 2010;36(Suppl 2):1010–1025.

24. Stimpson P, Hewitt R, Barnacle A, Roebuck DJ, Hartley B. Sodium tetradecyl sulphate sclerotherapy for treating venous malformations of the oral and pharyngeal regions in children. *Int J Pediatr Otorhinolaryngol.* 2012;76(4):569–573.

25. Gulsen F, Cantasdemir M, Solak S, Gulsen G, Ozluk E, Numan F. Percutaneous sclerotherapy of peripheral venous malformations in pediatric patients. *Pediatr Surg Int.* 2011;27(12):1283–1287.

26. Yamaki T, Nozaki M, Sakurai H, Takeuchi M, Soejima K, Kono T. Prospective randomized efficacy of ultrasound-guided foam sclerotherapy compared with ultrasound-guided liquid sclerotherapy in the treatment of symptomatic venous malformations. *J Vasc Surg.* 2008;47(3):578–584.

27. Hage AN, Chick JFB, Srinivasa RN et al. Treatment of venous malformations: The data, where we are, and how it is done. *Tech Vasc Interv Radiol.* 2018;21(2):45–54.

28. Forlee MV, Grouden M, Moore DJ, Shanik G. Stroke after varicose vein foam injection sclerotherapy. *J Vasc Surg.* 2006;43(1):162–164.

29. Li L, Feng J, Zeng X-Q, Li Y-H. Fluoroscopy-guided foam sclerotherapy with sodium morrhuate for peripheral venous malformations: Preliminary experience. *J Vasc Surg.* 2009;49(4):961–967.

30. Marrocco-Trischitta MM, Guerrini P, Abeni D, Stillo F. Reversible cardiac arrest after polidocanol sclerotherapy of peripheral venous malformation. *Dermatol Surg.* 2002;28(2):153–155.

31. Potter B, Gobeil F, Oiknine A, Laramée P. The first case of takotsubo cardiomyopathy associated with sodium tetradecyl sulphate sclerotherapy. *Can J Cardiol.* 2010;26(4):146–148.

32. Aronniemi J, Castrén E, Lappalainen K et al. Sclerotherapy complications of peripheral venous malformations. *Phlebology.* 2016;31(10):712–722.

33. Horbach SE, Rigter IM, Smitt JH, Reekers JA, Spuls PI, van der Horst CM. Intralesional bleomycin injections for vascular malformations: A systematic review and meta-analysis. *Plast Reconstr Surg.* 2016;137(1):244–256.

34. Lee BB, Baumgartner I, Berlien P et al. Guideline. Diagnosis and treatment of venous malformations. Consensus document of the International Union of Phlebology (IUP): Updated-2013. *Int Angiol.* 2015;34(2):97–149.

35. Scherer K, Waner M. Nd:YAG lasers (1064 nm) in the treatment of venous malformations of the face and neck: Challenges and benefits. *Lasers Med Sci.* 2007;22(2):119–126.

36. Eivazi B, Wiegand S, Teymoortash A, Neff A, Werner JA. Laser treatment of mucosal venous malformations of the upper aerodigestive tract in 50 patients. *Lasers Med Sci.* 2010;25(4):571–576.

37. Moreno-Arrones OM, Jimenez N, Alegre-Sanchez A, Fonda P, Boixeda P. Glomuvenous malformations: Dual PDL-Nd:YAG laser approach. *Lasers Med Sci.* 2018;33(9):2007–2010.

38. Murthy AS, Dawson A, Gupta D, Spring S, Cordoro KM. Utility and tolerability of the long-pulsed 1064-nm neodymium:yttrium-aluminum-garnet (LP Nd:YAG) laser for treatment of symptomatic or disfiguring vascular malformations in children and adolescents. *J Am Acad Dermatol.* 2017;77(3): 473–479.

39. Bittles M, Jodeh DS, Mayer JLR, Gallant M, Rottgers SA. Laser ablation of embryonic veins in children. *Pediatr Int.* 2019;61(4):358–363.

40. Patel PA, Barnacle AM, Stuart S, Amaral JG, John PR. Endovenous laser ablation therapy in children: Applications and outcomes. *Pediatr Radiol.* 2017; 47(10):1353–1363.

41. King K, Landrigan-Ossar M, Clemens R, Chaudry G, Alomari AI. The use of endovenous laser treatment in toddlers. *J Vasc Interv Radiol.* 2013;24(6):855–858.

42. Raju S, Neglén P. Stents for chronic venous insufficiency: Why, where, how and when—A review. *J Miss State Med Assoc.* 2008;49(7):199–205.

43. Neglén P. Stenting is the "method-of-choice" to treat iliofemoral venous outflow obstruction. *J Endovasc Ther.* 2009;16(4):492–493.

44. Park H, Kim JS, Park H et al. Venous malformations of the head and neck: A retrospective review of 82 cases. *Arch Plast Surg.* 2019;46(1):23–33.

45. Frumuseanu B, Balanescu R, Ulici A et al. A new case of lower extremity glomus tumor up-to date review and case report. *J Med Life.* 2012;5(2):211–214.

46. Chewning RH, Monroe EJ, Lindberg A et al. Combined glue embolization and excision for the treatment of venous malformations. *CVIR Endovasc.* 2018;1(1):22.

47. Tieu DD, Ghodke BV, Vo NJ, Perkins JA. Single-stage excision of localized head and neck venous malformations using preoperative glue embolization. *Otolaryngol Head Neck Surg.* 2013;148(4):678–684.

48. Kang GB, Bae YC, Nam SB, Bae SH, Sung JY. The usefulness of surgical treatment in slow-flow vascular malformation patients. *Arch Plast Surg.* 2017;44(4):301–307.

49. Uebelhoer M, Nätynki M, Kangas J et al. Venous malformation-causative TIE2 mutations mediate an AKT-dependent decrease in PDGFB. *Hum Mol Genet.* 2013;22(17):3438–3448.

50. Hammill AM, Wentzel M, Gupta A et al. Sirolimus for the treatment of complicated vascular anomalies in children. *Pediatr Blood Cancer.* 2011;57(6):1018–1024.

51. Boscolo E, Limaye N, Huang L et al. Rapamycin improves TIE2-mutated venous malformation in murine model and human subjects. *J Clin Invest.* 2015;125(9):3491–3504.

52. Alemi AS, Rosbe KW, Chan DK, Meyer AK. Airway response to sirolimus therapy for the treatment of complex pediatric lymphatic malformations. *Int J Pediatr Otorhinolaryngol.* 2015;79(12):2466–2469.

53. Triana P, Dore M, Cerezo VN et al. Sirolimus in the treatment of vascular anomalies. *Eur J Pediatr Surg.* 2017;27(1):86–90.

54. Hammer J, Seront E, Duez S et al. Sirolimus is efficacious in treatment for extensive and/or complex slow-flow vascular malformations: A monocentric prospective phase II study. *Orphanet J Rare Dis.* 2018;13(1):191.

55. Horbach SER, Lokhorst MM, Saeed P, de Goüyon Matignon de Pontouraude CMF, Rothová A, van der Horst CMAM. Sclerotherapy for low-flow vascular malformations of the head and neck: A systematic review of sclerosing agents. *J Plast Reconstr Aesthet Surg.* 2016;69(3):295–304.

35

Ethanol sclerotherapy: Is it gold standard for venous malformation management as well?

YOUNG SOO DO

Venous malformations (VMs) are the most common vascular malformations. The usual indications for treatment include pain, swelling, disfigured mass, and bleeding. Although there are various options in the treatment of VMs, sclerotherapy is generally accepted as the major therapeutic tool for focal or localized VMs, while extensive diffuse VMs of the extremities are often managed with compression garments.[1] Controlling the pain and growth of VM is the main goal of sclerotherapy, because a cure for venous malformation is difficult and usually not achieved. There are many different sclerosing agents, including ethanol, detergents (e.g., sodium tetradecyl sulfate, polidocanol, ethanolamine oleate), and antitumor agents (e.g., bleomycin, pingyangmycin, and OK 432). Among them, the most frequently used sclerosing agents for VMs are ethanol, sodium tetradecyl sulfate (STS), polidocanol, and bleomycin. They vary in their mode of action, relative toxicity, complication rate, and therapeutic effect.

Ethanol is known to be a most effective and potent sclerosing agent with respect to inducing permanent obliteration of the vessel lumen of the VM by vessel wall denudation and thrombus formation, resulting in the complete obliteration of the vessel lumen.[2,3] It has been reported that the effective rate of VM sclerotherapy with ethanol was 75%–95%,[4–6] but it is extremely painful on injection and thus is used under general anesthesia. Ethanol causes severe swelling, at its maximum about 24 hours after the injection. Skin necrosis and peripheral nerve injury are relatively common, even though most nerve injury recovers. Ethanol diffusion through the wall of the VM into surrounding tissue and skin is the cause of skin necrosis and nerve injury. Delayed complication of muscle fibrosis of calf muscle and contraction of the ankle was reported after ethanol sclerotherapy of calf muscle VM. Local complication rates as high as 12.4% per session and 27.9% per patients have been reported. But significant hemodynamic changes in the cardiopulmonary circulation are rare, because a relatively small amount of ethanol (less than 0.5 mL/kg of body weight) has been used

for VM sclerotherapy.[7] To prevent cardiopulmonary complications, a protocol of single bolus injection of ethanol less than 0.1 mL/kg, no more frequently than every 10 minutes, and total ethanol volume per session less than 0.5 mL/kg has been proposed.[8,9] Combination therapy, ethanol with STS or ethanol with bleomycin, can reduce the ethanol-related local complications by reducing the volume of ethanol.[10,11]

STS and polidocanol are best administered as foam, as it has been shown that a foamed agent is more effective in displacing the blood and penetrating the VM. Because the injection of foam sclerosing agent does not induce severe pain as ethanol, foam sclerotherapy can be performed safely on an outpatient basis with mild sedation. It causes less swelling, and the incidence of skin necrosis and nerve injury is less than that with ethanol sclerotherapy.[12] But the reported recurrence rate was about 13%, higher than that with ethanol.[7,12] This can be overcome by additional treatment sessions. More details about STS and polidocanol are discussed in Chapter 36.

Bleomycin is a cytotoxic antibiotic isolated from the gram-positive bacteria *Streptomyces verticillus*. Bleomycin inhibits DNA synthesis and is used as a chemotherapy agent. When used as a sclerosing agent, it induces an inflammatory reaction that subsequently causes fibrosis. It is very well tolerated with minimal swelling and pain after sclerotherapy.[4] In a systemic review and meta-analysis, the outcomes of intralesional bleomycin injection for VMs were studied in 12 articles including 690 patients. Good to excellent size reduction was reported in 87% of VMs without nerve injury.[13] Pulmonary fibrosis was not reported. Nausea, vomiting, and chills may occur soon after sclerotherapy. Treatment with bleomycin alone usually requires more procedures than other sclerosing agents.[4,13] A combination of bleomycin and other sclerosing agents (ethanol or foam sclerosing agents) shows better results with less complication rates. Because of concern for pulmonary fibrosis, the bleomycin dose is limited to 0.5 units/kg or 15 units per procedure, with a lifetime limit of 400 units.

The anatomical location of the VM is the most important factor in determining which sclerosing agent to use:

- *Superficial locations*: Superficial lesions with dermal involvement are at a higher risk of skin necrosis. For those lesions, bleomycin or 1% STS or 1% polidocanol foam is recommended to reduce skin necrosis. Ethanol should be reserved for the deeper VM.
- *Lesions near a nerve*: When the VM is located near a nerve, bleomycin or foam sclerosing agent is recommended, because high incidence of nerve injury was reported after ethanol sclerotherapy, especially for the forearm intramuscular VM.[7] The authors no longer recommend ethanol sclerotherapy for the intramuscular forearm VM.
- *Lesions near vital structures, like the airway or the orbital area*: Bleomycin causes the least amount of swelling after injection. For this reason, bleomycin is the most appropriate agent for treating sites where swelling is poorly tolerated, such as the orbit and the airway.[14,15]
- *Lesions with delayed muscle fibrosis and contracture*: When the VM is involved at the posterior part of the calf muscle, ethanol sclerotherapy of intramuscular VM can induce delayed muscle fibrosis and contracture of the ankle.[7,14] To avoid this complication, bleomycin is recommended in this area.

In conclusion, sclerotherapy of VM using ethanol is most effective but is associated with high local complications. Ethanol should be reserved for the deeper located lesion like intramuscular VM and lesions with no important nerves around. Sclerotherapy of VM with foam sclerosing agents or bleomycin is also effective and recommended for the superficial lesion, lesions near the nerve, lesions near the vital structures, and lesions prone to delayed muscle contracture.

REFERENCES

1. Lee BB, Baumgartner I, Berlien P et al. Diagnosis and treatment of venous malformations. Consensus document of the International Union of Phlebology (IUP): Updated 2013. *Int Angiol.* 2015;34(2):97–149.
2. Yun WS, Kim YW, Lee KB et al. Predictors of response to percutaneous ethanol sclerotherapy (PES) in patients with venous malformations: Analysis of patient self-assessment and imaging. *J Vasc Surg.* 2009;50:581–589.
3. Lee BB, Kim DI, Huh S et al. New experiences with absolute ethanol sclerotherapy in the management of a complex form of congenital venous malformation. *J Vasc Surg.* 2001;33:764–772.
4. Zhang J, Li HB, Zhou SY et al. Comparison between absolute ethanol and bleomycin for the treatment of venous malformation in children. *Exp Ther Med.* 2013;6:305–309.
5. Su L, Fan X, Zheng L, Zheng J. Absolute ethanol sclerotherapy for venous malformations in the face and neck. *J Oral Maxillofac Surg.* 2010;68:1622–1627.
6. Spence J, Krings T, TerBrugge KG, Agid R. Percutaneous treatment of facial venous malformations: A matched comparison of alcohol and bleomycin sclerotherapy. *Head Neck.* 2011;33:125–130.
7. Lee BB, Do YS, Byun HS et al. Advanced management of venous malformation with ethanol sclerotherapy: Mid-term results. *J Vasc Surg.* 2003;37:533–538.
8. Ko JS, Kim JA, Do YS et al. Prediction of the effect of injected ethanol on pulmonary arterial pressure during sclerotherapy of arteriovenous malformations: Relationship with dose of ethanol. *J Vasc Interv Radiol.* 2009;20:39–45.
9. Shin BS, Do YS, Cho HS et al. Cardiovascular effects and predictability of cardiovascular collapse after repeated intravenous bolus injections of absolute ethanol in anesthetized pigs. *J Vasc Interv Radiol.* 2010;21(12):1867–1872.
10. Gorman J, Zbarsky SJ, Courtemanche RJM et al. Image guided sclerotherapy for the treatment of venous malformations. *CVIR Endovascular.* 2018;1:2.
11. Jin Y, Lin X, Li W, Hu X, Ma G, Wang W. Sclerotherapy after embolization of draining vein: A safe treatment method for venous malformation. *J Vasc Surg.* 2008;47:1292–1299.
12. Park HS, Do YS, Park KB et al. Clinical outcome and predictors of treatment response in foam sodium tetradecyl sulfate sclerotherapy of venous malformations. *Eur Radiol.* 2015;26:1301–1310.
13. Horbach SE, Rigter IM, Smitt JH, Reekers JA, Spuls PI, van der Horst CM. Intralesional bleomycin injections for vascular malformations: A systematic review and metaanalysis. *Plast Reconstr Surg.* 2016;137(1):244–256.
14. Ozaki M, Kurita M, Kaji N et al. Efficacy and evaluation of safety of sclerosants for intramuscular venous malformations: Clinical and experimental studies. *J Plast Surg Hand Surg.* 2010;44:75–87.
15. Zheng JW, Yang XJ, Wang YA et al. Intralesional injection of Pingyangmycin for vascular malformations in oral and maxillofacial regions: an evaluation of 297 consecutive patients. *Oral Oncol.* 2009;45:872–876.

36

Foam sclerotherapy: First option for venous malformations?

KUROSH PARSI AND MINA KANG

INTRODUCTION

Sclerotherapy refers to the technique of injecting chemically ablative sclerosants into the target lesion to achieve endovascular fibrosis to ultimately occlude the vessel. There are three broad categories of sclerosants: detergents, osmotic agents, and chemical irritants. Sodium tetradecyl sulfate (STS) and polidocanol (POL) are the most popular detergent sclerosants used to treat venous incompetence and venous malformations. Hypertonic saline and dextrose are examples of osmotic agents used to treat telangiectasias. Ethanol and doxycycline are examples of chemical irritants commonly used in the treatment of arteriovenous and lymphatic malformations, respectively.

DETERGENT SCLEROSANTS

Detergent sclerosants are the most popular agents in current phlebology practice, owing to their unique chemical properties, enabling their conversion into a foam structure. The foam structure is produced by suspending the liquid detergent sclerosant in a gas such as room air, carbon dioxide (CO_2), or a combination of CO_2 and O_2.[1] Foam is commonly generated at bedside by physicians (physician-compounded foam [PCF]) using several techniques, the most popular of which is the Tessari technique.[2] The main advantage of foam sclerosants over the liquid agents is increased potency due to displacement of intravascular blood and clear visibility on ultrasound due to increased echogenicity.

Detergent sclerosants are derived from long-chain fatty acids and are chemically classified as surfactants.[3] They interfere with the extracellular lipid membranes and disrupt the endothelial lining, exposing the underlying collagen to induce endovascular fibrosis. STS is an anionic surfactant classified as a harsh detergent, manufactured as FIBRO-VEIN and SOTRADECOL (STD Pharma, Hereford, United Kingdom). POL is a nonionic surfactant alcohol classified as a mild detergent produced AETHOXYSKLEROL or

ASCLERA (Kreussler, Wiesbaden, Germany). Both STS and POL are manufactured as liquid agents converted to foam by physicians. VARITHENA (BTG Pharma, United Kingdom) is the only commercially available drug/delivery unit that produces POL 1% endovenous microfoam.[4]

Foam sclerosants are the agents of choice in the treatment of small VMs sized up to 2–3 mm in diameter or diffuse lesions where other modalities are not suitable. The authors prefer to treat larger lesions with endovenous laser ablation (EVLA) and n-butyl cyanoacrylate (n-BCA) glue. Ethanol has been mostly superseded by foam sclerosants in the management of VM and should only be used discriminately due to its significant complication profile. In experienced and expert hands, ethanol sclerotherapy is quite effective in treating a range of VMs, but it requires extensive training and monitoring, especially if large volumes are required. In our group's experience, we have not employed ethanol in the past 25 years to treat VMs. Surgical excision of VMs is associated with high recurrence rates and is not recommended. However, surgical debulking of the residual fibrofatty tissue following successful embolization can be indicated in cases where the remaining mass is causing symptoms.[5]

Foam sclerotherapy is performed under ultrasound or fluoroscopic guidance. Ultrasound-guided sclerotherapy (UGS) requires extensive training and is more than a simple method of producing and injecting foam into the target lesion. Foam sclerosants are introduced into target vessels by direct percutaneous injections or via catheter-guided delivery. The ideal lesion for foam sclerotherapy is one with a thin, nonfibrotic wall that is small in diameter. VMs presenting with thicker fibrotic walls and larger diameters are best treated with EVLA, which can achieve transmural damage to the lesion.

Foam sclerosants should not be mixed with intravascular blood, as they undergo significant deactivation that reduces the active concentration and hence efficacy. The clinical and biological efficacy of sclerosants is determined by the final therapeutic concentration in the target vessel, rather than the initial injected concentration. Both STS and

POL are neutralized and deactivated by circulating blood cell membranes, albumin, and other plasma proteins.[6–9] Deactivation of the sclerosant results in a significant reduction in the active concentration, which alters the coagulant profile of the agent from an anticoagulant one to a procoagulant one.[10] This activates platelets and triggers the release of procoagulant platelet-derived microparticles. Hence, lower concentrations of sclerosants adopt a procoagulant profile resulting in platelet activation and platelet microparticle release. Clinically, this results in thrombotic occlusion of the target lesion as opposed to a fibrotic occlusion. Thrombotic occlusion will lead to fibrinolysis and recanalization of the target vessel and hence treatment failure. In addition, it can result in thrombophlebitis and hyperpigmentation and other cosmetic complications. The aim of the treatment should be inducing fibrosclerosis rather than thrombosclerosis. The authors use STS at 1.5% foam for relatively larger and deeper subcutaneous lesions and POL at 0.5% foam for dermal and subdermal lesions.

CONCLUSION

Foam sclerotherapy is a safe and effective method to treat small, thin-walled VMs. The procedure requires training and familiarity with the agents.

REFERENCES

1. Parsi K, Exner T, Connor DE, Joseph JE, Fung DD. A convenient source of carbon dioxide for sclerosant foams. *Dermatol Surg.* 2006;32:1533–1534.
2. Tessari L, Cavezzi A, Frullini A. Preliminary experience with a new sclerosing foam in the treatment of varicose veins. *Dermatol Surg.* 2001;27:58–60.
3. Wong K, Chen T, Connor DE, Behnia M, Parsi K. Basic physiochemical and rheological properties of detergent sclerosants. *Phlebology.* 2015;30:339–349.
4. Star P, Connor DE, Parsi K. Novel developments in foam sclerotherapy: Focus on Varithena (polidocanol endovenous microfoam) in the management of varicose veins. *Phlebology.* 2017;33:150–162.
5. Parsi K, Kang M, Trimboli A. Ultrasound-guided TriVex-powered phlebectomy for debulking of peripheral vascular anomalies—A novel treatment technique. *Phlebology.* 2019;34:523–529.
6. Parsi K, Exner T, Connor DE, Herbert A, Ma DD, Joseph JE. The lytic effects of detergent sclerosants on erythrocytes, platelets, endothelial cells and microparticles are attenuated by albumin and other plasma components in vitro. *Eur J Vasc Endovasc Surg.* 2008;36:216–223.
7. Watkins MR. Deactivation of sodium tetradecyl sulphate injection by blood proteins. *Eur J Vasc Endovasc Surg.* 2011;41:521–525.
8. Tessari L, Cavezzi A, Izzo M, Zini F, Tessari M, Fanelli R. *In vivo* demonstration of sodium tetradecyl sulphate sclerosant foam binding with blood proteins. *13th Annual Meeting of the European Venous Forum.* Florence, Italy: Phlebology; 2012:307–326.
9. Connor DE, Cooley-Andrade O, Goh WX, Ma DD, Parsi K. Detergent sclerosants are deactivated and consumed by circulating blood cells. *Eur J Vasc Endovasc Surg.* 2015;49:426–431.
10. Parsi K, Exner T, Connor DE, Ma DD, Joseph JE. *In vitro* effects of detergent sclerosants on coagulation, platelets and microparticles. *Eur J Vasc Endovasc Surg.* 2007;34:731–740.

37

Considerations regarding feasibility, safety, and efficacy of N-butyl cyanoacrylate (n-BCA) and Onyx embolization for the treatment of venous malformations

JOVAN N. MARKOVIC AND CYNTHIA K. SHORTELL

Embolization, either alone or followed by surgical excision, is a successfully used treatment modality in patients with high-flow vascular malformations (HFVMs).[1,2] Currently, limited data are available regarding the use of embolization in patients with venous malformations (VMs). Initially, embolization was mostly considered as a preoperative treatment adjunct to surgery. In contrast to sclerotherapy, where percutaneous, intraluminal injection of a sclerosing agent causes chemical injury and disruption of the endothelial lining with subsequent endoluminal obliteration of the treated vessel, embolization includes intraluminal placement of material and/or agents (such as coils, plugs, and/or embolization glues and liquids), through a catheter into the lumen of the vessel to seal off the site where malformation connects to the feeding and/or draining blood vessels and/or to occupy the lumen of a malformation and therefore reduce the portion of malformation that can be filled with blood.[2] However, experience and data have shown that many arteriovenous malformations were successfully treated with embolization alone, and that surgical excision is primarily used for only well-localized lesions.[3,4]

The rationale for using combined glue embolization followed by immediate excision of VMs is to achieve a more hemostatic environment by selectively reducing the lumen of blood-filled, and frequently ill-defined VM and making a lesion more amenable to surgical excision, ideally, following embolization a complete excision can be achieved for focal VMs, which consequently reduces the potential for recurrent symptoms.

Although many embolization agents and devices have been used in the past, the principle of embolization is the same. It consists of percutaneous injection of embolic agents that polymerize rapidly upon contact with blood anions (via cascades of chemical reactions) and consequently solidifies and thus reduces or occludes the lumen of a lesion.[5] Based on biophysical characteristics, occlusive agents used for embolization can be classified into two major groups: adhesive or nonadhesive. The first commercially available adhesive agent was Eastman 910 Monomer (Eastman Corporation, Rochester, New York).[6] Chemically, it was a methyl cyanoacrylate, and it had a single carbon-ester group.[6] Following this, several other agents with four or six carbon ester groups became available. The first adhesive agent approved by the U.S. Food and Drug Administration (FDA) (September 2000) currently available in the United States is n-butyl cyanoacrylate (n-BCA) (Trufill, Cordis, Inc., Miami Lakes, Florida).

Onyx is a nonadhesive liquid embolic agent consisting of ethylene vinyl alcohol (EVOH) copolymer dissolved in various concentrations of dimethyl sulfoxide (DMSO).[7] To achieve adequate radio-opacity for visualization under fluoroscopy, this mixture is suspended in micronized tantalum powder. Onyx is commercially available in two concentrations: Onyx 18 (6% EVOH) and Onyx 34 (8% EVOH).[7] Onyx 18 has lower viscosity and will travel more distally and penetrate deeper into the nidus compared to Onyx 34.[7] With both concentrations, final solidification occurs within 5 minutes following intravascular injection.[7] Currently, Onyx is FDA approved for its use in the treatment of intracranial arteriovenous malformations, and it is used for the treatment of VMs as an "off-label" agent. Following intraluminal injection and contact with blood, DMSO rapidly diffuses from the mixture, which leads to *in situ* precipitation and causes solidification of the polymer, which in turn forms an embolus without adhesion to the vascular endothelium.[7] Due to its biochemical characteristics, Onyx was primarily used for the treatment of intracranial arteriovenous malformations. It is worth emphasizing that the cases of unexpected intraoperative flammability and combustion associated with Onyx (mixed with micronized tantalum [Ta] as radiopacifier) were reported when this embolic agent was used in conjunction with the mono-polar electro-cautery in the management of intracranial arteriovenous fistula.[8] Schirmer et al. recommend to rely on low- to medium-energy bipolar electrocautery when used near the Ta-opacified Onyx to mitigate this risk.[8]

Due to recent advancements in the management of congenital vascular malformations, both n-BCA and Onyx were evaluated in the management of patients with VMs. Data from several studies showed safety and efficacy of preoperative n-BCA embolization in VM patients. Tieu et al. evaluated 11 VMs treated with n-BCA embolization followed by surgical resection.[9] Data from this study showed that localized VMs in the head and neck can be completely removed without any major complications.[9] In 2018, Uller et al. showed that preoperative n-BCA embolization has the potential for reduction of intraoperative estimated blood loss (EBL) (which in turn can allow resection of large VMs) and shorter postoperative length of stay (LOS).[10] Data derived from 17 n-BCA embolizations performed in 14 pediatric patients (mean age: 5.5 years; range 0.1–16 years) showed the mean EBL of 70 mL (range 5–350 mL), mean LOS of 3.1 days (range 1–6 days), and uneventful immediate postprocedural recovery.[10] Authors reported that all of the patients had an improvement in symptoms at the mean follow-up time of 2.2 years (range: 0.2–4 years).[10] Long-term complications included one accessory (CN XI) nerve injury with resolution of symptoms over time. Residual malformation was seen in six patients. In these patients, VM was extending outside the area of surgical resection.[10]

Relatively recently, Holly et al. analyzed outcomes in 11 patients (age range: 2–47 years) treated with embolization followed by surgical resection of malformation.[11] Five patients had focal VMs, three had multifocal VMs, and three patients had diffuse VMs throughout the affected extremity.[11] A total of 27 VMs were treated. VM was located in the hand, the forearm, the elbow, and the wrist in ten, eight, six, and three cases, respectively. The mean volume of VMs was 9.4 mL (ranging from 0.95 to 43.5 mL).[11] The nerve involvement was reported in 75% of the lesions and tendon involvement in 25% of the patients. Subcutaneous, subcutaneous-intramuscular, intramuscular, and intramuscular-periosseous were reported in 25% (6 of 24), 29% (7 of 24), 29% (7 of 24), and 17% (4 of 24) cases, respectively.[11] Onyx was used to treat 19 of the 27 VMs, and n-BCA was used to treat eight VMs. The mean volume of Onyx was 3.9 mL (range, 0.5–14.9 mL) and mean volume of n-BCA was 2.4 mL (range, 0.6–5.5 mL).[11] Eighty percent of patients with focal VMs were followed for at least 12 months, and no further treatment was required. All three patients with diffuse VMs required ongoing treatment. Authors reported no major functional impairments and no major procedure-related complications. Estimated blood loss was minimal in all cases, and no patient required a blood transfusion.[11]

In summary, data from several studies showed that the multimodal approach of VMs, including preoperative embolization (with either n-BCA or Onyx), followed by surgical resection, appears to be a safe and effective treatment for focal VMs. More studies evaluated n-BCA than Onyx in the treatment of VMs. Data also showed that this treatment modality may not be adequate for patients with multifocal and diffuse lesions. Although initial results are promising, further studies with long-term follow-ups and larger groups of patients are needed to determine the safety and efficacy of this combined treatment modality as an alternative to the use of sclerotherapy and/or surgical resection, either alone or with adjunctive medical therapy in the management of patients with VMs.

REFERENCES

1. Lee BB. New approaches to the treatment of congenital vascular malformations (CVMs)—A single centre experience. *Eur J Vasc Endovasc Surg*. 2005; 30:184–197.
2. Marler JJ, Mulliken JB. Current management of hemangiomas and vascular malformations. *Clin Plast Surg*. 2005;32:99–116.
3. Lidsky ME, Markovic JN, Miller MJ Jr, Shortell CK. Analysis of the treatment of congenital vascular malformations using a multidisciplinary approach. *J Vasc Surg*. 2012;56(5):1355–1362.
4. Markovic JN, Shortell CE. Multidisciplinary treatment of extremity arteriovenous malformations. *J Vasc Surg Venous Lymphat Disord*. 2015;3(2):209–218.
5. Li YJ, Barthès-Biesel D, Salsac AV. Polymerization kinetics of n-butyl cyanoacrylate glues used for vascular embolization. *J Mech Behav Biomed Mater*. 2017;69:307–317.
6. Rosen RJ, Contractor S. The use of cyanoacrylate adhesives in the management of congenital vascular malformations. *Semin Intervent Radiol*. 2004; 21(1):59–66.
7. Siekmann R. Basics and principles in the application of onyx LD liquid embolic system in the endovascular treatment of cerebral arteriovenous malformations. *Interv Neuroradiol*. 2005;11(Suppl 1):131–140.
8. Schirmer CM, Zerris V, Malek AM. Electrocautery-induced ignition of spark showers and self-sustained combustion of onyx ethylene-vinyl alcohol copolymer. *Neurosurgery*. 2006 Oct;59(4 Suppl 2):ONS413–8.
9. Tieu DD, Ghodke BV, Vo NJ, Perkins JA. Single-stage excision of localized head and neck venous malformations using preoperative glue embolization. *Otolaryngol Head Neck Surg*. 2013;148:678–684.
10. Uller W, El-Sobky S, Alomari AI et al. Preoperative embolization of venous malformations using n-butyl cyanoacrylate. *Vasc Endovascular Surg*. 2018;52(4):269–274.
11. Holly BP, Patel YA, Park J et al. Preoperative epoxy embolization facilitates the safe and effective resection of venous malformations in the hand and forearm. *Hand (N Y)*. 2017;12(4):335–341.

Management: 2

38

Surgical therapy of venous malformation combined with embolo-/sclerotherapy: How much and when?

DIRK A. LOOSE

Venous malformations can be treated successfully in different ways:

1. Conservative
2. Nonsurgical
3. Surgical

The main characteristic of the venous malformation is the high recurrence after treatment, whatever treatment is done.[1,2] Another fact concerning venous malformation is that not every venous malformation has to be treated. An intervention is reserved for symptomatic lesions that, e.g., cause pain, cause deformity, or threaten vital anatomical structures.[3] A special indication for treatment is asymptomatic phlebectatic areas that are at risk for thromboembolism.

Experience has demonstrated that the different techniques of treatment have to be chosen based on the type and form of the venous malformation and also on the localization (face, hand, foot, extremity, location adjacent to an important nerve and/or neurovascular bundles).[4–6]

Two types of venous malformations are as follows:

1. Extra-truncal type:
   a. Superficial, circumscribed shape, epifascial
   b. Spongiform, infiltrating form, epifascial and subfascial

2. Truncal type
   a. Epifascial
   b. Subfascial

Extra-truncal type. The superficial form can be managed by laser, sclerotherapy, or surgery. The infiltrating form, epifascial or subfascial, can be treated by sclero-treatment or by surgery. If the very extensive infiltration form can be managed in one session by surgery, this technique is preferred (Figure 38.1).

If this infiltrating form has invaded a muscle completely, sclero-treatment could lead to a complete fibrosis (Figure 38.2) or even necrosis of the muscle and even at the extremity to a compartment syndrome.[7,8] To avoid such a situation, open surgery and over-and-over suture of the affected muscle, according to Loose (Figure 38.3), is the better solution, as it allows function of the muscle to be maintained, although complete obstruction of the infiltrated venous malformation is achieved.

In spite of precise sclerotherapy, more than 45% of the patients have partial recanalization. That is why a combination of sclerotherapy and resective vascular surgery is preferred. As neither sclerotherapy nor resective vascular surgery will be able to remove the malformation completely, it is mandatory to choose the better option for the patient at the right time.

We are not convinced that almost all venous malformations should have sclerotherapy before resective vascular surgery, because the opinion that this would facilitate resection is wrong. On the contrary, heavy scar formation complicates dissection of the different tissue layers (Figure 38.2). Our long-term study of quality of life after sclerotherapy as well as other comparable studies[9] have shown that patients are highly satisfied with the decline in previously reported complaints.

However, in our experience, many patients do not accept that numerous treatment sessions with sclerotherapy over many years would be required until dramatic symptom improvement occurs. We have seen young patients who have been treated with sclerotherapy (e.g., for more than 10 years) become discouraged and dissatisfied with treatment results, leading them to seek another treatment option and discovering for the first time that a surgical treatment is possible. It is worth emphasizing that traditionally the parents/guardians of patients with vascular malformation or the patients themselves are not sufficiently informed about treatment options (due to lack of expertise among

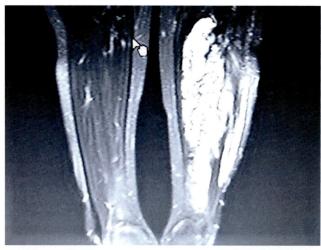

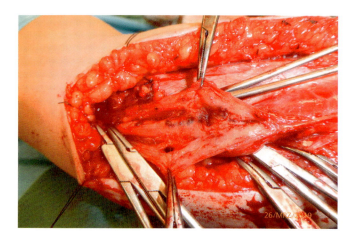

Figure 38.2 Complete fibrosis after sclerotreatment of the flexor carpi radialis muscle.

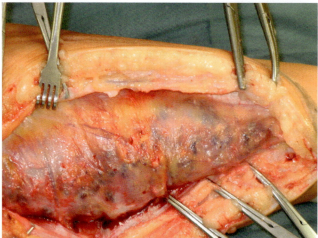

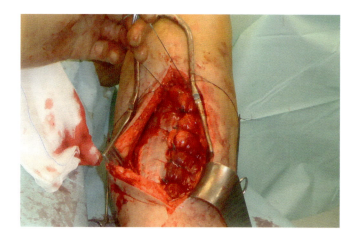

Figure 38.3 Complete suture closure (according to Loose) of extensive, isolated intramuscular malformation.

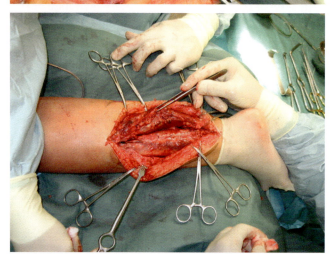

Figure 38.1 Extra-truncal extensive infiltration of the tibial muscle, partial resection.

medical providers). One of these patients was treated with surgical resection that provided (over 6 years follow-up) complete resolution of symptoms. After that, further individual sessions of sclerotherapy were required to maintain the achieved results, as recurrent venectasias were visible, and the patient wanted their removal.

Truncular type. The truncular type of VMs can involve the epifascial, marginal vein (see Chapter 41), which can be treated by surgery, endoluminal laser ablation, or radiofrequency ablation. The subfascial form, e.g., the sciatic vein or the accessory femoral vein (Figures 38.4 and 38.5), can be treated by interventional catheter techniques or by surgery. The control phlebography in this case after partial resection of the accessory vein and resection of the aneurysmal vein segment demonstrated malformations with aneurysms of the femoral vein that required further treatment. In this particular case, the inferior vena cava filter was placed for prophylaxis given that the patient had a history of pulmonary embolisms prior to aneurysm resection.

It is worth emphasizing that all of these patients are at high risk for thromboembolism. That is why many consider they are not ideal candidates for conventional sclerotherapy treatment, no matter which sclerosing agent is used, but rather are better candidates for surgery or for interventional catheter to obtain the occlusion of the malformed large veins.

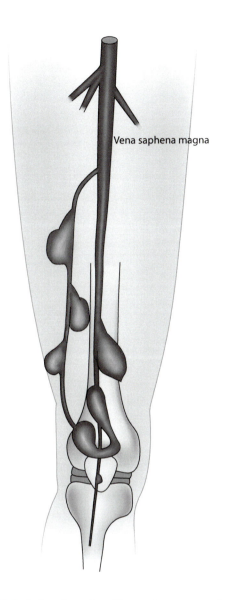

Figure 38.4 A drawing of malformed accessory femoral vein in a patient with medical history of three severe pulmonary emboli.

In some regions, a vascular surgeon experienced in the treatment of vascular malformations may be unavailable for vascular surgical treatment of a VM. In such a situation, one should never act according to the principle of *ut aliquid fiat* ("to do something") and carry out a dubious sclerosing treatment, but the therapeutic indication for the surgical procedure should be consistently followed. However, if there is a clear indication, the insurers, i.e., the payers, must give the affected patient the opportunity to seek treatment from remotely active specialists for ethical and medical reasons.

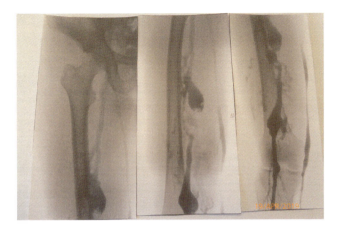

Figure 38.5 Recurrent venectasias were visible, and the patient wanted their removal. Phlebography after partial resection of the accessory femoral vein with two aneurysms demonstrating the highly malformed superficial femoral vein and with aneurysm.

REFERENCES

1. Lee BB, Do YS, Byun HS, Choo IW, Kim DI, Huh SH. Advanced management of venous malformation with ethanol sclerotherapy: Mid-term results. *J Vasc Surg.* 2003;37(3):533–538.
2. Gloviczki P, Stanson AW, Stickler GB et al. Klippel–Trenaunay syndrome: The risks and benefits of vascular interventions. *Surgery.* 1991;110(3):469–479.
3. Hage AN, Chick JFB, Sirinivasa RN et al. Treatment of venous malformations: The data, where we are, and how it is done. *Tech Vasc Interv Radiol.* 2018; 21(2):45–54.
4. Cabrera Garrido J, Rubia MV, Loose DA. Sclerotherapy in vascular malformations with polidocanol foam. In: Mattassi R, Loose DA, Vaghi M, eds. *Hemangiomas and Vascular Malformations.* 2nd ed. Rome, Italy: Springer; 2015:277–289.
5. Lee KB, Kim DI, Oh SK, Do YS, Kim KH, Kim YW. Incidence of soft tissue injury and neuropathy after embolo/sclerotherapy for congenital vascular malformation. *Vasc Surg.* 2008;48(5):1286–1291.
6. Loose DA. Surgical management of venous malformations. *Phlebology.* 2007;22(6):276–282.
7. Mendez-Echevarria A, Fernandez-Prieto A, de la Serna O et al. Acute lung toxicity after intralesional bleomycin sclerotherapy. *Pediatrics.* 2018;141(1):2016–1787.
8. Yakes WF, Baker R. Cardiopulmonary collapse: Sequelae of ethanol embolotherapy. *Radiology.* 1993;189:145.
9. Clemens RK, Baumann F, Husmann M et al. Percutaneous sclerotherapy for spongiform venous malformations—Analysis of patient-evaluated outcome and satisfaction. *VASA.* 2017;46(6):477–483.

39

How aggressive should management be of vascular bone syndrome caused by venous malformation?

RAUL MATTASSI

Vascular bone syndrome (VBS) is a limb length discrepancy (LLD) due to the effects of vascular anomalies (VAs), venous malformations (VMs), or arteriovenous malformations (AVMs), on the growth of the long bones of the limbs. VM may produce overgrowth but also growth inhibition, while AVM is responsible mainly for overgrowth.

In a 1993 study by Belov about LLD in a group of 251 patients affected by AVM or VM with limb overgrowth (angio-osteo-hypertrophy) or limb shortening (angio-osteo-hypotrophy), AVM was the main cause of overgrowth, while VM caused both hypertrophy and hypotrophy.[1] In a study about VM of the lower limbs in 69 cases, we also found no LLD in 50 cases (59%), overgrowth in 13 (19%), and limb shortening in 6 (7%).[2]

Before the knowledge of genetics was available for the vascular anomaly, the cause of overgrowth was considered as the effect of the AV connections in AVM and also the small AV connections, always existing in VM, while the reduced growth was considered to be due to the pressure on bones by periosteally located venous masses.

However, newer data found a significant relationship among the bone vasculature, bone growth, and molecules with both angiogenic and osteogenic activity, like vascular endothelial growth factor (VEGF), fibroblastic growth factor (FGF), transforming growth factor (TGF), bone morphogenetic proteins (BMP), and others.[3-5] Today, some mutations, like *PIK3CA*, are accepted as the cause of growth anomalies.[6] The mechanism by which mutations affect bone growth or if the vascular defect is the true cause of bone growth alteration is still under study. Nevertheless, the existence of a VA near the bone seems to influence bone growth.

The marginal vein, an abnormal, superficial, lateral limb vein, is also a defect that has proved to be associated with bone overgrowth but also with growth reduction. The marginal vein may be related to more or less small AV fistulas

involved in the vessel, especially in the case of deep vein aplasia, as reported by Belov since 1972.[7] The marginal vein should be removed in case of LLD, as it may be a cause of abnormal bone growth.[8]

The treatment of LLD in the presence of VM is based on vascular or orthopedic procedures.

Vascular treatment includes procedures on the abnormal vessels in order to remove or reduce as much as possible the abnormal vascular area that hemodynamically and/or mechanically affects bone growth.

Available techniques are as follows:

- *Surgical*: Removal of areas of VM, truncular or extra-truncular, especially if located near the bone growth/epiphyseal areas
- Percutaneous puncture of the malformation and occlusion of VM by alcohol injection or interstitial laser technique

These techniques can be combined and/or performed by steps; they can lead to spontaneous correction of the LLD when done early during the active bone growth period. Belov reported about surgical treatment in 59 children with VA and LLD with spontaneous correction in 26 cases after only surgical treatment on congenital vascular malformation (CVM) (44% of correction)[1] (Figures 39.1 and 39.2).

Orthopedic treatment is based on the procedures on the bone per se in order to stop growth during childhood or later to elongate or shorten an abnormal bone in adults. The main techniques are as follows:

- Blockade of bone growth by epiphysiodesis, temporary or permanent
- Bone elongation by Ilizarov technique or similar (Figure 39.3)
- Bone shortening by osteotomy

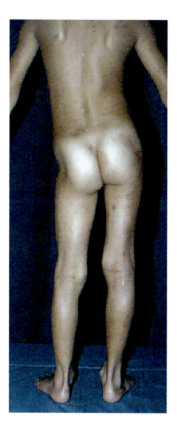

Figure 39.1 Limb length discrepancy of 5 cm in a child with arteriovenous malformation.

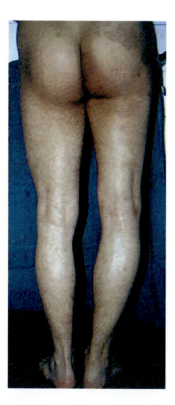

Figure 39.2 Partial spontaneous correction after 8 years to 2 cm limb length discrepancy after only vascular treatments.

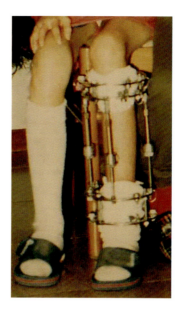

Figure 39.3 Ilizarov device for limb elongation. It can be placed on thigh or calf.

The treatment strategy is different in children and in adults, as bones grow only during childhood. In children, procedures to block or reduce bone growth may be considered in order to achieve progressive compensation of the length difference. Procedures are vascular but also orthopedic. In adults, bone growth has already been completed, so it is no longer possible to achieve a length compensation by removing the vascular cause of the defect or by blocking the growth with orthopedic procedures. Treatment of the vascular defect in an adult, therefore, may improve the symptoms, but no effect will be obtained on LLD. In other words, the use of other techniques, mainly orthopedic, may be needed, although more invasive techniques than those performed in childhood.

Because longitudinal growth is a limited event, the timing to proceed is a crucial point to obtain the best results. In children, a condition that is in evolution needs an early intervention, as the vascular defect will not regress by simply waiting. If a significant malformation exists and LLD is worsening, appropriate vascular procedures should be performed.

If there is a slight LLD (less than 2 cm), monitoring of the evolution of the condition is recommended. In addition, the epiphysiodesis is based on an individual decision and often should not be the first procedure, as successful vascular techniques alone may succeed in obtaining a complete correction. However, in cases with an extreme LLD that is quickly worsening, the epiphysiodesis may be added to the vascular techniques. In other cases with a diffuse and difficult lesion to treat, an orthopedic procedure alone could be the solution.

Timing to apply the epiphysiodesis is another crucial point, as the decision is based on growth preview curves in order to find out the best age to perform that operation. A treatment strategy in patients with VM and LLD should always be discussed in a multidisciplinary approach, including a discussion between the vascular surgeon and orthopedic surgeon.

In our experience, our strategy is as follows:

1. In children:
   - If LLD is recognized for the first time, a complete diagnosis on CVM is performed.
   - If no CVM is found, the patient is sent to orthopedics for further evaluation and management.
   - If CVM is recognized, LLD is less than 2 cm, and the patient has no symptoms, a periodic monitoring of the condition by the limb length measure (e.g., bone scanogram) and duplex ultrasonographic assessment are performed, usually every 6 months. In case of progressive increase of LLD, with a difference over 2 cm, specific treatment of the CVM is considered. In case of simple capillary superficial disease, which sometimes may also create LLD, epiphysiodesis is proposed to the patient.
   - If a symptomatic CVM is diagnosed, the treatment on vascular malformations only is immediately proposed.
   - If LLD does not reduce slowly or even progresses after the surgery intervention of the lesions, epiphysiodesis is performed.
   - In case of significant LLD at the first evaluation (<3–4 cm), vascular surgery and epiphysiodesis are performed simultaneously or in two steps in a short time period.
   - In case of angio-osteo-hypotrophy, our preference is to perform only treatment of the venous malformations, with all available techniques. Epiphysiodesis in early childhood on the healthy limb may reduce the final height of the patient. By monitoring the evolution of LLD after removing CVM (often the difference remains stable), it can be considered to block bone growth on the contralateral healthy limb only in the late growing period (adolescence).
2. In adults:
   - Correction of the CVM is considered as the first step, in order to allow further orthopedic surgery to be performed in relatively CVM-free tissue.
   - After completion of the treatment of CVM, the patient is sent for orthopedic surgery.
   - Angio-osteo hypertrophy is best corrected by the elongation procedure of the contralateral limb, using Ilizarov technique or a similar technique. Results of this operation are excellent.
   - Angio-osteo-hypotrophy is a much more difficult issue, because the hypotrophic bone may not be strong enough to guarantee acceptable healing after the elongation. A precise evaluation of bone structure is required before deciding the procedure. The first step is the treatment of the vascular malformation in order to get a bone as much as possible free of surrounding, dysplastic venous tissue. In significant LLD, a contralateral osteotomy can be considered.

In conclusion, management of LLD in VM should follow precise guidelines and should always be performed in accordance with an orthopedic specialist. A single approach, vascular or orthopedic, should be avoided.

REFERENCES

1. Belov St. Correction of lower limbs length discrepancy in congenital vascular bone diseases by vascular surgery performed during childhood. *Semin Vasc Surg.* 1993;6(4):245–251.
2. Mattassi R, Vaghi M. Vascular bone syndrome— Angio-osteodystrophy: Current concepts. *Phlebology.* 2007;22(6):287–290.
3. Bouletreau PJ, Warren SP, Spector JA et al. Hypoxia and VEGF up-regulate BMP-2 mRNA and protein expression in microvascular endothelial cells: Implications for fracture healing. *Plast Reconstr Surg.* 2002; 109:2384–2397.
4. Zelzer E, McLean W, Ng YS et al. Skeletal defects in VEGF (120/120) mice reveal multiple roles of VEGF in skeletogenesis. *Development.* 2002;129:1893–1904.
5. Deckers MM, van Bezooijen LL, van der Horst G et al. Bone morphogenetic proteins stimulate angiogenesis through osteoblast-derived vascular endothelial growth factor. *Endocrinology.* 2002;143: 1545–1553.
6. Keppler-Noreuil KM, Sapp JC, Lindhurst MJ et al. Clinical delineation and natural history of the PIK3CA-related overgrowth spectrum. *Am J Med Genet A.* 2014;164A(7):1713–1733.
7. Belov St. Congenital agenesia of the deep veins of the lower extremities: Surgical treatment. *J Cardiovasc Surg.* 1972;13:594–598.
8. Mattassi R, Vaghi M. Management of the marginal vein: Current issues. *Phlebology.* 2007;22:283–286.

40

To what extent should anticoagulation therapy be considered for venous malformations?

ALFONSO TAFUR, EVI KALODIKI, AND JAWED FAREED

INTRODUCTION

Venous thromboembolism (VTE) is a frequent complication among patients with venous malformations (VMs), occurring in over 20% of patients with extensive vascular malformations.[1,2] There is evidence of increased likelihood of coagulopathy among patients with palpable phleboliths or extensive areas of VM.[3] Patients with VMs often have localized intravascular coagulopathy (LIC). This entity is characterized by decreased fibrinogen along with increased D-dimer.[3] Platelet counts, however, usually remain normal or only slightly decreased. These patients will often have pain, a higher likelihood of thrombosis, and a higher propensity to have major bleeding. Rarely, disseminated intravascular coagulopathy (DIC) may complicate the presentation of patients with extensive VM.[4] There is, however, a paucity of consensus regarding coagulopathy screening and management in patients with vascular malformations.

The International Union of Angiology Consensus on vascular malformations provides a grade 1B recommendation to test D-dimer during the assessment of a vascular malformation (strong recommendation based on moderate quality of evidence). This chapter considers prevention, treatment, and extended prophylactic strategies as well as special scenarios among these patients with vascular malformations.

Anticoagulation for primary venous thromboembolism prevention in patients with venous malformations

The Caprini risk score is a thrombosis prediction score for patients undergoing surgery.[5] For surgical patients, the American College of Chest Physicians (ACCP) chest guidelines suggest using the Caprini score to decide which patients will benefit from preventive pharmacological prophylaxis.[6] Anchored in this stratification system, patients over 40 years of age with VMs who will be undergoing major surgery are expected to have a high risk of thrombosis and can benefit from postsurgical prophylaxis continued for 1–2 weeks.[7] Moreover, depending on additional risk factors, patients may benefit from extending prophylaxis for a full month. For general surgery, the best validated agent for nonorthopedic surgery remains low-molecular-weight heparin (LMWH). One of the proposed strategies for primary prophylaxis in surgery specific to vascular malformation would be to use LMWH starting 10 days prior to surgery, as well as consolidating chemoprevention before and after the surgical intervention.[8]

Patients who have not had a defined thrombotic event but suffer severe pain due to recurrent phleboliths (which represent localized thrombosis) may have improved symptom management with anticoagulation.[9] When pain is associated with elevated D-dimer, as an expert suggestion, we advocate initiation of therapy with LMWH.[3,10] Although limited, there is emerging data of efficacy of direct oral anticoagulants in improving the D-dimer and fibrinogen levels in patients with LIC, in the setting of low-flow vascular malformations.[11,12]

Hospital admission is also considered an opportunity for primary prevention in patients with VMs. The evidence for pharmacoprophylaxis in inpatient settings stems predominantly from three clinical trials of prophylaxis compared to placebo; the median duration of VTE prophylaxis administered during the studies was 7–14 days.[13–15] The eligibility criteria for all three trials included an age criterion, various definitions of degree of immobilization, and clinical criteria such as congestive heart failure (CHF) New York Heart Association (NYHA) class III/IV, acute respiratory illness, acute infection, acute rheumatic disorder, or inflamed bowel if at least one additional risk factor for VTE was present. The management of VMs in a hospitalized patient should be considered based on positive results of these studies and as the opportunity for prevention.

Anticoagulation in treatment of patients with VMs and VTE

A full review of anticoagulation in acute VTE is beyond the scope of this chapter. However, LMWH is the main pharmacological tool to treat patients with VMs and acute VTE. Conventionally, this will be followed by oral anticoagulation. Treatment with direct oral anticoagulants has been documented in the care of patients with VTE and VMs.[12,16,17] The use of vitamin K antagonist with proper anticoagulation bridging until international normalized ratio (INR) levels are therapeutic remains an option. However, note that among patients with an underlying coagulopathy, the INR levels may be misleading.[18] Thus, warfarin failure in the treatment of LIC is a recognized problem for patients with VMs.[19]

Extended prophylaxis

The value and recommendation of extended prophylaxis among patients with a history of VTE are anchored on the management of persistent risk factors. The nomenclature of provoked versus unprovoked events may be found misleading in patients with persistent risk factors.[20] Thus, the treating physician should discuss the potential value of extended therapy among patients with a prior VTE and persistent VM. Moreover, with the advent of low-dose direct oral anticoagulants, the therapeutic margin has been extended. In a trial of 2,486 patients with a first VTE who had completed 6–12 months of anticoagulation, the patients randomized to a low dose of apixaban of 2.5 mg two times a day had a rate of major bleeding comparable with that of placebo (difference of 0.2 percentage points; 95% confidence interval [CI], −0.3 to 0.8) and a relative risk of VTE recurrence no different than that of full-dose therapy (0.36 95% CI 0.25–0.53).[8] Similarly, results are also seen in a comparable 3,365-patient trial with rivaroxaban at a dose of 10 mg daily, compared to aspirin or to a rivaroxaban 20 mg once-daily dose. Notably, the authors did not exclude patients with a "provoked" event, yet the rates of recurrence were decreased with anticoagulation in this group as well, compared to aspirin. The rate of bleeding in patients with a 10 mg daily dosage of rivaroxaban was no different than that of aspirin (hazard ratio 1.6 95% CI 0.4–6.8).[21] Although there is neither a specific guideline nor a randomized trial specific to patients with VM and prior VTE, this practice is advocated in expert opinion.[9] Moreover, it is likely to be better accepted by patients relative to daily LMWH injections.

Considerations in patients with marginal vein

The marginal vein (MV) is a VM characterized by the absence of valves (avalvulia), and it can coexist with other vascular malformations in patients with Klippel–Trenaunay syndrome (KTS). The MV is associated with a high likelihood of VTE, as illustrated in numerous reports of fatal pulmonary embolisms. The MV runs in the lateral aspect of a leg, very superficially, and can be often mistaken as a varicose vein. The MV should be suspected when on a clinical exam a port-wine stain is seen adjacent to a large superficial lateral varicosity. Limb length discrepancy should also lead to the suspicion of this vascular malformation.

The MV, as an embryonic remnant, lacks maturity and also has deficient smooth muscle layers. Coupled with avalvulosis, these abnormalities cause patients to have severe venous stasis. While stasis and potential injury can lead to thrombosis, the absence of valves is plausibly another explanation for the prothrombotic state. The endothelial cells have a remarkable heterogeneity depending on the location; the valvular microenviroment plays a role in thromboresistance via lower expression of von Willebrand factor relative to lumen endothelium.[22–24]

Given a strong propensity toward thrombosis, anticoagulation is advocated as part of the management for the MV. Specifically, LMWH is usually recommended in the literature.[25]

The strong recommendation for primary anticoagulation is further stressed for those who have a hypoplastic or an absent iliofemoral venous system, which makes the MV the primary outflow system of the lower extremity.[8] Please refer to Chapter 83 for special consideration in KTS.

REFERENCES

1. Baskerville PA, Ackroyd JS, Lea Thomas M et al. The Klippel–Trenaunay syndrome: Clinical, radiological and haemodynamic features and management. *Br J Surg*. 1985;72(3):232–236.
2. Oduber CE, van Beers EJ, Bresser P et al. Venous thromboembolism and prothrombotic parameters in Klippel–Trenaunay syndrome. *Neth J Med*. 2013; 71(5):246–252.
3. Dompmartin A, Acher A, Thibon P et al. Association of localized intravascular coagulopathy with venous malformations. *Arch Dermatol*. 2008;144(7):873–877.
4. Zhuo K, Russell S, Wargon O et al. Disseminated intravascular coagulopathy in a child with extensive venous malformations. *J Paediatr Child Health*. 2017;53(3):320–321
5. Golemi I, Salazar-Adum J, Tafru A et al. Venous thromboembolism prophylaxis using the Caprini score. *Dis Mon*. 2019;65(8):249–298.
6. Gould MK, Garcia D, Wren S et al. Prevention of VTE in nonorthopedic surgical patients: Antithrombotic Therapy and Prevention of Thrombosis, 9th ed: American College of Chest Physicians Evidence-Based Clinical Practice Guidelines. *Chest*. 2012;141(2 Suppl):e227S–e277S.
7. Caprini J, Arcelus JI, Tafur A. Venous thromboembolic disease: Mechanical and pharmacologic prophylaxis. In: Sidawy A, Perler BA, eds. *Rutherford's Vascular Surgery and Endovascular Therapy*. 9th ed. Philadelphia, PA: Elsevier; 2019:1927–1935.

8. Agnelli G, Buller H, Cohen A et al. Apixaban for extended treatment of venous thromboembolism. *N Engl J Med.* 2013;368(8):699–708.

9. Lee BB, Antignani P, Baraldini V et al. ISVI-IUA consensus document diagnostic guidelines of vascular anomalies: Vascular malformations and hemangiomas. *Int Angiol.* 2015;34(4):333–374.

10. Dompmartin A, Ballieuw F, Thibon P et al. Elevated D-dimer level in the differential diagnosis of venous malformations. *Arch Dermatol.* 2009;145(11):1239–1244.

11. Mack JM, Richter GT, Crary SE. Effectiveness and safety of treatment with direct oral anticoagulant rivaroxaban in patients with slow-flow vascular malformations: A case series. *Lymphat Res Biol.* 2018;16(3):278–281.

12. Vandenbriele C, Vanassche T, Peetermans M et al. Rivaroxaban for the treatment of consumptive coagulopathy associated with a vascular malformation. *J Thromb Thrombolysis.* 2014;38(1):121–123.

13. Samama MM, Cohen AT, Darmon JY et al. A comparison of enoxaparin with placebo for the prevention of venous thromboembolism in acutely ill medical patients. Prophylaxis in medical patients with Enoxaparin Study Group. *N Engl J Med.* 1999;341(11):793–800.

14. Leizorovicz A, Cohen AT, Turpie AG et al. Randomized, placebo-controlled trial of dalteparin for the prevention of venous thromboembolism in acutely ill medical patients. *Circulation.* 2004;110(7):874–879.

15. Cohen AT, Davidson BL, Gallus AS et al. Efficacy and safety of fondaparinux for the prevention of venous thromboembolism in older acute medical patients: Randomised placebo controlled trial. *BMJ.* 2006;332(7537):325–329.

16. Yasumoto A, Ishiura R, Narushima M et al. Successful treatment with dabigatran for consumptive coagulopathy associated with extensive vascular malformations. *Blood Coagul Fibrinolysis.* 2017;28(8):670–674.

17. Ardillon L, Lambert C, Eeckhoudt S et al. Dabigatran etexilate versus low-molecular weight heparin to control consumptive coagulopathy secondary to diffuse venous vascular malformations. *Blood Coagul Fibrinolysis.* 2016;27(2):216–219.

18. Baumann Kreuziger LM, Datta YH, Johnson AD et al. Monitoring anticoagulation in patients with an unreliable prothrombin time/international normalized ratio: Factor II versus chromogenic factor X testing. *Blood Coagul Fibrinolysis.* 2014;25(3):232–236.

19. Mazoyer E, Enjolras O, Laurian C et al. Coagulation abnormalities associated with extensive venous malformations of the limbs: Differentiation from Kasabach–Merritt syndrome. *Clin Lab Haematol.* 2002;24(4):243–251.

20. Albertsen IE, Piazza G, Goldhaber SZ. Let's stop dichotomizing venous thromboembolism as provoked or unprovoked. *Circulation.* 2018;138(23): 2591–2593.

21. Weitz JI, Lensing A, Prins MH et al. Rivaroxaban or aspirin for extended treatment of venous thromboembolism. *N Engl J Med.* 2017;376(13):1211–1222.

22. Brooks EG, Trotman W, Wadsworth MP et al. Valves of the deep venous system: An overlooked risk factor. *Blood.* 2009;114(6):1276–1279.

23. Aird WC. Phenotypic heterogeneity of the endothelium: II. Representative vascular beds. *Circ Res.* 2007; 100(2):174–190.

24. Aird WC. Phenotypic heterogeneity of the endothelium: I. Structure, function, and mechanisms. *Circ Res.* 2007;100(2):158–173.

25. Lee BB. Marginal vein is not a varicose vein; it is a venous malformation. *Veins Lymphatics.* 2014;3:4050.

41

How to approach treatment of marginal vein combined with deep vein hypoplasia/aplasia?

DIRK A. LOOSE

The marginal vein, in the settings of a fully developed and patent deep venous system, should be treated in early childhood, e.g., by endoluminal laser ablation or by surgery. A sclerotreatment should not be performed due to a high risk of a potentially fatal pulmonary embolism. Also, a stripping technique should be avoided because this vein has many smaller arteriovenous (AV) fistulas, which cause a significant risk for bleeding. In the setting of the hypoplastic deep venous system, the marginal vein should be resected in stages so that the hypoplastic venous system can adapt slowly to the newly increasing venous backflow. A third anatomical and clinical scenario is the marginal vein in the setting of an absent (aplastic) deep venous system. In this scenario, the lateral marginal vein is called the *embryonic vein*, and it is the only draining vein of the affected extremity. This vein has no valves and is characterized by coexisting AV fistulas, which together provide the anatomical and hemodynamic environment for significant venous hypertension. For this reason, AV fistulas have to be ligated surgically in early childhood in a staged surgical fashion to significantly minimize the risk for venous hypertension and its associated symptoms.

The initial diagnostic step in evaluation of the marginal veins is performed by color duplex ultrasonography, which involves the acquisition of imaging of the entire venous drainage of the legs and, in particular, the clear and precise determination of whether a functional deep vein system is present or not.

The marginal vein (see Figures 41.1 and 41.2) is an atypical vein originating from the late embryonic period. It usually runs on the outside of the leg. A deep principal vein can be hypoplastic, but it is present.

In the embryonic phase, venous flow takes place through two embryonic vessels: the marginal vein and the sciatic vein. Both veins form early in gestation and represent primordial forms of veins that will differentiate into the mature venous system of the lower extremities. Sometimes, however, the marginal vein remains as an atypical valveless

and malformed vessel (Figure 41.3). This can lead to various disorders of venous drainage, causing discomfort due to venous hypertension, as mentioned previously.

If a treatment plan is to be developed, the exact phlebography recording of the entire vein system, the marginal vein itself, and its inflow and outflow is indispensable. The deep venous system is often difficult to visualize in imaging because of predominant flow in the superficial malformed veins. After removal of the lateral marginal vein, the deep venous system dilates, adapts, and is more easily seen radiographically.

Four different types of the marginal vein can be differentiated, as demonstrated in Figure 41.4.

The persistent marginal vein has many atypical connections to the deep veins, causing thromboembolism (estimated incidence of 4%–24%), and it always has small AV fistulas.[1-3]

Surgical resection or endovascular laser ablation of this vein is recommended in early childhood to remove any significant congestion symptoms. Often, the marginal vein is the cause of a difference in the lengths of the legs in children (Figure 41.5).

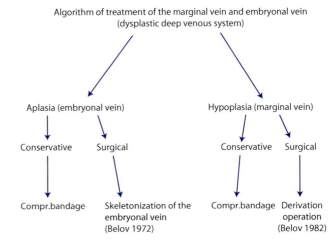

Figure 41.1 Algorithm of treatment of the marginal vein and embryonic vein with dysplastic deep venous system.

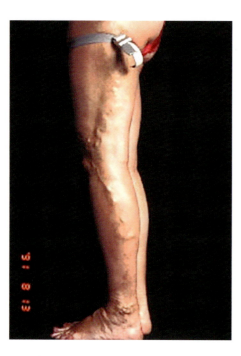

Figure 41.2 Clinical appearance of a marginal vein at the lateral part of the leg.

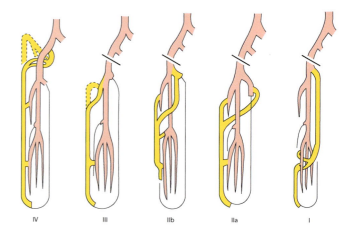

Figure 41.4 Persisting marginal vein. Segment and drainage types according to Weber and Daffinger (1995). (I) Lower leg type with anterior arch vein drainage to the saphenous vein. (IIa) Lower leg-knee type with main drainage via the posterior thigh circumflex vein. (IIb) Lower leg-knee-thigh type with main drainage via the anterior thigh circumflex vein. (III) Lower leg and thigh type with drainage to a "higher" deep femoral vein. (IV) Lower leg and thigh trunk with drainage to the lower, superior gluteal veins.

An early operative removal in childhood of the marginal vein and its associated AV fistulas can lead to a length compensation of the legs' size discrepancy over the years.[4-7]

A special type of a marginal vein is the *embryonic vein* (Figure 41.6). There is no other draining vein besides this marginal vein: the deep vein system is undeveloped and completely absent (Figure 41.7), and the venous drainage of the leg runs via this large embryonic vein only. This vein is functioning as a compensating collateral vein that runs via

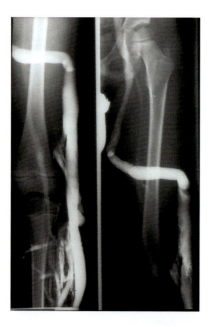

Figure 41.3 Phlebographic documentation of a marginal vein type III according to Weber and Daffinger (1995) (see Figure 41.4).

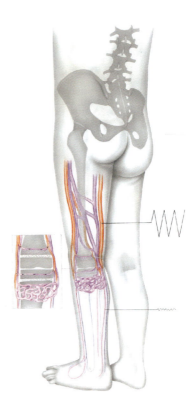

Figure 41.5 Pathophysiology of vascular bone syndrome: in the bone growth zones of the tibial bone, very small arteriovenous communications are caused by the venous hypertension, and they lead to a hypoxia in this zone. Thus, the osteoblasts are stimulated, and increased length growth is the consequence. The arterial pressure proximal to the zone with arteriovenous communications is high, and distally it is low.

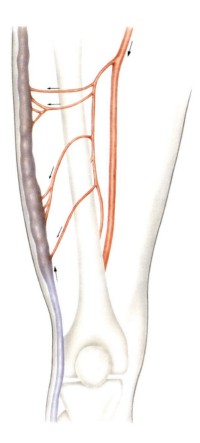

Figure 41.6 Embryonic vein and missing principal superficial femoral vein. Multiple arteriovenous communications—fistulas.

the suprapubic region to the contralateral pelvic veins. This is why this vein should never be removed. The embryonic vein has numerous AV fistulas (Figures 41.6 and 41.8). These are short circuits between arteries and veins, which lead to a pronounced venous hypertension and consequently to significant enlargements of venous segments (venous aneurysm [Figures 41.9 and 41.10]) of the embryonic vein.

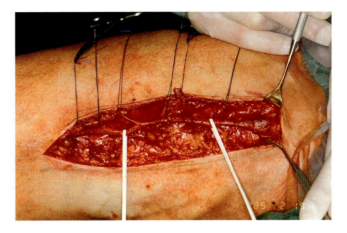

Figure 41.8 Documentation of AV fistulas at the embryonic vein before skeletonization procedure according to Belov.[3]

The additional influx from the arteries into the completely valveless and dysplastic embryonic vein results in venous hypertension with corresponding significant congestion symptoms. In order to reduce this hypertension, the operation of embryonic vein by skeletonization according to Belov[3] is indicated (Figure 41.11). During this procedure, all AV fistulas are surgically interrupted so that the venous pressure can be decisively reduced. The embryonic vein must of course be absolutely preserved.[8–11]

The opinion that one can easily remove any marginal vein or embryonic vein (regardless of the nomenclature) because "there are still some collateral veins somewhere," is completely wrong and absolutely contraindicated. This results from the previously mentioned remarks and also from findings of other studies.[12] In a case report, a patient with the marginal vein was treated by above-the-knee amputation of the affected lower extremity, which potentially could have been avoided if a diagnostic algorithm as the one outlined in this chapter was followed.

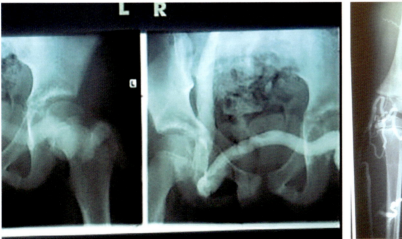
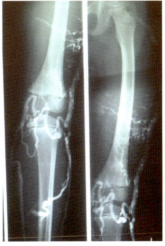

Figure 41.7 Phlebographic imaging of an embryonic vein in the left leg with suprapubic collateralization to the right pelvic veins. No principal veins.

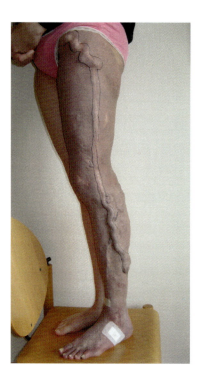

Figure 41.9 Clinical aspect of an embryonic vein 16 years after skeletonization procedure.

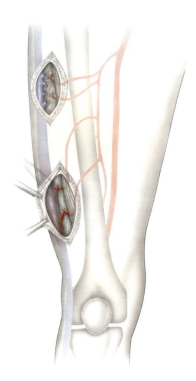

Figure 41.11 Embryonic vein: Surgical elimination of all AV fistulas: skeletonization procedure according to Belov on preservation of the embryonic vein.[3] Technique for elimination of venous hypertension in the embryonic vein.

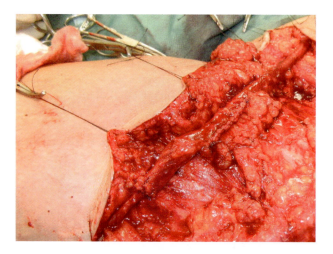

Figure 41.10 Embryonic vein after resection of multiple venous aneurysms 16 years after first treatment of the embryonic vein by skeletonization procedure.

REFERENCES

1. Soltész L. A végtagok veleszületett arterio-venosus sipolya. *Diss Budapest* 1963.
2. Soltész L, Solti F, Gloviczki P, Szlavi L, Entz L. Limb circulation in varicosity of various types. *Acta Med Acad Scien Hun.* 1982;39(1–2):63–67.
3. Belov St. Congenital agenesis of the deep veins of the lower extremity: Surgical treatment. *J Cardiovasc Surg.* 1972;13:594–598.
4. Loose DA, Funck I. Angeborene Venenfehler-Diagnostische und therapeutische Möglichkeiten. *Akt Chir.* 1995;30:329–340.
5. Belov St. Correction of lower limb length discrepancy in congenital vascular-bone disease by vascular surgery performed during childhood. *Semin Vasc Surg.* 1993;6(49):245–251.
6. Belov St. *Vascular Malformations—Diagnosis and Surgical Treatment.* Sofia, Medicina I fizkultura, 1982.
7. Hauert J, Loose DA. Orthopedic problems. In: Mattassi R, Loose DA, Vaghi M, eds. *Hemangiomas and Vascular Malformations.* 2nd ed. Milan, Italy: Springer; 2015:369–378.
8. Rathore A, Gloviczki P, Bjarnason H. Management of giant embryonic vein in Klippel–Trenaunay syndrome. *J Vasc Surg Venous Lymphat Disord.* 2018;(4): 523–525.
9. Greene AK. *Vascular Anomalies. Classification, Diagnosis and Management.* St. Louis, MO: Quality Medical Publishing; 2013.
10. Diehl S, Bruno R, Wikinson GA et al. Altered expression patterns of EphrinB2 and EphB2 in human umbilical vessels and congenital venous malformations. *Pediatr Res.* 2005;57(4):537–544.
11. Weber J, Daffinger H. Congenital vascular malformations; the persistence of marginal and embryonic veins. *VASA.* 2006;35(2):67–77.
12. Abdul-Rahman NR, Mohammed KF, Ibrahim S. Gigantism of the lower lateral marginal vein in KTS: Anatomy of the lateral marginal vein. *Singapore Med J.* 2009;50(6):e223–e225.

42

Indications for amputation in patients with extensive venous malformations

DIRK A. LOOSE

In the literature and from our experience, there are very seldom indications for an amputation in patients with venous malformations or in combined forms. However, very special indications for amputations have been shown. We have been able to differentiate between three indication groups: (a) sepsis, (b) bleeding, and (c) nonfunctioning (no stress possible, no movement, persistent pain).

It is important that indications for amputation in groups (a) and (b) are provided by a physician, while indications in group (c) primarily come from the patient, but in cooperation with the attending physician.

For every group, a clinical example is demonstrated.

Since the indications for an amputation in venous malformation are always very difficult and rare, there are only anecdotal reports in the literature. In their book, Browse et al.[1] report only occasional toe amputations: "because it enables the patient to wear a shoe of a normal size and to walk properly." Also emergency digital amputations are reported.[2] Some authors[3] are more aggressive in the indication for "amputation or synovectomy in knee arthropathy in patients with vascular malformations" (Klippel–Trenaunay syndrome). Belov et al.[4] published a case of a 7-year-old boy requiring an emergency amputation to save him from life-threatening bleeding. The same indication was met in a septic giant venous malformation complicated by bleeding.[5]

In our experience, three indication groups have formed due to the need for amputation in extra-truncular venous and hemolymphatic malformations:

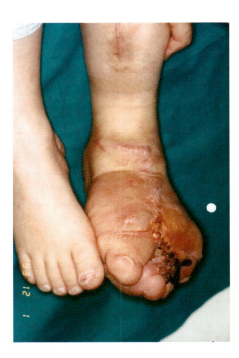

Figure 42.1 Hemolymphatic malformation of the left foot, acute septic, life-threatening situation originating in the foot (8-year-old girl).

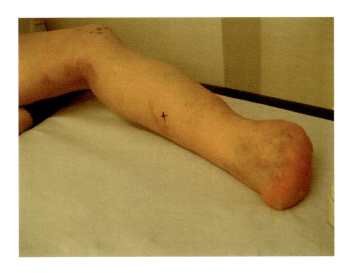

Figure 42.2 A Pirogoff amputation was performed.

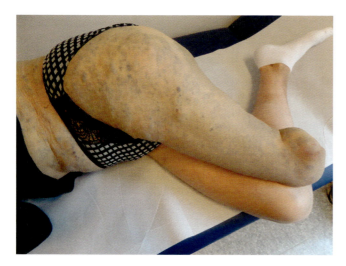

Figure 42.3 Situation after a knee joint exarticulation at the age of 12 years, when a life-threatening bleeding and a fracture of the tibial plateau occurred.

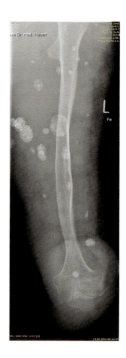

Figure 42.4 Same case as Figure 42.3. X-ray of the femoral bone with multiple phleboliths.

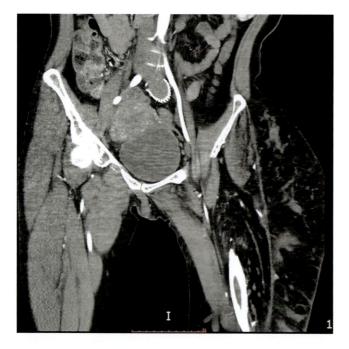

Figure 42.5 Magnetic resonance imaging of a young lady's pelvic region demonstrating an extensive venous malformation at the left thigh region. Situation after knee joint exarticulation after life-threatening bleeding at the age of 12 years.

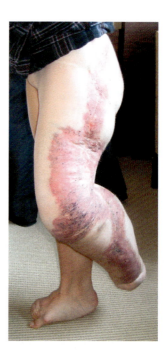

Figure 42.6 (Group c): 13-year-old girl with hemolymphatic malformation and after left foot amputation, contracture at the left knee joint, heavy congestion and rest pain at the left leg.

a. Uncontrollable septic disease (Figures 42.1 and 42.2)
b. Uncontrollable, life-threatening venous bleeding (Figures 42.3 through 42.5)
c. Functionless, useless, obstructive, painful limb (Figures 42.6 through 42.8)

In each group, we documented two (group a) to three (groups b and c) patients through the figures.

In groups (a) and (b), the indications are provided by the attending physicians.

Each patient of group (c) had a very long history, with more than 30 surgical procedures each. They requested an amputation or knee joint disarticulation because there was no other therapeutic alternative to ameliorating their situation and improving their quality of life.

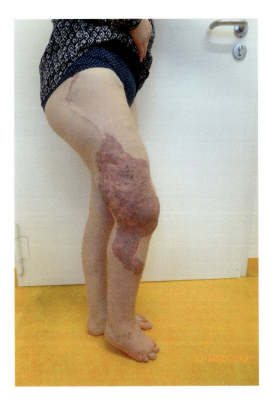

Figure 42.7 (Group c): 18-year-old girl, venous malformation of the right leg, several spontaneous fractures of the thigh and the tibial plateau as well as of the hip joint, femoral head necrosis, chronic luxation of the hip joint, chronic pain syndrome.

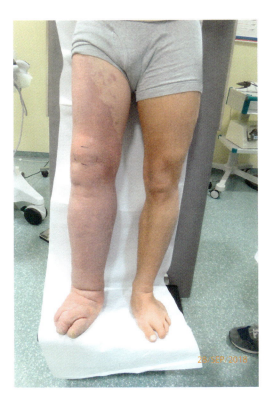

Figure 42.8 (Group c): Hemolymphatic malformation of the right leg with bone involvement, chronic erysipelas with many intensive care treatments since 20 years of age.

In rare emergencies, but also in elective, very selected cases, amputation may well be a proper therapeutic option, especially from the patient's perspective (see group c).

REFERENCES

1. Browse NL, Burnand KG, Irvine AT, Wilson NM. *Diseases of the Veins*. London, UK: Arnold Publisher; 1999:685. Einhorn Presse Verlag, Reinbek 1985.
2. Carlson B, Jones NF. Radical resection of a massive venous malformation of the thumb and immediate reconstruction with a microsurgical toe transfer. *J Hand Surg Am*. 2007;32(10):1587–1591.
3. Johnson JN, Shaughnessy WJ, Stans AA et al. Management of knee arthropathy in patients with vascular malformations. *J Pediatr Orthop*. 2009; 29(4):380–384.
4. Belov ST, Loose DA, Müller E. *Angeborene Gefäßfehler*. Reinbek, Germany: Einhorn Presse Verlag; 1985.
5. Tomita K, Watanabe E, Sadahiro T et al. Septic shock due to infected giant venous malformation complicated by massive bleeding. *Acute Med Surg*. 2016; 3(3):279–282.

43

How much pharmacological therapy can be incorporated in venous malformations management?

FRANCINE BLEI

This is a very relevant question, as pharmacological therapy holds promise for the treatment of patients with vascular malformations. Sclerotherapy and surgical procedures have been the mainstay of treatment for these disorders. Previous pharmacological agents were limited to anticoagulants, pain medications, and antibiotics. However, in conjunction with the identification of causative genetic mutations, inhibitors targeting the associated signaling pathways (including tyrosine kinase receptors, RAS/MAPK, and others) are becoming part of the multidisciplinary management of patients with vascular and lymphatic malformations. Phase I and II studies are being performed, and clinical trials are underway, to establish treatment protocols.

At this time, there are reports citing treatment with sirolimus/everolimus, miransertib (ARQ 092), alpelisib BYL719, taselisib, octreotide, brimonidine 0.33% gel, sildenafil, topical timolol maleate, propranolol, tetracycline derivatives, doxycycline, statins, bevacizumab/ranibizumab, thalidomide/pomalidomide, pazopanib, in patients with vascular malformations. As previously noted, the rationale for many of these therapies derives from the identification of somatic or genomic mutations in these disorders, with subsequent elucidation of the biological pathways. Targeted therapies are now a reality (Figure 43.1).

The first report documenting the efficacy of sirolimus in six patients with a range of vascular diagnoses[1] showed promise and was followed by a phase II trial of 61 patients treated for 6 months, demonstrating overall safety and efficacy during the duration of the study.[2] Previously, sirolimus had been shown to be promising for angiomyolipomas in patients with tuberous sclerosis complex or lymphangioleiomyomatosis.[3] Upregulation of mTor in vascular malformations had also been reported.[4] Thus, there was rationale for mTor inhibition in patients with vascular malformations. Boscolo et al. showed *in vitro* as well as clinical

efficacy of sirolimus for slow-flow vascular malformations.[5] Subsequently, a phase II study of 19 patients recalcitrant to prior therapies, treated for 12 months with sirolimus exhibited improved pain scores and D-dimer elevation over the course of treatment.[6]

Subsequent studies demonstrated effectiveness of sirolimus in many other *PIK3CA*-related disorders: generalized lymphatic anomaly, Gorham–Stout disease, blue rubber bleb nevus syndrome, fibroadipose vascular anomaly, kaposiform hemangioendothelioma, tufted angioma, lymphangioleiomyomatosis, and venous and lymphatic malformations.[5–13] The medication is generally well tolerated; however, there is an age-dependent drug clearance (due to differences in CYP3A metabolism and other factors); thus, dosing must be appropriately modified for infants and young children.[14–16] Appropriate patient/parent education and monitoring (sirolimus trough levels, adverse events, laboratory parameters) are required. Cases of pneumocystis pneumonia (due to the immunosuppressive effects of sirolimus) have been reported; many practitioners therefore recommend prophylactic antibiotics to prevent this infection.[17,18]

Biesecker et al., who identified a somatic activating mutation in *AKT1*, c.49G>A, pGlu17Lys, as causative of Proteus syndrome, later demonstrated suppression of AKT signaling by miransertib (ARQ 092) in cells and tissues from Proteus syndrome patients.[19] A recent publication by that group showed effectiveness of miransertib in six patients with Proteus syndrome. In this study, the primary endpoint was a 50% reduction of AKT phosphorylation in tissues from biopsies of treated patients.[20]

Venot and Canaud and colleagues published a promising study revealing the effectiveness of BYL719 (alpelisib) in 19 patients with *PIK3CA*-related overgrowth syndrome (PROS).[21] The authors studied a mouse model representative of CLOVES syndrome and showed that BYL719 prevented

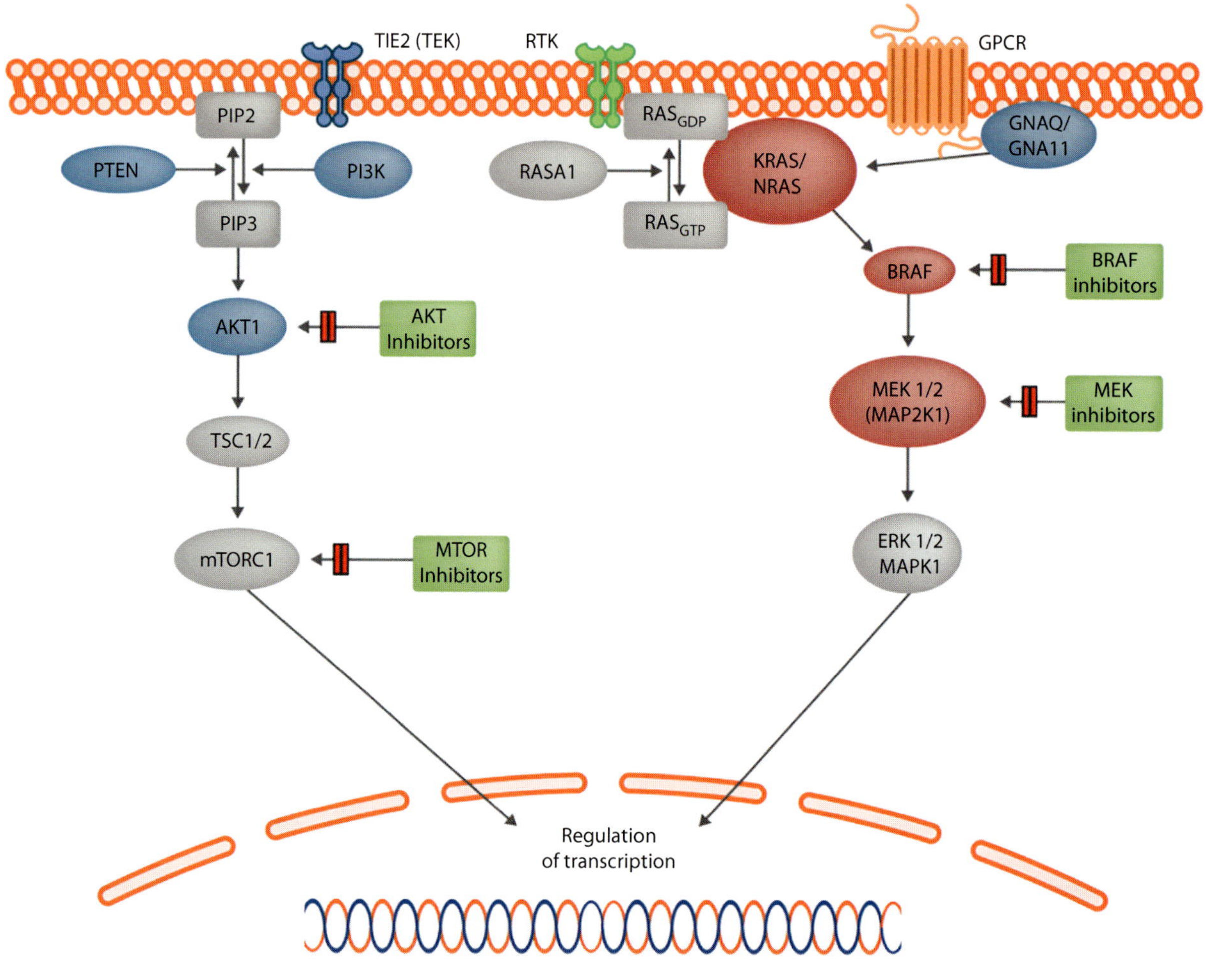

Figure 43.1 PI3K/AKT/MTOR and RAS/RAF/MEK/ERK signaling pathways in which genetic (somatic or genomic) mutations have been identified in patients with anomalies. (GPCR, G protein–coupled receptor; RTK, receptor tyrosine kinase.)

progression of the disease. Likewise, in the clinical trial, patients experienced improvement in overgrowth, vascular malformations, and other symptoms.

Al-Olabi and Kinsler et al. studied tissue samples from 160 patients with sporadic vascular malformations and identified mosaic activating genes in the RAS/MAPK pathway (*KRAS, NRAS, BRAF,* and *MAP2K1*). They found many high-flow lesions with these mutations, suggesting new pharmacological therapies for arteriovenous malformations may be identified.[22]

Hereditary hemorrhagic telangiectasia has been well studied, and several medical therapies have been proposed. Topical or systemic agents to prevent epistaxis and other sites of bleeding include thalidomide/pomalidomide, bevacizumab/ranibizumab, pazopanib, doxycycline (NCT03397004), propranolol, timolol, and other agents[23–25] (https://clinicaltrials.gov/ct2/results?cond=hht&term=&cntry=&state=&city=&dist=).

Further studies are necessary to establish appropriate dosing, define therapeutic endpoints, and monitor for long-term effects. Despite the array of medical therapies that are and will be available, interdisciplinary management with surgical and endovascular procedures will likely complement the medical interventions.

REFERENCES

1. Hammill AM, Wentzel M, Gupta A et al. Sirolimus for the treatment of complicated vascular anomalies in children. *Pediatr Blood Cancer.* 2011;57(6):1018–1024.
2. Adams DM, Trenor CC 3rd, Hammill AM et al. Efficacy and safety of sirolimus in the treatment of complicated vascular anomalies. *Pediatrics.* 2016;137(2):e20153257.
3. Bissler JJ, McCormack FX, Young LR et al. Sirolimus for angiomyolipoma in tuberous sclerosis complex or lymphangioleiomyomatosis. *N Engl J Med.* 2008;358(2):140–151.
4. Shirazi F, Cohen C, Fried L et al. Mammalian target of rapamycin (mTOR) is activated in cutaneous vascular malformations *in vivo. Lymphat Res Biol.* 2007; 5(4):233–236.
5. Boscolo E, Limaye N, Huang L et al. Rapamycin improves TIE2-mutated venous malformation in murine model and human subjects. *J Clin Invest.* 2015; 125(9):3491–3504.
6. Hammer J, Seront E, Duez S et al. Sirolimus is efficacious in treatment for extensive and/or complex slow-flow vascular malformations: A monocentric prospective phase II study. *Orphanet J Rare Dis.* 2018;13(1):191.

7. Ricci KW, Hammill AM, Mobberley-Schuman P et al. Efficacy of systemic sirolimus in the treatment of generalized lymphatic anomaly and Gorham–Stout disease. *Pediatr Blood Cancer.* 2019;66(5):e27614.

8. Yuksekkaya H, Ozbek O, Keser M et al. Blue rubber bleb nevus syndrome: Successful treatment with sirolimus. *Pediatrics.* 2012;129(4):e1080–e1084.

9. Unlusoy Aksu A, Sari S, Egritas Gurkan O et al. Favorable response to sirolimus in a child with blue rubber bleb nevus syndrome in the gastrointestinal tract. *J Pediatr Hematol Oncol.* 2017;39(2):147–149.

10. Erickson J, McAuliffe W, Blennerhassett L et al. Fibroadipose vascular anomaly treated with sirolimus: Successful outcome in two patients. *Pediatr Dermatol.* 2017;34(6):e317–e320.

11. Wang H, Guo X, Duan Y et al. Sirolimus as initial therapy for kaposiform hemangioendothelioma and tufted angioma. *Pediatr Dermatol.* 2018;35(5):635–638.

12. El-Chemaly S, Taveira-Dasilva A, Goldberg HJ et al. Sirolimus and autophagy inhibition in lymphangioleiomyomatosis: Results of a phase I clinical trial. *Chest.* 2017;151(6):1302–1310.

13. Strychowsky JE, Rahbar R, O'Hare MJ et al. Sirolimus as treatment for 19 patients with refractory cervicofacial lymphatic malformation. *Laryngoscope.* 2018;128(1):269–276.

14. Emoto C, Fukuda T, Mizuno T et al. Characterizing the developmental trajectory of sirolimus clearance in neonates and infants. *CPT Pharmacometrics Syst Pharmacol.* 2016;5(8):411–417.

15. Mizuno T, Emoto C, Fukuda T et al. Model-based precision dosing of sirolimus in pediatric patients with vascular anomalies. *Eur J Pharm Sci.* 2017;109S:S124–S131.

16. Mizuno T, Fukuda T, Emoto C et al. Developmental pharmacokinetics of sirolimus: Implications for precision dosing in neonates and infants with complicated vascular anomalies. *Pediatr Blood Cancer.* 2017;64(8).

17. Ying H, Qiao C, Yang X et al. A case report of 2 sirolimus-related deaths among infants with kaposiform hemangioendotheliomas. *Pediatrics.* 2018;141(Suppl 5):S425–S429.

18. Russell TB, Rinker EK, Dillingham CS et al. *Pneumocystis jirovecii* pneumonia during sirolimus therapy for kaposiform hemangioendothelioma. *Pediatrics.* 2018;141(Suppl 5):S421–S424.

19. Lindhurst MJ, Yourick MR, Yu Y et al. Repression of AKT signaling by ARQ 092 in cells and tissues from patients with Proteus syndrome. *Sci Rep.* 2015;5:17162.

20. Keppler-Noreuil KM, Sapp JC, Lindhurst MJ et al. Pharmacodynamic study of miransertib in individuals with Proteus syndrome. *Am J Hum Genet.* 2019;104(3):484–491.

21. Venot Q, Blanc T, Rabia SH et al. Targeted therapy in patients with *PIK3CA*-related overgrowth syndrome. *Nature.* 2018;558(7711):540–546.

22. Al-Olabi L, Polubothu S, Dowsett K et al. Mosaic RAS/MAPK variants cause sporadic vascular malformations which respond to targeted therapy. *J Clin Invest.* 2018;128(4):1496–1508.

23. Harrison L, Kundra A, Jervis P. The use of thalidomide therapy for refractory epistaxis in hereditary haemorrhagic telangiectasia: Systematic review. *J Laryngol Otol.* 2018;132(10):866–871.

24. Faughnan ME, Gossage JR, Chakinala MM et al. Pazopanib may reduce bleeding in hereditary hemorrhagic telangiectasia. *Angiogenesis.* 2019;22(1):145–155.

25. Kini SD, Yiu DW, Weisberg RA et al. Bevacizumab as treatment for epistaxis in hereditary hemorrhagic telangiectasia: A literature review. *Ann Otol Rhinol Laryngol.* 2019;128(5):467–471.

Lymphatic Malformations

Definition and Classification

44

Confusion on terminology: Primary lymphedema and lymphangioma (lymphatic malformation)

JAMES LAREDO AND BYUNG-BOONG LEE

INTRODUCTION

Primary lymphedema may be classified as a lymphatic malformation (LM) that develops during the late stages of lymphangiogenesis, ultimately resulting in hypoplasia, hyperplasia, or aplasia of lymph vessels.[1-3] Like all congenital vascular malformations (CVMs), LMs are further classified into two subgroups based on the embryological stage in which the developmental defect occurs. "Extra-truncular" lesions develop at an early stage of embryogenesis, and "truncular" lesions arise at a later stage. Truncular LM lesions produce primary lymphedema, and extra-truncular LM lesions produce lymphangiomas.[1,4] These two distinct LMs arising from different embryological stages may occur together and are often mistakenly identified as two different and unrelated disease entities.

EXTRA-TRUNCULAR LYMPHATIC MALFORMATION LESIONS

Extra-truncular lesions are the result of persistent, premature, embryonic tissue that fails to involute during the early reticular stage of lymphangiogenesis.[5,6] The cystic hygroma and cavernous lymphangioma are remnants of embryonic tissue that developed before the lymphatic and vascular trunks were formed. The extra-truncular LM may also be described as a pretruncal embryonic lesion.[1] Extra-truncular lesions maintain the unique embryonic characteristics of the mesenchymal cells with the potential to proliferate when provoked or stimulated by various conditions such as trauma, menarche, pregnancy, surgery, or hormonal changes. These lesions persist and are present throughout adult life and continue to grow.

Extra-truncular lesions present as diffuse infiltrating lesions without connections to the normal lymph conducting pathways and produce mechanical pressure on surrounding tissues and organs, including nerves and muscles (e.g., cystic hygroma).

TRUNCULAR LYMPHATIC MALFORMATION LESIONS

Truncular lesions are the result of developmental arrest that occurs in the later stage of embryogenesis during the formation of lymphatic trunks, vessels, and nodes long after the reticular stage of vascular development.[1,5,6] The truncular LM may also be described as a post-truncal embryonic lesion.[1] Truncular lesions no longer have the potential to proliferate with no risk of recurrence and have significant lymphodynamic effects on the lymph-transport system as a result of incomplete development of the axial or truncal lymphatic vessels. Lymphatic vessel aplasia, hypoplasia, or hyperplasia may occur, resulting in lymphatic obstruction or dilatation. Lymphatic vessel reflux occurs when the endoluminal valves are absent or defective.

LYMPHEDEMA

Lymphedema is an imbalance between lymphatic fluid formation and lymphatic fluid absorption, representing a high-output or low-output failure of the lymphatic system or a combination of both. The increase of interstitial fluid leads to a cascade of remodeling that leads to permanent changes in the tissues of the affected limb.[7-10]

High-output failure (also known as dynamic insufficiency) occurs when excessive lymphatic fluid formation exceeds the transport capacity of the intact lymphatic system. Increases in lymphatic fluid production may arise when Starling forces shift net pressure to favor flow of fluid into the interstitium. Increases in venous pressure result in

199

increased hydrostatic pressure within the venules, and capillaries increase the driving force for ultrafiltration.[7-9] Loss of oncotic pressure as seen in hypoproteinemic states such as malnutrition, has a similar effect. Elevated venous pressure occurs in patients with right heart failure, deep vein thrombosis, and venous insufficiency. Local inflammation increases capillary permeability, accelerating the loss of fluid and plasma proteins into the interstitium.[7-9]

In contrast, low-output failure (also known as mechanical insufficiency) occurs when there is injury or impairment of the lymphatic system due to paralysis, obstruction, or inadequacy of the lymphatics (e.g., lymphedema from filarial lymphatic obstruction or congenital hypoplasia).[7-9] As lymphatic obstruction progresses, tortuosity, dilatation, and pooling of lymphatic fluid give way to massive ectasia, valvular destruction, retrograde lymph flow, and lymph coagulation. Intrinsic truncal contractions fail, intraluminal valves give way, and hydrostatic pressure increases in the superficial valveless lymphatic watersheds. Chronic inflammation results in mast cell infiltration, disruption of the interstitial elastin fiber network, intense lymphangiogenesis and hemangiogenesis, fibrosis, and progressive fat deposits, and skin thickening.[7-9]

CLINICAL FEATURES

Dermal edema is the hallmark of lymphedema and represents the earliest clinical manifestation of lymphatic impairment.[7,8] The presence of dilated lymphatic vessels may also be evident. With prolonged lymphatic impairment, tissue changes include fibroplasia, hyperkeratosis, and increases in stromal cells. In addition, elastic tissue fragmentation, clumping, and loss of mature elastic fibers also occur. Abundant subcutaneous fat becomes a predominant component of the swelling seen in the affected limb.[9,10]

The inflammatory cells present in the edematous tissue contribute to the ongoing fibrosis. It is believed that the inflammatory cells fail to migrate to the lymph nodes due to impaired lymphatic transport and dysfunctional lymphangiogenesis, leading to worsening edema and further inflammation. This ultimately results in impaired immune trafficking and decreased clearance of pathogens.[7,8]

Lymphedema is a progressive and usually painless swelling of the limbs or genitals that is the result of decreased transport capacity of the lymphatic system. Lymphedema can be primary or secondary. Primary lymphedema is due to a defect in the lymph conducting pathways. Secondary lymphedema is due to an acquired cause that results in injury and impairment of the lymphatic system.[8-12]

PRIMARY LYMPHEDEMA

In patients with primary lymphedema, the cause of decreased lymphatic transport is due to an intrinsic defect or malfunction of the lymph-conducting elements, which is believed to be a genetically determined abnormality of lymph drainage.[8] The majority of lymphedemas classified as primary lymphedema have inborn abnormalities of the lymphatic system that manifest mostly with irregular or abnormal structural development caused by a gene mutation.[8,13] These abnormalities result in lymphatic hypoplasia, aplasia, numerical hyperplasia, or dilation (lymphangiectasia) with valvular incompetence.[8,13] Primary lymphedema is also classified as a CVM, specifically a truncular LM.

Primary lymphedemas have been classified into three groups depending on the age of onset: congenital (before age 2 years), praecox (onset between age 2 and 25 years), and tarda (after age 35 years). Lymphedema praecox is the most common form of primary lymphedema with a female-to-male ratio of 10:1. It is usually unilateral and often limited to the foot and calf in most patients.[8,12,13]

SECONDARY LYMPHEDEMA

Secondary lymphedema is far more common than primary lymphedema and represents 90% of cases of lymphedema. The most common causes of lower extremity lymphedema are tumor (e.g., lymphoma, prostate cancer, ovarian cancer), surgery involving the lymphatics, radiation therapy, trauma, and infection. Worldwide, infection with the parasitic nematode *Wuscheria bancrofti* (also known as filariasis), is the most common cause of lymphedema.[8,11,12]

LYMPHANGIOMA/LYMPHATIC MALFORMATIONS

Lymphangioma/lymphatic malformations are benign CVMs of the lymphatic system that can occur anywhere on the skin and mucous membranes. There are three distinct types of lymphangioma, each with their own symptoms and each distinguished by the depth and the size of abnormal lymphatic vessels.[14] Lymphangiomas/lymphatic malformations can be categorized as deep or superficial or as congenital or acquired.[15] The lymphangiomas/lymphatic malformations are classified as extra-truncular LMs by the Hamburg classification.[1]

The deep forms of lymphangioma/lymphatic malformations include two specific well-defined CVMs: cavernous lymphangiomas (=lymphatic malformations) and cystic lymphangiomas (=lymphatic malformations), which are also known as cystic hygromas.[16] Superficial forms of lymphangioma/lymphatic malformations include lymphangioma circumscriptum and acquired lymphangioma/lymphatic malformation, which is also referred to in the literature as lymphangiectasia.[14] Although both entities share similar clinical and histological features, the term *lymphangioma circumscriptum* describes lymphatic vessel dilation due to a LM; whereas, the term *lymphangiectasia*, or *acquired lymphangioma*, describes dilated lymphatic vessels of previously normal lymphatics that have become obstructed by an external cause.[14,17]

PATHOPHYSIOLOGY

Lymphangiomas/LMs result from congenital or acquired abnormalities of the lymphatic system. Congenital lymphangiomas are extra-truncular LMs that form due to blockage of the lymphatic system during fetal development.[1,14] Cystic lymphangiomas are associated with genetic disorders, including trisomies 13, 18, and 21, Noonan syndrome, Turner syndrome, and Down syndrome.[18] Analogous to secondary lymphedema, acquired lymphangiomas (also known as lymphangiectasias) occur as a sequela of any interruption of previously normal lymphatic drainage such as surgery, trauma, malignancy, and radiation therapy.

CLINICAL FEATURES

Clinically, lymphangioma circumscriptum appears as multiple, grouped or scattered, translucent or hemorrhagic vesicular papules that resemble frog-spawn.[14] Because the lesions consist of a combination of blood and lymph elements, purple areas can be seen scattered within the vesicle-like papules. In the genital area, the surface can be verrucous, and the lesions may be mistaken for warts.[14] Acquired lymphangiomas are most often found in the axilla, inguinal, and genital areas, and there is often coexisting lymphedema. Associated symptoms may include pruritus, pain, burning, lymphatic drainage, infection, and aesthetic concerns.[17]

Cavernous lymphangioma typically presents during infancy as a painless, ill-defined subcutaneous swelling with no changes of the overlying skin that can be several centimeters in size.[14] Rarely, an entire extremity may be affected. Patients may report tenderness on deep palpation of the area.[19] They are commonly mistaken for cysts or lipomas in clinical practice. Cystic hygromas are lymphatic malformations that are clinically more circumscribed than cavernous lymphangioma by old but popular terminology, and typically occur on the neck, axilla, or groin. On physical examination, they are soft, with varying sizes and shapes, and will typically grow if not surgically excised. When posterior neck lesions are present, there may be an association with Turner syndrome, hydrops fetalis, or other congenital abnormalities.[18] Lymphatic malformations can also present as central conducting lymphatic anomalies.[20-22]

REFERENCES

1. Lee BB, Villavicencio JL. Primary lymphoedema and lymphatic malformation: Are they the two sides of the same coin? *Eur J Vasc Endovasc Surg.* 2010; 39(5):646–653.
2. Rutkowski JM, Boardman KC, Swartz MA. Characterization of lymphangiogenesis in a model of adult skin regeneration. *Am J Physiol Heart Circ Physiol.* 2006;291:H1402–H1410.
3. Goldman J, Le TX, Skobe M, Swartz MA. Over-expression of VEGF-C causes transient lymphatic hyperplasia but not increased lymphangiogenesis in regenerating skin. *Circ Res.* 2005;96:1193–1199 (Comment: *Circ Res.* 2005;96:1132–1134).
4. Lee BB, Laredo J, Seo JM, Neville R. Treatment of lymphatic malformations. In: Mattassi R, Loose DA, Vaghi M, eds. *Hemangiomas and Vascular Malformations.* Milan, Italy: Springer-Verlag Italia; 2009:231–250 [Chapter 29].
5. Bastide G, Lefebvre D. Anatomy and organogenesis and vascular malformations. In: Belov St, Loose DA, Weber J, eds. *Vascular Malformations.* Reinbek, Germany: Einhorn-Presse Verlag GmbH; 1989:20–22.
6. Leu HJ. Pathoanatomy of congenital vascular malformations. In: Belov S, Loose DA, Weber J, eds. *Vascular Malformations.* Reinbek, Germany: Einhorn-Presse Verlag; 1989:37–46.
7. Dellinger MT, Bernas MJ, Witte MH. Lymphatic biology and pathobiology. In: Dieter RS, Dieter RA Jr, Dieter RA, eds. *Venous and Lymphatic Diseases.* New York, NY: McGraw-Hill; 2011:17–36.
8. Thanaporn PK, Rockson SG. Disease of the lymphatic vasculature. In: Dieter RS, Dieter RA Jr, Dieter RA, eds. *Venous and Lymphatic Diseases.* New York, NY: McGraw-Hill; 2011:569–594.
9. Rockson SG. Diagnosis and management of lymphatic vascular disease. *J Am Coll Cardiol.* 2008; 52(10):799–806.
10. Rooke TW, Felty C. Lymphedema: Pathophysiology, classification, and clinical evaluation. In: Gloviczki P, ed. *Handbook of Venous Disorders.* 3rd ed. London, UK: Hodder Arnold; 2009:629–634.
11. Tiwari A, Cheng KS, Button M, Myint F, Hamilton G. Differential diagnosis, investigation, and current treatment of lower limb lymphedema. *Arch Surg.* 2003;138(2):152–161.
12. Kerchner K, Fleischer A, Yosipovitch G. Lower extremity lymphedema update: Pathophysiology, diagnosis, and treatment guidelines. *J Am Acad Dermatol.* 2008;59(2):324–331.
13. Lee B, Andrade M, Bergan J et al. Diagnosis and treatment of primary lymphedema. Consensus document of the International Union of Phlebology (IUP)-2009. *Int Angiol.* 2010;29(5):454–470.
14. Miceli A, Stewart KM. *Lymphangioma.* StatPearls [Internet]. Treasure Island, FL: StatPearls Publishing; 2019.
15. Stewart CJ, Chan T, Platten M. Acquired lymphangiectasia ("lymphangioma circumscriptum") of the vulva: A report of eight cases. *Pathology.* 2009; 41(5):448–453.
16. Noia G, Maltese PE, Zampino G et al. Cystic hygroma: A preliminary genetic study and a short review from the literature. *Lymphat Res Biol.* 2019; 17(1):30–39.
17. Verma SB. Lymphangiectasias of the skin: Victims of confusing nomenclature. *Clin Exp Dermatol.* 2009; 34(5):566–569.

18. Sehgal VN, Sharma S, Chatterjee K, Khurana A, Malhotra S. Unilateral, Blaschkoid, large lymphangioma circumscriptum: Micro- and macrocystic manifestations. *Skinmed.* 2018;16(6):411–413.

19. Jiao-Ling L, Hai-Ying W, Wei Z, Jin-Rong L, Kun-Shan C, Qian F. Treatment and prognosis of fetal lymphangioma. *Eur J Obstet Gynecol Reprod Biol.* 2018;231:274–279.

20. Taghinia AH, Upton J, Trenor CC 3rd et al. Lymphaticovenous bypass of the thoracic duct for the treatment of chylous leak in central conducting lymphatic anomalies. *J Pediatr Surg.* 2019;54(3):562–568.

21. Biko DM, Reisen B, Otero HJ et al. Imaging of central lymphatic abnormalities in Noonan syndrome. *Pediatr Radiol.* 2019;49(5):586–592.

22. Connell FC, Gordon K, Brice G et al. The classification and diagnostic algorithm for primary lymphatic dysplasia: An update from 2010 to include molecular findings. *Clin Genet.* 2013;84(4):303–314.

45

Contemporary diagnosis of primary lymphedema and lymphatic malformation

STANLEY G. ROCKSON

Primary lymphedema results from an intrinsic developmental defect of anatomy or function of the lymphatic circulation.[1,2] The primary forms of lymphedema are thought to occur in approximately 1 of every 6–10,000 live births and are presumed to reflect heritable factors, even in the noncongenital presentations. Females are affected 2- to 10-fold more commonly than males.[3] Primary lymphedema represents a heterogeneous group of disorders. Patients with primary lymphedema can be classified by age of onset (congenital, pubertal, or late onset), functional anatomical attributes (lymphatic aplasia, hypoplasia, or hyperplasia),[4,5] and clinical presentation. The primary lymphedemas can often be characterized by associated clinical anomalies or associated physical attributes.[5]

The recognition and accurate diagnosis of primary lymphedema require consideration of all of these clinical variables but may also rely on a variety of imaging techniques, including radionuclide lymphoscintigraphy, computed axial tomography, magnetic resonance imaging, direct contrast lymphography, and/or near-infrared fluorescent lymphography.

In view of the nonprovoked nature of primary lymphedema, as well as the tendency for the congenital varieties to cluster within family cohorts, it is not unexpected that causal mutations have been identified in many of these disorders. Fourteen distinct genomic mutations have been identified in association with syndromic and nonsyndromic primary lymphedema (Table 45.1).[6,7] In general, recessive (autosomal or sex-linked) modes of inheritance in congenital lymphedema occur much less commonly than the dominant forms.

The list of heritable lymphedema-associated syndromes is long and growing.[6] Primary lymphedema has been described in association with some forms of chromosomal aneuploidy, such as Turner syndrome, with various dysmorphogenic-genetic anomalies such as Noonan syndrome and neurofibromatosis, and with various as yet unrelated disorders such as yellow nail syndrome[8] and congenital lymphangiectasia.[9]

Lymphatic vascular malformations present both in isolation and in more complex forms that might include peripheral lymphedematous components. In analogy to the primary lymphedemas, the diagnosis of lymphatic vascular malformations is initially based on the historical presentation and the physical examination. Subsequent diagnostic investigations include Doppler ultrasonography and magnetic resonance imaging and may also include assessment of D-dimer and fibrinogen levels in order to identify a venous component and/or to exclude a coagulation abnormality.[10]

In many patients with lymphatic malformation, genetic evaluation is warranted (see Chapter 8).[11] For a large and growing list of the complex vascular anomalies, with and without lymphatic components, causal somatic activating mutations have been identified. Lymphatic malformations are thought to be caused by mosaic activating mutation in *PIK3CA*, with increased mTOR/AKT signaling.[12–14]

The decision to pursue a genetic assessment in these cases entails tissue biopsy; thus, testing eligibility criteria for combined vascular lesions and large lymphatic malformations have been established.[15] Known mutations can be quickly and inexpensively screened by droplet digital polymerase chain reaction (PCR).[16] Gene-focused next-generation sequencing (NGS), using single-molecule molecular inversion probes, has identified additional *PIK3CA* mutations. NGS technology has revolutionized the ability to analyze mutational aberrations.[17]

Table 45.1 Identified gene mutations responsible for various presentations of primary lymphedema

ADAMTS3	GJC2
CCBE1	HGF
EPHB4	KIF11
FAT4	PIEZO1
FLT4	RASA1
FOXC2	SOX18
GATA2	VEGFC

Several of the more complex presentations of lymphatic vascular malformation merit focused attention. The *PIK3CA*-related overgrowth spectrum (PROS) reflects a broad array of somatic disease (Chapter 8) caused by activating mutations in *PIK3CA*.[18] This constellation includes CLOVES (congenital lipomatous overgrowth, vascular malformations, linear keratinocytic epidermal nevi, and skeletal/spinal anomalies as well as isolated lymphatic malformations) syndrome.[15,19]

Generalized lymphatic anomalies (GLAs) entail multiple sites of lymphatic malformation with involvement, serous effusions, and evidence of disease burden in soft tissues, liver, spleen, and bones. Evidence of the lymphatic nature of these lesions can be acquired through immunohistochemistry of tissue biopsy, and the causal somatic mutation may be confirmed to be *PIK3CA*.

In kaposiform lymphangiomatosis (KLA), the involvement of viscera, including bone and spleen, often resembles GLA. In addition, KLA is characterized by severe coagulopathy, with components of hypofibrinogenemia and thrombocytopenia.[11] Lymphatic channel defects may also be present.[20,21] Distinctive histological features include abnormal lymphatic components accompanied by poorly defined clusters or sheets of spindle cells.[11] Somatic *NRAS* mutation may be identified.

Central conducting lymphatic anomalies (CCLAs) are characterized progressive disorders caused by reflux and leakage of lymphatic fluid into the peritoneum, pleura, pericardium, lungs, bone, and soft tissues.[22] The large recurrent ascites and pleuropericardial effusions can be accompanied by severe edema, hypoproteinemia, recurrent infection, and organ dysfunction. CCLA reflects dysfunction of the thoracic duct and cisterna chyli, which can be documented through a variety of procedures that permit direct lymphangiographic visualization of these central lymphatic channels.[23] Genetic evaluation may disclose a germline mutation of *EPHB4*.[24]

Klippel–Trenaunay syndrome (KTS) is a vascular malformation overgrowth syndrome that can more properly be classified as a capillary lymphaticovenous malformation.[25] There is variable overgrowth of soft tissue and bone.[11] This condition can be considered to represent an aspect of the PROS[19]: upon genetic testing, *PIK3CA* mutations may be detected in the biopsied involved tissue.

REFERENCES

1. Brouillard P, Boon L, Vikkula M. Genetics of lymphatic anomalies. *J Clin Invest.* 2014;124:898–904.
2. Ho B, Gordon K, Mortimer PS. A genetic approach to the classification of primary lymphoedema and lymphatic malformations. *Eur J Vasc Endovasc Surg.* 2018;56:465–466.
3. Rockson SG. Lymphedema. *Am J Med.* 2001;110:288–295.
4. Kinmonth JB, Taylor GW, Tracy GD, Marsh JD. Primary lymphoedema; Clinical and lymphangiographic studies of a series of 107 patients in which the lower limbs were affected. *Br J Surg.* 1957;45:1–9.
5. Rockson S. Syndromic lymphedema: Keys to the kingdom of lymphatic structure and function? *Lymph Res Biol.* 2003;1:181–183.
6. Mortimer PS, Gordon K, Brice G, Mansour S. Hereditary and familial lymphedemas. In: Lee BB, Rockson SG, Bergan J, eds. *Lymphedema: A Concise Compendium of Theory and Practice.* 2nd ed. London, UK: Springer; 2018:29–43.
7. Connell FC, Gordon K, Brice G et al. The classification and diagnostic algorithm for primary lymphatic dysplasia: An update from 2010 to include molecular findings. *Clin Genet.* 2013;84(4):303–314.
8. Cousins E, Cintolesi V, Vass L et al. A case-control study of the lymphatic phenotype of yellow nail syndrome. *Lymphat Res Biol.* 2018;16:340–346.
9. Yuan SM. Congenital pulmonary lymphangiectasia: A disorder not only of fetoneonates. *Klin Padiatr.* 2017;229:205–208.
10. Wassef M, Vanwijck R, Clapuyt P, Boon L, Magalon G. Vascular tumours and malformations, classification, pathology and imaging. *Ann Chir Plast Esthet.* 2006;51:263–281.
11. Adams DM, Ricci KW. Vascular anomalies: Diagnosis of complicated anomalies and new medical treatment options. *Hematol Oncol Clin North Am.* 2019;33:455–470.
12. Boscolo E, Coma S, Luks VL et al. AKT hyper-phosphorylation associated with PI3 K mutations in lymphatic endothelial cells from a patient with lymphatic malformation. *Angiogenesis.* 2015;18:151–162.
13. Osborn AJ, Dickie P, Neilson DE et al. Activating PIK3CA alleles and lymphangiogenic phenotype of lymphatic endothelial cells isolated from lymphatic malformations. *Hum Mol Genet.* 2015;24:926–938.
14. Queisser A, Boon LM, Vikkula M. Etiology and genetics of congenital vascular lesions. *Otolaryngol Clin North Am.* 2018;51:41–53.
15. Keppler-Noreuil KM, Rios JJ, Parker VE et al. PIK3CA-related overgrowth spectrum (PROS): Diagnostic and testing eligibility criteria, differential diagnosis, and evaluation. *Am J Med Genet A.* 2015;167A:287–295.
16. Luks VL, Kamitaki N, Vivero MP et al. Lymphatic and other vascular malformative/overgrowth disorders are caused by somatic mutations in PIK3CA. *J Pediatr.* 2015;166:1048–1054.e1–5.
17. Giardina T, Robinson C, Grieu-Iacopetta F et al. Implementation of next generation sequencing technology for somatic mutation detection in routine laboratory practice. *Pathology.* 2018;50:389–401.

18. Nathan N, Keppler-Noreuil KM, Biesecker LG, Moss J, Darling TN. Mosaic disorders of the PI3 K/PTEN/AKT/TSC/mTORC1 signaling pathway. *Dermatol Clin.* 2017;35:51–60.

19. Keppler-Noreuil KM, Sapp JC, Lindhurst MJ et al. Clinical delineation and natural history of the PIK3CA-related overgrowth spectrum. *Am J Med Genet A.* 2014;164A:1713–1733.

20. Croteau SE, Kozakewich HP, Perez-Atayde AR et al. Kaposiform lymphangiomatosis: A distinct aggressive lymphatic anomaly. *J Pediatr.* 2014;164: 383–388.

21. Ozeki M, Fujino A, Matsuoka K, Nosaka S, Kuroda T, Fukao T. Clinical features and prognosis of generalized lymphatic anomaly, Kaposiform lymphangiomatosis, and Gorham–Stout disease. *Pediatr Blood Cancer.* 2016;63:832–838.

22. Trenor CC 3rd, Chaudry G. Complex lymphatic anomalies. *Semin Pediatr Surg.* 2014;23:186–190.

23. Krishnamurthy R, Hernandez A, Kavuk S, Annam A, Pimpalwar S. Imaging the central conducting lymphatics: Initial experience with dynamic MR lymphangiography. *Radiology.* 2015;274:871–878.

24. Li D, Wenger TL, Seiler C et al. Pathogenic variant in *EPHB4* results in central conducting lymphatic anomaly. *Hum Mol Genet.* 2018;27:3233–3245.

25. Blatt J, Finger M, Price V, Crary SE, Pandya A, Adams DM. Cancer risk in Klippel–Trenaunay syndrome. *Lymphat Res Biol.* 2019. https://doi.org/10.1089/lrb.2018.0049

46

Clinical staging of lymphedema: How practical is it for clinical management of primary lymphedema?

SANDRO MICHELINI, ALESSANDRO FIORENTINO, ALESSANDRO FAILLA, AND GIOVANNI MONETA

Staging of lymphedema is a perennial topic for discussion within national and international congresses. To be universally accepted, the requirements of simplicity, recognizability, and worldwide utilization must be met. Clinical staging is very important for clinical management of primary lymphedema. For each clinical stage, there are specific diagnostic and therapeutic indications. Although there are guidelines of international scientific societies (International Society of Lymphology [ISL], International Union of Phlebology [IUP]), which show the same clinical staging, in many countries and by many schools, "personalized" classifications continue to be used. The ISL's classification, however, which identifies four stages (from subclinical stage, to complicated elephantiasis) of lymphedema is very practical.

Primary lymphedema has different clinical stages of evolution, in part mutually reversible, that influence affected patients differently from the physical, emotional, and psychological points of view. Achieving common acceptance of stages of lymphedema, as in other diseases, seems to be a problem that cannot be postponed further for reasons of "scientific communication" and for the undoubted legal medical and social impact. In more advanced clinical stages, the condition takes on the characteristics of a real "social disease" with costs generated both from medical care and from loss of productive capacity. The clinical staging, reported in the Consensus Document of the ISL,[1] currently includes four clinical stages (Table 46.1); it initially included three clinical stages (I, II, and III) but recently highlighted the importance of including the "subclinical" aspect of primary lymphedema, potentially progressive (e.g., subject with blood relation with patient suffering from primary lymphedema), and the subclinical stage (stage 0) was included. Stage 0 refers to a latent or subclinical condition, where swelling is not evident despite impaired lymph transport. Stage I represents an early accumulation of fluid,

Table 46.1 ISL Clinical staging—Clinical stage evidence

0	Subclinical with possible clinical evolution (Figure 46.1)
I	Edema regressing with treatments with positive pitting test (Figure 46.2)
II	Edema partially regressing with treatments with negative pitting test (Figure 46.3)
III	Elephantiasis with cutaneous complications and recurrent infections (Figure 46.4)

relatively high in protein content, that subsides with limb elevation. Pitting may occur. Stage II signifies that limb elevation alone rarely reduces tissue swelling; pitting is manifested. Stage III encompasses lymphostatic elephantiasis where pitting is absent and trophic skin changes, such as acanthosis, fat deposits, and warty overgrowths, develop. The severity of the stages is based on the volume differences: minimal (<20% increase), moderate (20%–40% increase), and severe (>40% increase). These stages refer only to the physical condition of the extremities.

Some health-care workers examining disability utilize the World Health Organization's guidelines for the *International Classification of Functioning, Disability, and Health* (ICF). Quality of life issues (social, emotional, physical inabilities, etc.) may also be addressed by individual clinicians and can have a favorable impact on therapy and compliance.[2]

The "German School" proposed four clinical stages,[3] adding to those reported in the previous "Consensus Document" a "stage 0," which represents all cases of subclinical lymphedema but with a significant risk of clinical progression (e.g., lymphoscintigraphy strongly predictive) (Table 46.2).

Since 1997,[4–8] five clinical stages have been recognized in Italy (Table 46.3). This system emphasizes the importance of

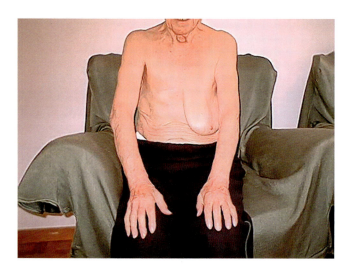

Figure 46.1 ISL Clinical Staging—Clinical stage evidence: 0 Subclinical with possible clinical evolution.

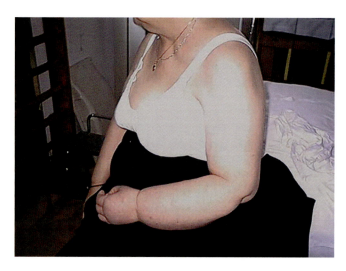

Figure 46.3 ISL Clinical Staging—Clinical stage evidence: II Edema partially regressing with treatments with negative pitting test.

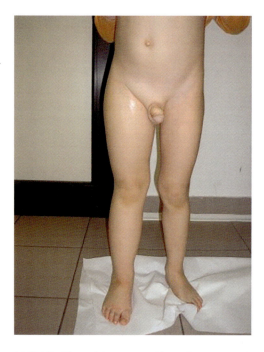

Figure 46.2 ISL Clinical Staging—Clinical stage evidence: I Edema regressing with treatments with positive pitting test.

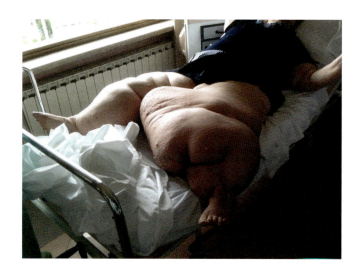

Figure 46.4 ISL Clinical Staging—Clinical stage evidence: III Elephantiasis with cutaneous complications and recurrent infections.

subclinical cases at risk of evolution (in stage I) and cases of elephantiasis with major chronic inflammatory and infectious complications and risk of neoplastic tissue degeneration (stage V). Depending on the stage, it is also possible to direct the therapeutic treatment toward the corresponding preventive options.[8]

The Japan School heightened sensitivity to infectious complications in cutaneous and subcutaneous tissues of lymphedema and proposed four stages involving inspection and palpation of the affected areas and assessment of the frequency of the infectious episodes and inflammatory complications; based on the developmental stage, it is possible to obtain prognostic information (Table 46.4). This is obviously a staging with a more strictly dermatologic point of view.

Table 46.2 German clinical staging—Clinical stage evidence

0	No edema, but evidence of a risk condition for evolution
I	Edema regressing with treatments (positive pitting test)
II	Edema partially regressing with treatments (negative pitting test)
III	Elephantiasis with cutaneous complications and recurrent infections

Source: Reprinted from Foldi M, Foldi E, Kubik S. *Foldi's Textbook of Lymphology.* Munchen, Germany. Copyright 2004, with permission from Elsevier.

Table 46.3 Italian clinical staging (Michelini-Campisi)—
Clinical stage evidence

I	No edema in individuals at risk (subclinical)
II	Edema spontaneously regressing with elevation of arm and night rest
III	Edema that does not regress spontaneously (or only partially by the treatments)
IV	Elephantiasis (abolition of tendon and bone projections)
V	Elephantiasis complicated by cutaneous and recurrent infections and impairment of deep body structures (muscles, joints)

Source: Campisi C et al. Eur J Lymphol. 1999;7(25):27–31.

Table 46.4 Japanese clinical staging

I	Normal Pitting ++ Absent Temporary
II	Thin skin increase in thickness, pitting + Absent Permanent
III	Cutaneous lichenification. Increase in thickness, pitting
IV	Verrucosis pitting absent, very often worsening

Source: Ohkuma, M. Eur J Lymphol Relat Probl. 2003;11:1–2.

The Brazilian School, in addition to taking into account the importance of preclinical cases at risk of development in infectious and degenerative complications, also analyzes the functional effects of edema on the limb with impairment of one, two, or three major joints. This aspect also permits better definition of the commitments of global functional rehabilitation, the degree of care needed by the patient, and impairment in activities of daily living (Table 46.5). This classification thus utilizes both clinical and functional criteria for patient assessment.[9]

The respective positions of the "experts" on such a delicate and transitional moment for both public and private health systems in different countries also stems from the need to redefine welfare parameters for these highly prevalent diseases. At more advanced stages of disease, in fact, lymphedema can be identified as a "social disease" for which the health system must provide incentives and normative facilitations, comparable to the other chronic

Table 46.5 Brazilian clinical staging

Stage 0	No edema in individuals, no joint impairments at risk (subclinical)
Stage I	Lymphedema stage I (involvement of one major joint)
Stage II	(Involvement of two major joints of the limb)
Stage III	(Involvement of three major joints of the limb)
Stage IV	(Cutaneous infections and inflammatory complications of the limb)

Source: Abstract book of XX Congress of International Society of Lymphology. Sociedade Brasileira de Linfologia. Salvador Bahia; 2005:46.

diseases. It is pointless to say that, currently, many national health-care systems provide therapies to patients with primary lymphedema in an equitable manner, with poor distribution of health-care resources. In most countries, the costs of materials, elastic garments, and drugs are charged to the patient.[2]

The synthesis of the different proposals was provided by the last version of the Consensus Document of the ISL. This staging provides important indications also under therapeutic and prognostic points of view; in detail, in stage 0 (subclinical), genetic study is essential with the segregation studies of the patient's family to identify those at risk (with subsequent confirmation by mean of the lymphoscintigraphy) and adopt more appropriate principles of prevention and therapy (wear the elastic garment in risk conditions, and respect rules of hygiene in order to avoid clinical development).

In stage I, the early diagnosis (in lots of cases, still today, too much too late) is essential, and timely physical treatment and wearing of the elastic garment in the daytime are also mandated; in selected cases, it is also possible to imply appropriate surgery (e.g., derivative/bypass microsurgery or super microsurgery). But, a concrete indication for the intervention among the candidates still must be better defined to ensure clinical success.

In stage II, complex decongestive physical treatment must also include treatments for fibrosis (ultrasound, radial shock waves, Linfotaping), in addition to applying bandages with short elasticity with the appropriate mesh nets specific for underbandaging in correspondence to the fibrotic zones. In this stage, the prevention of derma-lymphangio-adenitis (DLA) is essential, and patients should wear the flat knitted elastic garment in the daytime.

In stage III, the physical treatment, both for the involvement of large joints and also for removal of dystrophic lesions with high interstitial protein content, often requires hospitalization, especially during "acute" treatment. Acute treatment often requires close monitoring for 24 hours, especially in patients over the age of 65 years, for possible complications such as heart failure or temporary and reversible renal insufficiency, which can be caused by the obstruction of the renal tubules due to the high concentrations of proteins removed from the tissues in a short time.[8]

Nevertheless, the treatment should be personalized to meet individual needs and also adjusted based on the patient's response. For example, in advanced clinical stages, rapid reabsorption of the protein component of edema may result in cardiac overload by increased preload and should be anticipated. Hence, it is necessary to monitor both the condition of the heart (NT-proBNP level) as well as renal status (e.g., possible impairment at tubular level). And it may be necessary to modify the decongestive treatment, splitting it over time, and eventually, associating it with a short period of diuretic therapy to avoid possible complications and to allow better compliance of the patient.

REFERENCES

1. International Society of Lymphology. The diagnosis and treatment of peripheral lymphedema: 2013 Consensus Document of the International Society of Lymphology. *Lymphology*. 2013;46:1–11.
2. World Health Organization (WHO). *International Classification of Functioning, Disability and Health*. Geneva, Switzerland: WHO; 2001.
3. Foldi M, Foldi E, Kubik S. *Foldi's Textbook of Lymphology*. Munchen, Germany: Elsevier; 2004.
4. Michelini S, Campisi C, Ricci M et al. Linee Guida Italiane sul Linfedema. *Eur Med Phys*. 2007;43(Suppl 1–3): 34–41.
5. Michelini S, Campisi C, Failla A et al. Staging of lymphedema: Comparing different proposals. *Eur J Lymphol*. 2006;16(46):7–10.
6. Michelini S, Failla A. Linfedemi: Inquadramento diagnostico clinico e strumentale. *Minerva Cardioangiol*. 1997;45(6 Suppl I):11–15.
7. Campisi C, Michelini S, Boccardo F. Lymphology in medical and surgical practice. Italian guidelines looking towards Europe and World. *Eur J Lymphol*. 2004;14(42):26–28.
8. Campisi C, Michelini S, Boccardo F, Zilli A, Borrelli V. Modern stadiation of lymphedema and corresponding preventive options. *Eur J Lymphol*. 1999;7(25): 27–31.
9. Abstract book of XX Congress of International Society of Lymphology. Sociedade Brasileira de Linfologia. Salvador Bahia; 2005:46.

47

Laboratory (lymphoscintigraphic) staging guideline?

BYUNG-BOONG LEE AND JAMES LAREDO

Throughout the last century, chronic lymphedema had been considered a simple "static" condition of lymph fluid stasis following the failure of lymphatic transport by the lymph vessels. This old concept has now become obsolete, due to our much-improved understanding of the nature of chronic lymphedema. Chronic lymphedema is now considered a "dynamic" condition with constant interplay between the lymphatic system and the surrounding soft tissue.[1-4]

Lymphedema is now correctly understood as a progressive condition of chronic degenerative and inflammatory process involving the lymphatic system as well as the entire skin and soft tissue, resulting in fibrotic changes following recurrent episodes of dermato-lympho-adenitis.[5,6] Such a steadily progressing condition throughout the surrounding soft tissue will eventually result in a disabling and distressing condition to many when left alone, portending significant disability throughout the patient's life.

This is, therefore, a serious condition involving the tissues beyond the lymphatics and lymph nodes, often associated with many potentially serious complications: local/regional/systemic sepsis caused by bacterial and fungal infection, dermato-lipo-fibrosis, immunodeficiency-related various phenomena, and malignancy (e.g., Kaposi sarcoma, lymphangiosarcoma).[7,8]

Chronic lymphedema is now fully perceived as the beginning of serious complex systemic disease to warrant proper diagnosis in its earliest possible stage in order to provide an effective treatment regimen based on accurate staging.

Currently available staging systems of lymphedema, proposed by quite a few leading societies, have shown only limited value despite substantial efforts over several decades to provide proper clinical staging, including the International Society of Lymphology (ISL) staging system.[9,10]

Most of the staging systems limit the assessment guidelines to the physical examination (e.g., tissue turgor and limb shape) and neglect many other critical clinical elements (e.g., number of major joints with changes in tissue composition), including the limitations on physical activity that impair quality of life (QoL) and socioeconomic status by less productive as well as less adaptive conditions.[11,12]

So far, none of the current staging systems, mostly based on the clinical findings alone, are able to provide sufficient guidelines for improved management of lymphedema in different stages. Hence, new proposals put forth to compensate for such liability include the Lymph CEAP classification and also a staging system combining clinical and radiographic data based on separate clinical staging and laboratory staging with the lymphoscintigraphic findings.[13,14] Laboratory staging, as proposed[13] (Table 47.1), is based on the functional study of the lymphatic system with radionuclide lymphoscintigraphy (LSG)[15,16] using 99mTc-labeled human serum albumin or 99mTc-labeled sulfur colloid. Radionuclide LSG is able to monitor the movement status of the colloid from the injection site based on: the transition time to the knee, groin, or axilla; absence or presence of major lymphatic collectors; number and size of vessels and nodes (e.g., popliteal nodes); presence of collaterals and reflux; and symmetrical activity with the opposite side.[17,18]

LSG fulfills the critical role as a precise method of evaluation of lymphatic function status based on the direct visualization of lymphatics, lymph nodes, and dermal backflow in addition to semiquantitative data on radiotracer (lymph) transport. LSG is now well accepted as a new gold standard for the assessment of lymphedema, visualizing structural and functional changes in lymphatic flow dynamics; it is well proven to be safe, noninvasive, easy to perform, and harmless to the lymphatic endothelial lining (cf. conventional lymphography with oil-based contrast).[1-4,16]

LSG-based laboratory staging would be able to provide a much more accurate condition of chronic lymphedema when combined with clinical staging, especially when reconstructive or ablative surgical therapy is considered as a supplement in a patient who has failed to respond to basic care with decongestive lymphatic therapy (DLT).[16]

Table 47.1 Laboratory (lymphoscintigraphic) staging

Grade/Stage I
  Lymph node uptake (LN): decreased (±)
  Dermal backflow (DBF): none (−)
  Collateral lymphatics (CL): good visualization (+)
  Main lymphatics (ML): decreased visualization (±)
  Clearance of radioisotope from injection site (CR):
    decreased lymphatic transport (±)
Grade/Stage II[a]
  LN: Decreased to none (−)
  DBF: Visualization (+)
  CL: Decreased visualization (±)
  ML: Poor to no visualization (±)
  CR: More decreased (±)
Grade/Stage III
  LN: No uptake (−)
  DBF: Visualization (+)
  CL: Poor visualization (−)
  ML: No visualization (−)
  CR: No clearance (−)
Grade/Stage IV
  LN: None (−)
  DBF: Poor to no visualization (−)
  CL: No visualization (−)
  ML: No visualization (−)
  CR: No clearance (−)

[a] IIA, extent of DBF does not exceed half of each limb; IIB, exceed half of each limb.

In our own limited experience,[13,16,19] the addition of laboratory staging based on the status of lymph node uptake, dermal backflow, collateral lymphatics and main lymphatics, and clearance of radioisotope from injection site (CR) to currently available clinical staging system with further modification has improved the overall predictability of treatment outcome and progression of the lymphedema.

For example, among the patients in the same clinical stage, the one with the more advanced laboratory stage has shown a tendency to progress faster so that this newly added laboratory stage has been used as one of the criteria to determine which lymphedema patients would benefit to proceed to incorporate additional treatment modalities with no delay, particularly surgical therapy before further disease deterioration.[13]

This new approach based on a combined clinical and laboratory staging system allowed for earlier determination of treatment failure among patients with minimal clinical improvement with DLT, so optimal timing of surgical therapies was not lost and timely supplements to failed DLT were added before being too late to achieve the goal. Indeed, this combined approach is able to provide critical information on the decision-making process for supplemental surgical therapy to choose the appropriate timing of surgical intervention before irreversible progression of disease occurs.[19–22]

Hence, this new approach incorporating laboratory/lymphoscintigraphic staging should be accepted as a more reliable and objective method to guide proper treatment and management than the conventional approach solely based on the clinical staging.[1–4]

REFERENCES

1. Lee BB, Andrade M, Bergan J et al. Diagnosis and treatment of primary lymphedema—Consensus document of the International Union of Phlebology (IUP)-2009. *Int Angiol.* 2010;29(5):454–470.
2. Lee BB, Andrade M, Antignani PL et al. Diagnosis and treatment of primary lymphedema. Consensus document of the International Union of Phlebology (IUP)-2013. *Int Angiol.* 2013;32(6):541–574.
3. Lee BB, Antignani PL, Baroncelli TA et al. IUA-ISVI consensus for diagnosis guideline of chronic lymphedema of the limbs. *Int Angiol.* 2015;34(4):311–332.
4. Lee BB. State of art in lymphedema. Management: Part 1. *Phlebolymphology.* 2018;25(2):160–171.
5. Lee BB. State of art in lymphedema. Management: Part 2. *Phlebolymphology.* 2018;25(3):189–200.
6. Lee BB. Chronic lymphedema, no more stepchild to modern medicine! *Eur J Lymphol.* 2004;14(42):6–12.
7. Consensus document of the International Society of lymphology. The diagnosis and treatment of peripheral lymphedema. *Lymphology.* 2009;42:51–60.
8. International Lymph Framework. *Best Practice for the Management of Lymphoedema.* 2nd ed. 2012. https://www.lympho.org
9. Michelini S, Campisi C, Gasbarro V et al. National guidelines on lymphedema. *Lymphology.* 2007;55: 238–242.
10. ISL. Consensus documents on the diagnosis and treatment of peripheral lymphedema. *Lymphology.* 2016;49:170–184.
11. Michelini S, Failla A, Moneta G. Lymphedema: Epidemiology, disability and social costs. *Lymphology.* 2002;35:169–171.
12. Michelini S, Failla A, Moneta G et al. Lymphedema and occupational therapy. *Lymphology.* 2007;55: 243–246.
13. Lee BB, Bergan JJ. New clinical and laboratory staging systems to improve management of chronic lymphedema. *Lymphology.* 2005;38(3):122–129.
14. Gasbarro V, Michelini S, Antignani PL, Tsolaki E, Ricci M, Allegra C. The CEAP-L classification for lymphedemas of the limbs: The Italian experience. *Int Angiol.* 2009;28(4):315–324.
15. Gloviczki P, Calcagno D, Schirger A et al. Noninvasive evaluation of the swollen extremity: Experiences with 190 lymphoscintigraphy examinations. *J Vasc Surg.* 1989;9:683–689; discussion 690.
16. Lee BB, Laredo J. Contemporary role of lymphoscintigraphy: We can no longer afford to ignore! Editorial. *Phlebology.* 2011;26:177–178.

17. Guidelines 6.2.0. on lymphoscintigraphy and lymphangiography. In: Gloviczki P, ed. *Handbook of Venous Disorders: Guidelines of the American Venous Forum*. 3rd ed. London, UK: A Hodder Arnold; 2009:647 [Chapter 58].

18. Burnand KM, Glass DM, Sundaraiya S, Mortimer PS, Peters AM. Popliteal node visualization during standard pedal lymphoscintigraphy for a swollen limb indicates impaired lymph drainage. *Am J Roentgenol*. 2011;197:1443–1448.

19. Lee BB, Kim DI, Whang JH, Lee KW. Contemporary management of chronic lymphedema—Personal experiences. *Lymphology*. 2002;35(Suppl):450–455.

20. Lee BB, Laredo J, Neville R. Reconstructive surgery for chronic lymphedema: A viable option, but. *Vascular*. 2011;19(4):195–205.

21. Lee BB, Laredo J, Neville R. Current status of lymphatic reconstructive surgery for chronic lymphedema: It is still an uphill battle! *Int J Angiol*. 2011;20(2):73–79.

22. Lee BB. Current issue in management of chronic lymphedema: Personal reflection on an experience with 1065 patients. *Lymphology*. 2005;38:28.

Diagnosis

48

Ultrasonographic assessment of lymphatic malformations—Lymphangioma and primary lymphedema: A new role for diagnosis?

ERICA MENEGATTI AND SERGIO GIANESINI

LYMPHATIC MALFORMATION MORPHOLOGY AND HEMODYNAMIC CHARACTERISTICS USEFUL FOR ULTRASONOGRAPHIC ASSESSMENT

Extra-truncular lymphatic malformations

Lymphangioma is more accurately termed a lymphatic malformation[1] (LM), and it is the second most common type of vascular malformation after the venous type.[2] From the histological point of view, it is possible to characterize LMs like a collection of anomalous lymphatics vessels, often combined to small blood vessels, lined by a quiescent endothelium without cellular hyperplasia.[3] LMs involve the lymphatic system and circulation resulting in sequestered lymphatic sacs that fail to communicate with peripheral draining channels.[4] Over 50% of LM cases are frequently located in the head and neck soft tissues, while around 40% are those of the trunk and limbs.[5]

LMs can be subdivided into two different types: macrocystic (cystic or cystic lymphangioma) constituted by larger cysts of variable sizes, and microcystic composed of multiple cysts smaller than 2 mm in a background of a solid matrix.[2] The two forms are often associated, especially when they involve the face and mouth regions or are found in visceral localizations. Most of these lesions are already present at birth or appear within 2 years of life. Unlike venous malformations, LMs are generally known to be noncompressible,[5] but they also can be compressible and transilluminate. However, they do not fill with Valsalva or the dependent position, as do venous malformations. Ultrasound (US) is a valuable and effective tool to differentiate vascular and LMs that are both classified according to the flow dynamics among low-flow lesions.[5]

Truncular lymphatic malformations

Lymphedema presents structural abnormalities of the lymphatic trunks resulting in an impaired lymphatic transport with localized form of tissue swelling, which in turn causes increased limb volume.[2] Primary lymphedema is sporadic, rarely familial or associated with complex developmental malformative or genetic disorders.

Chronic lymphedema is characterized by skin thickening and tissue fibrosis; it presents signs of inflammation and nonpitting skin texture.[7] Despite lymphedema being primarily a clinical diagnosis, further diagnostic techniques can be used to exclude other causes of extremity swelling.[8] Lymphoscintigraphy is a "gold standard" imaging study to confirm the delayed transit time to the regional lymph nodes, dermal backflow, or formation of collateral lymphatic channels.[8] Other imaging modalities such as magnetic resonance imaging and computed tomography are neither sensitive nor specific for diagnosing lymphedema.[2,8,9] Duplex US is actually considered a nonspecific tool in lymphedema diagnosis, but it can be used to detect associated venous disorders such as deep venous obstruction and/or reflux that may occur simultaneously.[8]

HIGH-RESOLUTION B-MODE ULTRASOUND EVALUATION

The US characterization of LMs can be done on appearance from macrocystic to microcystic type. The former presents as multilocular cystic masses with large thin-walled cysts containing variable echogenicity. Some of the internal septa may have variable thickness or show some vessels[6,8] (Figure 48.1). The latter are usually shown as hyperechoic masses as a result of the multiple interfaces constituted by the small

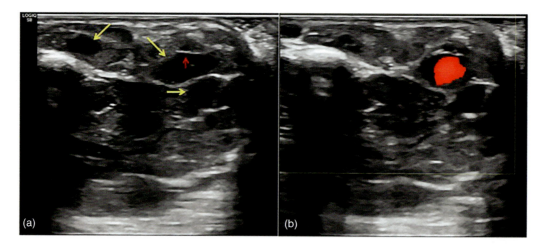

Figure 48.1 Macrocystic lymphatics malformation in young boy involving the back of the hand, and it extends also to the distal part of the forearm. **(a)** B-mode characterization of multilobular cystic masses (yellow arrows), while the red arrow indicates a septum dividing the cyst into two different cavities. **(b)** Color Doppler coding enhance the presence of flow when the operator compresses with the US probe.

cysts. In these lesions, poor arterial and venous flows are seen (Figure 48.2). Regarding lymphedema, the high-resolution B-mode US of tissue layers in the edematous limb can provide information on the etiology and severity of the disease.[10]

This technique allows an accurate evaluation of soft tissue, such as measurement of the skin thickness and supra- and subfascial compartments, as well as identification of fluid collections and fibrotic areas.[11,12] A detailed description of imaging milestones has been recently published, and it can be helpful during lymphedema US investigation[13]:

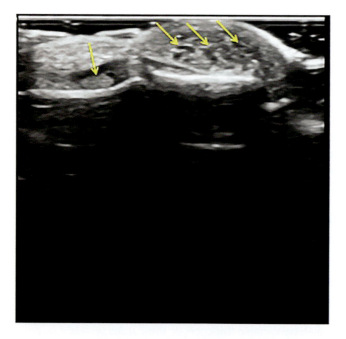

Figure 48.2 B-mode ultrasound image of microcystic lymphatic malformation on index finger in a young girl; the yellow arrows show small cystic formation with hyperechoic structure inside.

Figures 48.1 through 48.3 demonstrate the various anatomical features that can be identified with US of LMs:

- The presence of the "lymphatic lakes" (Figure 48.3a)
- Ectasia of the lymphatic trunks and/or collectors (Figure 48.3b)
- Lymph node visualization (Figure 48.3c)
- Deep and/or superficial venous system involvement (Figure 48.3d–f)

Since one of the most common lymphedema complications is deep skin infections, high-resolution B-mode evaluation can identify the presence of fluid collections, edema, or soft tissue stranding indicating inflammation. Usually, signs of a deeper infection, perifascial fluid accumulation and subcutaneous emphysema, may also be apparent via US imaging.[14]

The use of US can also influence treatment decisions and can provide an objective measurement of the response to therapy by determining the thickness of each of the tissue elements in the limb before and after treatment.[10,14]

DOPPLER EQUIPMENT

The most modern US devices certainly allow a thorough examination and an accurate echographic characterization of LM and lymphedema.

The linear array transducer, with frequency ranging from 7 to 12 MHz, is suitable for this study.

Higher frequencies reduce the US beam penetration but increase the resolution; therefore, for skin and subcutis layers investigation, the best diagnostic accuracy is given by the 18–20 MHz probes.[15]

As demonstrated by Nauori et al., high-resolution US (using a 20 MHz transducer) allows also to differentiate lymphedema from lipedema. In lymphedema, the thickness of the skin and dermal hypoechogenicity are increased, especially in the distal part of the extremities for primary

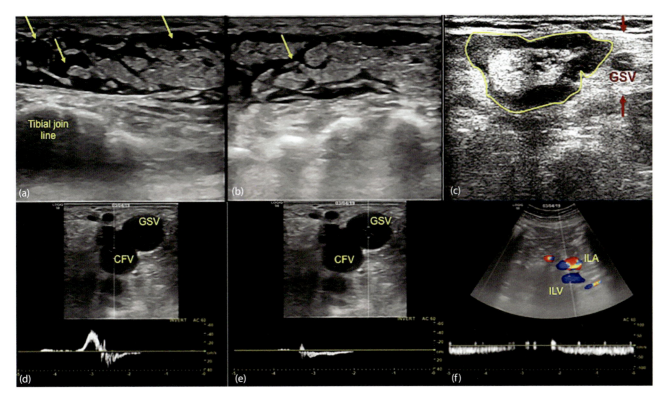

Figure 48.3 A case of a 63-year-old man affected by monolateral lower limb lymphedema. **(a)** High-resolution US B-mode (12 MhZ linear array transducer) showing the presence of the "lymphatic lakes" (yellow arrows) just above the tibial join line distal part. **(b)** Moving toward the thigh, the yellow arrow indicates lymphatic trunk ectasia. **(c)** Groin region just below the sapheno-femoral junction, a noticeable increased lymph node (encircled in yellow) next to the great saphenous vein (GSV) between the superficial and deep muscular facia. **(d)** Spectral Doppler investigation of common femoral vein (CFV) that shows no deep reflux (<1 second). **(e)** To the contrary, spectral Doppler analysis performed on GSV presents a superficial venous reflux (>0.5 second) verifying an associated involvement of superficial venous system. **(f)** Investigation of common iliac vein (ILV) with 7.5 MhZ convex transducer, aimed to exclude a deep vein obstruction upstream sapheno-femoral junction. The flow is always present and phasic with patient breath.

lymphedema, to the contrary in lipedema, which is due to an increase in hypodermal tissue with no true dermal edema; dermal echogenicity is similar to normal skin.[16]

Disadvantages of conventional high-frequency US with an upper frequency of 15–18 MHz include operator dependency (i.e., the pressure of the probe on the skin can cause artificial deformation of underlying structure) and the difficulty in distinguishing the lymphatic vessels from the subcutaneous structures (veins or the nerves) when lymphatic vessels are smaller than 0.3 mm.

More updated ultrahigh-resolution US systems provide frequencies as high as 70 MHz and resolution capability as fine as 30 μm, which could allow for more precise imaging of the lymphatic vessels and of small anatomical structures.[17]

COLOR DOPPLER ULTRASOUND AND SPECTRAL WAVE ANALYSIS

Such lesions must be qualified according to their vascularization pattern using color Doppler US and/or spectral analysis.

In malformations with very low-flow velocities such as LMs, showing no flow signal at rest, the use of a maneuver evoking color-shift signal is represented by the compression

of the lesion with the US probe[2,18] (Figure 48.1b). Moreover, some venous and less often arterial signals can be detected in about 60% of cyst walls; however, cysts of typical LMs are not detectably perfused; to the contrary, if flow signal is detected, the veno-lymphatic malformation should be suspected.[19]

The use of spectral analysis and/or color Doppler in lymphedema is restricted to the detection of the frequently associated impairments of the venous system. Duplex US must be useful to evaluate valve function in case of primary venous reflux, and to exclude deep vein thrombosis or post-thrombotic syndrome as a cause or contributing factor of edema.[20,21]

REFERENCES

1. Wassef M, Blei F, Adams D et al. ISSVA Board and Scientific Committee. Vascular anomalies classification: Recommendations from the International Society for the Study of Vascular Anomalies. *Pediatrics.* 2015;136(1):e203–e214.
2. Lee BB, Antignani PL, Baraldini V et al. ISVI-IUA consensus document diagnostic guidelines of vascular anomalies: Vascular malformations and hemangiomas. *Int Angiol.* 2015;34(4):333–374.

3. Mulliken JB, Glowacki J. Hemangiomas and vascular malformations in infants and children: A classification based on endothelial characteristics. *Plast Reconstr Surg.* 1982;69(3):412–422.

4. Maguiness SM, Frieden JI. Vascular birthmarks: Tumors and malformation. In: Schachner L, Hansen R, eds. *Pediatric Dermatology.* 4th ed. London, UK: Mosby; 2011:1135–1181.

5. McCafferty IJ, Jones RG. Imaging and management of vascular malformations. *Clin Radiol.* 2011;66:1208–1218.

6. Madani H, Farrant J, Chhaya N et al. Peripheral limb vascular malformations: An update of appropriate imaging and treatment options of a challenging condition. *Br J Radiol.* 2015;88(1047):20140406.

7. Grada AA, Phillips TJ. Lymphedema: Pathophysiology and clinical manifestations. *J Am Acad Dermatol.* 2017;77(6):1009–1020.

8. Grada AA, Phillips TJ. Lymphedema: Diagnostic workup and management. *J Am Acad Dermatol.* 2017; 77(6):995–1006.

9. Maclellan RA, Greene AK. Lymphedema. *Semin Pediatr Surg.* 2014;23(4):191–197.

10. O'Donnell TF Jr, Rasmussen JC, Sevick-Muraca EM. New diagnostic modalities in the evaluation of lymphedema. *J Vasc Surg Venous Lymphat Disord.* 2017;5(2):261–273.

11. Doldi SB, Lattuada E, Zappa MA, Pieri G, Favara A, Micheletto G. Ultrasonography of extremity lymphedema. *Lymphology.* 1992;25(3):129–133.

12. Kim W, Chung SG, Kim TW, Seo KS. Measurement of soft tissue compliance with pressure using ultrasonography. *Lymphology.* 2008;41:167–177.

13. Cavezzi A. Duplex ultrasonography In: Lee BB, Rockson GS, Bergan J, eds. *Lymphedema Compendium.* 2nd ed. New York, NY: Springer International Publishing; 2018:315–329.

14. O'Rourke K, Kibbee N, Stubbs A. Ultrasound for the evaluation of skin and soft tissue infections. *Mo Med.* 2015;112:202–205.

15. Hayashi A, Yamamoto T, Yoshimatsu H et al. Ultrasound visualization of the lymphatic vessels in the lower leg. *Microsurgery.* 2016;36:397–401.

16. Naouri M, Samimi M, Atlan M et al. High-resolution cutaneous ultrasonography to differentiate lipedema from lymphedema. *Br J Dermatol.* 2010;163(2): 296–301.

17. Hayashi A, Giacalone G, Yamamoto T et al. Ultra high-frequency ultrasonographic imaging with 70 MHz scanner for visualization of the lymphatic vessels. *Plast Reconstr Surg Glob Open.* 2019;7(1): e2086.

18. Gruber H, Peer S. Ultrasound diagnosis of soft tissue vascular malformations and tumours. *Curr Med Imaging Rev.* 2009;5:55–61.

19. Paltiel HJ, Burrows PE, Kozakewich HPW, Zurakowski D, Mulliken JB. Soft tissue vascular anomalies: Utility of US for diagnosis. *Radiology.* 2000;214:747–754.

20. Lee BB, Andrade M, Antignani PL et al. Diagnosis and treatment of primary lymphedema. Consensus document of the International Union of Phlebology (UIP)-2013. *Int Angiol.* 2013;32(6):541–574.

21. Thomis S. New diagnostic modalities in lymphedema. *Phlebolymphology.* 2017;24:152–160.

49

Radionuclide lymphoscintigraphy—Gold standard for assessment of lymphatic malformation: Lymphangioma and primary lymphedema or both?

VAUGHAN KEELEY

BACKGROUND

Radionuclide lymphoscintigraphy (LSG) demonstrates lymphatic function and was felt to be the gold standard investigation for diagnosing primary lymphedema in the International Union of Phlebology (IUP) guidelines (2013).[1] This technique involves the injection of 99mTc-labeled human serum albumin or sulfur colloid into the web spaces of the toes or fingers. Subsequently, a series of images are obtained using a γ-camera, and from these, features such as the speed of movement of tracer from the injection site to the regional lymph nodes, the presence of abnormal collateral flow pathways, e.g., through the popliteal nodes or dermal backflow, and the appearance of the lymph nodes can be assessed.

VARIATIONS IN TECHNIQUE

There is no internationally agreed standard technique for carrying out LSG. For example, there is variation in the tracer used, the site of injection (intradermal versus subcutaneous), and the timing of imaging.[2] Although a series of qualitative images can provide a measure of function, quantitative methods to determine the flow of tracer, e.g., by measuring the uptake of tracer in the regional lymph nodes compared with the amount injected distally at a fixed time point, may improve the diagnostic accuracy of the technique. A recent study emphasized the importance of this method and that delayed flow may be the only abnormality seen in some cases of lymphedema.[3] There is, however, no internationally agreed standardized quantitative LSG

protocol, making comparisons between reports from different institutions difficult.

ROLE IN PHENOTYPING OF PRIMARY LYMPHEDEMA

The St. George's Hospital, London, classification of primary lymphedema by phenotype has facilitated the discovery of genetic mutations responsible for different types of the condition.[4] LSG, if used routinely in the diagnosis of primary lymphedema, can contribute to the phenotyping process, as it has become recognized that the pattern of lymph flow may be different in the various types of primary lymphedema (Figures 49.1 and 49.2).

In Milroy lymphedema, there is what may be described as a functional dysplasia where the tracer injected into the feet is not absorbed into the initial lymphatics and therefore remains at the injection site for long periods of time. Quantitative imaging demonstrates very reduced uptake by the ilioinguinal lymph nodes. In lymphedema distichiasis, the injected tracer travels rapidly up to the regional lymph nodes but refluxes to the skin giving the appearance of dermal backflow due to the lymphatic valvular incompetence typical of this condition. In Meige lymphedema, there is usually delayed flow, dermal backflow, and the visualization of popliteal nodes suggesting rerouting of the injected tracer through the deep lymphatic system (Figure 49.2).

Carrying out LSG in young children may require a prolonged general anesthetic for images to be taken at different time points; many centers may defer carrying out LSG until the child is older, e.g., at least 8 years of age.

221

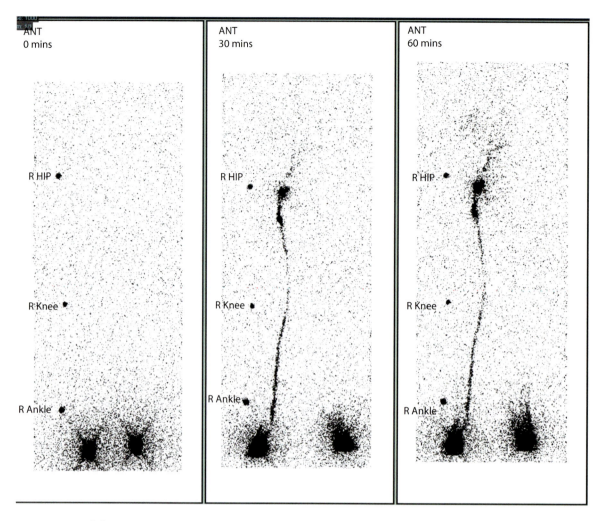

Figure 49.1 Patient with late-onset unilateral primary lymphedema of the left leg. Lymphoscintigraphy shows a normal pattern in unaffected right leg but delayed flow and dermal backflow in the left foot.

SENSITIVITY AND SPECIFICITY OF LYMPHOSCINTIGRAPHY

In a recent study of 227 patients with possible lymphedema, which was diagnosed clinically in 169 patients, the sensitivity and specificity of LSG were measured using intradermal injections of tracer and qualitative imaging.[5] The sensitivity was 96% and the specificity 100%.

In those who did not have lymphedema, the causes of limb swelling included vascular malformations, overgrowth syndromes, and conditions such as lipedema. This study suggests that LSG is very good at diagnosing lymphedema but not necessarily helpful in the assessment of vascular malformations including lymphatic malformations.

Interestingly, those patients with false-negative LSG were all felt to have primary lymphedema. In two patients, repeat LSG was carried out after 1 year and was abnormal. This suggests that in some cases of early primary lymphedema, qualitative LSG may not detect any abnormalities. However, it is possible that quantitative methods may be helpful in these cases. Alternatively, considering repeat qualitative LSG at a future date may be appropriate to facilitate defining the type of primary lymphedema.

COMPARISON OF LYMPHOSCINTIGRAPHY WITH OTHER TECHNIQUES

In a study of magnetic resonance lymphangiography (MRL) compared with LSG in 46 patients with leg lymphedema, MRL had a sensitivity of 68%, specificity 91%, positive predictive value 82%, and negative predictive value 83%.[6]

In another study, indocyanine green (ICG) lymphography was compared with LSG in 169 limbs with secondary lymphedema and 65 limbs with suspected primary lymphedema.[7] In those with secondary lymphedema, the sensitivity was 97% and specificity 55%. In those with suspected primary lymphedema, the sensitivity was 97% and the specificity 78%. The authors suggest that ICG lymphography could be a useful tool for screening for primary lymphedema. If positive, then LSG was recommended to provide more detailed information, but if negative it was suggested that no further investigation is required.

Although ICG lymphography is a relatively new and valuable technique in assessing superficial lymphatic function and anatomy, the main limitation in the context of diagnosing primary lymphedema is that the technique only visualizes lymphatics within 10 mm of the skin surface.

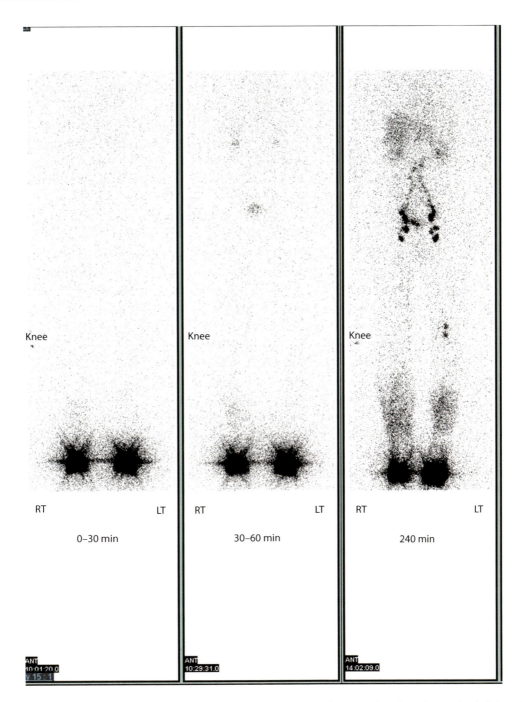

Knee

Knee

Knee

RT   LT

RT   LT

RT   LT

0–30 min

30–60 min

240 min

Figure 49.2 Meige lymphedema. Bilateral delayed flow and dermal backflow. Popliteal nodes in the left leg demonstrating rerouting through the deep subfascial lymphatics.

It may, however, have a role in the further phenotyping of lymphatic abnormalities in primary lymphedema.

LIMITATIONS OF LYMPHOSCINTIGRAPHY

LSG is not a useful tool in imaging the deeper central conducting lymphatics such as the thoracic duct and related structures. These can be affected in some complex types of primary lymphedema and in some lymphatic malformations. As reported earlier, LSG may not be helpful in patients with vascular malformations and overgrowth syndromes, although there may be a lymphatic component to these.

LSG may not contribute to the assessment of macrocystic, microcystic, or mixed lymphatic malformations, whereas magnetic resonance imaging (MRI) has a significant role.[8]

VISUALIZATION OF THE CENTRAL CONDUCTING LYMPHATICS

A recently developed technique (dynamic contrast-enhanced [DCE] magnetic resonance [MR] lymphangiography/nodal MR lymphangiography) involving the intranodal injection of gadolinium into the inguinal nodes enables visualization of the central conducting lymphatics.[9] It can be used to assess patients with chylous reflux and central lymphatic malformations; in turn, this has led, in some cases, to the use of interventional radiology techniques to seal leaks and prevent reflux.

CONCLUSIONS

LSG remains the gold standard investigation for the diagnosis of primary lymphedema affecting the limbs. Nevertheless, the development of an internationally recognized standard protocol for quantitative LSG is likely to improve its diagnostic accuracy and allow comparison of images between institutions and in research reports. New imaging techniques such as nodal MR lymphangiography are helpful in the assessment of abnormalities of the central conducting lymphatics and have a role in facilitating interventional radiological treatment of these. LSG does not contribute greatly to the imaging of lymphatic malformations, where MRI is the preferred modality.

REFERENCES

1. Lee BB, Andrade M, Antignani P et al. Diagnosis and treatment of primary lymphedema. Consensus document of the International Union of Phlebology (IUP)-2013. *Int Angiol.* 2013;32:541–574.
2. Bourgeois P. Radionuclide lymphoscintigraphies. In: Lee BB, Rockson S, Bergan J, eds. *Lymphedema.* 2nd ed. Cham, Switzerland: Springer International Publishing AG; 2018:257–327. https://doi.org/10.1007/978-3-319-52423-8_22.
3. Keramida G, Winterman N, Wroe E et al. Importance of accurate ilio-inguinal quantification in lower extremity lymphoscintigraphy. *Nucl Med Commun.* 2017;38: 209–214.
4. Connell FC, Gordon K, Brice G et al. The classification and diagnostic algorithm for primary lymphatic dysplasia: An update from 2010 to include molecular findings. *Clin Genet.* 2013;84(4):303–314.
5. Hasseinen A, Maclellan R, Grant F et al. Diagnostic accuracy of lymphoscintigraphy for lymphedema and analysis of false-negative tests. *Plast Reconstr Surg Glob Open.* 2017;5:e1396; doi: 10.1097/GOX.0000000000001396.
6. Weiss M, Burgard C, Baumeister R et al. Magnetic resonance imaging versus lymphoscintigraphy for the assessment of focal lymphatic transport disorders of the lower limb: First experiences. *Nuklearmedizin.* 2014;53:190–196.
7. Akita S, Mitsukawa N, Kazama T et al. Comparison of lymphoscintigraphy and indocyanine green lymphography for the diagnosis of extremity lymphoedema. *J Plast Reconstr Aesthet Surg.* 2013;66:792–798.
8. Flors L, Leiva-Salinas C, Maged IM et al. MR imaging of soft-tissue vascular malformations: Diagnosis, classification, and therapy follow-up. *RadioGraphics.* 2011;31:1321–1340.
9. Itkin M, Nadolski GJ. Modern techniques of lymphangiography and interventions: Current status and future development. *Cardiovasc Intervent Radiol.* 2018;41(3):366–376.

50

Magnetic resonance imaging and magnetic resonance lymphangiography of primary lymphedema: A new gold standard?

NINGFEI LIU

Primary lymphedema is defined as edema caused by lymphatic dysplasia or/and dysfunction due to congenital[1] or unknown factors. The clinical manifestations of primary lymphedema are variable. It most commonly occurs in one lower extremity but may affect both lower limbs. The relatively rare types of primary lymphedema are: unilateral lymphedema of an upper extremity, facial, and isolated external genital lymphedema. In general, external genital lymphedema is associated with edema of the lower limb(s). In very rare cases, lymphedema occurs in multiple sites, such as the ipsilateral face, upper and lower limbs, or contralateral upper and lower extremities.

The lymphatic system is composed of pre-collecting, collecting lymph vessels (afferent and efferent) and lymph nodes.[2] Luminal valves, essential for preventing retrograde lymph flow, are a special feature of collecting vessels. The pre-collecting vessel is between the capillary vessels and collecting vessels. The lymphatic malformations in primary lymphedema can occur at any level of the lymphatic system. Those anomalies of lymph vessels can occur alone or in combination. Thus, it may account for the diversity of clinical signs of the disease.

Currently, lymphedema, especially primary lymphedema, remains an "incurable" condition until a causal genetic defect is properly corrected or compensated. The treatment adopted in general can only slow the progression of the disease. The lack of effective treatment is due largely to lack of precise diagnostic modality to understand the pathological changes of the lymphatic system. The commonly used lymphoscintigraphy (LSG) with isotopic contrast agent has insufficient resolution to accurately outline the internal anatomy of the lymph node and lymphatic vessels.[3] Newly emerging lymphatic imaging techniques such as noncontrast three-dimensional (3D) magnetic resonance imaging (MRI) and contrast magnetic resonance lymphangiography (MRL) are useful in evaluating lymphatic system malformations,[4-6] as their high-resolution picture and dynamic real-time observation make both anatomical and functional diagnoses possible.

Three-dimensional MRI is special in detecting dilated and stagnant lymphatics, when the lymph flow is impaired and the channels dilated and filled with stagnated lymph. A 3D heavily T2-weighted MRI with an optimized protocol is performed for imaging stationary fluid to obtain high signal intensity. Under heavy T2-weighted imaging, the static or motionless fluid (lymph in the vessels and edema fluid in the tissues) displays high signals. When the background is saturated, lymph flow itself may act as a contrast medium to highlight the path of the lymphatic channels. Three-dimensional MRI can provide imaging of a quality similar to that of direct lymphangiography. The enlarged lymphatic vessels with channels (approximately 1 mm or more) and local dilated lesions can be clearly depicted. A special advantage of 3D MRI over LSG is its ability to display deep lymphatic trunks, i.e., abnormalities of the inguinal, iliac, and lumbar branches with increased channels (Figure 50.1).

Contrast MRL is now a routine assessment tool in the author's clinic since 2007, and more than 3,000 patients have been examined. Gd-BOPTA with a gadolinium (Gd) concentration of 0.5 mol/L was injected intradermally into the dorsal aspect of each foot or hand in the region of the four interdigital webs. 3D fast spoiled gradient-recalled echo T1-weighted images with a fat saturation technique (T1 high-resolution isotropic volume excitation, THRIVE) are acquired. To outline lymphatic vessels, maximum intensity projection (MIP) reconstruction images are calculated as well.

The enhancement of these lymphatic pathways persisted throughout the examination time, around 40 minutes. On the initial images, the enhancement of lymphatic channels may be light and discontinued. But the signal intensity increased, and the channels gradually became totally opacified with time. The lymphatic vessels in the edematous limbs

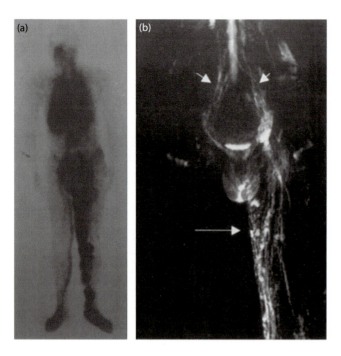

Figure 50.1 A 34-year-old man with lymphatic hyperplasia of the left leg. **(a)** Lymphoscintigraphy shows an intensive radioactive signal along the medial part of the left lower extremity and in the pelvis, groin, and scrotum. **(b)** Three-dimensional magnetic resonance imaging depicts enlarged lymphatics in the thigh (arrow). The estimated diameter of the lymphatics is 2–5 mm. Clusters of dilated inguinal, iliac, scrotum, and lumbar trunks (arrowhead) are also visualized.

are irregular in shape or uneven diameter and twisted, the characteristics making it easily distinguished from venous channels. The number of contrast-enhanced lymphatics in lymphedematous limbs varied from single to numerous. The diameters of visualized lymphatics ranged from 1.2 to 8 mm. The identical patterns of the lymphatic pathway in primary limb lymphedema are diverse[7]: radiating arranged enhanced vessels in the lower leg assemble to the medial portion of the knee and went up to the thigh, discontinued and lightly enhanced but dilated vessels in the medial portion of the lower limb; bunches of extremely dilated and significantly highlighted lymphatic located mainly in the media and less in the lateral portion of the thigh; and remarkably dilated and opacified lymphatic went from lower leg directly to the inguinal node with few branches (Figure 50.2).

About 17% of primary lymphedema is caused by lymph node abnormalities.[7] The morphological changes of lymph nodes including nodal size, internal lymph node architecture, and lymph node borders are evaluated. The shape of inguinal lymph node in the contralateral side of healthy volunteers are spherical or oval, numbered from 2–3 to 7–8 with a diameter around 1 cm. Compared with contralateral limbs, the morphological abnormalities of inguinal nodes in edematous limbs observed in the present study are as follows: absence of node, single large or multiple small fibrotic nodes, small nodules, nodes with irregular borders and homogeneous structure; irregular nodal outline with homogeneous architecture, markedly enlarged nodes with increased number. Dynamic

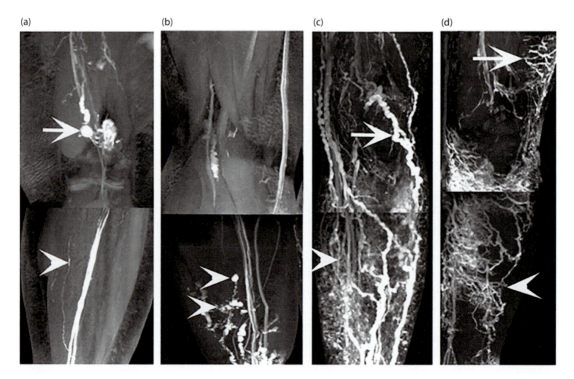

Figure 50.2 Composition images of magnetic resonance lymphangiogram shows various lymphatic drainage pathways in primary lymphedematous limbs. **(a)** Single deep lymph vessel (arrowhead) and popliteal nodes (arrow) were enhanced with the absence of superficial lymph vessel. **(b)** Enhanced lymph vessels with cystic dilatation (arrowhead) in the distal part of the leg. **(c)** Both superficial lymphatics (arrowhead) and deep lymph vessels and popliteal nodes (arrow) were involved. **(d)** A crisscross network of hyperplastic vessels in the thigh (arrow) and the calf (arrowhead).

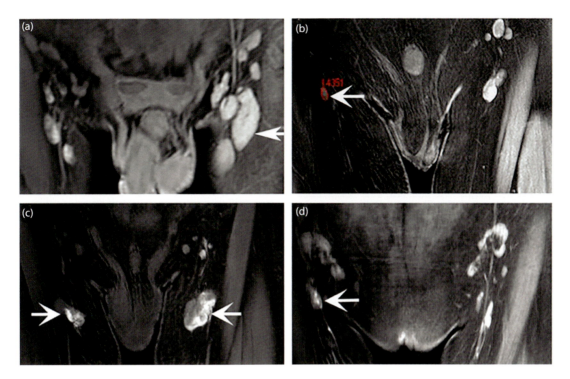

Figure 50.3 Diverse inguinal node abnormalities of primary lymphedematous displayed on magnetic resonance lymphangiograms. **(a)** Enlarged inguinal lymph nodes (arrow) with homogeneous texture in the left side in contrast with lymph nodes of normal size in the right side. **(b)** Single small node in a limb (arrow) with lymphatic hypoplasia and lymphedema is compared with lymph nodes in a limb without lymphedema. **(c)** Partially contrast-enhanced inferior inguinal nodes (arrow) in bilateral lymphedema with secondary lymphatic dilatation. **(d)** Small nodes that are irregularly shaped (small arrow) in a limb with lymphangiectasia (large arrow).

MR demonstrated abnormal patterns of contrast filling in the draining inguinal nodes. Postcontrast MRL images, however, displayed more structural abnormalities as (1) no contrast enhancement in the nodes, which may indicate total fibrosis of the nodes; (2) uneven nodal enhancement, which may indicate structural anomalies; and (3) partial enhancement within the nodes, which may be a congenital pathology of the nodes (Figure 50.3).

MRL can also detect the lymphatic function. The rapid transportation of contrast agent by draining lymphatic and regional lymph nodes ensures a consecutive and real-time inspection of the transporting function of lymphatic and lymph node within a reasonable length of time. Tracing the movement of enhanced flow within the lymphatic vessel allowed quantitative assessment of abnormal lymph flow kinetics. Inspection of the enhancement of contrast in inguinal nodes by comparison of the time—signal intensity curves allows for clarification of delayed or declined transport of lymph in an individual node and for quantitative assessment of abnormal nodal lymph flow kinetics.

The combination of the lymphatic and lymph node images may then outline the integral picture of the affected lymphatic system. On the MRL images, lymphatic abnormalities fell into two major categories: aplasia/hypoplasia or hyperplasia. Lymph node abnormalities fell into three major categories: aplasia/hypoplasia, or hyperplasia or structural abnormalities. MRL classification of the lymphatic system in primary lymphedema based on MRL imaging is proposed as follows:

1. Lymph nodes affected only with structurally abnormal node
2. Lymph vessel affected only with lymphatic aplasia/hypoplasia, lymphatic hyperplasia, or lymphatic dysfunction
3. Lymph vessel and lymph node affected with subgroups: (a) lymphatic and nodal aplasia/hypoplasia, (b) lymphatic aplasia/hypoplasia + nodal hyperplasia, (c) lymphatic aplasia/hypoplasia + nodal structural abnormalities, (d) lymphatic and nodal hyperplasia, (e) lymphatic hyperplasia + nodal aplasia/hypoplasia, (f) lymphatic hyperplasia + nodal structural abnormalities
4. Lymphatic dysfunction

The malformations of lymphatic vessels are not always concordant with those of lymph nodes in primary lymphedema. The lymph vessel and lymph node may be affected together or alone and may express different types of anatomical anomalies.[7] The advantage of MRL is that it can detect the precise anatomy of lymphatic vessels and lymph nodes in lymphedematous limbs. It also provides information concerning the functional status of lymph flow transport in the lymphatic vessels and lymph nodes of these limbs.

REFERENCES

1. Ferrell RE, Levinson KL, Esman JH et al. Hereditary lymphedema: Evidence for linkage and genetic heterogeneity. *Hum Mol Genet.* 1998;7:2073–2078.
2. Földi M, Földi E, Kubik S, eds. *Textbook of Lymphology: For Physicians and Lymphoedema Therapists.* San Francisco, CA: Urban and Fischer; 2003.
3. Liu NF, Lu Q, Wu XF. Comparison of radionuclide lymphoscintigraphy and dynamic magnetic resonance lymphangiography for investigating extremity lymphoedema. *Br J Surg.* 2010;97:359–365.
4. Liu NF, Lu Q, Jiang ZH. Anatomic and functional evaluation of lymphatics and lymph nodes in diagnosis of lymphatic circulation disorders with contrast magnetic resonance lymphangiography. *J Vasc Surg.* 2009;49:980–987.
5. Lu Q, Xu J, Liu N. Chronic lower extremity lymphedema: A comparative study of high- resolution interstitial MR lymphangiography and heavily T2-weighted MRI. *Eur J Radiol.* 2010;73:365–373.
6. Liu NF, Wang BS. Functional lymphatic collectors in breast cancer-related lymphedema arm. *Lymphat Res Biol.* 2014;12:232–237.
7. Liu NF, Yan ZX. Classification of lymphatic system malformations in primary lymphoedema based on MR lymphangiography. *Eur J Vascu Endo Surg.* 2012; 44:345–349.

51

Indocyanine green fluorescent lymphography: Clinical implementation

TAKUMI YAMAMOTO

Evaluation of lymph circulation is essential for the management of vascular malformations affecting the lymphatic system. Near-infrared fluorescent lymphography using indocyanine green (ICG) is a minimally invasive lymph imaging procedure, without radiation exposure, which allows real time clear visualization of superficial lymph flow.[1–5] Although deep lymph flow cannot be visualized directly, ICG lymphography is becoming popular with its clinical usefulness for clinical classification, severity staging, prediction of prognosis, and consideration of indications of several treatments.[1–4,6–10]

ICG lymphography is performed by injecting ICG intradermally or subcutaneously into the affected region—at the foot for lower extremity, at the hand for upper extremity, and at the midline in the face for head and neck lymph flow evaluation.[1,2,4] Using a near-infrared camera, fluorescent images are obtained in real time. ICG lymphography findings are largely classified into normal "linear" and abnormal "dermal backflow (DB)" patterns; DB patterns can be subdivided into "reticular," "splash," "stardust," and "diffuse" patterns.[3,7]

In a transient phase, immediately after ICG injection, linear and/or reticular patterns can be seen. In a plateau phase, several hours later, the reticular pattern changes to a splash, stardust, or diffuse pattern[2,7] (Figure 51.1). Since a lymphatic vessel's pathological characteristics are different according to ICG lymphography patterns, the differentiation of DB patterns is critical; as ICG lymphography findings change from linear to splash, stardust, and finally to diffuse pattern, collecting/pre-collecting lymphatic vessels become sclerotic with smaller lumen, while dermal capillary lymphatic vessels become dilated to work as collateral lymph pathways.[3,7–10] ICG lymphography findings should be evaluated at a plateau phase. Based on ICG lymphography findings, primary lymphedema can be classified into four types: proximal DB (PDB), distal DB (DDB), less enhancement (LE), and no enhancement (NE) types[6] (Figure 51.2).

In the PDB pattern, DB patterns extend distally from the proximal lymph flow obstruction site as seen in secondary lymphedema following cancer treatments. Lymph flow obstruction due to lymphatic malformation in the trunk is suspected as an etiology of primary lymphedema with a PDB pattern.[1,2,6] In the DDB pattern, DB patterns are seen only in the distal region but not in the proximal region. Localized distal malformation or lymphatic valve malformation are suspected as causes. Patients with DDB pattern usually have a past history of cellulitis attacks.[6,11] In the LE pattern, the linear pattern is seen only in the distal region, and no ICG enhancement is detected in the proximal region. The hypoplastic superficial lymphatic system and aging-related pump dysfunction are considered as causes. Most patients with LE pattern suffer from mild lymphedema.[6] In the NE pattern, no ICG enhancement is detected other than in the injected sites; no linear pattern or DB pattern is shown. Localized lymphatic aplasia and severe lymph malabsorption are suspected as causes. Most patients with NE pattern

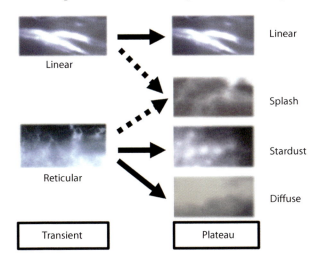

Figure 51.1 Indocyanine green lymphography findings at transient and plateau phase. At the transient phase, linear, and/or reticular patterns are seen. At the plateau phase, the reticular pattern extends and changes to splash, stardust, and/or diffuse patterns.

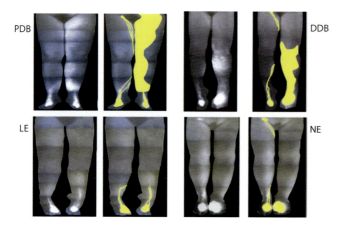

Figure 51.2 Indocyanine green lymphography classification for primary lymphedema.

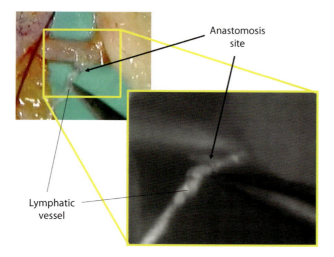

Figure 51.3 Indocyanine green lymphography navigation for lymphedema surgery. The lymphatic vessel can be easily identified, and lymph flow can be evaluated intraoperatively. Lymph flows into venous circulation via the anastomosis.

are congenital and suffer from severe lymphedema.[6,12] As ICG lymphography visualizes superficial lymph flows very clearly, ICG lymphography navigation is applied in various lymphedema treatments.[12–17] Manual lymph drainage can be guided under ICG navigation; the most effective massage/maneuver can be confirmed with real-time ICG lymphography.[16] In lymphatic bypass surgery, collecting lymphatic vessels can be easily detected under ICG lymphography navigation and efficiently bypassed to lymphatic or venous circulation with intact flows[13,14,17] (Figure 51.3). To maximize safety in vascularized lymph node transfer, ICG lymphography is used to map donor site lymph flows—reverse lymphatic mapping.[12,15] Although a relatively novel modality for lymph imaging, ICG lymphography is becoming popular in daily practice and research in the fields of lymphedema and lymph-related diseases with its convenience for real-time evaluation without a risk of radiation

exposure. With an increasing number of clinical research publications, ICG lymphography is becoming a useful option for the evaluation of lymph-related diseases.[3,6,8,10,18–20]

The major limitations of ICG lymphography are that there are many protocols for ICG injection and fluorescent image observation and that it does not allow direct visualization of deep lymph flows.[1–3,5,16,18,19] Further studies are warranted to clarify an optimal protocol of ICG lymphography and to compare ICG lymphography findings and deep lymph flow image findings.

ACKNOWLEDGMENT

Preparation of this chapter is supported, in part, by NCGM Biobank Fund (29-2004).

REFERENCES

1. Yamamoto T, Narushima M, Doi K et al. Characteristic indocyanine green lymphography findings in lower extremity lymphedema: The generation of a novel lymphedema severity staging system using dermal backflow patterns. *Plast Reconstr Surg.* 2011;127(5):1979–1986.
2. Yamamoto T, Yamamoto N, Doi K et al. Indocyanine green (ICG)-enhanced lymphography for upper extremity lymphedema: A novel severity staging system using dermal backflow (DB) patterns. *Plast Reconstr Surg.* 2011;128(4):941–947.
3. Yamamoto T, Matsuda N, Doi K et al. The earliest finding of indocyanine green (ICG) lymphography in asymptomatic limbs of lower extremity lymphedema patients secondary to cancer treatment: The modified dermal backflow (DB) stage and concept of subclinical lymphedema. *Plast Reconstr Surg.* 2011;128(4):314e–321e.
4. Yamamoto T, Iida T, Matsuda N et al. Indocyanine green (ICG)-enhanced lymphography for evaluation of facial lymphoedema. *J Plast Reconstr Aesthet Surg.* 2011;64(11):1541–1544.
5. Unno N, Inuzuka K, Suzuki M et al. Preliminary experience with a novel fluorescence lymphography using indocyanine green in patients with secondary lymphedema. *J Vasc Surg.* 2007;45(5):1016–1021.
6. Yamamoto T, Yoshimatsu H, Narushima M, Yamamoto N, Hayashi A, Koshima I. Indocyanine green lymphography findings in primary leg lymphedema. *Eur J Vasc Endovasc Surg.* 2015;49:95–102.
7. Yamamoto T, Yamamoto N, Furuya M, Hayashi A, Koshima I. Genital lymphedema score: Genital lymphedema severity scoring system based on subjective symptoms. *Ann Plast Surg.* 2016;77(1):119–121.
8. Yamamoto T, Yamamoto N, Yoshimatsu H, Narushima M, Koshima I. Factors associated with lymphosclerosis: An analysis on 962 lymphatic vessels. *Plast Reconstr Surg.* 2017;140(4):734–741.

9. Yamamoto T, Narushima M, Koshima I. Lymphatic vessel diameter in female pelvic cancer-related lower extremity lymphedematous limbs. *J Surg Oncol.* 2018;117:1157–1163.

10. Yamamoto T, Yamamoto N, Fuse Y, Narushima M, Koshima I. Optimal sites for supermicrosurgical lymphaticovenular anastomosis: An analysis of lymphatic vessel detection rates on 840 surgical fields in lower extremity lymphedema. *Plast Reconstr Surg.* 2018;142:924e–930e.

11. Yamamoto T, Koshima I. Supermicrosurgical anastomosis of superficial lymphatic vessel to deep lymphatic vessel for a patient with cellulitis-induced chronic localized leg lymphedema. *Microsurgery.* 2015;35(1):68–71.

12. Yamamoto T, Yoshimatsu H, Yamamoto N. Complete lymph flow reconstruction: A free vascularized lymph node true perforator flap transfer with efferent lymphaticolymphatic anastomosis. *J Plast Reconstr Aesthet Surg.* 2016;69(9):1227–1233.

13. Yamamoto T, Narushima M, Yoshimatsu H et al. Minimally invasive lymphatic supermicrosurgery (MILS): Indocyanine green lymphography-guided simultaneous multi-site lymphaticovenular anastomoses via millimeter skin incisions. *Ann Plast Surg.* 2014;72(1):67–70.

14. Yamamoto T, Yamamoto N, Azuma S et al. Near-infrared illumination system-integrated microscope for supermicrosurgical lymphaticovenular anastomosis. *Microsurgery.* 2014;34(1):23–27.

15. Yamamoto T, Iida T, Yoshimatsu H, Fuse Y, Hayashi A, Yamamoto N. Lymph flow restoration after tissue replantation and transfer: Importance of lymph axiality and possibility of lymph flow reconstruction using free flap transfer without lymph node or supermicrosurgical lymphatic anastomosis. *Plast Reconstr Surg.* 2018;142:796–804.

16. Lopera C, Worsley PR, Bader DL, Fenlon D. Investigating the short-term effects of manual lymphatic drainage and compression garment therapies on lymphatic function using near-infrared imaging. *Lymphat Res Biol.* 2017;15(3):235–240.

17. Yamamoto T, Yoshimatsu H, Koshima I. Navigation lymphatic supermicrosurgery for iatrogenic lymphorrhea: Supermicrosurgical lymphaticolymphatic anastomosis and lymphaticovenular anastomosis under indocyanine green lymphography navigation. *J Plast Reconstr Aesthet Surg.* 2014;67(11):1573–1579.

18. Narushima M, Yamamoto T, Ogata F, Yoshimatsu H, Mihara M, Koshima I. Indocyanine green lymphography findings in limb lymphedema. *J Reconstr Microsurg.* 2016;32:72–79.

19. Brahma B, Yamamoto T. Breast cancer treatment-related lymphedema (BCRL): An overview of the literature and updates in microsurgery reconstruction. *Eur J Surg Oncol.* 2019;45:1138–1145.

20. Kato M, Watanabe S, Iida T, Watanabe A. Flow pattern classification in lymphatic malformations by indocyanine green lymphography. *Plast Reconstr Surg.* 2019;143(3):558e–564e.

52

Oil contrast lymphangiography: New role for the surgical candidate?

FRANCESCO BOCCARDO, SARA DESSALVI, CORRADO CESARE CAMPISI, AND CORRADINO CAMPISI

In order to reach positive results in the treatment of lymphatic and chylous disorders, especially when it is possible to use microsurgical solutions, an accurate diagnostic assessment is of utmost importance. Standard lymphangiography (LAG) uses ultrafluid liposoluble contrast medium (Lipiodol Ultra Fluid) injected after isolation and cannulation of the lymphatics of the dorsum of the foot. If coupled with a computed tomography (CT) scan, LAG allows for a more accurate assessment of disease extension, as well as the site of the obstacle and source of chylous leakage.[1] Conventional LAG can be performed in two different ways: (1) by injecting Lipiodol Ultra Fluid after isolation and cannulation of the lymphatics of the dorsum of the foot with microsurgical technique[2]; although LAG performed with bipodal microsurgical technique allows to assess also lower limb lymphatics and nodes, it is a demanding technique that requires microsurgical expertise. (2) Intranodal LAG is faster and technically easier but can cause lymph node disruption.

The main indications to the use of direct oil contrast LAG are represented by the preoperative assessment of patients affected by chylous disorders: chyloperitoneum, chylothorax, chylous cysts, mediastinal chyloma or chylomediastinum, chylopericardium, chyluria, chylo-colpometrorrhea, chyloedema of external genitalia and of lower extremities with chylo-lymphostatic verrucosis and subsequent chylolymphorrhea, and chylous joint effusion.[3–9] In the past, it was also used for the staging of Hodgkin's disease, as it supplied a morphological and structural evaluation of subdiaphragmatic and mediastinal lymph nodes.

TECHNIQUE

In local anesthesia with Carbocaine 2%, the blue dye is injected at the first two interdigital spaces of the foot bilaterally in order to delineate the transit site of the main lymphatic collectors and, therefore, to perform a 1 cm skin incision just at the medial third of the intermalleolar line, looking for a viable lymphatic vessel suitable for the cannulation[10] (Figure 52.1a). Carbocaine is also useful for its sympatholytic effect that permits managing a possible lymphangiospasm of the lymphatic vessels. The isolation of the lymphatic collector from the surrounding tissues is performed under the operative microscope (25×). A lymphatic collector is accurately prepared trying to avoid disruption of the surrounding tissue and lymphatics, which can cause a very troublesome lymphorrhea and be a source of infections, especially in cases of obstructive lymphedema (Figure 52.1b). A 27G needle is introduced into the lymphatic vessels again under the guide of the microscope. This technique reduces the risk of the oil contrast leaking at the site of the puncture (Figure 52.1c). Once the lymphatic vessel is cannulated, the needle is connected to a manual injector, and two vials of Lipiodol Ultra Fluid (20 cc combined) are injected. The manual technique allows for assessment of the proper pressure of injection for the whole time of the investigation, avoiding excessively high pressure and consequent damage to the lymphatic structures. During the procedure, fluoroscopic assessment is performed (Figure 52.1d) in order to identify possible lymphatic-venous fistulas, which would become evident radiologically like an image of "caviar eggs," and to avoid the risk of pulmonary microembolism. In case of complications, the manual injection can be suddenly stopped.

After completing the contrast medium injection, the needle is removed from the lymphatics, and the surgical wound is closed. A CT investigation is performed 30 minutes after the surgical procedure. This investigation allows for the study of lymphatics and lymph nodes of the iliac, lumbo-aortic, retroperitoneal regions, the chylocyst and the thoracic duct up to its end into the jugular vein. An accurate assessment of the extension of the disease as well as the site of the obstacle or reflux and sources of chylous leakage (Figure 52.2a and b) is therefore performed. A three-dimensional

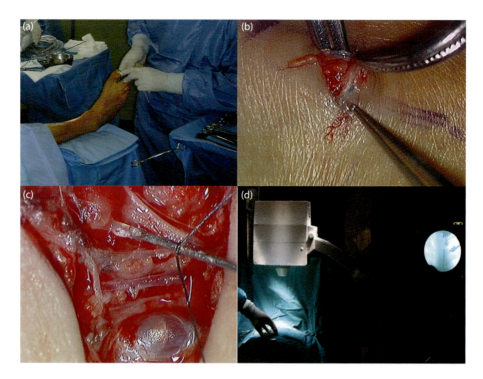

Figure 52.1 Technique. **(a)** 1 cm skin incision just at the medial third of the intermalleolar line is made to identify a viable lymphatic vessel suitable for the cannulation. **(b)** Operative microscope (25×) is used for the visualization during isolation of the lymphatic collector from the surrounding tissues. **(c)** A 27G needle is introduced into the lymphatic vessels under microscope guidance. **(d)** A fluoroscopic assessment is performed during the procedure to detect possible lymphatic-venous fistulas—to avoid the risk of pulmonary microembolism.

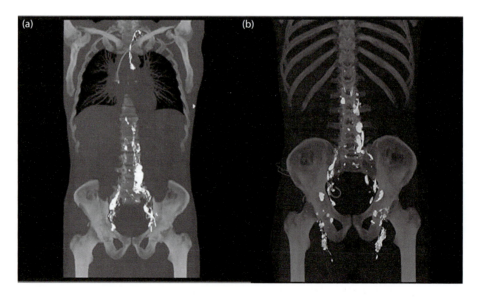

Figure 52.2 **(a)** and **(b)** A computed tomography investigation is performed 30 minutes after the surgical procedure. Assessment of the extension of the disease as well as the site of the obstruction or reflux and sources of chylous leakage is performed.

(3D) CT scan allows relations between lymphatic-lymph nodal structures and skeletal apparatus to be pointed out, bringing precise information about the site of chylous dysplasia and/or fistulas (Figure 52.3). For better recognition of chyliferous vessels, a fatty meal (60 g of butter in 200 mL of milk) is administered 4–5 hours before surgery.

In the literature, it is reported that the Lipiodol Ultra Fluid can also have sclerosing effects on lymphatics, causing the closure of lymphatic fistulas in some patients with chylous ascites or chylothorax. The possible resolution of prolonged chylous leakage by performing lymphangiography should encourage its use in such clinical cases.[11] Notwithstanding

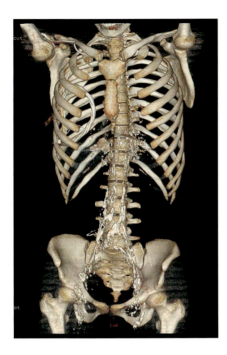

Figure 52.3 A three-dimensional computed tomography scan is performed to determine the site of chylous dysplasia and/or fistulas.

the clinical findings, the lymphangiographic sclerosis effect has to be studied more closely. This effect surely depends on the high or low output of the fistula and its etiology, being more possible in secondary cases than in primary dysplastic ones. But it was found that even in the secondary cases, there was anatomo-functional congenital anomalies, and that is why the sclerosing effect of LAG is so rare.

From the etiopathological point of view, primary forms of chyloperitoneum are basically correlated with congenital dysplasic alterations and more or less extended malformations of chyliferous vessels, cisterna chyli, and/or of the thoracic duct, as well as of regional lymph nodes in the affected areas. These conditions account for approximately 70% of all cases. Conversely, "secondary" forms due to mechanical causes or obstructions of various types or disruptions, including trauma, are less common.[12-17]

It should be pointed out that from a pathophysiological point of view, malformation-related dysplasic alterations act as actual obstacles to antigravity lymphatic drainage, just like mechanical obstruction. A malformation affecting the thoracic duct, Pecquet cyst, and/or chyliferous vessels illustrates this concept and represents a significant obstacle to lymph drainage and, in particular, to intestinal drainage. Accordingly, chyliferous vessels along the walls of the small intestine and of the mesentery become significantly dilated and abnormally stretched due to chylous stasis. The disease also features lymphatic megacollectors with more or less extensive chylous lymphangiectasia, chylous cysts, often associated with lymphangiomyomatosis. These are located not only right below the visceral peritoneal layer

with a mesh-like arrangement but also throughout the small intestine and more specifically at the level of intestinal villi. Hence, dysplastic chyliferous megalymphatics may break due to a localized swelling (the "mesentery chylous cyst") or anywhere along the wall of extremely ectatic collectors, sometimes through a two-step process. Once the peritoneum layer is opened up by chyle with subsequent development of a "chyloma," chyle begins to flow into the abdominal cavity. Also, in other cases, the chyliferous vessel at the center of the villus breaks into the intestinal lumen, thereby causing loss of proteins, lymphocytes, immunoglobulins, lipids, lipoproteins, and even calcium and glucose, which leads to metabolic disorders that are typical of "protein losing enteropathy" (PLE).[18-23]

Owing to the direct link between the septic intestinal environment and the inner lining of chyliferous vessels, there may be recurrent attacks of acute infections and acute mesenteric lympho-angioadenitis which, in some cases, may even lead to septic shock or to a chronic process, a sort of vicious circle with further worsening of the intestinal lymphatic drainage.

Chyloperitoneum and PLE may often be combined. Also, it should not be forgotten that, apart from intestinal lymphatics, lumbar lymphatics—collecting the lymph from the lower limbs, external genitalia, intra-abdominal organs, kidneys, adrenal gland, and abdominal wall—flow into the cisterna chyli. Furthermore, considering the thoracic-mediastinal catchment basin of the thoracic duct and that lymphatic dysplasias can affect even one or more extraabdominal sites, due to bizarre malformation combinations, chyloperitoneum can also be associated with a whole range of different pathological pictures: chylothorax; chylous cyst, mediastinal chyloma, or chylomediastinum; chyloperidium; chyluria; chylo-colpometrorrhea; chyloedema of external genitalia and/or of one or both lower limbs, with chylo-lymphostatic verrucosis and subsequent chylo-lymphorrhea; and chylous joint effusion.

The wide-ranging extension of the foregoing malformations and the complexity of their association with dysplasia of chylo-lymphatic vessels, thoracic duct, and chylous cyst explain why, in the newborn, they are sometimes incompatible with life. Furthermore, upon clinical onset of the most severe cases, effective treatment may be difficult to achieve later in life, thereby leading to more or less complex prognostic implications involving *quoad valetudinem* as well as *quoad vitam* issues.

Chylous thoracic and/or abdominal disorders can affect patients even at birth for primary forms or be related to oncological operations with lymphatic injuries. The only possibility to accurately assess the pathological condition is offered by LAG, which represents the only diagnostic investigation that can supply precise topographic information about the site and cause of the pathology (Figure 52.4). On the basis of LAG findings, the proper therapeutic management is planned.

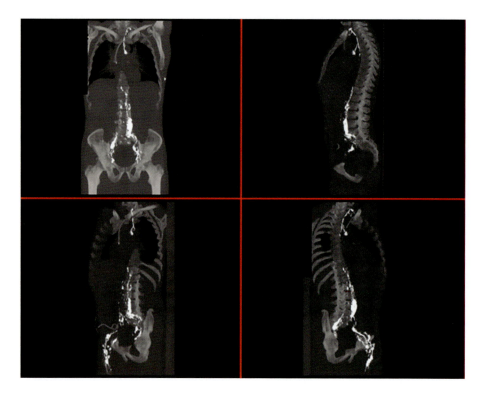

Figure 52.4 Lymphangiography represents the only diagnostic investigation that can provide precise topographic information regarding the site and cause of the pathology.

REFERENCES

1. Dessalvi S, Boccardo F, Molinari L, Spinaci S, Campisi C, Ferrari GM. Chyloperitoneum: Diagnostic and therapeutic options. *Lymphology.* 2016;49(1):1–7.
2. Dessalvi S, Boccardo F, Campisi CC et al. Lesion of thoracic duct: Clinical case report. *Eur J Lymphol Relat Probl.* 2017;29(77):29–31.
3. Cruikshank W. *The Anatomy of the Absorbing Vessels.* 2nd ed. London, England: G Nicol Pall Mall; 1790.
4. Busey SC. *Congenital Occlusion and Dilation of Lymph Channels.* New York, NY: William Wood and Co.; 1878.
5. Campisi C, Boccardo F, Zilli A et al. Chylous reflux pathologies: Diagnosis and microsurgical treatment. *Int Angiol.* 1999;18:10.
6. Campisi C, Da Rin E, Bellini C et al. Pediatric lymphedema and correlated syndromes: Role of microsurgery. *Microsurgery.* 2008;28:138.
7. Giampalmo A. *Patologia delle Malformazioni Vascolari.* Rome, Italy: Società Ed. Universo; 1972.
8. Jamal S, Kumaraswami V, Witte MH et al. Lymphatic abnormalities in microfilaraemics by lymphoscintigraphy, in *Progress in Lymphology XIV*, edited by MH Witte, CL Witte. *Lymphology.* 1994;27(Suppl):357.
9. Jamal S. Failure in lymphedema treatment (filarial). The patient factor. *Lymphology.* 1998;31(Suppl):403.
10. Boccardo F, Campisi C, Zilli A, Casaccia M. Direct lymphography with microsurgical technique: Indications and results. *Lymphology.* 1998;31(Suppl):559–561.
11. Mullins JK, Pierorazio PM, Hyams ES, Mitchell SE, Allaf ME. Lymphangiography with sclerotherapy: A novel therapy for refractory chylous ascites. *Can J Urol.* 2012;19(3):6250–6254.
12. Bellini C, Boccardo F, Campisi C et al. Pulmonary lymphangiectasia. *Lymphology.* 2005;38:111.
13. Bellini C, Boccardo F, Campisi C et al. Congenital pulmonary lymphangiectasia. *Orphanet J Rare Dis.* 2006;30(1):43.
14. Bellini C, Boccardo F, Bonioli E et al. Lymphodynamics in the fetus and newborn. *Lymphology.* 2006;39:110.
15. Bellini C, Hennekam RC, Boccardo F et al. Nonimmune idiopathic hydrops fetalis and congenital lymphatic dysplasia. *Am J Med Genet (Part A).* 2006;140:678.
16. Bellini C, Boccardo F, Campisi C et al. Lymphatic dysplasias in newborns and children: The role of lymphoscintigraphy. *J Pediatr.* 2008;152:587.
17. Belov St, Loose DA, Weber J. Vascular malformations. *Periodica Angiologica 16 - Einhorn, Presse Verlag* 1989;16.
18. Rutigliani M, Boccardo F, Campisi C et al. Immunohistochemical studies in a hydroptic fetus with pulmonary lymphangiectasia and trisomy 21. *Lymphology.* 2007;40:114.
19. Case TC, Witte CL, Witte MH et al. Magnetic resonance imaging in human lymphedema: Comparison with lymphangioscintigraphy. *Magn Reson Imaging.* 1992;10:549.

20. Browse N, Burnard KG, Mortimer PS, eds. *Diseases of the Lymphatics*. London, England: Arnold Publishers; 2003.
21. Boccardo F, Bellini C, Eretta C et al. The lymphatics in the pathophysiology of thoracic and abdominal surgical pathology: Immunological consequences and the unexpected role of microsurgery. *Microsurgery*. 2007;27:339.
22. Gruwez J. Lymphoedema, basic mechanism, clinical problems, indications for therapy, chylous reflux. *Proceedings of the 4th ISL Congress*, Tucson, Arizona, 1973.
23. Gruwez JA, Lerut T, Rahardjo T, Van Elst F. The lymphatics in angiodysplastic syndromes. *Progress in Lymphology, Proc. VIIth Int. Congr. ISL*, Florence, Italy, 1979, Avicenum Czechoslovak, Medical Press, Prague, 1981.

53

Fluorescent microlymphangiography: Controversy, confusion, and neglected problems

CLAUDIO ALLEGRA, MICHELANGELO BARTOLO, AND SALVINO BILANCINI

The venous and the lymphatic systems work together; they are connected by tiny lymphovenous anastomoses that are activated when the pressure in the lymphatic system rises.[1] Persistent venous stasis will lead to functional overload in the lymphatic system, which may result in dynamic insufficiency because the fluid overload exceeds transport capacity of the lymphatics. In these conditions, lymphangiopathy develops, which, in turn, exacerbates edema, which is no longer only of venous but also of lymphatic origin.[1,2] Modern imaging modalities and technology allow visualization of the lymphatics in any part of the body and are used to evaluate the lymphatic system more accurately.

Microlymphatic vessel morphology, diameter and permeability, number of microlymphatic loops, and extension of the contrast halo from the injection site can be determined by injecting contrast into microlymphatics. This contrast enhancement technique involves subdermal injection of FITC-dextran 150000 (0.01 mL) using a microsyringe (ca. 0.2 mm).[1–4] Following the subdermal contrast injection, the images are acquired on a videocassette and subsequently images are digitally processed to analyze data.

Microlymphography determines the following parameters:

1. Number of open or available lymphatic vessels
2. Morphology of open or available lymphatic vessels
3. Permeability of available lymphatic vessels
4. Superficial diffusion of contrast material from the injection site (mm)
5. Diameter of available lymphatic vessels (μm)
6. Intralymphatic pressure (mm Hg)
7. Interstitial pressure (mm Hg)

When the data from dynamic capillaroscopy and capillary blood velocity (CBV) are combined with microlymphography, a more complete picture can be obtained for understanding the pathophysiology of a microcirculatory system.[5,6]

MEASUREMENT OF MICROLYMPHATIC PRESSURE

During the 1960s, microcirculatory pressure was measured directly using micropipettes (at least 15 μm in diameter). With this passive method, the time needed to measure pressure was about 10 seconds.[7,8] The major limitation of this technique was extreme difficulty in acquiring an accurate measurement, as the large micropipettes when used on the skin could change the delicate pressure balance inside the microlymphatics leading to false measurements.

A significant advance in measuring intramicrolymphatic pressure came in the 1970s when Marcos Intaglietta created the servo-nulling system, a device that permitted active pressure measurement with real-time response (0.05 seconds).[7,8] The micropipettes used in this system had diameter less than half compared to the previously used (mentioned earler) micropipettes (about 7 μm). With additional improvements of the servo-nulling system implemented in a Model 5a (that was created in 1990), which had added on a preamplifier near the micropipette, much smaller pipettes (about 1 μm in diameter) were used for pressure measurement.[8,9] The introduction of micropipettes of only 1 μm in diameter made a very detailed study of intramicrolymphatic pressure possible. After resting for 30 minutes, a patient is placed in supine position and pressure is measured for at least 1 minute. Data from numerous studies that used the previously described system and measuring protocol have improved our knowledge of the pathophysiology of the lymphatic circulation in healthy subjects and in patients with chronic venous disease, lymphedema, and other vascular conditions.[5,9–11,16] Besides intramicrolymphatic pressure,

Table 53.1 Interstitial pressure

	CVI II stage (C3 C4)	Lymphedema	Controls
Interstitial pressure (mm Hg)	1.47 ± 1.7	4.33 ± 1.7	0.65 ± 1.6

Source: Allegra C et al. *Int Angiol.* 1997;16(3)(Suppl. 1).

this method can be used to measure interstitial pressure in healthy individuals and in those with chronic venous disease and lymphedema[16] (Table 53.1).

There are two controversial, confusing, and neglected problems:

1. Use of the intralymphatic, tissue pressure and measurement of the lymphatic flow velocity on the microlymphatic.
2. Not taking into consideration the blocking structures (anatomy structures, found inside or around the microvessel, which can cause opening or closing of the vessel lumen). These anatomical structures are important to determine the lymph distribution and the relationship between the superficial and deep lymphatic systems.

It is worth emphasizing that only a few practitioners use the servo-nulling pressure system[9,10,12,15] and to the best of our knowledge measuring of the interstitial tissue pressure and measuring of the lymph velocity have not been utilized to date.

Measurement of the interstitial tissue pressure is simple, because we have to use the same instrument used for measurement of the intralymphatic pressure. These data are very important to compare the variations of the tissue pressure according to the oncotic-hydrostatic balance and according to the activation of the initial microlymphatic system that depends on tissue pressure gradients. Variations in tissue pressure lead to variations in microlymphatic pressure (and vice versa).

The spread (distribution) of the dye in the lymphatic capillaries does not reflect the real velocity of the microlymphatic flow; until our research on the microlymphatic flow velocity, the only method to measure the lymphatic flow was the spread velocity of the dye,[3,15] but now for the first time we can visualize and measure the flow dynamics[3] (Figure 53.1) and increasing velocity of flow, as well as the functioning of blocking anatomical structures[13] (Figure 53.2).

LYMPHATIC VASOMOTION AND LYMPHATIC FLOW MOTION

Several important findings were discovered accidentally. After having recorded thousands of microlymphographs and fast-forwarded several images, we noticed that it was sometimes possible to recognize, even with the naked eye, flow movement inside the microlymphatics. We digitized

several microlymphographs and observed and measured lymphatic flow. For the first time, the velocity of lymphatic flow was visualized and measured *in vivo* in a human. We noted two different types of intramicrolymphatic flow: (1) a very slow granular flow that we termed *lymphatic flow motion* (about $10 \pm 4\ \mu/s$); (2) a pulsating, "stop-and-go" flow pattern, which was faster than lymphatic flow motion (about $91 \pm 58\ \mu/s$), with periodic accelerations that we termed *lymphatic vasomotion*. The periodicity of the flow accelerations was about 1 min $\pm$ 25 sec (mean $\pm$ standard deviation). We were unable to visualize either type of previously mentioned flow pattern in healthy subjects; however,

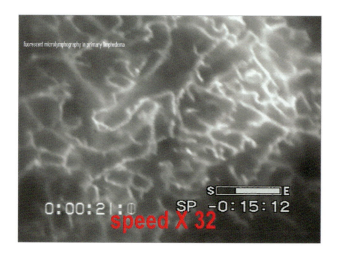

Figure 53.1 Fluorescent microlymphography in primary lymphedema with the lymphatic flow increasing × 32 the speed of the recorder.

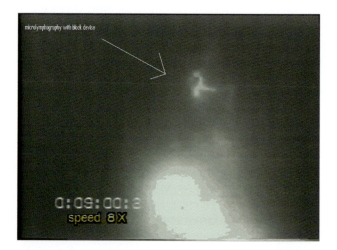

Figure 53.2 Fluorescent microlymphography with the block device.

in patients with chronic venous disorders (CVDs) (CEAP 2,3), we sometimes found a pulsating flow (lymphatic vasomotion) in the proximity of the pre-collectors but never granular flow (lymphatic flow motion). In patients with soft edema, we more often found a granular flow pattern but rarely a periodic flow pattern in the proximity of the pre-collectors. That granular flow pattern is visible only in a setting of soft lymphedema but not in patients with CVD or healthy subjects. This flow pattern may be associated with an increase in the superficial flow that compensates for obstruction of normal deep flow.[1]

In the settings of lymphedema, the presence of a pulsating flow (lymphatic vasomotion) is related to deep drainage due to the opening of the pre-collectors, probably resulting from critical pressure levels.[1] In patients with CVDs, the pulsating flow pattern is related to similar dynamics, even if the underlying pathophysiological mechanism is failure of the microlymphatic system and increased interstitial pressure due to capillary stasis.[10–12,14] In healthy subjects, neither flow pattern is detected since the lymph flows not in the superficial but rather in the deep network through the collectors and therefore cannot be visualized.

Recent developments in monitoring and studying lymphatic flow have provided insights into the pathophysiology of lymphatic circulation. The parameters such as lymph velocity, interstitial pressure, and block devices can provide knowledge of the microcirculation system that we can measure.

REFERENCES

1. Bartolo M Jr, Allegra C. Image: Can we see lymphatics? *Int J Micr Clin Exp.* 1994;14(Suppl 1):191.
2. Bollinger A, Fagrell B. *Clinical Capillaroscopy.* Lewiston, NY: Hogrefe and Huber; 1990.
3. Allegra C, Bartolo M Jr., Bonifacio M, Carioti B, Cassiani D, Criscuolo A. Interstitial pressure: our experience. *Int Angiol.* 1997;16(3)(Suppl. 1).
4. Lauchli S, Haldimann L, Leu AJ, Franzeck UK. Fluorescence microlymphography of the upper extremities. Evaluation with a new computer programme. *Int Angiol.* 1999;18(2):145–148.
5. Allegra C, Carlizza A. Rheopletysmography and laser-Doppler velocimetry in the study of microcirculatory flow variability. In: Allegra C, Intaglietta M, Messmer K, eds. *Vasomotion and Flowmotion. Progress in Applied Microcirculation.* Vol. 20. Basel, Switzerland: Karger; 1991.
6. Allegra C. Microcirculatory techniques and assessment of chronic venous insufficiency. *Medicographia.* 1996;18:30.
7. Intaglietta M. Pressure measurements in the microcirculation with active and passive transducers. *Microvasc Res.* 1973;5:317–323.
8. Intaglietta M, Tompkins WR. Simplified micropressure measurements via bridge current feedback. *Microvasc Res.* 1990;39:386–389.
9. Bollinger A, Amann-Vesti BR. Fluorescence microlymphography: Diagnostic potential in lymphedema and basis for the measurement of lymphatic pressure and flow velocity. *Lymphology.* 2007;40:52–62.
10. Bartolo M Jr, Carioti B, Cassiani D, Allegra C. Lymphatic capillary pressure in human skin of patients with chronic venous insufficiency. *Int J Micr Clin Exp.* 1994;14(Suppl 1):191.
11. Allegra C, Bartolo M Jr. Haemodynamic modifications induced by elastic compression therapy in CVI evaluated by microlymphography. *Phlebology.* 1995;95:9–17.
12. Allegra C, Bartolo M Jr, Sarcinella R. Morphologic and functional changes of the microlymphatic network in patients with advanced stages of primary lymphedema. *Lymphology.* 2002;35:114–120.
13. Allegra C, Carlizza A. Oedema in chronic venous insufficiency: Physiopathology and investigation. *Phlebology.* 2000;15:122–125.
14. Allegra C. Lymphatics of the skin in primary lymphoedemas. *Int J Micr Clin Exp.* 1996;16(Suppl 1):114.
15. Husmann MJ, Barton M, Vesti BR, Franzeck UK. Postural effects on interstitial fluid pressure in humans. *J Vasc Res.* 2006;43(4):321–326.
16. Lee BB, Bergan J, Rockson SG. *Lymphedema; a Concise Compendium of Theory and Practice.* London, UK: Springer-Verlag London Limited; 2011:191–197.

54

Can indocyanine green replace role of lymphoscintigraphy?

TAKUMI YAMAMOTO

Indocyanine green (ICG) lymphography visualizes superficial lymph flows more clearly than lymphoscintigraphy (LSG) (Figure 54.1). However, it is impossible to directly visualize deep lymph flows; the maximum depth for visualization is 1.5–2 cm from the skin surface.[1-4] LSG is a gold standard for lymph flow imaging study, which allows systemic objective lymph flow evaluation including deep lymph flows.[5,6] Especially for evaluation of primary lymphedema or lymphatic malformation, LSG or other deep lymph flow imaging such as magnetic resonance (MR) lymphography is critical, because diseases may affect not only the superficial lymphatic system but also the deep lymphatic system.[5-7]

Therefore, ICG lymphography alone is not adequate for evaluation of primary lymphedema or lymphatic malformation and will never replace the role of LSG.[3,5,6] Systemic whole-body thorough lymph flow imaging should be done with LSG or single photon emission computed tomography (SPECT)/computed tomography (CT). ICG lymphography should be used in combination with LSG to complement the drawbacks in LSG: obscure image, low sensitivity to detect abnormal lymph circulation, and non-real-time imaging.

Because of its obscure image, LSG is not good at detecting a very slight lymph flow abnormality, especially in a small region such as the face and the genitalia[4,8-11] (Figure 54.2). ICG lymphography is better at early diagnosis and at evaluation of facial and genital lymphedema.[1,3,4,11]

Since ICG lymphography allows real-time lymph flow imaging, medical staffs can observe real-time lymph flow changes before and after manual lymph drainage or compression treatment, and surgeons can operate lymphatic surgeries under lymph flow navigation.[9,10,12-16] ICG lymphography maximizes the safety and efficacy of lymphedema treatments based on individual lymph flow imaging, allowing tailor-made lymphedema management.

Although ICG lymphography never replaces the role of LSG, it plays an important role in lymph flow imaging as a complement to LSG.

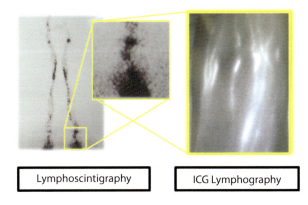

Figure 54.1 Indocyanine green lymphography visualizes superficial lymph flows more clearly than lymphoscintigraphy.

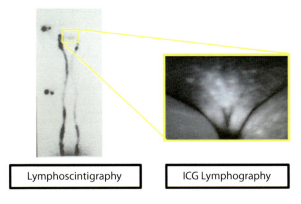

Figure 54.2 Indocyanine green lymphography clearly demonstrates abnormal lymph flow (stardust pattern), whereas lymphoscintigraphy hardly shows abnormality.

ACKNOWLEDGMENT

Preparation of this chapter is supported, in part, by NCGM Biobank Fund (29-2004).

243

REFERENCES

1. Yamamoto T, Yamamoto N, Doi K et al. Indocyanine green (ICG)-enhanced lymphography for upper extremity lymphedema: A novel severity staging system using dermal backflow (DB) patterns. *Plast Reconstr Surg.* 2011;128(4):941–947.

2. Yamamoto T, Narushima M, Doi K et al. Characteristic indocyanine green lymphography findings in lower extremity lymphedema: The generation of a novel lymphedema severity staging system using dermal backflow patterns. *Plast Reconstr Surg.* 2011;127(5):1979–1986.

3. Yamamoto T, Yoshimatsu H, Narushima M, Yamamoto N, Hayashi A, Koshima I. Indocyanine green lymphography findings in primary leg lymphedema. *Eur J Vasc Endovasc Surg.* 2015;49:95–102.

4. Yamamoto T, Yamamoto N, Yoshimatsu H, Hayami S, Narushima M, Koshima I. Indocyanine green lymphography for evaluation of genital lymphedema in secondary lower extremity lymphedema patients. *J Vasc Surg Venous Lymphat Disord.* 2013;1(4):400–405.

5. Zhibin Y, Quanyong L, Libo C et al. The role of radionuclide lymphoscintigraphy in extremity lymphedema. *Ann Nucl Med.* 2006;20:341–344.

6. Tartaglione G, Pagan M, Morese R et al. Intradermal lymphoscintigraphy at rest and after exercise: A new technique for the functional assessment of the lymphatic system in patients with lymphoedema. *Nucl Med Commun.* 2010;31:547–551.

7. Case TC, Witte CL, Witte MH et al. Magnetic resonance imaging in human lymphedema: Comparison with lymphangioscintigraphy. *Magn Reson Imaging.* 1992;10:549–558.

8. Yamamoto T, Iida T, Matsuda N et al. Indocyanine green (ICG)-enhanced lymphography for evaluation of facial lymphoedema. *J Plast Reconstr Aesthet Surg.* 2011;64(11):1541–1544.

9. Yamamoto T, Narushima M, Yoshimatsu H et al. Indocyanine green velocity: Lymph transportation capacity deterioration with progression of lymphedema. *Ann Plast Surg.* 2013;71(5):591–594.

10. Yamamoto T, Narushima M, Yoshimatsu H et al. Dynamic indocyanine green lymphography for breast cancer-related arm lymphedema. *Ann Plast Surg.* 2014;73(6):706–709.

11. Yamamoto T, Matsuda N, Doi K et al. The earliest finding of indocyanine green (ICG) lymphography in asymptomatic limbs of lower extremity lymphedema patients secondary to cancer treatment: The modified dermal backflow (DB) stage and concept of subclinical lymphedema. *Plast Reconstr Surg.* 2011;128(4):314e–321e.

12. Yamamoto T, Narushima M, Yoshimatsu H et al. Minimally invasive lymphatic supermicrosurgery (MILS): Indocyanine green lymphography-guided simultaneous multi-site lymphaticovenular anastomoses via millimeter skin incisions. *Ann Plast Surg.* 2014;72(1):67–70.

13. Yamamoto T, Yamamoto N, Azuma S et al. Near-infrared illumination system-integrated microscope for supermicrosurgical lymphaticovenular anastomosis. *Microsurgery.* 2014;34(1):23–27.

14. Yamamoto T, Yoshimatsu H, Koshima I. Navigation lymphatic supermicrosurgery for iatrogenic lymphorrhea: Supermicrosurgical lymphaticolymphatic anastomosis and lymphaticovenular anastomosis under indocyanine green lymphography navigation. *J Plast Reconstr Aesthet Surg.* 2014;67(11):1573–1579.

15. Yamamoto T, Yoshimatsu H, Yamamoto N. Complete lymph flow reconstruction: A free vascularized lymph node true perforator flap transfer with efferent lymphaticolymphatic anastomosis. *J Plast Reconstr Aesthet Surg.* 2016;69(9):1227–1233.

16. Yamamoto T, Iida T, Yoshimatsu H, Fuse Y, Hayashi A, Yamamoto N. Lymph flow restoration after tissue replantation and transfer: Importance of lymph axiality and possibility of lymph flow reconstruction using free flap transfer without lymph node or supermicrosurgical lymphatic anastomosis. *Plast Reconstr Surg.* 2018;142(3):796–804.

55

How to differentiate between lymphedema and lipedema: How to rule out lipedema

GYŐZŐ SZOLNOKY

DEFINITION

Lipedema is a disproportional obesity with presumed endocrinological and genetic backgrounds consisting of bilateral, symmetrical, stove-pipe-shaped fatty swelling of the legs or arms.[1-3] The estimated incidence of lipedema is uncertain; however, according to multicentric observations, up to 18.8% of all patients referred to lymphedema clinics had lipedema.[2] Lipedema, especially in advanced stages, is quite frequently combined with lymphatic or venous insufficiency that may strongly modify the original limb shape resembling the features of identical vascular affection (lymph- or/and phlebedema).[2]

CLASSIFICATION

In stage I, the skin looks flat and on palpation feels like "Styrofoam balls in a plastic bag." In stage II, the overlying skin has an irregular surface ("mattress phenomenon") in conjunction with walnut-to-apple-sized indurations. Stage III shows robust lobular fat deposits.[2] There is also a location-related classification: predominantly buttocks (type I), buttocks to knees (type II), buttocks to ankles (type III), mainly arms (type IV), and rather lower legs (type V).[2]

EVOLUTION

Manifestations of lipedema usually begins after puberty or with the initiation of hormonal contraceptives. Lipidema may improve in menopause. Weight gain inevitably worsens clinical symptoms.[2,3]

CLINICAL DIAGNOSIS

In most cases, lipedema can be easily diagnosed by patient history and clinical examination;[1-3] however, there is no absolutely unambiguous pathognomonic diagnostic test for lipedema.[3] The following clinical differential diagnostic criteria facilitate assessment.

CUFFING SIGN

Pure lipedema always spares the feet; the abnormal fat deposition often creates a ring of fatty tissue overlapping the top of the feet (cuffing sign).[2,3]

RETROMALLEOLAR FAT PADS

Fat pads behind the ankles are present in lipedema in its pure form, and absent in primary lymphedema.[2,3]

STEMMER SIGN

This is absent in pure lipedema and usually present in primary lymphedema.[2,3]

TENDERNESS OF SKIN AND SUBCUTANEOUS FAT

This is a true hallmark of lipedema, and absent in primary lymphedema. The pinch test is the simplest method for pain detection.[4] Lipedematous pain is complicated to describe, however, a 30-item questionnaire facilitates the characterization. A four-grade scale was assigned to each item, and adjunctives with the highest grades referred to the most characteristic descriptions.[5] In a comparative clinical trial, the 10 best-fitting items as well as a special numerical analog scale (from 0 to 10), the pain rating scale and Wong Baker face pain scale were used for pain assessment.[4]

EXAMINATION

Physical examinations

WAIST-TO-HEIGHT RATIO

Of the anthropometric measurements, the waist-to-height ratio may give reasonable results in lipedema.[6]

STREETEN TEST

The patient consumes 20 mL water/body-weight kg, then the patient remains in an upright position for 4 hours while urine is collected. The leg volume is measured both before and after the test. Normal healthy nonlipedematous persons excrete more than 60% of the ingested water and the leg volume does not increase with more than 350 mL/kg.[7] This test has rather historical importance rather than of practical importance.

CAPILLARY FRAGILITY ASSESSMENT

Bruising is attributed to increased capillary fragility,[1-3] and lipedema is associated with easy bruising.[8] Measurement is done with a vacuum suction chamber (Parrot angiosterrometer) exerting an adjustable suction to the skin. Determination of capillary fragility is based on the count of viable petechiae. There is no available comparative study between lipedema and lymphedema; however, noncomplicated lipedema was associated with a significantly higher count of petechiae compared with ordinary obesity.[9] Nevertheless, the absence of easy bruising is generally known in lymphedema,[10] thus capillary fragility could be a differential diagnostic criterion from this aspect, too.

Imaging techniques

TISSUE DIELECTRIC CONSTANT MEASUREMENT

Tissue dielectric constant (TDC) measurement serves for the quantification of local tissue water content. This device may aid in differentiating lipedema from lymphedema.[11]

DUAL-ENERGY X-RAY ABSORPTIOMETRY

Dual-energy x-ray absorptiometry (DXA) measures regional body composition including the extension of adipose tissue. DXA is, of course, a useful tool helping clinicians in differential diagnosis and also in the assessment of the efficacy of various invasive or noninvasive interventions.[12]

Ultrasound examination

High-resolution duplex sonography can distinguish lipedema from phlebedema or lymphedema with a high level of sensitivity.[13,14]

Lipedematous subcutaneous tissue is definitely enlarged with higher echogenicity ("snowfall sign") without echo-loosing spaces or channels. Subcutaneous septae are thickened having increased echogenicity. Conversely, lymphedema has thickened subcutaneous tissue with small, <1 mm echo-loosing spaces as initial dilated lymphatic vessels and larger, longer echo-loosing spaces and channels with echo-rich margins as lymphatic collectors under congestion. The mean dermal to subcutaneous fat echogenicity ratio is decreased in those with lymphedema compared to lipedema.

COMPUTED TOMOGRAPHY SCANS, MAGNETIC RESONANCE IMAGING

Computed tomography (CT)[15] and magnetic resonance imaging (MRI)[16,17] are rather indicated for scientific purposes or subtle cases and show that true edema is limited, and limb swelling is mostly attributed to bilateral enlargement of the subcutaneous fat.

LYMPHOSCINTIGRAPHY AND FLUORESCENT MICROLYMPHOGRAPHY

Adiposity of the predilection areas is presumably linked with microangiopathy and altered microcirculation leading to an increasing amount of interstitial fluid. Therefore, in less advanced forms of lipedema, increased lymph flow may be visualized by lymphoscintigraphy. Conversely, slower lymph transport is associated with advanced forms.[18] Interestingly, a recent study of lymphoscintigraphy showed alterations (low or low-moderate grades) in nearly 50% of patients with noncomplicated lipedema.[19] Fluorescent microlymphography displays lymphatic microaneurysms and dilated vessels of the uppermost lymphatic network, indicating that lymph vessels are also involved.[20]

ASSESSMENT OF AORTIC DISTENSIBILITY AND STIFFNESS IN LIPEDEMA

In a clinical trial where women with noncomplicated lipedema were compared with healthy age and body mass index (BMI)-matched individuals, lipedema was associated with notably higher aortic stiffness.[21]

ASSESSMENT OF CARDIAC MORPHOLOGY AND FUNCTION IN LIPEDEMA

In another clinical trial where women with noncomplicated lipedema were compared with age- and BMI-matched healthy individuals and lymphedema patients, lipedema was associated with a high incidence of altered left ventricular (LV) standard two-dimensional (2D) echocardiographic parameters (end-diastolic and end-systolic volumes, transmitral flow velocity) and rotational changes (significantly lower LV apical rotation and twist) detected by three-dimensional speckle-tracking echocardiography (3DSTE).[22]

REFERENCES

1. Szél E, Kemény L, Groma G, Szolnoky G. Pathophysiological dilemmas of lipedema. *Med Hypotheses*. 2014;83(5):599–606.
2. Forner-Cordero I, Szolnoky G, Forner-Cordero A, Kemény L. Lipedema: An overview of its clinical manifestations, diagnosis and treatment of the disproportional fatty deposition syndrome—systematic review. *Clin Obes*. 2012;2(3–4):86–95.

3. Torre YS, Wadeea R, Rosas V, Herbst KL. Lipedema: Friend and foe. *Horm Mol Biol Clin Investig.* 2018;33(1):20170076.

4. Szolnoky G, Varga E, Varga M, Tuczai M, Dósa-Rácz E, Kemény L. Lymphedema treatment decreases pain intensity in lipedema. *Lymphology.* 2011;44(4):178–182.

5. Schmeller W, Meier-Vollrath J. Schmerzen beim Lipödem. *LymphForsch.* 2008;12(1):8–12.

6. Herpertz U. Adipositas-Diagnostik in der Lymphologie. *LymphForsch.* 2009;13(2):90–93.

7. Streeten DH. Idiopathic edema. Pathogenesis, clinical features, and treatment. *Endocrinol Metab Clin North Am.* 1995;24(3):531–547.

8. Szolnoky G, Nagy N, Kovács RK et al. Complex decongestive physiotherapy decreases capillary fragility in lipedema. *Lymphology.* 2008;41(4):161–166.

9. Szolnoky G, Ifeoluwa A, Tuczai M et al. Measurement of capillary fragility: A useful tool to differentiate lipedema from obesity? *Lymphology.* 2017;50(4):203–209.

10. van Esch-Smeenge J, Damstra RJ, Hendrickx AA. Muscle strength and functional exercise capacity in patients with lipoedema and obesity: A comparative study. *J Lymphoedema.* 2017;12(1):23–31.

11. Birkballe S, Jensen MR, Noerregaard S, Gottrup F, Karlsmark T. Can tissue dielectric constant measurement aid in differentiating lymphoedema from lipoedema in women with swollen legs? *Br J Dermatol.* 2014;170(1):96–102.

12. Dietzel R, Reisshauer A, Jahr S, Calafiore D, Armbrecht G. Body composition in lipoedema of the legs using dual-energy x-ray absorptiometry: A case-control study. *Br J Dermatol.* 2015;173(2):594–596.

13. Iker E, Mayfield CK, Gould DJ, Patel KM. Characterizing lower extremity lymphedema and lipedema with cutaneous ultrasonography and an objective computer-assisted measurement of dermal echogenicity. *Lymphat Res Biol.* 2019. doi: 10.1089/lrb.2017.0090.

14. Naouri M, Samimi M, Atlan M et al. High resolution cutaneous ultrasonography to differentiate lipoedema from lymphoedema. *Br J Dermatol.* 2010;163(2):296–301.

15. Monnin-Delhom ED, Gallix BP, Achard C, Bruel JM, Janbon C. High resolution unenhanced computed tomography in patients with swollen legs. *Lymphology.* 2002;35(3):121–128.

16. Tiwari A, Cheng KS, Button M, Myint F, Hamilton G. Differential diagnosis, investigation, and current treatment of lower limb lymphedema. *Arch Surg.* 2003;138(2):152–161.

17. Lohrmann C, Foeldi E, Langer M. MR imaging of the lymphatic system in patients with lipedema and lipo-lymphedema. *Microvasc Res.* 2009;77:335–339.

18. Brauer WJ. Altersbezogene Funktionslymphszintigraphie beim Lipödem und Lipolymphödem. *LymphForsch.* 2000;4:74–77.

19. Forner-Cordero I, Oliván-Sasot P, Ruiz-Llorca C, Muñoz-Langa J. Lymphoscintigraphic findings in patients with lipedema. *Rev Esp Med Nucl Imagen Mol.* 2018;37(6):341–348.

20. Zetzmann K, Ludolph I, Horch RE, Boos AM. Imaging for treatment planning in lipo-and lymphedema. *Handchir Mikrochir Plast Chir.* 2018;50(6):386–392.

21. Szolnoky G, Nemes A, Gavallér H, Forster T, Kemény L. Lipedema is associated with increased aortic stiffness. *Lymphology.* 2012;45(2):71–79.

22. Nemes A, Kormanyos A, Domsik P et al. Left ventricular rotational mechanics differ between lipedema and lymphedema: Insights from the three-dimensional speckle tracking echocardiographic MAGYAR-path study. *Lymphology.* 2018;51(3):102–108.

Management: 1—Primary Lymphedema

56

Manual lymphatic drainage: Myth?

ISABEL FORNER-CORDERO AND JEAN-PAUL BELGRADO

The management of lymphedema involves decongesting lymphatic pathways in order to reduce the size of the limb, encouraging the development of collateral drainage routes and stimulating the function of remaining patent routes so as to control swelling in the long term. Traditionally, treatment has followed a "two-phase" approach—an intensive phase and a maintenance phase—and most guidelines follow this model of treatment.[1-4] Decongestive lymphatic therapy (DLT) is backed by long-standing experience, and it consists of multicomponent bandages, range-of-motion active mobilization underneath the bandage, manual lymphatic drainage (MLD), skin care, and sometimes intermittent compression therapy (sequential intermittent pneumatic compression [SIPC]).[5] When all these ingredients are combined, the efficacy of the above interventions to reduce limb volume has been achieved,[6-12] being the reported average of volume reduction of 50%–70%.[13-15] Multicomponent bandages (MBs) and MLD are highly intra- and interoperator dependent. Until a few years ago, no real-time feedback existed to help the practitioner to evaluate and adapt his or her technique during the treatment. However, now micropressure sensors and near-infrared fluorescence lymphatic imaging (NIRFLI) enable monitoring of the effectiveness of these techniques. Despite the widely used MLD techniques for many years, there are few robust randomized clinical trials and/or studies that demonstrate their efficacy. The term *MLD* covers a large variation in parameters and applications.

The treatment of lymphedema is difficult, costly, and time consuming. An annual average cost of 890USD per patient has been reported by Kärki[16]; the more recent study of Gutknecht found a cost of 6439USD per patient and year,[17] enhancing the need for optimization of resources.

There is a great deal of controversy as to which components of a physical treatment program are the most effective in reducing edema.[18] While MLD is the core of DLT, few randomized studies focused on the clinical effect of the volume reduction have been performed, and they have failed to report any extra benefit with historical MLD techniques.[19-24] It is unclear if there is a "placebo effect" contributing to an improved quality of life. We also need to highlight the accuracy of the measurement instruments and clarify the cut-off of the presence or absence of edema. A Cochrane review published in 2004 states that MLD may offer additional benefit to compression bandaging for reduction; and the patients with mild-to-moderate BCRL may be the ones who benefit from adding MLD to compression bandaging.[25] MLD needs a more accurate assessment through randomized studies.[18,26] Studies on the basis of the actual knowledge in lymphatic physiology and historical concept of the MLD technique must be performed; for example, the controversy on the forces, the pressure to be applied on the skin by the hand of the therapist during MLD.[27]

To assess the efficacy of MLD, pneumatic massage (PM), and SIPC in DLT, in the Lymphedema Unit of Hospital La Fe, we conducted a randomized, comparative single-blind study in patients with lymphedema.[28] Patients were randomized to receive 20 sessions of the following regimens: Branch A: MLD, SIPC with multi-compartmental pump and MB; Branch B: PM, SIPC and MB; Branch C: SIPC and MB. The end point was the "percentage reduction in excess volume (PREV)" and was assessed by a blinded evaluator. At the end, 174 patients were included, and we found that no significant differences were seen between the groups of treatment. The global mean of PREV was 72.2% that was in the high range of the published results.[14,18,29] MLD did not add any benefit to SIPC followed by MBs in terms of reduction of excess volume. As Yamamoto et al. reported,[30] we observed that results were already reached with 10 sessions of DLT. Gradalski et al. reported in a randomized trial that MLD may not be needed in DLT to obtain edema reduction. Choosing MLD-sparing DLT as a standard procedure in moderate-to-severe lymphedema can remarkably diminish time consumption and thus therapy costs.[31]

Are we saying that MLD is not useful in lymphedema patients? The primary outcome chosen in the studies was reduction of volume, but this quantitative result does not reflect the entire effect of MLD, so this is one of the limitations of our study. With new imaging techniques such as NIRFLI, Lopera demonstrated that MLD improved lymph function. In that study, the authors found an increase of the velocity of transient lymph packets from a median of 6.7 mm/s at baseline to 13.3 mm/s after MLD in healthy volunteers.[32] This effect may not be as evident in lymphedema patients. NIRFLI could enhance the diagnosis and treatment of lymphedema, allowing the observation of changes in lymphatic function, the evaluation of the MLD methods with real-time feedback, and the implementation of targeted physical therapy.[33]

REFERENCES

1. Eliska O, Benda K, Houdova H et al. The founding and development of the Czech Lymphology Society. Brief guidelines of the Czech Lymphology Society. *Eur J Lymphol Relat Probl.* 2006;16(47):1–6.

2. Lee BB, Andrade M, Antignani PL et al. Diagnosis and treatment of primary lymphedema. Consensus document of the International Union of Phlebology (IUP)-2013. *Int Angiol.* 2013;32(6):541–574.

3. Campisi C, Michelini S, Boccardo F; Societá Italiana di Linfangiologia. Guidelines of the Societá Italiana di Linfangiologia: Excerpted sections. *Lymphology.* 2004;37(4):182–184.

4. The Swedish Council on Technology Assessment in Health Care. Manual lymph drainage combined with compression therapy for arm lymphedema following breast cancer treatment. In: SBU alert [database online]. Stockholm, Sweden: SBU; 2005. SBU alert report no 2005–04. http://www.sbu.se/upload/Publikationer/Content0/3/Manual_Lymph_Drainage_Compression_Arm_Lymphedema_Breast_Cancer_200504.pdf

5. Executive Committee. The diagnosis and treatment of peripheral lymphedema: 2016 consensus document of the International Society of Lymphology. *Lymphology.* 2016;49(4):170–184.

6. Szuba A, Cooke JP, Yousuf S, Rockson SG. Decongestive lymphatic therapy for patients with cancer-related or primary lymphedema. *Am J Med.* 2000;109(4):296–300.

7. Williams AF, Vadgama A, Franks PJ, Mortimer PS. A randomized controlled crossover study of manual lymphatic drainage therapy in women with breast cancer-related lymphoedema. *Eur J Cancer Care (Engl).* 2002;11(4):254–261.

8. Kim SJ, Park YD. Effects of complex decongestive physiotherapy on the oedema and the quality of life of lower unilateral lymphoedema following treatment for gynecological cancer. *Eur J Cancer Care (Engl).* 2008;17(5):463–468.

9. Mondry TE, Riffenburgh RH, Johnstone PA. Prospective trial of complete decongestive therapy for upper extremity lymphedema after breast cancer therapy. *Cancer J.* 2004;10(1):42–48.

10. Hamner JB, Fleming MD. Lymphedema therapy reduces the volume of edema and pain in patients with breast cancer. *Ann Surg Oncol.* 2007;14(6):1904–1908.

11. Kim SJ, Yi CH, Kwon OY. Effect of complex decongestive therapy on edema and the quality of life in breast cancer patients with unilateral lymphedema. *Lymphology.* 2007;40(3):143–151.

12. Fu MR, Deng J, Armer JM. Putting evidence into practice: Cancer-related lymphedema. *Clin J Oncol Nurs.* 2014;18(Suppl):68–79.

13. Yamamoto R, Yamamoto T. Effectiveness of the treatment-phase of two-phase complex decongestive physiotherapy for the treatment of extremity lymphedema. *Int J Clin Oncol.* 2007;12(6):463–468.

14. Ko DS, Lerner R, Klose G, Cosimi AB. Effective treatment of lymphedema of the extremities. *Arch Surg.* 1998;133:452–458.

15. Koul R, Dufan T, Russell C et al. Efficacy of complete decongestive therapy and manual lymphatic drainage on treatment-related lymphedema in breast cancer. *Int J Radiat Oncol Biol Phys.* 2007;67(3):841–846.

16. Kärki A, Anttila H, Tasmuth T, Rautakorpi UM. Lymphoedema therapy in breast cancer patients: A systematic review on effectiveness and a survey of current practices and costs in Finland. *Acta Oncol.* 2009;48(6):850–859.

17. Gutknecht M, Herberger K, Klose K et al. Cost-of-illness of patients with lymphoedema. *J Eur Acad Dermatol Venereol.* 2017;31(11):1930–1935.

18. Badger C, Preston N, Seers K, Mortimer P. Physical therapies for reducing and controlling lymphoedema of the limbs. *Cochrane Database Syst Rev.* 2004;(4):CD003141.

19. Anderson L, Hojris I, Erlandsen M, Anderson J. Treatment of breast-cancer-related lymphedema with or without manual lymphatic drainage: A randomized study. *Acta Oncol.* 2000;39:399–405.

20. Johansson K, Lie E, Ekdahl C, Lindfeldt J. A randomized study comparing manual lymph drainage with sequential pneumatic compression for treatment of postoperative arm lymphedema. *Lymphology.* 1998;31(2):56–64.

21. McNeely ML, Magee DJ, Lees AW et al. The addition of manual lymph drainage to compression therapy for breast cancer related lymphedema: A randomized controlled trial. *Breast Cancer Res Treat.* 2004;86:95–106.

22. Devoogdt N, Christiaens MR, Geraerts I et al. Effect of manual lymph drainage in addition to guidelines and exercise therapy on arm lymphoedema related to breast cancer: Randomised controlled trial. *BMJ.* 2011;343:d5326. doi: 10.1136/bmj.d5326.

23. Finnane A, Janda M, Hayes SC. Review of the evidence of lymphedema treatment effect. *Am J Phys Med Rehabil.* 2015;94(6):483–498.

24. Huang TW, Tseng SH, Lin CC et al. Effects of manual lymphatic drainage on breast cancer-related lymphedema: A systematic review and meta-analysis of randomized controlled trials. *World J Surg Oncol.* 2013;11:15.

25. Ezzo J, Manheimer E, McNeely ML et al. Manual lymphatic drainage for lymphedema following breast cancer treatment. *Cochrane Database Syst Rev.* 2015;5:CD003475.

26. Lasinski BB, McKillip Thrift K, Squire D et al. A systematic review of the evidence for complete decongestive therapy in the treatment of lymphedema from 2004 to 2011. *PM&R.* 2012;4(8):580–601.

27. Belgrado JP, Vandermeeren L, Vankerckhove S et al. Near-infrared fluorescence lymphatic imaging to reconsider occlusion pressure of superficial lymphatic collectors in upper extremities of healthy volunteers. *Lymphat Res Biol.* 2016;14(2):70–77.

28. Forner-Cordero I, Muñoz-Langa J, DeMiguel-Jimeno JM, Rel-Monzó P. Physical therapies in the decongestive treatment of lymphedema: A phase III, multicenter, randomized, controlled study. In: *Abstracts of the 23rd ISL Congress*; September 19–23, 2011; Malmö, Sweden.

29. Lawenda BD, Mondry TE, Johnstone PA. Lymphedema: A primer on the identification and management of a chronic condition in oncologic treatment. *CA Cancer J Clin.* 2009;59:8–24.

30. Yamamoto T, Todo Y, Kaneuchi M et al. Study of edema reduction patterns during the treatment phase of complex decongestive physiotherapy for extremity lymphedema. *Lymphology.* 2008;41(2):80–86.

31. Gradalski T, Ochalek K, Kurpiewska J. Complex decongestive lymphatic therapy with or without Vodder II manual lymph drainage in more severe chronic postmastectomy upper limb lymphedema: A randomized noninferiority prospective study. *J Pain Symptom Manage.* 2015;50(6):750–757.

32. Lopera C, Worsley PR, Bader DL, Fenlon D. Investigating the short-term effects of manual lymphatic drainage and compression garment therapies on lymphatic function using near-infrared imaging. *Lymphat Res Biol.* 2017;15(3):235–240.

33. Giacalone G, Belgrado JP, Bourgeois P et al. A new dynamic imaging tool to study lymphedema and associated treatments. *Eur J Lymphol Relat Probl.* 2011;22:10–14.

57

Compression therapy: Optimal pressure? Bandage versus stocking

ISABEL FORNER-CORDERO AND JEAN-PAUL BELGRADO

KEY POINTS ARE AS FOLLOWS

- Compression is the cornerstone of lymphedema management.
- Multicomponent bandages and elastic sleeves are *complementary*, they have different mechanical behavior, and thermic insulation effect.
- During decongestive lymphatic therapy (DLT), multicomponent bandages are used 2–24 hours, with supplemental layers above after ½ hour and more of the application.
- For maintenance treatment, custom-made, flat tissue garments, Compression Class 3 (ccl3), are used during the day. Overlapping different garments can improve the doff and donning and can be useful to increase the pressure.
- Because geometry of an edematous limb has its own specificity, customized sleeves are recommended.
- When the patient is in the orthostatic position, because of loss or reduction of the venulo-arteriolar reflex in lymphedema (this edema shows a flagrant pitting sign), the pressure at the distality of the limb must be increased. A second sleeve should be placed, covering the distal segment (Figure 57.1).

COMPRESSION IS CORNERSTONE OF LYMPHEDEMA MANAGEMENT

Although the pathophysiology of edema varies, static and dynamic compression are the cornerstone of lymphedema management. However, the evidence base for the optimal application, duration, and intensity of compression therapy is lacking.[1,2] Different scientific groups have tried to summarize the recommendations for prescribing compression.[3,4]

In a few years, progress in technology can give us better information thanks to new communication systems, miniaturization, and price reduction of the pressure sensors, accelerometer, and other sensors, placed at the interface skin/bandages. The systematic review performed by the International Compression Club provides a degree of recommendation 1B to bandages and intermittent pneumatic compression in the treatment of lymphedema.[1]

Therapies to treat or manage lymphedema have limited evidence, partly because objective lymphatic measures are scarce. The use of near-infrared fluorescence lymphatic imaging (NIRFLI) in evaluating interventions can change this reality.[5]

WHAT TYPE OF COMPRESSION SYSTEM TO CHOOSE?

At the first phase, *intensive decongestive lymphatic treatment* (DLT) aims to reduce the limb volume, as the multicomponent bandages can be adapted better to the changing volume and geometry of the limb.

Short-stretch bandages associated with foam of specific viscoelasticity have shown their efficacy in reducing the volume of the limb,[6,7] with the highest level of recommendation.[4] Patients' adherence was one of the most important predictive factors of response to DLT.[8]

Despite the findings that a two-layer bandage was better tolerated than a short-stretch bandage by healthy volunteers,[9] short-stretch bandages showed a higher static stiffness index and a greater pressure difference between muscle contraction and relaxation; thus, they are expected to be more efficient in improving the muscle pump.[10] As the interface pressure drops after 2 hours,[11] bandaging again over the bandage can improve the results of DLT.

The two-layer bandage with a similar level of subbandage pressure than a four-layer system, maintained over 1 week, was partially better than short-stretch bandaging and was better tolerated by the patients.[9]

Short-stretch bandages showed a higher static stiffness index and a greater pressure difference between muscle contraction and relaxation in tip-toe and knee-bending exercises than long-stretch bandages and short-stretch stockings. The authors conclude that short-stretch bandages

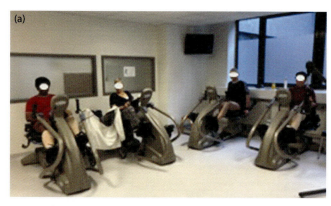

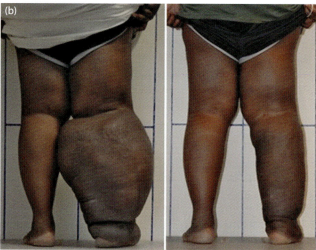

Figure 57.1 Reduction of a primary lymphedema in 3 weeks: treatment performed with multicomponent bandages. Patient mobilized the leg, wearing the bandage. During night, the bandage is released for better sleep and quality of life during intensive treatment. (Lymphology Research Unit, Université libre de Bruxelles, Belgium, JP Belgrado, K. Dusart, L. Vandermeeren.)

can be expected to have more benefits for augmenting muscle pump than long-stretch bandages and short-stretch stockings (Table 57.1).[10]

Skin pressures were always highest at the ankle and on the anterior side of the leg in all positions. Extension and flexion of the knee influence significantly the skin pressure at the anterior and posterior aspects of the leg, especially with the knee flexion at 90°. Body postures may be one of the most important factors influencing the skin pressure profiles applied by compression stockings as demonstrated by Liu et al. in 2007.[12]

The pressure targeted with short-stretch bandages of 50–60 mm Hg was only achieved in 10% of the cases, during nursing training courses, and 77% of the bandages were applied with pressure that was too low (<30 mm Hg).[13] Reapplication of the bandage can be done twice a day, or placement of a layer above the current bandage can efficiently restore the pressure (Figure 57.2).

An option situated between multicomponent bandages and elastic sleeves can be the adjustable compression wrap devices handled by the patients themselves that can produce pressure following the reduction of the circumference of the edema. This option can be more convenient and can deliver more consistent pressure.[14,15] Other than the benefits in the maintenance of the pressure, these devices can reduce trips to the hospital, as external treatment is easier, and can facilitate the treatment of patients with wounds. More robust studies must be done to clarify the best management of those adjustable elastic sleeves.

Maintenance phase

For maintenance treatment, compression garment prescription is essential for long-term management.[3] The best results are obtained with custom-made, flat tissue garments, ccl3—pressure range 34–46 mm Hg, used during the day. Overlapping different garments can improve the doffing and donning and can be useful to increase the pressure.

Yasuhara[16] and Vignes[17] have shown that the use of compression garments was the only therapy that was effective in maintaining the volume of the limb, and nonadherence to it was associated with negative results. The pressure under the stocking drops after 8 hours, due to fatigue of the elastic material, but the pressure amplitude remains the same.[18]

The difficulty in prescribing garments is conditioned by the patient's characteristics. A voluminous abdomen or hand's osteoarthritis can be an obstacle for prescribing a flat-knitted pantyhose, so we can prescribe a Capri garment and below-knee stockings to make it easier for the patient to be adherent to it. Overlapping different garments can improve putting on and taking off a garment and can be useful to increase the pressure. A seamless gauntlet can be better tolerated for babies and children with primary lymphedema. In severe cases, nightly compression can be useful by the means of self-multilayer bandages or with self-adjusted Velcro devices[19] (Figure 57.3).

DOSE OF COMPRESSION

There is a high level of evidence that high pressure (obtained with bandages and strong compression stockings 30–40 mm Hg) is effective for lymphedema management. The differing effects of elastic and short-stretch compression are also little understood.[1] Muscle contraction induces high-pressure variation at the limb/bandage interface, and for that reason, patients are invited to do cycling, rowing, and running while wearing the multicomponent bandage (Figure 57.4).

After the work of Zaleska et al., which sought to determine the pressures that should be generated to evacuate the stagnant fluid, in 20 patients with lower limb lymphedema,[20] visualized by lymphangiography, the threshold to mobilize edema was determined to be 40 mm Hg on the tissue. Data also showed that higher pressures were ineffective.[21] The working pressure would be adequate with 60–90 mm Hg, and above 50–60 mm Hg it is rather counterproductive.[22]

Table 57.1 Bandages versus stockings

Bandages	Stockings
Effects: Reduce edema volume—aim to change physical tissue conditions, inducing evacuation of the edema components	**Effects:** Maintain the reduction obtained with multicomponent bandages—aim to reduce filtration
Composition: Cotton Jersey + foam with specific thickness and viscoelastic properties, acting as numerous springs and short elastic bands to squeeze the foam and acting as a semi-rigid cast.	**Composition:** Elastane fibers—Cotton fibers—Silk fibers • Fibers knitted in circular way: standard • Fibers knitted in a flat way: customized
Advantages: • Application changes every day or more • Adaptation to the current volume • Good-to-extremely good efficacy in reducing the volume • Generate high-amplitude pressure variation at the interface skin-bandage, with a low basal pressure • "Increased" skin temperature reaching ±36°C[26]	**Advantages:** • Comfortable • "Easy" to put on and to wear • Easy to wear underneath clothes • Colors suit with fashion • No or low operator dependence • Not time-consuming • Rewashable
Disadvantages: • Difficult to perform • Need long learning curve • They lose pressure when the volume reduces, then must be adapted or changed after 2 hours • Uncomfortable in wet and warm climate • Not cosmetic and voluminous • Rolling down if not well placed • Highly intra- and interoperator dependent	**Disadvantages:** • Not effective if volume changes • Measurements need training • They lose pressure when the volume reduces • They lose compression when they lose stiffness • Expensive • Squeeze the initial lymphatic network, that helps fluid to leave the limb, when the proximal fixation is too small, creating a relative tourniquet

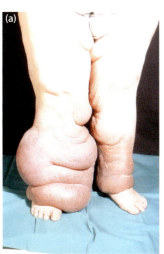
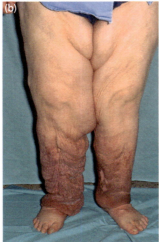

Figure 57.2 Patient with primary chronic lymphedema treated only with multicomponent bandages in Lymphedema Unit of Hospital Universitari i Politecnic La Fe of Valencia, Spain.

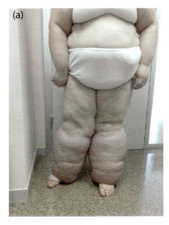
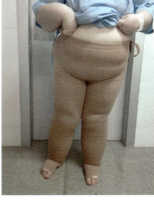

Figure 57.3 A 25-year-old woman with primary lymphedema. The perimeter for her calf reduced from 90 cm to 60 cm with decongestive lymphatic therapy. For maintenance treatment, two garments were prescribed, a legging pantyhose in flat-knitted ccl3 and overlapped stockings in ccl2 (Lymphedema Unit of Hospital Universitari i Politecnic La Fe of Valencia, Spain.)

WHY DOES IT WORK?

Sugisawa et al. have shown that compression stockings can elevate the pumping lymph pressure in the leg and ameliorate the edema, and this effect was more striking with pressures of 20 mm Hg than 10 mm Hg.[23] Trying to identify the basic mechanisms of lymphatic contraction, it has been shown that wearing compression stockings may raise the wall shear stress in lymphatic vessels and consequently induce nitric oxide production and modulate contractions via the cyclic-guanosine-monophosphate-dependent protein-kinase G pathway.[24] Another mechanism is the reduction of capillary filtration.[25]

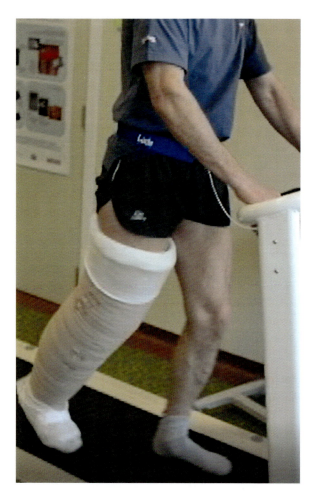

Figure 57.4 Wearing the multicomponent bandage, the patient performs exercises to generate high-pressure variation underneath the bandage.

REFERENCES

1. Partsch H, Flour M, Smith PC; International Compression Club. Indications for compression therapy in venous and lymphatic disease consensus based on experimental data and scientific evidence. *Under the auspices of the IUP. Int Angiol.* 2008;27(3):193–219.
2. Stout N, Partsch H, Szolnoky G et al. Chronic edema of the lower extremities: International consensus recommendations for compression therapy clinical research trials. *Int Angiol.* 2012;31(4):316–329.
3. Executive Committee. The diagnosis and treatment of peripheral lymphedema: 2016 consensus document of the International Society of Lymphology. *Lymphology.* 2016;49(4):170–184.
4. Lymphoedema Framework. *Best Practice for the Management of Lymphoedema. International Consensus.* London, UK: MEP Ltd; 2006.
5. Giacalone G, Belgrado JP, Bourgeois P et al. A new dynamic imaging tool to study lymphedema and associated treatments. *Eur J Lymphol Relat Probl.* 2011;22:10–14.
6. Partsch H, Clark M, Mosti G et al. Classification of compression bandages: practical aspects. *Dermatol Surg.* 2008;34(5):600–609.
7. Damstra RJ, Brouwer ER, Partsch H. Controlled, comparative study of relation between volume changes and interface pressure under short-stretch bandages in leg lymphedema patients. *Dermatol Surg.* 2008;34(6):773–778.
8. Forner-Cordero I, Muñoz-Langa J, Forner-Cordero A, Demiguel-Jimeno JM. Predictive factors of response to decongestive therapy in patients with breast-cancer-related lymphedema. *Ann Surg Oncol.* 2010;17(3):744–751.
9. Jünger M, Ladwig A, Bohbot S, Haase H. Comparison of interface pressures of three compression bandaging systems used on healthy volunteers. *J Wound Care.* 2009;18(11):476–480.
10. Hirai M, Niimi K, Iwata H et al. A comparison of interface pressure and stiffness between elastic stockings and bandages. *Phlebology.* 2009;24(3):120–124.
11. Damstra RJ, Brouwer ER, Partsch H. Controlled, comparative study of relation between volume changes and interface pressure under short-stretch bandages in leg lymphedema patients. *Dermatol Surg.* 2008;34(6):773–778.
12. Liu R, Kwok YL, Li Y et al. Skin pressure profiles and variations with body postural changes beneath medical elastic compression stockings. *Int J Dermatol.* 2007;46(5):514–523.
13. Heyer K, Protz K, Augustin M. Compression therapy—Cross-sectional observational survey about knowledge and practical treatment of specialised and non-specialised nurses and therapists. *Int Wound J.* 2017;14:1148–1153.
14. Partsch H. Reliable self-application of short stretch leg compression: Pressure measurements under self-applied, adjustable compression wraps. *Phlebology.* 2018;34(3):208–213.
15. Mosti G, Cavezzi A, Partsch H et al. Adjustable Velcro compression devices are more effective than inelastic bandages in reducing venous edema in the initial treatment phase: A randomized controlled trial. *Eur J Vasc Endovasc Surg.* 2015;50:368–374.
16. Yasuhara H, Shigematsu H, Muto T. A study of the advantages of elastic stockings for leg lymphedema. *Int Angiol.* 1996;15(3):272–277.
17. Vignes S, Porcher R, Arrault M, Dupuy A. Long-term management of breast cancer-related lymphedema after intensive decongestive physiotherapy. *Breast Cancer Res Treat* 2007;101(3):285–290.
18. van der Wegen-Franken CP, Tank B, Nijsten T, Neumann HA. Changes in the pressure and the dynamic stiffness index of medical elastic compression stockings after having been worn for eight hours: A pilot study. *Phlebology* 2009;24(1):31–37.

19. Langhaus-Nixon J, Forner-Cordero I, Rubio-Maicas C et al. An easy device for night compression in the maintenance treatment of lymphedema. In: Abstracts of the XXXIX ESL Congress; 2013 June 6–8; Valencia, Spain. *Eur J Lymphol Relat Probl* 2013;24(67–68):23.

20. Zaleska MT, Olszewski WL, Durlik M et al. Tonometry of deep tissues for setting effective compression pressures in lymphedema of limbs. *Lymphat Res Biol.* 2018;16(2):193–200.

21. Zaleska MT, Olszewski WL. Indocyanine green near-infrared lymphangiography for evaluation of effectiveness of edema fluid flow under therapeutic compression. *J Biophotonics.* 2018;11:e201700150.

22. Piller NB, Green T, Parkinson L et al. Feeling the pressure? How can we be sure we are getting it right? *J Lymphoedema.* 2019;14(1):52–55.

23. Sugisawa R, Unno N, Saito T et al. Effects of compression stockings on elevation of leg lymph pumping pressure and improvement of quality of life in healthy female volunteers: A randomized controlled trial. *Lymphat Res Biol.* 2016;14(2):95–103.

24. Dixon JB, Greiner ST, Gashev AA et al. Lymph flow, shear stress, and lymphocyte velocity in rat mesenteric prenodal lymphatics. *Microcirculation.* 2006;13:597–610.

25. Wollina U, Abdel-Naser MB, Mani R. A review of the microcirculation in skin in patients with chronic venous insufficiency: The problem and the evidence available for therapeutic options. *Int J Low Extrem Wounds.* 2006;5:169–180.

26. Belgrado JP, Baudier C, Natoli G et al. The skin temperature under multilayer bandages. *Eur J Lymphol Relat Probl.* 2006;16(47):17–20.

58

Sequential intermittent pneumatic compression: Rationale? How much can it be incorporated into compression therapy?

ISABEL FORNER-CORDERO AND JEAN-PAUL BELGRADO

Sequential intermittent pneumatic compression (SIPC) is one of the physical therapies available for primary lymphedema. SIPC consists in the application of a force on an edema in order to evacuate its components as much as possible toward the physiological drainage pathways: venous, lymphatics, and interstitium.[1] Its use as a component of decongestive lymphatic therapy (DLT) is extended but controversial. SIPC is used by professionals integrated into a multitherapeutic approach as adjuvant therapy or as a unique therapy; nevertheless, no consensus has been attained among the users concerning the appropriate protocol of SIPC, concerning the time and the pressure applied.[2,3]

EFFECTS OF SEQUENTIAL INTERMITTENT PNEUMATIC COMPRESSION

- Evacuation of the liquid phase[4] through the extracellular matrix is undisputable, by pushing fluid and macromolecule just proximal to the pneumatic sleeve.
- SIPC does not facilitate the reabsorption of the radiocolloid into the initial lymphatics in lymphoscintigraphy and it is not efficient to evacuate the protein part of lymphedema.[1,5,6]
- Near-infrared-fluorescence imaging (NIRFLI)[7] enables the qualitative observation and a semi-quantification of changes in lymphatic transport with SIPC using transparent pneumatic sleeves.[7] There is limited evidence that SIPC can increase lymph activity,[8] in all lymphedema-affected extremities.[9]
- With lymphoscintigraphy and immunohistopathology of tissue biopsies, Zaleska et al. showed that compression of lymphedema tissues leads to the formation of "tissue channels" as pathways for the evacuation of edema fluid. Pneumatic compression replaces the missing lymphatic function by providing fluid a moving force, subsequently enhancing the channel formation

process and in effect facilitating evacuation of fluid containing excess cytokines, among them upregulating collagen synthesis. The fibrosis process is slowed down, and subsequently there is no constriction of fluid channels, what may be seen in very advanced stages of lymphedema.[10]
- During SIPC sessions, the patient is at rest in the lying position, which means that the lymph nodes are not solicited by joint mobilization.
- During SIPC sessions, forces acting on the skin surface are perpendicular, never tangential. A combination of both favors the transfer of fluid and macromolecules from the interstitium into the lymph collectors. Consequently, lymph collectors cannot be filled with lymph during SIPC. However, when the lymph collectors are already filled with lymph, SIPC can empty the collectors, applying only perpendicular forces.

CLINICAL EFFECTS OF SEQUENTIAL INTERMITTENT PNEUMATIC COMPRESSION

- SIPC is useful in reducing the limb volume,[11,12] and improving the results of DLT.[13] It seems better to begin a DLT session by SIPC, then place the multicomponent bandages followed by MLD and skin care.
- The effect of SIPC with pressures of 30–80 mm Hg are to aid venous return, reduce edema, and even help to increase arterial flow.[14] In addition to the effects on microcirculation decreasing blood capillary filtration,[6] SIPC releases anticoagulant mediators' anti-inflammatory and vasoactive substances.[15]
- SIPC was associated with a favorable impact on the rate of hospitalizations, clinic visits, cellulitis, and the use of physical therapy, all of which represent important

clinical and therapeutic endpoints that reflect patient health status and quality of life.[16]

- SIPC can be recommended as an adjuvant therapy, particularly for patients with a compromised capacity for exercise.[17]

SAFETY

- Despite the report of increased genital lymphedema with IPC,[18] other studies have demonstrated its safety and lack of adverse effects with a controlled program.[19–21] The relationship between cause and effect is complex, notably because of the long duration between the SIPC sessions/treatment and genital edema development. But reasonably, we have to be careful with the interpretation of this observation. It is clear that fluids from the edema are pushed into the root of the limb. Regarding the lower limb, those fluids reach the groin, the iliac fossa, and also the pubic area. When the patient stands up after a SIPC session, due to gravity, part of the fluid drains into the external genitals. If the drainage of that specific anatomical territory is limited, repeated SIPC procedures can progressively induce a genital edema when no external genital compression is performed.
- The use of SIPC in pediatric lymphedema has shown volume reduction without notable adverse effects.[22]
- Trying to answer if the volume reduction is dose dependent, Vanscheidt and his group proved in subjects with chronic venous edema of the lower extremity that pneumatic compression was safe and well tolerated.[23]
- No complications in limb tissues were observed with long-term, high-pressure SIPC, long inflation timed therapy can be safely recommended to patients with lower limb lymphedema.[24]

TYPE OF DEVICE

The use of a multichambered pump has shown the best results.[25] By using continuous pressure during 6 hours, higher pressure is associated with greater volume reduction of the limb.[23] The work of Zaleska et al. aimed to know the pressures that should be generated to evacuate the stagnant fluid in lower limb lymphedema.[26] They found that the threshold pressures were 80 mm Hg in the compression device and >40 mm Hg in the tissue, but in some cases, it was ineffective despite applying higher compression forces.[26]

TAKE-HOME MESSAGE

- SIPC is safe, preferably accomplished with multichamber pumps, when applied in a controlled setting.
- It can improve volume reduction and enhance lymphatic channel formation.
- It can improve the DLT results when adjuvant to a multidisciplinary therapeutic program.

REFERENCES

1. Belgrado JP, Bourgeois P, Röh N et al. Intermittent pneumatic compression in the treatment of lymphedema: Current state of knowledge. *Eur J Lymphol Relat Probl.* 2007;17(50):4–10.
2. Klein MJ, Alexander MA, Wright JM et al. Treatment of adult lower extremity lymphedema with the Wright linear pump: Statistical analysis of a clinical trial. *Arch Phys Med Rehabil.* 1988;69(3):202–206.
3. Theys S, Deltombe T, Jamart J et al. A 30 or 90 mm Hg—manual or pneumatic—drainage in primary limb lymphedema: A comparative plethysmographic study. *Eur J Lymphol Relat Probl.* 2004;41:3.
4. Delis KT, Husmann MJ, Szendro G et al. Haemodynamic effect of intermittent pneumatic compression of the leg after infrainguinal arterial bypass grafting. *Br J Surg.* 2004;91(4):429–434.
5. Weissleder H. Lymphedema treatment: Any value in using intermittent pneumatic compression? Review of international literature. *Lymphol Forsch Prax.* 2003;7(1):15–18.
6. Miranda F Jr, Perez MC, Castiglioni ML et al. Effect of sequential intermittent pneumatic compression on both leg lymphedema volume and on lymph transport as semiquantitatively evaluated by lymphoscintigraphy. *Lymphology.* 2001;34(3):135–141.
7. Giacalone G, Belgrado JP, Bourgeois P et al. A new dynamic imaging tool to study lymphedema and associated treatments. *Eur J Lymphol Relat Probl.* 2011;22:10–14.
8. Adams KE, Rasmussen JC, Darne C et al. Direct evidence of lymphatic function improvement after advanced pneumatic compression device treatment of lymphedema. *Biomed Opt Expr.* 2010;1:114–125.
9. Aldrich MB, Gross D, Morrow JR et al. Effect of pneumatic compression therapy on lymph movement in lymphedema-affected extremities, as assessed by near-infrared fluorescence lymphatic imaging. *J Innov Opt Health Sci.* 2017;10(2):1650049.
10. Zaleska M, Olszewski WL, Cakala M et al. Intermittent pneumatic compression enhances formation of edema tissue fluid channels in lymphedema of lower limbs. *Lymphat Res Biol.* 2015;13(2):146–153.
11. Richmand DM, O'Donnell TF Jr, Zelikovski A. Sequential pneumatic compression for lymphedema. A controlled trial. *Arch Surg.* 1985;120(10):1116–1119.
12. Dini D, Del Mastro L, Gozz A et al. The role of pneumatic compression in the treatment of postmastectomy lymphedema. A randomized phase III study. *Ann Oncol.* 1998;9:187–191.
13. Szuba A, Achalu R, Rockson SG. Decongestive lymphatic therapy for patients with breast carcinoma-associated lymphedema. A randomized, prospective study of a role for adjunctive intermittent pneumatic compression. *Cancer.* 2002;95:2260–2267.

14. Partsch H. Understanding the pathophysiological effects of compression. In: *European Wound Management Association. Understanding Compression Therapy.* London, UK: Medical Education Partnership Ltd; 2003:2–4.

15. Partsch H, Flour M, Smith PC, International Compression Club. Indications for compression therapy in venous and lymphatic disease consensus based on experimental data and scientific evidence. Under the auspices of the IUP. *Int Angiol.* 2008;27(3): 193–219.

16. Brayton KM, Hirsch AT, O Brien PJ et al. Lymphedema prevalence and treatment benefits in cancer: impact of a therapeutic intervention on health outcomes and costs. *PLOS ONE.* 2014;9(12):e114597.

17. Lee BB. State of art in lymphedema management: Part 1. *Phlebolymphology.* 2018;25(2):160–171.

18. Boris M, Weindorf S, Lasinski BB. The risk of genital edema after external pump compression for lower limb lymphedema. *Lymphology.* 1998;31(1): 15–20.

19. Pappas CJ, O'Donnell TF. Long-term results of compression treatment for lymphedema. *J Vasc Surg.* 1992;16:555–562.

20. Klein MJ, Alexander MA, Wright JM et al. Treatment of adult lower extremity lymphedema with the Wright linear pump: Statistical analysis of a clinical trial. *Arch Phys Med Rehabil.* 1988;69:202–206.

21. Zanolla R, Monzeglio C, Balzarini A et al. Evaluation of the results of three different methods of post-mastectomy lymphedema treatment. *J Surg Oncol.* 1984;26:210–213.

22. Hassall A, Graveline C, Hilliard P. A retrospective study of the effects of Lymphapress pump on lymphedema in a pediatric population. *Lymphology.* 2001; 34(4):156–165.

23. Vanscheidt W, Ukat A, Partsch H. Dose-response of compression therapy for chronic venous edema--higher pressures are associated with greater volume reduction: Two randomized clinical studies. *J Vasc Surg.* 2009;49(2):395–402.

24. Zaleska M, Olszewski WL, Durlik M. The effectiveness of intermittent pneumatic compression in long-term therapy of lymphedema of lower limbs. *Lymphat Res Biol.* 2014;12(2):103–109.

25. Bergan JJ, Sparks S, Angle N. A comparison of compression pumps in the treatment of lymphedema. *Vasc Endovascular Surg.* 1998;32(5):455–462.

26. Zaleska MT, Olszewski WL. Indocyanine green near-infrared lymphangiography for evaluation of effectiveness of edema fluid flow under therapeutic compression. *J Biophotonics.* 2018;11:e201700150.

59

Reconstructive surgery: Lymphovenous anastomosis versus lymph node transplantation—Can they stay as independent therapy options?

CORRADINO CAMPISI, FRANCESCO BOCCARDO, MELISSA RYAN, MICHELE MARUCCIA, FABIO NICOLI, PIETRO DI SUMMA, AND CORRADO CESARE CAMPISI

The development, within the last 50 years, of newer surgical techniques to restore lymphatic flow in patients with lymphedema offers a treatment that targets more than symptomatic relief, providing a functional repair of the underlying problem of lymph-stasis. Initial surgical methods were ablative and employed in the advanced stages of disease with significant levels of fibrotic tissue. However, these were often characterized by significant scarring, poor wound healing, and infection, and have largely been abandoned as microsurgical techniques arose.[1-3]

Initial microsurgical procedures involved lymph nodal-venous shunts, but these had a high failure rate due to the thrombogenic effect of the lymph node pulp entering the venous system and re-endothelization of the lymph node surface.[4] Subsequent approaches involved anastomosing lymphatic vessels directly to collateral veins (lymphatic-venous anastomoses [LVA]) or to venular vessels (lymphatic-venular anastomoses; supermicrosurgery).[5,6] These modifications improved the long-term outcome of lymphatic microsurgery, but the efficacy, in terms of volume reduction and long-term stability, remains highly variable between surgical centers worldwide.[2]

In the 1990s, vascularized lymph node transfers (VLNTs) were developed based on the idea to transfer working lymph nodes into the area of lymph stasis, in the hopes of restoring some lymphatic flow.[7] VLNTs are performed by harvesting a lymph node or several lymph nodes along with their vascular supply from a donor site and transferring this vascularized tissue to the affected extremity as a free tissue transfer or pedicled flap. The concept was first examined in animal models and then transferred to humans, largely in small case studies. The long-term efficacy has not yet been established in large sample sizes or in multisite trials.[8-10]

LYMPHATIC MICROSURGERY—LYMPHATIC-VENOUS ANASTOMOSES IN SINGLE AND MULTIPLE SURGICAL SITES

Lymphatic microsurgery performed in Genoa, Italy, consists of multiple lymphatic venous anastomoses (MLVA) performed at a single incisional site. Some surgeons performing lymphatic microsurgery have adopted other techniques of making multiple incisions distally down the lymphedematous limb and performing a lymphatic-venular anastomosis at each incision (supermicrosurgery).[11-16] While this is technically impressive due to the diameter of the vessels involved, only the most superficial lymphatic vessels are used, just subdermal, and these are prone to closure by compression and thrombosis. In addition, recent research suggests that only a small minority of lymphedema cases involve only the superficial vessels.[17] The majority of patients also have deep vessel abnormalities, which are not treated by a supermicrosurgical multisite approach.[17,18]

The rationale behind using a single-site technique is twofold. First, a proximal single-site surgery likely lowers the risk of infection, as there is less surface area for bacteria to breach the skin barrier. This is particularly relevant for advanced stages of disease with significant lymph stasis.[19-23] In addition, in our clinical experience, the majority of infections occur distally (in the feet or hands of the affected limb), perhaps due to difficulty of the immune system in mobilizing dendritic cells through the thickened tissue to the lymph nodes.[24-26] Second, the caliber of the lymphatic vessels increases proximally. Not only are these vessels easier to use to create anastomoses, but they also allow a greater amount of lymph to flow through the anastomosis. This is important when trying to redress the balance of fluid in and out of a limb.[27,28] Supermicrosurgery using small-caliber vessels requires meticulous surgical technique but may not be sufficient to restore lymphatic flow in a limb, especially in late-stage lymphedema.[27]

There is the argument against the use of larger-caliber vessels, however, that the pressure difference in such cases between the venous and lymphatic systems is too great to prevent thrombosis of the anastomoses.[13,29] The Genoa MLVA technique takes measures to overcome this pressure difference by creating the anastomoses in close proximity to a valve in the vein. In this way, the valvular pumping creates a suction that pulls the lymph immediately through the anastomosis to prevent thrombosis. The end-to-end approach utilized in lymphatic-venular anastomoses (supermicrosurgery) instead allows the close contact of lymph and blood without this additional suction and may therefore lead to thrombosis of the anastomoses. With MLVA the lymphatic vessels have the perilymphatic tissue intact ensuring that these vessels are well-functioning, and this also helps to prevent thrombosis (Figure 59.1).

LVA can achieve up to an average of 86% excess volume reduction, and the MLVA concept, in particular, has shown to give stable reductions for more than 20 years of follow-up, particularly in the earlier stages of disease (Figure 59.2).[30-32] LVAs are applicable for both primary and secondary forms of lymphedema in the both the early and more advanced stages, provided that there is not complete lymph node or vessel aplasia.[33] Complication rates reported in the literature are negligible. Most importantly, LVAs are associated with a significant reduction in the incidence of cellulitis and lymphangitis, postoperatively.[31,34]

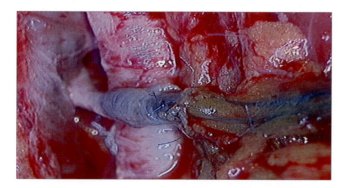

Figure 59.1 Multiple lymphatic venous anastomoses: multiple lymphatic vessels, stained blue, still encased in the perilymphatic tissue can be seen entering the vein branch. The passage of blue lymph into the vein branch, as seen under the operating microscope, verifies the patency of the anastomosis.

VASCULARIZED LYMPH NODE TRANSFER

Lymph nodes are harvested from a donor site with their supporting artery and vein and transferred to the recipient site of an affected area. The mechanism of action of this surgery is through two proposed hypotheses: physiological drainage and lymphangiogenesis.[9] One theory is that lymphatic vessel angiogenesis occurs due to cytokines (primarily vascular endothelial growth factor, VEGF-C) from the transplanted lymph node flap, establishing new lymphatic vessels between the flap and the surrounding tissue. Another hypothesis is that the transferred lymph nodes act by a pumping mechanism, whereby the nodes, as low-pressure systems (lower oncotic pressure than blood), collect lymphatic fluid and shift it into the venous system, also using Starling forces.[35,36] However, these theories are largely speculative, and it is unknown how VLNT works and how effective it may be over the long term.

The optimal donor site for VLNT is still an area of considerable debate. There are a number of possible donor sites: submental, supraclavicular, cervical, lateral thoracic, groin, and the omentum; the choice depends on patient characteristics, such as the location of swelling, previous lymphadenectomy, and other factors like scar visibility and risk of complications.[37] One of the more popular donor sites was the groin flap, as it can be combined with a deep inferior epigastric perforator (DIEP) abdominal flap to allow for simultaneous breast reconstruction for secondary upper limb lymphedema.[38] However, iatrogenic lymphedema at the donor site is a significant concern, which is not entirely eliminated even with the use of sentinel node techniques (reverse lymphatic mapping) to try to avoid harvesting nodes that drain the lower limb.[39-41] Rates of iatrogenic lymphedema after groin VLNT have been as high as 23%.[39] Other complications that can occur are seroma, lymphocele, flap loss, nerve damage, and delayed wound healing.[42]

Each donor site has particular characteristics that are advantageous or potentially negative.[37] As noted earlier, the groin flap, while advantageous with its well-concealed scar, is concerning for its potential for iatrogenic lymphedema. The supraclavicular lymph node flap has a lower risk of lymphedema but requires meticulous surgical skill to avoid the many vital structures in the supraclavicular region including the carotid artery, internal jugular vein, thoracic duct, and phrenic nerve.[43] Likewise, use of the submental donor site requires careful dissection to avoid injuring the marginal mandibular nerve, which runs superficial to the facial vessels. Injury to this nerve can lead to facial movement asymmetries, which are noticeable during mouth opening, smiling, or grimacing.[44]

Recently, the omentum, which is a rich source of lymphatic tissue, has gained popularity as a VLNT due to the lowered risk for donor site lymphedema.[10] It is also possible to harvest a smaller VLNT based on the right gastroepiploic vessels instead of the whole omentum (Figure 59.3). Plastic surgeons can safely take the right gastroepiploic artery and surrounding 3 cm of tissue to include two or three lymph

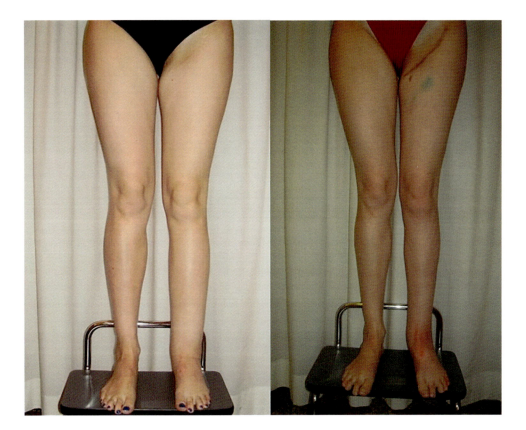

Figure 59.2 Pre- and immediately post multiple lymphatic venous anastomoses in patient with left lower limb lymphedema secondary to oncological treatment.

nodes.[45,46] Moreover, an extended flap based on the right gastroepiploic vessels can be harvested and divided into two halves for a "double-level" transfer on the affected limb. The use of minimally invasive surgery techniques for flap harvest (laparoscopic or robotic) reduces the donor site morbidity. Initial studies have shown reduction in volume of the effective limb with the omentum flap. Harvesting of the omentum has little to no risk of iatrogenic lymphedema; however, it does require an intra-abdominal approach, leading to risk of adhesions and subsequent bowel obstruction or incisional hernias.

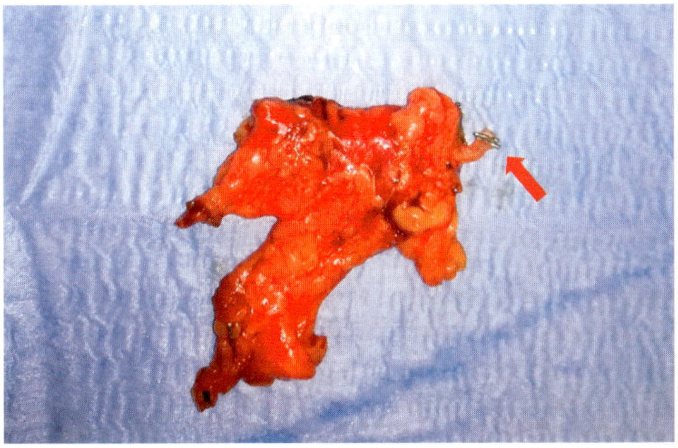

INDICATIONS FOR SURGERY

A problem in monitoring the success of surgical interventions is that there is no standard for measuring the degree of lymphedema and no standardized conservative treatment protocol before or after surgery. In addition, often the research studies varied in their outcome units and so it is difficult to compare between studies.[9,42] Scaglioni et al. report improvements after VLNT ranging from 30% to 100% "improvement" but noted a huge inconsistency in reporting.[42] Simple volume reduction measurements can also be misleading: sometimes small reductions in excess volume are clinically significant for patients if it allows them to reduce the levels of compression garments or means freedom from infection. Lymphedema can be a difficult disease to manage and is prone to progression without adequate treatment. In response to this, some surgical centers are now combining LVA and VLNT with other procedures such as liposuction or a modified Charles procedure.[47,48] Unfortunately, this further muddies the water, as a successful outcome is difficult to interpret: is it due to the combined approach, or would it have been obtained by a single technique if applied in isolation? Until we have standardization in our research methods, we cannot begin to move forward to delineate the nuances of which surgery for which lymphedema patient.[49]

Figure 59.3 Right gastroepiploic lymph node flap. The arrow points to the vascular pedicle (right gastroepiploic artery and vein).

REFERENCES

1. Fujita T. Optimizing surgical treatment for lymphedema. *J Am Coll Surg.* 2013;216:169–170.
2. Mehrara B, Zampell JC, Suami H et al. Surgical management of lymphedema: Past, present, and future. *Lymphat Res Biol.* 2011;9:159–167.
3. Ryan M, Campisi CC, Boccardo F, Campisi C. Surgical treatment for lymphedema: Optimal timing and optimal techniques. *J Am Coll Surg.* 2013;216:1221–1223.
4. Dellachà A, Boccardo F, Zilli A, Napoli F, Fulcheri E, Campisi C. Unexpected histopathological findings in peripheral lymphedema. *Lymphology.* 2000;33:62–64.
5. O'Brien BM. Replantation and reconstructive microvascular surgery. Part II. *Ann R Coll Surg.* 1976;58:171–182.
6. Campisi C, Boccardo F. Lymphedema and microsurgery. *Microsurgery.* 2002;22:74–80.
7. Chen HC, O'Brien BM, Rogers IW, Pribaz JJ, Eaton CJ. Lymph node transfer for the treatment of obstructive lymphoedema in the canine model. *Br J Plast Surg.* 1990;43(5):578–586.
8. Ozturk CN, Ozturk C, Glasgow M et al. Free vascularized lymph node transfer for treatment of lymphedema: A systematic evidence based review. *J Plast Reconstr Aesthet Surg.* 2016;69(9):1234–1247.
9. Garza R, Skoracki R, Hock K, Povoski SP. A comprehensive overview on the surgical management of secondary lymphedema of the upper and lower extremities related to prior oncologic therapies. *BMC Cancer.* 2017;17:468.
10. Gould DJ, Mehrara BJ, Neligan P, Cheng MH, Patel KM. Lymph node transplantation for the treatment of lymphedema. *J Surg Oncol.* 2018;118(5):736–742.
11. Koshima I, Nanba Y, Tsutsui T, Takahashi Y, Itoh S. Long-term follow-up after lymphaticovenular anastomosis for lymphedema in the leg. *J Reconstr Microsurg.* 2003;19:209–215.
12. Koshima I, Nanba Y, Tsutsui T, Takahashi Y, Itoh S, Fujitsu M. Minimal invasive lymphaticovenular anastomosis under local anesthesia for leg lymphedema: Is it effective for stage III and IV? *Ann Plast Surg.* 2004;53:261–266.
13. Nagase T, Gonda K, Inoue K. Treatment of lymphedema with lymphaticovenular anastomoses. *Int J Clin Oncol.* 2005;10:304–310.
14. Mihara M, Hayashi Y, Murai N et al. Regional diagnosis of lymphoedema and selection of sites for lymphaticovenular anastomosis using elastography. *Clin Radiol.* 2011;66:715–719.
15. Maegawa J, Yabuki Y, Tomoeda H, Hosono M, Yasumura K. Outcomes of lymphaticovenous side-to-end anastomosis in peripheral lymphedema. *J Vasc Surg.* 2012;55:753–760.
16. Mihara MM, Hara H, Narushima M et al. Lower limb lymphedema treated with lymphatico-venous anastomosis based on pre- and intraoperative ICG lymphography and non-contact vein visualization: A case report. *Microsurgery.* 2012;32:227–230.
17. Campisi CC, Ryan M, Villa G et al. Rationale for study of the deep subfascial lymphatic vessels during lymphoscintigraphy for the diagnosis of peripheral lymphedema. *Clin Nucl Med.* 2019;44(2):91–98.
18. Villa G, Campisi CC, Campisi C et al. Procedural recommendations for lymphoscintigraphy in the diagnosis of peripheral lymphedema: The Genoa Protocol. *Nuclear Medicine and Molecular Imaging.* 2019;53:47–56.
19. Rutkowski JM, Davis KE, Scherer PE. Mechanisms of obesity and related pathologies: The macro- and microcirculation of adipose tissue. *FEBS J.* 2009;276:5738–5746.
20. Olszewski WL, Engeset A, Romaniuk A, Grzelak I, Ziolkowska A. Immune cells in peripheral lymph and skin of patients with obstructive lymphedema. *Lymphology.* 1990;23(1):23–33.
21. Rockson SG. Lymphedema. *Am J Med.* 2001;110(4):288–295.
22. Beilhack A, Rockson SG. Immune traffic: A functional overview. *Lymphat Res Biol.* 2003;1(3):219–234.
23. Szolnoky G, Dobozy A, Kemény L. Decongestion improves cell-mediated immunity in postmastectomy arm lymphoedema: A pilot study. *J Eur Acad Dermatol Venereol.* 2013;27(12):1579–1582.
24. Angeli V, Randolph GJ. Inflammation, lymphatic function, and dendritic cell migration. *Lymphat Res Biol.* 2006;4:217–228.
25. Hwang ST. Homeward bound: How do skin dendritic cells find their way into the lymph system? *J Invest Dermatol.* 2012;132:1070–1073.
26. Swartz M, Hubbell JA, Reddy ST. Lymphatic drainage function and its immunological implications: From dendritic cell homing to vaccine design. *Semin Immunol.* 2008;20:147–156.
27. Suami H, Chang DW. Overview of surgical treatments for breast cancer–related lymphedema. *Plast Reconstr Surg.* 2010;26:1853–1863.
28. Koshima I, Kawada S, Moriguchi T, Kajiwara Y. Ultrastructural observations of lymphatic vessels in lymphedema in human extremities. *Plast Reconstr Surg.* 1996;97:397–405.
29. Penha TR, Ijsbrandy C, Hendrix NAM et al. Microsurgical techniques for the treatment of breast cancer-related lymphedema: A systematic review. *J Reconstr Microsurg.* 2013;29(2):99–106.
30. Campisi CC, Ryan M, Boccardo F, Campisi C. A single-site technique of multiple lymphatic venous anastomoses for the treatment of peripheral lymphedema: Long-term clinical outcomes. *J Reconstr Microsurg.* 2016;32(1):42–49.
31. Carl HM, Walia G, Bello R et al. Systematic review of the surgical treatment of extremity lymphedema. *J Reconstr Microsurg.* 2017;33(6):412–425.
32. Campisi C, Ryan M, Campisi CS, Boccardo F, Campisi CC. Lymphatic venous anastomosis applied in the surgical management of peripheral lymphedema: From prophylaxis to advanced disease. In: Chen H-C,

Ciudad P, Chen S-H, Tang YB, eds. *Lymphedema Surgical Approaches and Specific Topics.* 2nd ed. New York, NY: Elsevier; 2018:55–70.

33. Campisi C, Boccardo F, Campisi CC, Ryan M. Reconstructive microsurgery for lymphedema: While the early bird catches the worm, the late riser still benefits. *J Am Coll Surg.* 2013;216(3):506–507.

34. Maclellan RA, Couto RA, Sullivan JE et al. Management of primary and secondary lymphedema: Analysis of 225 referrals to a center. *Ann Plast Surg.* 2015;75:197–200.

35. Raju A, Chang DW. Vascularized lymph node transfer for treatment of lymphedema: A comprehensive literature review. *Ann Surg.* 2015;261(5):1013–1023.

36. Cheng MH, Huang JJ, Wu CW et al. The mechanism of vascularized lymph node transfer for lymphedema: Natural lymphaticovenous drainage. *Plast Reconstr Surg.* 2014;133(2):192e–198e.

37. Schaverien MV, Badash I, Patel KM, Selber JC, Cheng MH. Vascularized lymph node transfer for lymphedema. *Semin Plast Surg.* 2018;32(1):28–35.

38. Scaglioni MF, Suami H. Lymphatic anatomy of the inguinal region in aid of vascularized lymph node flap harvesting. *J Plast Reconstr Aesthet Surg.* 2015;68(3):419–427.

39. Vignes S, Blanchard M, Yannoutsos A, Arrault M. Complications of autologous lymph-node transplantation for limb lymphoedema. *Eur J Vasc Endovasc Surg.* 2013;45(5):516–520.

40. Viitanen TP, Mäki MT, Seppänen MP, Suominen EA, Saaristo AM. Donor-site lymphatic function after microvascular lymph node transfer. *Plast Reconstr Surg.* 2012;130(6):1246–1253.

41. Sulo E, Hartiala P, Viitanen T, Mäki M, Seppänen M, Saarikko A. Risk of donor-site lymphatic vessel dysfunction after microvascular lymph node transfer. *J Plast Reconstr Aesthet Surg.* 2015;68(4):551–558.

42. Scaglioni MF, Arvanitakis M, Chen YC, Giovanoli P, Chia-Shen Yang J, Chang EI. Comprehensive review of vascularized lymph node transfers for lymphedema: Outcomes and complications. *Microsurgery.* 2018;38(2):222–229.

43. Ooi ASH, Chang DW. 5-step harvest of supraclavicular lymph nodes as vascularized free tissue transfer for treatment of lymphedema. *J Surg Oncol.* 2017;115(1):63–67.

44. Steinbacher J, Tinhofer IE, Meng S et al. The surgical anatomy of the supraclavicular lymph node flap: A basis for the free vascularized lymph node transfer. *J Surg Oncol.* 2017;115(01):60–62.

45. Howell AC, Gould DJ, Hassani C, Patel KM. Anatomic basis of the gastroepiploic vascularized lymph node transfer: A radiographic evaluation using computed tomography angiography (CTA). *Plast Reconstr Surg Glob Open.* 2017;5:73.

46. Ciudad P, Maruccia M, Socas J et al. The laparoscopic right gastroepiploic lymph node flap transfer for upper and lower limb lymphedema: Technique and outcomes. *Microsurgery.* 2017;37(3):197–205.

47. Yamamoto T, Yoshimatsu H, Yamamoto N. Complete lymph flow reconstruction: A free vascularized lymph node true perforator flap transfer with efferent lymphaticolymphatic anastomosis. *J Plast Reconstr Aesthet Surg.* 2016;69(9):1227–1233.

48. Ciudad P, Agko M, Huang TCT et al. Comprehensive multimodal surgical treatment of end-stage lower extremity lymphedema with toe management: The combined Charles,' Homan's, and vascularized lymph node transfer (CHAHOVA) procedures. *J Surg Oncol.* 2019;119(4):430–438.

49. Campisi CC, Jiga LP, Ryan M, di Summa PG, Campisi C, Ionac M. Mastering lymphatic microsurgery: A new training model in living tissue. *Ann Plast Surg.* 2017;79(3):298–303.

60

Excisional surgery: When and how much it can be incorporated

JUSTIN CHIN-BONG CHOI, JAMES LAREDO, AND BYUNG-BOONG LEE

Chronic lymphedema is a "steadily progressive condition that affects the entire soft tissue," resulting in irreversible damage.[1,2] It is traditionally managed with complex decongestive therapy (CDT) and/or compression therapy.[3–5] However, as the lymphedema reaches its end stages (stages IV–V), these traditional means of management become less effective as the compression bandages are more difficult to apply properly to highly disfigured and swollen limbs.[6] As the condition worsens, patients become more prone to developing bacterial and fungal infections with subsequent sepsis, dermatolipofibrosclerosis, immunodeficiency and wasting phenomena, and malignancies such as Kaposi sarcoma and lymphangiosarcoma.[6–9]

Surgical debulking of chronic lymphedema has been described since the early 1900s, including procedures by Charles (1912), Sistrunk (1918), Homans (1936), and Thompson (1962).[10–15] While these operations removed scarred and disfigured lymphedema tissue from the limb, they were performed without adequate patient selection and resulted in high morbidity and mortality, bringing their effectiveness into question. During the last 10 years, modifications of these once-abandoned operations (e.g., modified Auchincloss and Homans procedures) have become of interest as potential palliative operations for chronic end-stage lymphedema and resulted in improved outcomes.[10,16,17]

The indications for excisional/debulking surgery should include progression of the lymphedema to end stage despite maximal CDT, increased frequency and/or severity of sepsis episodes, and failure to implement proper care at end-stage chronic lymphedema.[2,19,20] However, long-term success is highly dependent on patient compliance to maintain postoperative CDT.[6,21,22] Surgery alone will likely fail in the long term.[6] While surgery is a viable option to supplement CDT, there is no consensus on the optimal timing of operative intervention or the choice of procedure.[18,19]

Liposuction is another debulking technique that aims to obliterate the epifascial compartment by using a "circumferential" suction-assisted lipectomy instead of resecting the entire soft tissue, thus making it a less radical approach compared to excisional surgery. It also avoids morbidity and mortality associated excision.[23–25] However, because liposuction removes only fat, it should not be performed before CDT is implemented, as it will need to transform pitting edema to nonpitting edema. Patients who benefit the most are those who develop excess fat accumulation due to secondary lymphedema of the upper limb after breast cancer treatment.[23,24] Like with excisional surgery, CDT should be continued after liposuction. Patients need to be informed that life-long, continuous use of compression garments is required postoperatively for liposuction to be efficient. Some authors advocate for preoperative assessment of patients' readiness to comply with compression garment therapy and use this criterion to exclude patients from liposuction consideration if they do not demonstrate readiness to commit to life-long postoperative garment compression therapy (see Chapter 67 for more details).

While liposuction has been shown to be effective in significant long-term volume reduction in secondary lymphedema,[26] its efficacy has not yet been proven for primary lymphedema as there are limited studies. This is likely because primary lymphedema mostly affects the lower extremities, and there is no proven evidence of selective overgrowth of adipose tissue in that group.[27–30] Furthermore, primary lymphedema is manifested by truncular lymphatic malformation with a high risk of combined extra-truncular lymphatic malformation. Liposuction in the setting of coexisting extra-truncular lymphatic malformations has been shown to worsen the condition by stimulating rapid growth of mesenchymal cells.[31–33] A recent study by Lamprou et al., however, showed that 47 patients with primary lymphedema that were treated with liposuction appeared to be effective, with a 79% reduction in leg volume 2 years after surgery.[34]

REFERENCES

1. Lee BB, Laredo J. Pathophysiology of primary lymphedema. In: Neligan PC, Piller NB, Masia J, eds. *Complete Medical and Surgical Management*. Boca Raton, FL: CRC Press; 2016:177–188.

2. Lee BB, Andrade M, Antignani PL et al.; IUP. Diagnosis and treatment of primary lymphedema. *Int Angiol*. 2013;32(6):541–574.

3. Hwang JH, Lee KW, Chang DY et al. Complex physical therapy for lymphedema. *J Korean Acad Rehabil Med*. 1998;22:224–229.

4. Bastien MR, Goldstein BG, Lesher JL Jr, Smith JG Jr. Treatment of lymphedema with a multicompartmental pneumatic compression device. *J Am Acad Dermatol*. 1989;20(5 Pt 1):853–854.

5. Hwang JH, Kim TU, Lee KW, Kim DI, Lee BB. Sequential intermittent pneumatic compression therapy in lymphedema. *J Korean Acad Rehabil Med*. 1997;21:146–153.

6. Lee BB, Kim YW, Kim DI, Hwang JH, Laredo J, Neville R. Supplemental surgical treatment to end stage (stage VI-V) of chronic lymphedema. *Int Angiol*. 2008;27(5):389–395.

7. Olszewski WL. Episodic dermatolymphangioadenitis (DLA) in patients with lymphedema of the lower extremities before and after administration of benzathine penicillin: A preliminary study. *Lymphology*. 1996;29:126–131.

8. Lee BB, Bergan JJ. New clinical and laboratory staging systems to improve management of chronic lymphedema. *Lymphology*. 2005;38:122–129.

9. Lee BB. Current issue in management of chronic lymphedema: Personal reflection on an experience with 1065 patients. *Lymphology*. 2005;38:28–31.

10. Kim DI, Huh S, Lee SJ, Hwang JH, Kim YI, Lee BB. Excision of subcutaneous tissue and deep muscle fascia for advanced lymphedema. *Lymphology*. 1998;31:190–194.

11. Dellon AL, Hoopes JE. The Charles procedure for primary lymphedema. Long-term clinical results. *Plast Reconstr Surg*. 1977;60:589–595.

12. Sistrunk WE. Further experiences with the Kondoleon operation for elephantiasis. *JAMA*. 1918;71:800.

13. Homans J. The treatment of elephantiasis of the legs. *N Engl J Med*. 1936;215:1099.

14. Weiss JM, Spray BJ. The effect of complete decongestive therapy on the quality of life of patients with peripheral lymphedema. *Lymphology*. 2002;35:46.

15. Kinmonth JB, Patrick J, II, Chilvers AS. Comments on operations for lower limb lymphedema. *Lymphology*. 1975;8:56–61.

16. Lee BB. State of art in lymphedema management: Part 1. *Phlebolymphology*. 2018;25(2):160–171.

17. Huh SH, Kim DI, Hwang JH, Lee BB. Excisional surgery in chronic advanced lymphedema. *Surg Today*. 2003;34:434–435.

18. Brorson H. Liposuction in lymphedema treatment. *J Reconstr Microsurg*. 2016;32:56–65.

19. Lee BB. State of art in lymphedema management: Part 2. *Phlebolymphology*. 2018;25(2):189–200.

20. Lee BB, Andrade M, Bergan J et al.; IUP. Diagnosis and treatment of primary lymphedema. *Int Angiol*. 2010;29(5):454–470.

21. Lee BB, Kim DI, Whang JH, Lee KW. Contemporary issues in management of chronic lymphedema—Personal reflection on an experience with 1065 patients. Commentary. *Lymphology*. 2005;38:28–31.

22. Lee BB. Contemporary issues in management of chronic lymphedema: Personal reflection on an experience with 1065 patients. *Lymphology*. 2005;38(1):28–31.

23. Brorson H, Svensson H. Liposuction combined with controlled compression therapy reduces arm lymphedema more effectively than controlled compression therapy alone. *Plast Reconstr Surg*. 1998;102(4):1058–1067.

24. Brorson H, Svensson H, Norrgren K, Thorsson O. Liposuction reduces arm lymphedema without significantly altering the already impaired lymph transport. *Lymphology*. 1998;31(4):156–172.

25. Brorson H. From lymph to fat: Complete reduction of lymphoedema. *Phlebology*. 2010;25(Suppl 1):52–63.

26. Brorson H. Liposuction in arm lymphedema treatment. *Scand J Surg*. 2003;92(4):287–295.

27. Lee BB, Kim YW, Seo JM et al. Current concepts in lymphatic malformation (LM). *Vasc Endovascular Surg*. 2005;39(1):67–81.

28. Lee BB. Lymphedema-angiodysplasia syndrome: A prodigal form of lymphatic malformation. *Phlebolymphology*. 2005;47:324–332.

29. Lee BB, Villavicencio JL. Primary lymphedema and lymphatic malformation: Are they the two sides of the same coin? *Eur J Vasc Endovasc Surg*. 2010;39(5):646–653.

30. Lee BB, Laredo J, Neville R. Primary lymphedema as a truncular lymphatic malformation. In: Lee BB, Bergan J, Rockson SG, eds. *Lymphedema: A Concise Compendium of Theory and Practice*. London, UK: Springer-Verlag; 2011:419–426.

31. Lee BB, Laredo J, Lee TS, Huh S, Neville R. Terminology and classification of congenital vascular malformations. *Phlebology*. 2007;22(6):249–252.

32. Lee BB, Laredo J, Kim YW, Neville R. Congenital vascular malformations: General treatment principles. *Phlebology*. 2007;22(6):258–263.

33. Lee BB. All congenital vascular malformations should belong to one of two types: "Truncular" or "extra-truncular", as different as apples and oranges! *Phlebol Rev*. 2015;23(1):1–3.

34. Lamprou DA, Voesten HG, Damstra RJ, Wikkeling OR. Circumferential suction-assisted lipectomy in the treatment of primary and secondary end-stage lymphoedema of the leg. *Br J Surg*. 2017;104(1):84–89.

61

Multidisciplinary approach with liposuction in primary lymphedema: Is there a difference compared to patients with secondary lymphedema?

ROBERT J. DAMSTRA AND HÅKAN BRORSON

INTRODUCTION

Lymphedema is clinical condition due to impaired fluid transport through the lymphatic system due to either an impaired lymphatic system or a disbalance between filtration and fluid transport capacity and can be divided into primary and secondary forms.[1] Fluid stasis due to decreased transport capacity of the lymphatics is called *mechanical insufficiency* or *low-output failure* (raised afterload), while an overload of filtration within a normal lymph system leading to fluid stasis is called *dynamic insufficiency* or *high-output failure* (raised preload). This distinction is important because it influences the choice of treatment algorithm (Figures 61.1 through 61.3).

In dynamic insufficiency, decreasing the filtration of fluid is essential and mandatory instead of stimulating lymphatics, which is already functioning at its highest capacity. Examples to reduce filtration are compression garments, reduction of weight, or downregulation of inflammation, e.g., by antibiotics in case of infection or by compression.[2] Raised afterload can be addressed by stimulation of lymphatic pump function by compression therapy, exercises, and perhaps reconstructive surgery and manual lymph drainage.

Traditionally, the treatment of choice for lymphedema was empirical conservative management with decongestive lymphatic treatment (DLT) including manual lymph drainage (MLD), compression therapy, skin care, and exercises.[3] During the last decades, many separate components of DLT have been studied more scientifically; the role of MLD became controversial since its effect is unclear, and MLD is not considered to be effective and time consuming.[4–9]

The most common etiology for lymphatic impairment is infection, trauma, and/or iatrogenic injury (e.g., secondary to cancer treatment by surgical resection and/or radiation therapy). The prevalence of lymphatic filariasis and neoplastic diseases alone implies a large global burden of lymphatic disease.[10]

Primary lymphedema due to an inborn defect of lymphatic transport is considered a rare disease affecting 1/100,000 children.[4] Primary lymphedema represents a heterogeneous group including sporadic, hereditary, and syndromal forms (e.g., Noonan syndrome, Turner, or overgrowth syndromes).[5] A number of genetic aberrations are identified that underline pathophysiological mechanisms that lead to the development of primary lymphedema.

Modern treatment of lymphedema is more integrated (in secondary lymphedema, e.g., monitoring and early diagnostics, secondary prevention) and interdisciplinary as medical specialists, physiotherapists, edema therapists, compression specialists, and social workers are involved. It also takes chronic care models (CCMs)[11] as well as the *International Classification of Functioning, Disability, and Health* (ICF)[12] and risk stratification into account. CCM focuses more on the ability of a patient to be self-effective with self-management techniques, to participate in the care for their chronic condition, and to become as much as possible independent from a health-care provider during the maintenance phase[13–15]). The ICF model includes five domains of a patient's functionality profile, such as biomedical aspects, activities in daily life, participation in society, and personal and environmental factors, and uses validated clinical metrics for these domains for monitoring the result of a treatment program.

273

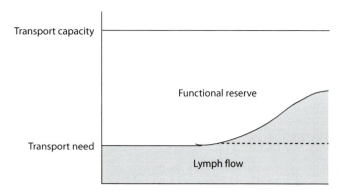

Figure 61.1 The *lymphatic safety factor* implies that the normal lymph vascular system is able for a time to handle an increased lymphatic protein and water load and thus prevent edema. It is not until the lymph flow is reduced by 80% that lymph starts to accumulate in the interstitium.

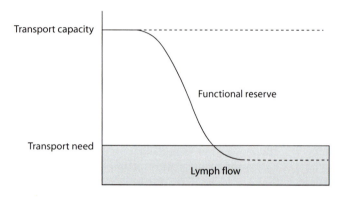

Figure 61.2 Mechanical insufficiency or low-output failure.

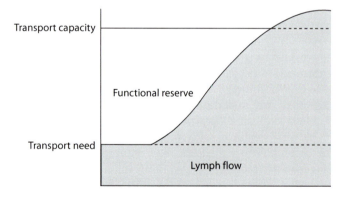

Figure 61.3 *Dynamic insufficiency* or *high-output failure* arises if the lymphatic load exceeds the lymphatic transport capacity. This is typically caused by venous obstruction, simply leading to an excess of tissue fluid with a low protein content.

The Dutch Guidelines for lymphedema are based on these concepts.[16] Liposuction for end-stage lymphedema fits nicely in this concept and has great and long-lasting results.[17,18]

EFFECTIVENESS OF LIPOSUCTION FOR LYMPHEDEMA

In end-stage lymphedema, long-lasting lymph stasis leads to excess adipose tissue formation[19–21] caused by

inflammation.[22–24] In 1998, Idy-Peretti et al.[25] described the increase of suprafascial fat formation in primary and secondary lymphedema as well as to a small extent in muscles.[26,27] As liposuction is an effective technique for adipose tissue removal,[28–30] the thought to remove adipose tissue by this procedure is rational. Since the first publication in 1987 by Teimourian[31] and Apesos et al.[29] in 1997 for liposuction in breast cancer–related lymphedema, many publications followed. Two recent publications by Schaverien et al.[18] and by Hoffner et al.[17] showed that there is a significant scientific basis that circumferential suction-assisted lipectomy (CSAL) liposuction for advanced stages of lymphedema is safe, gives complete reduction of volume, and provides long-lasting results when proper compression is maintained.[17,32] The technique should be practiced in a multidisciplinary setting.[33,34]

PRIMARY LYMPHEDEMA AND LIPOSUCTION

Liposuction in advanced lymphedema is most frequent in secondary lymphedema of the arms due to breast cancer treatment or of the legs in oncological therapy of the pelvis. As primary lymphedema is a rare disease, only two case reports[35,36] and two studies of 29 and 47 patients, with primary leg lymphedema and a follow-up of 10 and 2 years, respectively, have been published.[37,38]

Brorson et al. presented 27 patients with secondary lymphedema following cancer therapy and 29 with primary lymphedema with a follow-up at most of 10 years with an excess volume of 3935 mL and achieved complete reduction

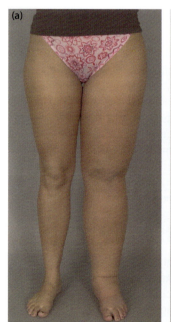
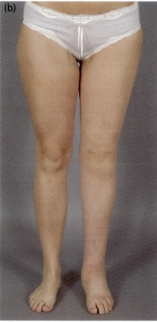

Figure 61.4 Preoperative excess volume 6630 mL in a patient with primary lymphedema **(a)**. Complete reduction at 2 years **(b)**. (Reproduced from Brorson H, Ohlin K, Svensson B. *J Lymphoedema* 2008;1:38–47.)

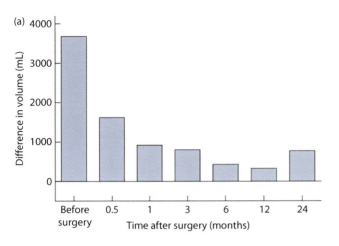 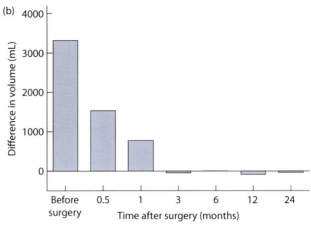

Figure 61.5 Median volume differences between affected and unaffected leg during 2 years of follow-up. **(a)** Primary lymphoedema. **(b)** Secondary lymphoedema.

after 1 year, which was maintained during the 10-year follow-up with constant use of compression garments (Figure 61.4).[37]

Lamprou et al.[38] compared CSAL in 88 patients with primary lymphedema ($n = 47$: 17 men, 30 women) and secondary lymphedema ($n = 41$: 4 men, 37 women) of the legs. The indication was in all patients made by the same multidisciplinary team, and the pre-, peri-, and postoperative protocols were the same.[38] Most striking were differences in prevalence of men in both groups. There was no statistically significant difference in duration of the procedure, ($p = 0.610$), preoperative body mass index ($p = 0.209$) or age between groups. The duration of operation was the same in both groups, but in primary lymphedema in men the CSAL was physically more strenuous as mentioned by the surgeons. There was no statistical difference in the amount of aspirated adipose tissue between primary and secondary lymphedema (3750 and 3975 mL, respectively). Multivariable regression analysis of data from this study demonstrated that preoperative volume difference and gender were two predicting factors for treatment efficacy. Male patients with primary lymphedema had a statistically significant volume reduction compared to females in the same group with respective median volumes of 1629 and 275 mL ($p < 0.001$). Figure 61.5 shows the data of a follow-up at 2 years.

Follow-up showed[38] that men were less coherent and compliant than women but were more satisfied with the end result even if there was still a positive excess volume. The authors hypothesized that perhaps primary lymphedema in men leads to more fibrosis related to a different pathophysiology between both types of lymphedema or sex-linked factors.

Another explanation can be a gender difference of the inner structure of the skin and subcutaneous tissues clinically observed as cellulite, which is recognized by de la Casa Almeida et al. as a physiological phenomenon and characteristic in women.[39]

CONCLUSIONS

In *advanced* stages of lymphedema that is resistant to conservative treatment, a further volume reduction can improve the efficacy of the overall management, and CSAL is the first-choice/option treatment. CSAL should be performed in a multidisciplinary setting combined with life-long proper compression therapy, exercise, and weight control. An overview study by Schaverien et al.[18] showed a significant amount of convincing evidence that this applies to secondary lymphedema (of the arms and legs); consequently, data support that this statement is also valid for primary lymphedema of the legs, although there are minor differences in outcome.

REFERENCES

1. Rockson SG. Update on the biology and treatment of lymphedema. *Curr Treat Options Cardiovasc Med*. 2012;14:184–192.
2. Beidler SK, Douillet CD, Berndt DF, Keagy BA, Rich PB, Marston WA. Inflammatory cytokine levels in chronic venous insufficiency ulcer tissue before and after compression therapy. *J Vasc Surg*. 2009; 49(4):1013–1020.
3. Rockson SG, Miller LT, Senie R et al. American Cancer Society Lymphedema Workshop. Workgroup III: Diagnosis and management of lymphedema. *Cancer*. 1998;83(12 Suppl American):2882–2885.
4. Smeltzer DM, Stickler GB, Schirger A. Primary lymphedema in children and adolescents: A follow-up study and review. *Pediatrics*. 1985;76: 206–218.
5. Connell FC, Gordon K, Brice G et al. The classification and diagnostic algorithm for primary lymphatic dysplasia: An update from 2010 to include molecular findings. *Clin Genet*. 2013;84:303–314.
6. Tambour M, Holt M, Speyer A, Christensen R, Gram B. Manual lymphatic drainage adds no further volume reduction to Complete Decongestive Therapy on breast cancer-related lymphoedema: A multicentre, randomised, single-blind trial. *Br J Cancer*. 2018;119:1215–1222.

7. Müller M, Klingberg K, Wertli MM, Carreira H. Manual lymphatic drainage and quality of life in patients with lymphoedema and mixed oedema: A systematic review of randomised controlled trials. *Qual Life Res.* 2018;27:1403–1414.

8. Devoogdt N, Van Kampen M, Geraerts I, Coremans T, Christiaens M-R. Different physical treatment modalities for lymphoedema developing after axillary lymph node dissection for breast cancer: A review. *Eur J Obstet Gynecol Reprod Biol.* 2010; 149:3–9.

9. Huang T-W, Tseng S-H, Lin C-C et al. Effects of manual lymphatic drainage on breast cancer-related lymphedema: A systematic review and meta-analysis of randomized controlled trials. *World J Surg Oncol.* 2013;11:15.

10. Rockson SG, Rivera KK. Estimating the population burden of lymphedema. *Ann N Y Acad Sci.* 2008; 1131:147–154.

11. Wagner EH. Chronic disease management: What will it take to improve care for chronic illness? *Eff Clinical Practice.* 1998;20:2–4.

12. Stucki G, Cieza A, Ewert T, Kostanjsek N, Chatterji S, Ustün TB. Application of the International Classification of Functioning, Disability and Health (ICF) in clinical practice. *Disabil Rehabil.* 2002;24:281–282.

13. Damstra RJ. Self-management in lymphedema. *Veins Lymphat.* 2018;7:134.

14. Ridner SH, Fu MR, Wanchai A, Stewart BR, Armer JM, Cormier JN. Self-management of lymphedema: A systematic review of the literature from 2004 to 2011. *Nurs Res.* 2012;61:291–299.

15. Barlow J, Wright C, Sheasby J, Turner A, Hainsworth J. Self-management approaches for people with chronic conditions: A review. *Patient Educ Couns.* 2002;48:177–187.

16. Damstra RJ, Halk AB; Dutch Working Group on Lymphedema. The Dutch lymphedema guidelines based on the International Classification of Functioning, Disability, and Health and the chronic care model. *J Vasc Surg Venous Lymphat Disord.* 2017;5:756–765.

17. Hoffner M, Ohlin K, Svensson B, Manjer J, Hansson E, Troëng T, Brorson H. Liposuction gives complete reduction of arm lymphedema following breast cancer: A 5 years' follow-up. *Plast Reconstr Surg Glob Open.* 2018;6:e1912.

18. Schaverien M, Munnoch D, Brorson H. Liposuction Treatment of Lymphedema. *Semin Plast Surg.* 2018;32:42–47.

19. Brorson H, Ohlin K, Olsson G, Nilsson M. Adipose tissue dominates chronic arm lymphedema following breast cancer: An analysis using volume rendered CT images. *Lymphat Res Biol.* 2006;4:199–210.

20. Brorson H, Ohlin K, Olsson G, Karlsson MK. Breast cancer-related chronic arm lymphedema is associated with excess adipose and muscle tissue. *Lymphat Res Biol.* 2009;7:3–10.

21. Schneider M, Conway EM, Carmeliet P. Lymph makes you fat. *Nat Genet.* 2005;37:1023–1024.

22. Zampell JC, Aschen S, Weitman ES et al. Regulation of adipogenesis by lymphatic fluid stasis: Part I. Adipogenesis, fibrosis, and inflammation. *Plast Reconstr Surg.* 2012;129:825–834.

23. Aschen S, Zampell JC, Elhadad S, Weitman E, De Brot M, Mehrara BJ. Regulation of adipogenesis by lymphatic fluid stasis: Part II. Expression of adipose differentiation genes. *Plast Reconstr Surg.* 2012;129:838–847.

24. Levi B, Glotzbach JP, Sorkin M et al. Molecular analysis and differentiation capacity of adipose-derived stem cells from lymphedema tissue. *Plast Reconstr Surg.* 2013;132:580–589.

25. Idy-Peretti I, Bittoun J, Alliot FA, Richard SB, Querleux BG, Cluzan RV. Lymphedematous skin and subcutis: In vivo high resolution magnetic resonance imaging evaluation. *J Invest Dermatol.* 1998;110:782–787.

26. Hoffner M, Peterson P, Månsson S, Brorson H. Lymphedema leads to fat deposition in muscle and decreased muscle/water volume after liposuction: A magnetic resonance imaging study. *Lymphat Res Biol.* 2018;16:174–181.

27. Trinh L, Peterson P, Brorson H, Månsson S. Assessment of subfascial muscle/water and fat accumulation in lymphedema patients using magnetic resonance imaging. *Lymphat Res Biol.* 2019;17(3):340–346.

28. Nava VM, Lawrence WT. Liposuction on a lymphedematous arm. *Ann Plast Surg.* 1988;21:366–368.

29. Apesos J, Chami R. Functional applications of suction-assisted lipectomy: A new treatment for old disorders. *Aesth Plast Surg.* 1991;15:73–79.

30. Brorson H, Svensson H. Complete reduction of lymphoedema of the arm by liposuction after breast cancer. *Scand J Plast Reconstr Surg Hand Surg.* 1997;31: 137–143.

31. Teimourian B. *Suction Lipectomy and Body Sculpturing,* 1st edition. St. Louis, MO: Mosby; 1987: 656–684, ISBN-10: 0801649234.

32. Brorson H, Svensson H. Liposuction combined with controlled compression therapy reduces arm lymphedema more effectively than controlled compression therapy alone. *Plast Reconstr Surg.* 1998;102:1058–1067.

33. Damstra RJ, Voesten HGJM, Klinkert P, Brorson H. Circumferential suction-assisted lipectomy for lymphoedema after surgery for breast cancer. *Br J Surg.* 2009;96:859–864.

34. Boyages J, Kastanias K, Koelmeyer LA et al. Lipo-suction for advanced lymphedema: A multidisci-plinary approach for complete reduction of arm and leg swelling. *Ann Surg Oncol.* 2015;22(Suppl 3):S1263–S1270.

35. Brorson H, Ohlin K, Svensson B, Svensson H. Controlled compression and liposuction treatment for lower extremity lymphedema. *Lymphology.* 2008;41:52–63.

36. Espinosa-de-los-Monteros A, Hinojosa CA, Abarca L, Iglesias M. Compression therapy and liposuction of lower legs for bilateral hereditary primary lymphedema praecox. *J Vasc Surg.* 2009; 49:222–224.

37. Brorson H. Liposuction normalizes lymphedema induced adipose tissue hypertrophy in elephantiasis of the leg—A prospective study with a ten-year follow-up. *Plast Reconstr Surg.* 2015;36(4S Suppl):133–134.

38. Lamprou D-AA, Voesten HGJ, Damstra RJ, Wikkeling ORM. Circumferential suction-assisted lipectomy in the treatment of primary and secondary end-stage lymphoedema of the leg. *Br J Surg.* 2017;104:84–89.

39. de la Casa Almeida M, Suarez Serrano C, Rebollo Roldán J, Jiménez Rejano JJ. Cellulite's aetiology: A review. *J Eur Acad Dermatol Venerol.* 2013;27:273–278.

40. Brorson H, Ohlin K, Svensson B. The facts about lipo-suction as a treatment for lymphoedema. *J Lymphoe-dema.* 2008;1:38–47.

62

How much pharmacological therapy can be incorporated in primary lymphedema management?

VAUGHAN KEELEY AND NEIL PILLER

BACKGROUND

Primary lymphedema arises as a result of an inherent, probably genetically caused abnormality of the lymphatic system, whereas secondary lymphedema is due to damage to an apparently normal lymphatic system, e.g., by surgery, radiotherapy, and/or infection. In both types, lymph stasis results in long-term changes in the skin and subcutaneous tissues as a result of chronic inflammation and also a vulnerability to infection, particularly bacterial cellulitis, due, at least in part, to a locally impaired immune response.

The role of pharmacological therapy in the management of lymphedema has, to date, predominantly focused on secondary lymphedema, but these approaches may be relevant to the management of the effects of lymph stasis in primary lymphedema as well.

This chapter focuses on possible pharmacological therapy for primary lymphedema but also considers drugs relevant to both primary and secondary lymphedema.

PRIMARY LYMPHEDEMA

The understanding of the genetic causes of some types of primary lymphedema has grown considerably over the last 20 years. A classification of the types of primary lymphedema by phenotype developed by the St. George's team in London, United Kingdom, has facilitated this process and is also recommended for use in clinical practice.[1] Using this approach, a number of gene mutations that cause primary lymphedema have been discovered. Many of these affect the vascular endothelial growth factor receptor-3 (VEGFR3) signaling pathway and also downstream of other tyrosine kinase receptors.[2] It is hoped that an understanding of the molecular mechanisms by which these mutations cause lymphedema may lead to new pharmacological/gene therapy treatments.

GENE THERAPY

The potential value of this approach has been shown using a mouse model of primary lymphedema of the Milroy type (caused by heterozygous inactivating missense mutations of the *FLT4* gene, which regulates VEGFR3 expression) and virus-mediated VEGFC gene therapy (VEGFC is the natural ligand of VEGFR3).[3] The gene therapy led to the generation of functional lymphatic vessels.

This concept is currently being investigated in secondary lymphedema. Lymfactin (Herantis), an adenovirus gene transfer vector carrying the human VEGFC gene, causes local gene expression for about 2 weeks in the tissues where it is injected. In a phase 2 randomized, double-blind, placebo-controlled study of 40 patients with breast cancer–related lymphedema, it is being used in combination with vascularized lymph node transfer (from the patient's abdominal wall or the inguinal area to the axillary region of the affected upper extremity) to try to improve lymph vessel regeneration and lymph node function (AdeLE study).[4] The estimated completion date for this study is December 2024, designed to provide 5-year follow-up data. As yet, however, there are no current studies of this type in primary lymphedema.

BENZOPYRONES AND FLAVONOIDS

Benzopyrones, such as coumarin, is the only group of drugs that have evidence to indicate a benefit in reducing all forms of high protein edemas, i.e., both primary and secondary lymphedema. They reduce the volume of any high protein edema by the stimulation of proteolysis by tissue macrophages. By removing the protein, there is less osmotic force holding the fluids; thus, they are freed to leave the accumulation sites, reducing associated chronic inflammation, fibrosis formation, and risk of secondary infection.[5]

However, in a Cochrane review in 2004, it was not possible to draw conclusions about the effectiveness of benzopyrones in reducing limb volume, pain, or discomfort in lymphedematous limbs due to the heterogeneity of the trials published at the time.[6]

There is also concern about the use of coumarin clinically due to reported hepatotoxicity. However, this may potentially be overcome through pharmacogenomics studies to target its use to those with a functional CYP2A6. A reduction of CYP2A6 results in the shunting of coumarin into other metabolic pathways, which can result in the production of cytotoxic metabolites such as o-hydroxy-phenylacetaldehyde rather than the beneficial 7-hydroxycoumarin, leading to hepatotoxicity.[7,8]

Similar preparations such as micronized purified flavonoid fractions of diosmin and hesperidin may be beneficial when there are associated chronic venous disorders presenting along with the primary lymphedema.[9]

However, there have not been any recent new trials of benzopyrones in primary lymphedema, and they are not used routinely in clinical practice.

CILOSTAZOL

Cilostazol is an antiplatelet agent and vasodilator. In a clinical case report, there was a reduction of lymph leakage in a patient with lymphatic filariasis following its use.[10]

In mouse lymphedema models and in vitro studies of human lymphatic endothelial cells (LECs), cilostazol has been shown to improve lymph flow and lymphedema and promote the growth of LECs, respectively.[11] This suggests a possible role for cilostazol in the treatment of human lymphedema. However, there have been no clinical trials to date.

RETINOIC ACID

In in vitro and animal studies, 9-cis retinoic acid has been found to promote lymphangiogenesis by activating fibroblast growth factor receptor signaling and promotes lymphatic regeneration in an experimental lymphedema model.[12] Furthermore, in a mouse model of secondary lymphedema, 9-cis retinoic acid was found to have a significant effect in preventing the development of lymphedema by increasing lymphatic clearance and lymphangiogenesis.[13]

However, there is concern about the potential cancer-promoting effects of drugs, which stimulate lymphangiogenesis, when they are used to treat lymphedema secondary to cancer treatment.[14] However, a role in the treatment of primary lymphedema may be possible. As yet, no clinical trials have been reported.

ANTI-INFLAMMATORY DRUGS

In a mouse model of secondary lymphedema, ketoprofen was found to improve lymphatic function and edema.[15] It was proposed that this effect was mediated by the inhibition of leukotriene B4 (LTB4). Low levels of LTB4 stimulate lymphangiogenesis, but high levels as are observed in established lymphedema are harmful to lymphatic repair mediated by inhibition of the VEGFR3 and Notch pathways.

In two pilot studies in human primary and secondary lymphedema, ketoprofen was found to improve lymphatic function.[16] One of these (that enrolled patients from 2011 to 2015) was a small double-blind, placebo-controlled study ($n = 34$); 16 patients received ketoprofen, and 18 patients received placebo treatment. There were no serious adverse effects. One ketoprofen-treated patient with a history of hemorrhoids had an episode of rectal bleeding, and a second patient in the same group had nonhemorrhagic dyspepsia.

The drug ubenimex inhibits LTB4 synthesis and has been investigated in a phase 2, double-blind, placebo-controlled study with a 6-month treatment period, in adults with primary and secondary lymphedema (ULTRA study, Eiger). Unfortunately, the study demonstrated no improvement of ubenimex over placebo in the primary endpoint of skin thickness and secondary endpoints of limb volume and bioimpedance.[17]

ANTI-T-CELL DRUGS

In mouse models of lymphedematous skin, there is evidence of upregulation of many T-cell-related networks, and depletion of CD4$^+$ T cells has been shown to improve lymphedema.[18] Regulatory T cells (Tregs) are a subpopulation of T cells that modulate the immune system, maintain tolerance to self-antigens, and prevent autoimmune disease. Tregs suppress activation, proliferation, and cytokine production of CD4$^+$ and CD8$^+$ T cells. In the mouse model, increasing the number of Treg cells reduced lymphedema development, and adoptively transferred Tregs reduced edema, inflammation, and fibrosis and increased lymphatic drainage in established lymphedema.

T-helper 2 (Th2) cell differentiation has also been shown to be important in the development of fibrosis and lymphatic dysfunction in the mouse model.[19] In this study, inhibition of Th2 differentiation using interleukin-4 (IL-4) or IL-13 blockade prevented initiation and progression of lymphedema by decreasing tissue fibrosis and significantly improving lymphatic function.

Furthermore, topical therapy in the mouse model with the anti-T-cell immunosuppressive drug, tacrolimus, prevented lymphedema development and improved established lymphedema.[20] There was reduced swelling, T-cell infiltration, and tissue fibrosis, but increased formation of lymphatic collaterals. There was minimal systemic absorption of the drug.

These studies raise the possibility of the use of drugs like tacrolimus in the treatment of secondary lymphedema, but they may also have a place in the management of primary lymphedema. Studies in humans are awaited.

LYMPHATIC MALFORMATIONS AND ROLE OF MTOR INHIBITORS

Sporadic lymphatic malformations and those associated with overgrowth syndromes, such as CLOVES (congenital, lipomatous, overgrowth, vascular malformations, epidermal nevi, and spinal/skeletal anomalies and/or scoliosis) syndrome, may result from somatic activating mutations in the PI3 K/AKT/mTOR pathway.[2] mTOR inhibitors, such as sirolimus, may be an effective treatment for patients with extensive lymphatic malformations,[21] but at present, randomized controlled trials are lacking, and there is no information on the dosage, duration, and possible long-term side-effects of this treatment. Sirolimus is an immunosuppressive drug and can lead to sepsis.

Furthermore, sirolimus has been reported to cause lymphedema in some patients[22] and therefore is unlikely to be of value in the management of primary lymphedema except in those cases, which may be associated with lymphatic malformations due to somatic activating mutations in the PI3K/AKT/mTOR pathway.

ANTIBIOTICS

Patients with all types of lymphedema including primary lymphedema are vulnerable to recurrent episodes of bacterial cellulitis, probably mainly caused by β-hemolytic streptococci. Acute infections can be serious and lead to sepsis. Recurrent episodes of cellulitis may lead to worsening lymphedema and an increased risk of further infections.

Intravenous or oral treatment with antibiotics such as flucloxacillin is recommended for acute cellulitis.[23] Recurrent episodes of cellulitis can be reduced by the use of prophylactic antibiotics such as oral phenoxymethylpenicillin in conjunction with improved management of the lymphedema and treatment of skin conditions. A recent Cochrane review reported a moderate level of evidence to support the use of antibiotic prophylaxis in recurrent cellulitis of the leg.[24]

DIURETICS

It has long been recognized that diuretics do not have a significant role to play in the management of edema, which is primarily of lymphatic origin.[25] They reduce capillary filtration and therefore may have a transient effect when used initially but have no impact on lymphatic drainage. Furthermore, their long-term use can cause problems such as hyponatremia and impaired renal function.

In cases of chronic edema of mixed cause such as those, which may include an element of heart failure, diuretics may have a role to play. In primary lymphedema, however, they are only likely to be of value in rarer syndromes where primary lymphedema may be associated with cardiac abnormalities.

ANALGESICS

Although the feelings of heaviness and swelling are commonly associated with lymphedema, severe pain is not usually due to the edema itself but may be associated with other comorbidities, e.g., those that cause back pain and may result in nerve root compression. Pain from the swelling itself, particularly in those where there is a component of venous hypertension, is often relieved by the use of compression garments.

Pain can be a feature of cellulitis and in this situation analgesia is appropriate. The British Lymphology Society guidelines recommend the use of simple analgesics such as paracetamol/acetaminophen.[23]

There has been some suggestion in the past that the use of nonsteroidal anti-inflammatory drugs (NSAIDs) may be a risk factor for the development of the more severe infection of necrotizing fasciitis.[26] There is even evidence that in varicella infections in children, the use of NSAIDs may predispose to cellulitis. However, a more recent study of ibuprofen in cellulitis did not show an increased incidence of necrotizing fasciitis associated with its use.[27]

ANTIFUNGALS

Skin conditions, which reduce the natural barrier function of the skin, predispose to the development of cellulitis in people with lymphedema. Therefore, treating these with topical preparations, e.g., topical steroid ointments for eczema, may help to reduce the risk of cellulitis.

One of the more common conditions encountered in all types of lymphedema is the fungal infection tinea pedis (athlete's foot). A Cochrane review has shown that terbinafine cream is an effective treatment.[28] The usual recommended dose is twice-daily application to the web spaces for 2 weeks.

For fungal nail infections, oral preparations are more effective than topical preparations. A recent Cochrane review has reported that oral terbinafine is the preferred treatment.[29]

CONCLUSIONS

Although there have been some important developments in understanding the genetics of primary lymphedema and the pathophysiology of lymphedema in general in recent years, which may lead to potential drug treatments in the future, there is still no established drug treatment for primary lymphedema at present. Perhaps the most important drugs that can be used in managing primary lymphedema, for which there is a good evidence base, are prophylactic antibiotics to reduce the risk of recurrent cellulitis in those at high risk.

REFERENCES

1. Connell FC, Gordon K, Brice G et al. The classification and diagnostic algorithm for primary lymphatic dysplasia: An update from 2010 to include molecular findings. *Clin Genet*. 2013;84(4):303–314.
2. Brouillard P, Boon L, Vikkula M. Genetics of lymphatic anomalies. *J Clin Invest*. 2014;124(3):898–904.

3. Karkkainen M, Saaristo A, Jussila L et al. A model for gene therapy of human hereditary lymphedema. *PNAS*. 2001;98(22):12677–12682.

4. AdeLE study protocol. Available at www.clinicaltrials.gov; Trial no. NCT03658967 accessed 13.4.19.

5. Casley-Smith JR, Morgan RG, Piller NB. Treatment of Lymphoedema of the arms and legs with 5–6 Benzo-α-pyrone. *N Engl J Med*. 1993;329:1158–1163.

6. Badger C, Preston N, Seers K et al. Benzopyrones for reducing and controlling lymphedema of the limbs. *Cochrane Database Syst Rev*. 2004;(2):CD003140.

7. Farinola N, Piller NB. CYP2A6 Polymorphisms: Is there a role for pharmacogenomics in preventing coumarin-induced hepatotoxicity in lymphoedema patients? *Pharmacogenomics*. 2007;8(2):151–158.

8. Hu M, Piller NB. Strategies for avoiding benzopyrone hepatotoxicity in lymphoedema management: The role of pharmacogenetics, metabolic enzyme gene identification and patient selection. *Lymphatic Res Biol*. 2017;15(4):317–323.

9. Hnatek L. Therapeutic potential of micronized purified flavonoid fraction (MPFF) of diosmin and hesperidin in the treatment of chronic venous disorders. *Vnitr Lek*. 2015;61(9):807–814.

10. Kimura E, Itoh M. Filariasis in Japan some 25 years after its eradication. *Trop Med Health*. 2011;39(1 Suppl 2):57–63. Case quoted from Masuzawa M, Hara H et al. Severe lymphorrhea and lymphedema caused by filariasis: The efficacy of oral treatment with cilostazol. *Jpn J Dermatol*. 2001;111:179–183.

11. Kimura T, Hamazaki TS, Sugaya M et al. Cilostazol improves lymphatic function by inducing proliferation and stabilization of lymphatic endothelial cells. *J Dermatol Sci*. 2014;74:150–158.

12. Choi I, Lee S, Chung HK et al. 9-cis retinoic acid promotes lymphangiogenesis and enhances lymphatic vessel regeneration: Therapeutic implications of 9-cis retinoic acid for secondary lymphedema [published correction appears in *Circulation*. 2015;131(14):e401–e402]. *Circulation*. 2012;125(7):872–882.

13. Bramos A, Perrault D, Yang S et al. Prevention of postsurgical lymphedema by 9-cis retinoic acid. *Ann Surg*. 2016;264:353–361.

14. Cooke JP. Lymphangiogenesis: A potential new therapy for lymphedema? *Circulation*. 2012;125(7):853–855.

15. Tian W, Rockson S, Jiang X et al. Leukotriene B4 antagonism ameliorates experimental lymphedema. *Sci Transl Med*. 2017;9:eaal3920.

16. Rockson S, Tian W, Jiang X et al. Pilot studies demonstrate the potential benefits of antiinflammatory therapy inhuman lymphedema. *JCI Insight*. 2018; 3(20):e123775.

17. ULTRA study, Eiger Pharmaceuticals. http://www.eigerbio.com/eiger-biopharmaceuticals-announces-phase-2-ultra-results-of-ubenimex-in-lower-leg-lymphedema-study-did-not-meet-primary-or-secondary-endpoint.

18. Gousopoulos E, Proulx ST, Bachmann SB et al. Regulatory T cell transfer ameliorates lymphedema and promotes lymphatic vessel function. *JCI Insight*. 2016;1(16):e89081.

19. Avraham T, Zampell J, Yan A et al. Th2 differentiation is necessary for soft tissue fibrosis and lymphatic dysfunction resulting from lymphedema. *FASEB J*. 2013;27(3):1114–1126.

20. Gardenier J, Kataru R, Hespe G et al. Topical tacrolimus for the treatment of secondary lymphedema. *Nat Commun*. 2017;8:14345.

21. Wiegand S, Wichmann G, Dietz A. Treatment of lymphatic malformations with the mTOR inhibitor sirolimus: A systematic review. *Lymphat Res Biol*. 2018;16(4):330–339.

22. Desai N, Heenan S, Mortimer P. Sirolimus-associated lymphoedema: Eight new cases and a proposed mechanism. *Br J Dermatol*. 2009;160(6):1322–1326.

23. British Lymphology Society, 2017. Consensus guidelines on the management of cellulitis in lymphedema. Available at https://www.thebls.com.

24. Dalal A, Eskin-Schwartz M, Mimouni D et al. Interventions for the prevention of recurrent erysipelas and cellulitis Cochrane Systematic Review—Intervention Version published: 20 June 2017 Cochrane Database of Systematic Reviews. https://doi.org/10.1002/14651858.CD009758.pub2.

25. Mortimer PS. Therapy approaches for lymphedema. *Angiology*. 1997;48:87–91.

26. Voss L. Necrotising fasciitis associated with non-steroidal anti-inflammatory drugs. Prescriber Update 20: 4–7 November 2000. Medsafe. New Zealand Medicines and Medical Devices Safety Authority.

27. Davis JS, Mackrow C, Binks P et al. A double-blind randomized controlled trial of ibuprofen compared to placebo for uncomplicated cellulitis of the upper or lower limb. *Clin Microbiol Infect*. 2017;23(4):242–246.

28. Crawford F, Hollis S. Topical treatments for fungal infections of the skin and nails of the foot. *Cochrane Database Syst Rev*. 2007;(3):CD001434.

29. Kreijkamp-Kaspers S, Hawke K, Guo L et al. Oral antifungal medication for toenail onychomycosis. *Cochrane Database Syst Rev*. 2017;(7):CD010031.

63

What is difference in management of primary lymphedema between adults and children, and how much?

CRISTOBAL M. PAPENDIECK AND MIGUEL A. AMORE

Lymphedema in pediatrics deserves special consideration due to its etiopathogenesis, which is completely different from lymphedema in adults. In pediatrics, 80% of lymphedema cases are primary. Based on data from genetic studies, lymphedema is considered to be a part of 144 different syndromes—life-conditioning syndromes, or syndromes for the whole life. For this reason, only part of primary lymphedema is expressed in adults. Terminology used to diagnose this disorder as congenital lymphedema (early and late) is semantic and not etiopathogenesis based[1] (Figures 63.1 through 63.3).

The underlying pathogenesis of primary lymphedema may be due to aberrations of the lymphatic system caused by congenital lymphatic malformations. They may present as interstitial lymphatic endothelial dysfunction, lymphangiodysplasias (avalvulation, disvalvulation, lymphangioneurosis, lymphangiomatosis, lymphangioleiomyomatosis, etc.), and/or lymphadeno-dysplasias (nodal lymphangiomatosis, nodal angiomatosis, nodal venous malformation, capsular fibrosis, hypoplasia or nodal hyperplasia). Nevertheless, since the agenesis of the lymphatic system is incompatible with life, the aplasia/agenesis cannot exist in reality. However, the question remains that if lymphedema has the same characteristics in all the syndromes or different, as other malformations can have different hemodynamic, morphological, and pathophysiological characteristics[1-4] (Figure 63.4).

The functionality of the lymphatic system must be established in primary lymphedema, as what previously did not exist cannot be rehabilitated. Functionality may be established by triggering structural changes to the lymphatic system on the cellular level by using VEGF, for example. This concept is valid as long as it is not out of control. The use of VEGF in lymphatic malformations generates more malformation and therefore augments the dysfunction.[1,3,4]

Vascular/lymphatic rehabilitation (e.g., manual lymphatic drainage [MLD]-based complex decongestive therapy [CDT]) in primary lymphedema is similar to all other lymphatic rehabilitation, like the Vodder method with its variables (e.g., Leduc, Foldi, and others). This treatment modality requires continuous use and is associated with insufficient efficacy.[1,3]

Microsurgery can be performed in the pediatrics patient population. But the main concern is based on a fact that a vessel of these sizes can provide variable degrees of the transport capacity of that system. It would be necessary to do many anastomoses and also to consider performing it on malformed vessels if it is technically feasible, or with a deficient muscle (leiomyomatosis). The lymph node–vein anastomosis can be done, but the drawback is to achieve a lymphovenous pressure gradient that remains persistent in time at the level of the anastomosis. The vascularized lymph node transfer is also technically possible and also useful, but it is risky or insufficient if the lymphatic pathology is a systemic condition.[1,5-7]

Interstitial hypertension, as it happens in lymphedema, can also cause adipose overgrowth with chronic inflammation that leads to fibrosis. For this reason, the drugs suggested and used (although without a consensus) are curcumin/boswellia serratia as an anti-inflammatory and anti-edematous agents, diosmin for edema treatment (lymphovenous), and rapamycin as an antiangiogenic. Ultimately, however, hyperadipogenesis can be reduced or limited if the interstitial hypertension is reduced or limited. Aims for the rehabilitation by manual maneuver MLD-based CDT and/or surgery are to create new pathways for drainage[1,3,4] (Figure 63.5).

Although the oncological risk of primary lymphedema remains unknown, cases of progression to oncological disorders have been reported in adults. Therefore, this argument should be used to indicate an early efficient treatment of lymphedema whenever feasible.

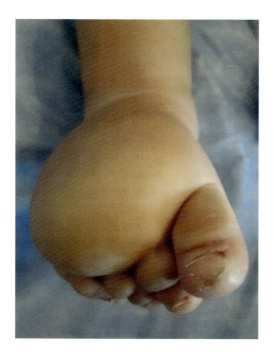

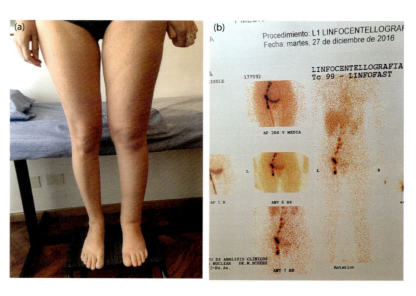

Figure 63.3 **(a)** Adult primary lymphedema. **(b)** Lymphoscintigraphy.

Figure 63.1 Right foot in an infant with primary lymphedema.

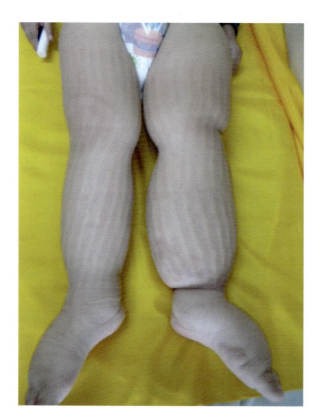

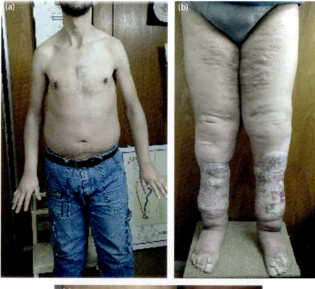

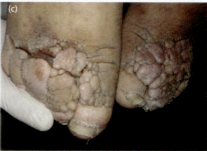

Figure 63.2 Lower extremities. Asymmetric bilateral primary lymphedema.

Figure 63.4 Primary lymphedema. **(a)** Upper extremities lymphedema, **(b)** lower extremities lymphedema, **(c)** feet papillomatosis.

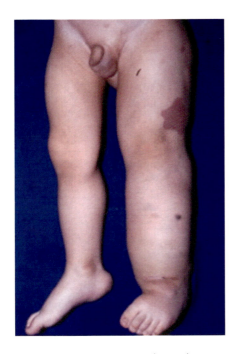

Figure 63.5 Lipomatous overgrowth syndrome, with vascular malformation. Primary lymphedema.

In conclusion, all lymphedema, whether primary or secondary, requires the attempt of early treatment, even if it is insufficient to deliver satisfactory results, because it can make the patient at an older age eligible for other therapeutic alternatives, if necessary, which are also associated with variable degrees of efficacy.

REFERENCES

1. Papendieck CM, Amore MA. An atlas of neonatal and infantile lymphedema. In: Lee BB, Rockson S, Bergan J, eds. *Lymphedema A Concise Compendium of Theory and Practice*. New York, NY: Springer; 2018: 777–798.
2. Lee BB, Andrade M, Antignani P et al. Diagnosis and treatment of primary lymphedema consensus document of up 2013. *Int Angiol*. 2013;32(6):541–574.
3. Papendieck CM, Amore MA. Treatment strategy on neonatal and infant CVMs. In: Young Wook K, Byung Boong L, Wayne Y, Young SD, eds. *Congenital Vascular Malformations*. New York, NY: Springer; 2017: 349–367.
4. Hennekam RC. Syndromic lymphatic maldevelopment. *4 International Conference National Lymphedema Network*, Florida, 2000. Abstract 11–12.
5. The Diagnosis and Treatment of Peripheral Lymphedema: 2016. Consensus document of the International Society of Lymphology. *Lymphology*. 2016;49(4):170–184.
6. Becker C. Vascularized lymph node transfer. In: Neligan P, Masia J, Piller N, eds. *Lymphedema, Complete Medical and Surgical Management*. Boca Raton, FL: CRC Press; 2016:487–493.
7. Papendieck CM, Barbosa ML, Amore MA et al. A new combined operative technique using crossed inguinal lymphatic rescue for pediatric patients with mixed lymphatic and venous malformations. *Lymphology*. 2017;50:141–147.

64

How to manage lipedema involved with primary lymphedema?

GYŐZŐ SZOLNOKY

The combination of lipedema and primary lymphedema is a rare condition. However, comprehensive management should be tailored to affect each component, including noninvasive and invasive therapeutical approaches.

WEIGHT CONTROL

Weight loss or at least weight control in patients with high body mass index (BMI) represents a cornerstone in the conservative management of both lipedema and primary lymphedema, as high BMI is a known aggravating factor of lipedema[1,2] and also worsens lymphedema.[3]

Long-term stability of body weight in the majority of lipedema patients is not confirmed by a recently published single-center experience.[4] In the long run, many patients with this diagnosis exhibit a constant weight gain. Weight gain in lipedema patients mostly loads and feeds typical lipedematous adipose tissue predilection sites, such as the buttocks, thighs, and upper arms. In this view, the progression of lipedema could be more likely explained with BMI increase than with the natural course of the disease.[4-6]

According to the general myth supported by literature data based on only anecdotal evidence, lipedema usually fails to adequately respond to dietary approaches with calorie restriction[1,2]; thus, gluteofemoral and arm adipose tissues are found to lag behind fat tissues localized elsewhere in terms of diet-induced reduction. There is no clear explanation to this phenomenon owing to the insufficient knowledge on lipedema pathophysiology; however, low metabolic activity of gluteofemoral adipose tissue proven in women without lipedema might be a key physiological factor.[7,8] Furthermore, gluteofemoral subcutaneous adipose tissue imparts protection against diet-induced metabolic derangement. This type of adiposity usually reacts by hyperplasia formation when exposed to calorie excess. Nevertheless, these concepts remain a subject of debate in lipedema; hence, there is no available clinical trial data regarding the assessment of the response of lipedematous adipose tissue to any kind of diet. These studies are needed to further elucidate the previously mentioned correlation between calorie intake and lipedema.

Bariatric surgery may be beneficial for obese patients who have coexisting lymphedema[9] with high BMI, whose weight loss attempts do not succeed in a prolonged period, or morbidly obese patients with or without obesity-related comorbidities; however, the most effective form of this kind of surgery has remained unspecified. This surgical intervention is occasionally applied in lipedema and most results of anecdotal observations are recorded; however, a single clinical trial consisting of two case reports showed its efficacy.[10]

The real potency of bariatric surgery cannot be evaluated in the absence of multicentric clinical studies with a larger number of patients and long-term follow-ups.

Future directions that stem from obesity studies should be constructed toward the evaluation of the role of dietary approaches and bariatric surgery in lipedema.

INTENSIVE DECONGESTION

Decongestive lymphatic therapy incorporating manual lymphatic drainage and compression bandaging could generate significant ($p < 0.05$) but moderate volume reduction (<10%)[11] and is also efficient in pain reduction[12] and contributes to less frequent bruising.[13] This kind of physiotherapy is an integrated part of the conservative approach to primary lymphedema, so both diseases could get certain benefit from this noninterventional therapy. Intermittent pneumatic therapy has no adjunctive role in lipedema care in terms of volume reduction,[11] and its use is rather supported in primary lymphedema; however, medical personnel must be cautious because genital lymphedema might be one of the side effects of pneumatic pumps.[14]

LIPOSUCTION

Liposuction is reported to be currently the best treatment for lipedema[15,16]; however, endurance of the results (volume reduction, decrease of subjective complaints and capillary fragility) and the necessity of supplementary, continuous decongestive physiotherapy have now been critically reviewed.[17]

Nevertheless, patients with lipedema show consistent results regarding significant reductions in spontaneous pain, sensitivity to pressure, feeling of tension, and bruising in the postoperative follow-up.[16] The same holds true for patient self-assessment of cosmetic appearance, quality of life, and overall impairment.[16]

Liposuction in primary lymphedema has also gained a noteworthy adjunctive role in decongestion and the evacuation of excess adipose tissue.[18,19]

MAINTENANCE WITH COMPRESSION GARMENTS

In maintenance therapy, compression garments stabilize volume reduction yielded through intensive decongestion and/or liposuction. The best-fitting material to both primary lymphedema and lipedema is the flat knit one, as the limb shape irregularity could be under appropriate control of these disease-modifying garments.[20] Since both disorders usually affect the whole limb, panty-hoses should be recommended for leg involvement. The old dogma as patients with lipedema tolerate only stockings with relatively low compression pressure has been rejected, so compression garments with high pressures can also be applied.[21]

REFERENCES

1. Szél E, Kemény L, Groma G, Szolnoky G. Pathophysiological dilemmas of lipedema. *Med Hypotheses*. 2014;83:599–606.
2. Torre YS, Wadeea R, Rosas V, Herbst KL. Lipedema: friend and foe. *Horm Mol Biol Clin Investig*. 2018;33(1): 20170076.
3. Shaw C, Mortimer P, Judd PA. A randomized controlled trial of weight reduction as a treatment for breast cancer-related lymphedema. *Cancer*. 2007;110(8):1868–1874.
4. Bertsch T, Erbacher G. Lipödem—mythen und fakten teil 1. *Phlebologie*. 2018;47:84–92.
5. Bertsch T, Erbacher G. Lipödem—mythen und fakten teil 2. *Phlebologie*. 2018;47(04):120–126.
6. Bertsch T, Erbacher G. Lipödem—mythen und fakten teil 3. *Phlebologie*. 2018;47(04):188–198.
7. Hill JH, Solt C, Foster MT. Obesity associated disease risk: The role of inherent differences and location of adipose depots. *Horm Mol Biol Clin Investig*. 2018;33(2). doi: 10.1515/hmbci-2018-0012.
8. Krotkiewski M, Billing-Marczak K. Different types of obesity. Can some types of obesity be protective? *Pol Merkur Lekarski*. 2014;37(219):175–180.
9. Fife C, Carter M. Lymphoedema in bariatric patients. *J Lymphoedema*. 2009;2:29–37.
10. Pouwels S, Huisman S, Smelt HJM, Said M, Smulders JF. Lipoedema in patients after bariatric surgery: Report of two cases and review of literature. *Clin Obes*. 2018;8(2):147–150.
11. Szolnoky G, Borsos B, Barsony K, Balogh M, Kemeny L. Complete decongestive physiotherapy of lipedema with or without pneumatic compression: A pilot study. *Lymphology*. 2008;41:50–52.
12. Szolnoky G, Nagy N, Kovacs RK et al. Complex decongestive physiotherapy decreases capillary fragility in lipedema. *Lymphology*. 2008;41:54–56.
13. Szolnoky G, Varga E, Varga M, Tuczai M, Dósa-Rácz É, Kemény L. Complex decongestive physiotherapy decreases pain intensity in lipedema. *Lymphology*. 2011;44:178–182.
14. Boris M, Weindorf S, Lasinski BB. The risk of genital edema after external pump compression for lower limb lymphedema. *Lymphology*. 1998;31:15–20.
15. Wollina U, Heinig B. Treatment of lipedema by low-volume micro-cannular liposuction in tumescent anesthesia: Results in 111 patients. *Dermatol Ther*. 2019;32(2):e12820.
16. Baumgartner A, Hueppe M, Schmeller W. Long-term benefit of liposuction in patients with lipoedema: A follow-up study after an average of 4 and 8 years. *Br J Dermatol*. 2016;174(5):1061–1067.
17. Bertsch T, Erbacher G, Torio-Padron N. Lipödem—mythen und fakten teil 4. *Phlebologie*. 2019;48(1): 47–56.
18. Stewart CJ, Munnoch DA. Liposuction as an effective treatment for lower extremity lymphoedema: A single surgeon's experience over nine years. *J Plast Reconstr Aesthet Surg*. 2018;71(2):239–245.
19. Lamprou DA, Voesten HG, Damstra RJ, Wikkeling OR. Circumferential suction-assisted lipectomy in the treatment of primary and secondary end-stage lymphoedema of the leg. *Br J Surg*. 2017;104(1):84–89.
20. Wagner S. Lymphedema and lipedema-an overview of conservative treatment. *VASA*. 2011;40(4):271–279.
21. Flour M, Clark M, Partsch H et al. Dogmas and controversies in compression therapy. Report of an International Compression Club (ICC) meeting, May 2011, Brussels. *Int Wound J*. 2012;10(5):516–526.

65

How to assess response/efficacy of manual lymphatic drainage and compression therapy

GYŐZŐ SZOLNOKY

VOLUMETRY

The most common approach to assessing the efficacy of decongestive therapy is limb volumetry or in case of unilateral swelling edema, volume measurement (volume of affected minus volume of unaffected limb).[1]

Water displacement volumetry as a direct method is generally considered to be the gold standard[2,3] for the objective assessment of treatment efficacy.

Indirect methods of lower limb volume assessment consist of leg circumference measurement with a tape[2,3] or "Leg-O-Meter."[2] These are reliable and standardized instruments that allow for simple and rapid measurements to be obtained. Leg circumference measurements can also be implemented to estimate leg volume by either frustrum or disc modeling.[2,3] Based on the most recent data, calculated volume based on arm circumferences seems to be the most reliable form of measurements with the least limitations, lowest cost, and technical simplicity.[3]

For direct measurement, optoelectronic devices offer fast measurement acquisitions and easily reproducible results; however, outcome variation needs to be minimized with accurate limb positioning. A perometer could accomplish measurements in vertical or horizontal positions.[4] An Image-3D digital imaging system can be used to produce a three-dimensional image of the leg after the patient stands on a platform with 360° turns, in a relatively rapid way.[5] Their limitation resides in their high cost.

Computed tomography (CT),[6] magnetic resonance imaging (MRI),[7] and dual x-ray absorptiometry (DXA)[8] give reliable results; however, limb volume calculation is time consuming and demands experienced personnel. These methods and perometry are capable of measuring different segments of the limbs with or without the foot or hand volumes.

TISSUE COMPOSITION

Tissue composition can be determined with bioimpedance, ultrasound imaging, while DXA, CT, and MRI are also applicable for this particular purpose due to their multimodality. One of the earliest signs of lymphatic failure is subtle fluid accumulation in the affected limb. Subclinical lymphedema without relevant change in limb size may lead to false-negative diagnosis. Bioimpedance is useful for fluid content measurement and gives early proof of an increased amount of extracellular fluid.[9] There are also radiofrequency-based devices that are capable of identifying segmental fluid accumulation based on tissue dielectric constants.[10] As late stages of lymphedema are associated with fibrosis and the enlargement of subcutaneous adipose tissue, DXA is of practical importance for fat and lean mass calculation. CT and MRI could also give reliable quantification of the amount of adipose tissue.

JOINT MOVEMENT

Range of motion (ROM) is a measurement of the distance and direction a joint can move to its full potential. In lymphedema, ROM is often found to be restricted and therefore serves as a good indicator of therapeutic efficacy.[11]

TISSUE CONSISTENCY AND FIBROTIC INDURATION

Pitting is a sign that results from the displacement of subcutaneous fluid by external pressure.[12] Once pressure is released, fluid reequilibrates and flows back. Based on the expertise of experienced therapists, it is recommended to perform the test with longer duration, higher pressure, and a larger contact area.

The sign of the thickened cutaneous fold (Stemmer sign) of the second toe is typical for the early and differential diagnosis of a primary ascending lymphedema without false-positive findings. It reflects the thicker epidermis. This sign was first described by Mór Kaposi and nearly 100 years later by Robert Stemmer.[13]

Tonometry is a simple method that measures the resistance of the tissues to compression and is a potential indicator of underlying fibrosis. A similar measurement can be performed with an indurometer, and cross-validation has also been undertaken; however, they are not entirely interchangeable in terms of function.[14] Variations in fibrotic tissues can be further analyzed by ultrasound, CT, or MRI.

MEASUREMENT OF SUBJECTIVE PERCEPTION: GENERAL AND DISEASE-SPECIFIC QUALITY OF LIFE

In the management of lymphedema, especially when swelling is the consequence of cancer treatment, the improvement of QOL is nearly always at least as important as the effective decongestion and the clearance of fibrosis, since lymphedema is a lifelong stigma causing frustration and a psychologically debilitating condition.

The assessment of subjective parameters consists of general and lymphedema-related assessment of variables. The most commonly used general QOL tests include Psychology General Well-being Scale[15]; Nottingham Health Profile[16]; Disability of Arm, Shoulder and Hand DEMMI-joint mobility index[17]; Lower Extremity Functional Scale (LEFS)[18]; Visual Analogue Scale (VAS)[15]; SF-12[19]; or 36 scales.[20] Disease-specific devices are also available to precisely detect and follow the changes of QOL (e.g., FLQA-LS,[21] Lymphedema Quality of Life Measurement [LYMQOL],[18] International Classification of Functioning, Disability and Health Core Sets [ICF]).[22]

MEASUREMENT OF STRUCTURAL CHANGES OF LYMPHATIC SYSTEM

Ultrasound is useful to determine morphological changes (e.g., the thicknesses of skin layers, fascias, the presence of "lymphatic lakes" in the epifascial compartment or subcutaneously, the location and extension of fibrotic alterations).[23] It is also capable of visualizing and identifying deep lymphatic collectors. Lymph node visualization, size measurement, and structural analysis are also part of the lymphatic network assessment.

As another ultrasound-related modality, the sonoelastography[24] provides an excellent opportunity to estimate soft tissue stiffness and to follow its change along lymphedema therapy. Its role is supposed to be essential in the preliminary phase, where other techniques fail to detect lymphatic impairment.

Single photon emission computed tomography (SPECT)/CT, CT, MRI may offer higher accuracy, but cost and availability preclude their application except for scientific purposes.[25]

MEASUREMENT OF FUNCTIONAL CHANGES OF LYMPHATIC SYSTEM

Lymphoscintigraphy is considered to be the most powerful diagnostic tool to describe superficial and deep lymphatic function.[26,27] Qualitative assessment comprises the visualization of functioning collaterals, connections between superficial and deep lymphatic networks, the area of dermal backflow, and the location of lymph flow blockade. In terms of quantitative aspects, the location, distribution, and density of the radiotracer, the time of arrival, and the rate of uptake of lymphatic nodes provide functional information. Lymphoscintigraphy could be combined with other imaging techniques to improve accuracy.

Magnetic resonance lymphography is an upgrade of conventional MRI with lymphangiogram.[28] Its main advantage over classic lymphangiography is better display of anatomical structures.

Near-infrared fluorescent lymphography is a nonradioactive method using indocyanine green contrast medium and is popularly applied to detect superficial lymphatic morphology and function.[29]

REFERENCES

1. Stout N, Partsch H, Szolnoky G et al. Chronic oedema of the lower extremities; International consensus recommendations for compression therapy clinical research trials. *Int Angiol*. 2012;31:316–329.
2. Rabe E, Carpentier P, Maggioli A. Understanding lower leg volume measurements used in clinical studies focused on venous leg edema. *Int Angiol*. 2018;37(6):437–443.
3. De Vrieze T, Gebruers N, Tjalma WA et al. What is the best method to determine excessive arm volume in patients with breast cancer-related lymphoedema in clinical practice? Reliability, time efficiency and clinical feasibility of five different methods. *Clin Rehabil*. 2019;33(7):1221–1232.
4. Szolnoky G, Nemes-Szabó D, Molnár G, Varga E, Varga M, Kemény L. Comparison of Mediven ulcer kit and Mediven Plus compression stockings: Measurement of volume, interface pressure and static stiffness index changes. *Veins Lymphat*. 2013;2:e13.
5. Rapprich S, Dingler A, Podda M. Liposuction is an effective treatment for lipedema-results of a study with 25 patients. *J Dtsch Dermatol Ges*. 2011;9(1):33–40.
6. Yoo JS, Chung SH, Lim MC et al. Computed tomography-based quantitative assessment of lower extremity lymphedema following treatment for gynecologic cancer. *J Gynecol Oncol*. 2017;28(2):e18.
7. Gardner GC, Nickerson JP, Watts R, Nelson L, Dittus KL, O'Brien PJ. Quantitative and morphologic change associated with breast cancer-related lymphedema. Comparison of 3.\0T MRI to external measures. *Lymphat Res Biol*. 2014;12(2):95–102.

8. Gjorup CA, Hendel HW, Zerahn B et al. Volume and tissue composition changes measured with dual-energy x-ray absorptiometry in melanoma-related limb lymphedema. *Lymphat Res Biol.* 2017;15(3):274–283.

9. van Zanten M, Piller N, Ward LC. Inter-changeability of impedance devices for lymphedema assessment. *Lymphat Res Biol.* 2016;14(2):88–94.

10. Mayrovitz HN. Assessing lower extremity lymphedema using upper and lower extremity tissue dielectric constant ratios: Method and normal reference values. *Lymphat Res Biol.* 2019;17(4):457–464.

11. Gianesini S, Tessari M, Bacciglieri P et al. A specifically designed aquatic exercise protocol to reduce chronic lower limb edema. *Phlebology.* 2017;32(9):594–600.

12. Sanderson J, Tuttle N, Box R, Reul-Hirche HM, Laakso EL. The pitting test: An investigation of an unstandardized assessment of lymphedema. *Lymphology.* 2015;48(4):175–183.

13. Stemmer R. Stemmer's sign—Possibilities and limits of clinical diagnosis of lymphedema. *Wien Med Wochenschr.* 1999;149(2–4):85–86.

14. Vanderstelt S, Pallotta OJ, McEwen M, Ullah S, Burrow L, Piller N. Indurometer vs. tonometer: Is the indurometer currently able to replace and improve upon the tonometer? *Lymphat Res Biol.* 2015; 13(2):131–136.

15. Herberger K, Blome C, Heyer K, Ellis F, Münter KC, Augustin M. Quality of life in patients with primary and secondary lymphedema in the community. *Wound Repair Regen.* 2017;25(3):466–473.

16. Sitzia J, Sobrido L. Measurement of health-related quality of life of patients receiving conservative treatment for limb lymphoedema using the Nottingham Health Profile. *Qual Life Res.* 1997;6(5):373–384.

17. Jans MP, Slootweg VC, Boot CR, de Morton NA, van der Sluis G, van Meeteren NL. Reproducibility and validity of the Dutch translation of the de Morton Mobility Index (DEMMI) used by physiotherapists in older patients with knee or hip osteoarthritis. *Arch Phys Med Rehabil.* 2011;92(11):1892–1899.

18. Lee TS, Morris CM, Czerniec SA, Mangion AJ. Does lymphedema severity affect quality of life? Simple question. Challenging answers. *Lymphat Res Biol.* 2018;16(1):85–91.

19. Brown JC, Lin LL, Segal S et al. Physical activity, daily walking, and lower limb lymphedema associate with physical function among uterine cancer survivors. *Support Care Cancer.* 2014;22(11):3017–3025.

20. Hoffner M, Bagheri S, Hansson E, Manjer J, Troëng T, Brorson H. SF-36 shows increased quality of life following complete reduction of postmastectomy lymphedema with liposuction. *Lymphat Res Biol.* 2017;15(1):87–98.

21. Augustin M, Conde Montero E, Hagenström K, Herberger K, Blome C. Validation of a short-form of the Freiburg Life Quality Assessment for lymphoedema (FLQA-LS) instrument. *Br J Dermatol.* 2018;179(6):1329–1333.

22. Viehoff PB, Heerkens YF, Van Ravensberg CD et al. Development of consensus International Classification of Functioning, Disability and Health (ICF) core sets for lymphedema. *Lymphology.* 2015;48(1): 38–50.

23. Suehiro K, Morikage N, Murakami M, Yamashita O, Samura M, Hamano K. Significance of ultrasound examination of skin and subcutaneous tissue in secondary lower extremity lymphedema. *Ann Vasc Dis.* 2013;6(2):180–188.

24. Erdogan Iyigun Z, Agacayak F, Ilgun AS et al. The role of elastography in diagnosis and staging of breast cancer-related lymphedema. *Lymphat Res Biol.* 2019;17(3):334–339.

25. Baulieu F, Bourgeois P, Maruani A et al. Contributions of SPECT/CT imaging to the lymphoscintigraphic investigations of the lower limb lymphedema. *Lymphology.* 2013;46(3):106–119.

26. Keo HH, Gretener SB, Staub D. Clinical and diagnostic aspects of lymphedema. *VASA.* 2017;46(4):255–261.

27. Devoogdt N, Van den Wyngaert T, Bourgeois P et al. Reproducibility of lymphoscintigraphic evaluation of the upper limb. *Lymphat Res Biol.* 2014;12(3):175–184.

28. Olszewski WL, Liu NF. Magnetic resonance lymphography (MRL): Point and counter-point. *Lymphology.* 2013;46(4):202–207.

29. O'Donnell TF Jr, Rasmussen JC, Sevick-Muraca EM. New diagnostic modalities in the evaluation of lymphedema. *J Vasc Surg Venous Lymphat Disord.* 2017;5(2):261–273.

66

How to assess efficacy of lipedema management involved in lymphedema

GYŐZŐ SZOLNOKY

As lipedema is definitely not a true edema but the peculiar enlargement of adipose tissue, measurement of the changes of adipose tissue should be stressed; however, a variable degree of fluid accumulation is associated with lipedema.[1] The most recent findings show increased density of dilated capillaries and angiogenesis in the absence of improvement in lymphatic transport capacity and lymphangiogenesis allowing consecutively higher amounts of interstitial fluid, which may further stimulate adipogenesis, inflammation, and fibrosis, especially among obese lipedema patients.[2]

The rationale behind decongestive therapy is directed toward generating higher interstitial pressure and reducing excess interstitial fluid by improving the fluid transport capacity of lymphatics.[2] In this regard, volumetric measurements of the affected limb and its fluid content are preferred.

When adipose tissue reduction is targeted by dietary approach, exercise, bariatric surgery, and/or liposuction, the measurements of the amount of adipose tissue and tissue composition are of primary importance. Assessments of quality of life (QOL), pain, and bruising are useful tools, regardless of which of the previously mentioned treatment modalities are used.

VOLUMETRY

As reviewed in Chapter 65, for various methods of assessment of primary lymphedema, the most common approach to assess the efficacy of decongestive therapy for the lipedema involved with the lymphedema is also a limb volume measurement.[3]

The water displacement method is the gold standard for direct measurement of upper or lower limb volume,[4,5] and a simple and rapid indirect method of limb volume assessment comprises leg circumference measurements with a centimeter tape or "Leg-O-Meter."[4] Whole limb volume is calculated using either the frustrum or disc model on the basis of girth variables,[6] as mentioned in Chapter 65.

Popular optoelectronic devices offer fast measuring acquisition and easily reproducible results in an indirect way. The Perometer is an optoelectronic system that uses infrared wavelengths to measure the limb and calculates the volume electronically using a mathematical formula.[7,8] The Image-3D digital imaging system is also applicable to yield a three-dimensional image of the affected lower extremity.[8]

Other techniques such as computed tomography (CT),[9] magnetic resonance imaging (MRI),[10] and dual x-ray absorptiometry (DXA)[11] also give reliable results; however, limb volume calculation is slow and requires experienced personnel. Optoelectronic, CT, MRI, and DXA techniques are eligible to measure different segments of the limbs with or without the foot or hand volumes.

TISSUE COMPOSITION

Tissue composition is measurable with different techniques including bioimpedance,[11] ultrasound imaging, DXA, CT, and MRI, as described in Chapter 65. Radiofrequency-based devices are capable of identifying fat tissue enlargement based on tissue dielectric constants.[12] Sonographic findings are able to differentiate lymphedema and lipedema and measure the thickness and echogenicity of subcutaneous fat.[13] DXA is suitable for fat and lean mass calculation. Besides limb volume assessment, CT and MRI could give reliable quantification of the amount of adipose tissue.

PAIN

The pinch test is the easiest but nonquantitative method for pain detection. Lipedematous pain could be precisely described with a 30-item questionnaire containing adjectives that describe pain qualities.[14] For each item, patients are asked to grade pain qualities using a four-grade scale ("Fits exactly," "Fits fairly well," "Fits to a limited extent," or "Does not fit"), and the highest grades were assigned to the most severe complaints. In a comparative clinical trial, the 10 most fitting items as well as a special numerical analogue scale (from 0 to 10) called the Numeric Pain Rating Scale and Wong-Baker FACES scale were applied for pain assessment.[15] The classical visual analog scale (VAS) is also appropriately eligible for pain evaluation.[16]

BRUISING

Bruising is attributed to increased capillary fragility in lipedema.[17,18] Capillary fragility measurement corresponding to the count of viable petechiae subsequent to the use of vacuum suction chamber (Parrot angiosterrometer).[17] There is no comparative study between lipedema and lymphedema; however, noncomplicated obesity appeared to be distinguishable from noncomplicated lipedema since lipedema was associated with a significantly higher count of petechiae.

QUALITY OF LIFE MEASUREMENT

The outcomes of perceived changes between pre- and post-treatment conditions are also important in the assessment of lipedema-related therapeutic success. We recommend that QOL measurement receive more attention from the medical community than it currently has, since even subtle differences can be easily pointed out.

There are a limited number of surveys discussing lipedema; however, the Psychology General Well-being Scale, QOL (WHOQOL-BREF), satisfaction with life scale (SWLS), psychological flexibility (Acceptance and Action Questionnaire-II), social connectedness (Social Connectedness Scale-Revised),[19] appearance-related distress (Derriford Appearance Scale 24), Lower Extremity Functional Scale (LEFS),[20] multimodal EQ-5D-3L[21] comprising mobility, self-care, usual activities, pain/discomfort, and anxiety/depression assessment have been approved to fulfill the criteria of global assessment, while SF-12 and SF-36 scales could also fit the goals of QOL analysis. Disease-specific health-related QOL estimation implicates the use of the FLQA-L (Freiburg Life Quality Assessment in Lymphedema).[22]

REFERENCES

1. Szél E, Kemény L, Groma G, Szolnoky G. Pathophysiological dilemmas of lipedema. *Med Hypotheses.* 2014;83(5):599–606.
2. Al-Ghadban S, Cromer W, Allen M et al. Dilated blood and lymphatic microvessels, angiogenesis, increased macrophages, and adipocyte hypertrophy in lipedema thigh skin and fat tissue. *J Obes.* 2019;2019:8747461.
3. Stout N, Partsch H, Szolnoky G et al. Chronic edema of the lower extremities: International consensus recommendations for compression therapy clinical research trials. *Int Angiol.* 2012;31(4):316–329.
4. Rabe E, Carpentier P, Maggioli A. Understanding lower leg volume measurements used in clinical studies focused on venous leg edema. *Int Angiol.* 2018;37(6):437–443.
5. De Vrieze T, Gebruers N, Tjalma WA et al. What is the best method to determine excessive arm volume in patients with breast cancer-related lymphoedema in clinical practice? Reliability, time efficiency and clinical feasibility of five different methods. *Clin Rehabil.* 2019;33(7):1221–1232.
6. Adriaenssens N, Buyl R, Lievens P, Fontaine C, Lamote J. Comparative study between mobile infrared optoelectronic volumetry with a Perometer and two commonly used methods for the evaluation of arm volume in patients with breast cancer related lymphedema of the arm. *Lymphology.* 2013;46(3):132–143.
7. Szolnoky G, Nemes-Szabó D, Molnár G, Varga E, Varga M, Kemény L. Comparison of Mediven ulcer kit and Mediven Plus compression stockings: Measurement of volume, interface pressure and static stiffness index changes. *Veins Lymphat.* 2013;2:e13.
8. Rapprich S, Dingler A, Podda M. Liposuction is an effective treatment for lipedema-results of a study with 25 patients. *J Dtsch Dermatol Ges.* 2011;9(1):33–40.
9. Monnin-Delhom ED, Gallix BP, Achard C, Bruel JM, Janbon C. High resolution unenhanced computed tomography in patients with swollen legs. *Lymphology.* 2002;35(3):121–128.
10. Tiwari A, Cheng KS, Button M, Myint F, Hamilton G. Differential diagnosis, investigation, and current treatment of lower limb lymphedema. *Arch Surg.* 2003;138(2):152–161.
11. Ibarra M, Eekema A, Ussery C, Neuhardt D, Garby K, Herbst KL. Subcutaneous adipose tissue therapy reduces fat by dual x-ray absorptiometry scan and improves tissue structure by ultrasound in women with lipoedema and Dercum disease. *Clin Obes.* 2018;8(6):398–406.
12. Birkballe S, Jensen MR, Noerregaard S, Gottrup F, Karlsmark T. Can tissue dielectric constant measurement aid in differentiating lymphoedema from lipoedema in women with swollen legs? *Br J Dermatol.* 2014;170(1):96–102.
13. Iker E, Mayfield CK, Gould DJ, Patel KM. Characterizing lower extremity lymphedema and lipedema with cutaneous ultrasonography and an objective computer-assisted measurement of dermal echogenicity. *Lymphat Res Biol.* 2019. doi: 10.1089/lrb.2017.0090.
14. Schmeller W, Meier-Vollrath J. Schmerzen beim Lipödem. *LymphForsch.* 2008;12(1):8–12.
15. Szolnoky G, Varga E, Varga M, Tuczai M, Dósa-Rácz E, Kemény L. Lymphedema treatment decreases pain intensity in lipedema. *Lymphology.* 2011;44(4):178–182.

16. Dadras M, Mallinger PJ, Corterier CC, Theodosi-adi S, Ghods M. Liposuction in the treatment of lipedema: A longitudinal study. *Arch Plast Surg.* 2017;44(4):324–331.

17. Szolnoky G, Nagy N, Kovács RK et al. Complex decongestive physiotherapy decreases capillary fragility in lipedema. *Lymphology.* 2008;41(4):161–166.

18. Szolnoky G, Ifeoluwa A, Tuczai M et al. Measurement of capillary fragility: A useful tool to differentiate lipedema from obesity? *Lymphology.* 2017;50(4):203–209.

19. Dudek JE, Białaszek W, Ostaszewski P. Quality of life in women with lipoedema: A contextual behavioral approach. *Qual Life Res.* 2016;25(2):401–408.

20. Dudek JE, Białaszek W, Ostaszewski P, Smidt T. Depression and appearance-related distress in functioning with lipedema. *Psychol Health Med.* 2018;23(7):846–853.

21. Romeijn JRM, de Rooij MJM, Janssen L, Martens H. Exploration of patient characteristics and quality of life in patients with lipoedema using a survey. *Dermatol Ther (Heidelb).* 2018;8(2):303–311.

22. Blome C, Augustin M, Heyer K et al. Evaluation of patient-relevant outcomes of lymphedema and lipedema treatment: Development and validation of a new benefit tool. *Eur J Vasc Endovasc Surg.* 2014;47(1):100–107.

67

Pathophysiology behind adipose tissue deposition in lymphedema and how liposuction can completely reduce excess volume

HÅKAN BRORSON

EXCESS SUBCUTANEOUS ADIPOSITY AND CHRONIC LYMPHEDEMA

Liposuction is the only method to completely reduce a non-pitting chronic lymphedema where the excess volume is dominated by adipose tissue.[1-3] The incidence of postmastectomy arm lymphedema varies between 8% and 80%, depending in part on whether axillary lymph nodes have been removed and postoperative radiation has been given.[4,5] The sentinel node technique had decreased the incidence of postoperative lymphedema to an estimated incidence of approximately 6%–8%.[6]

The outcome of the surgical procedure as well as of the radiation of the tissue often results in destruction of lymphatic vessels. When this is combined with the removal of lymph nodes and tissue scarring, the lymphatic vessels that remain are likely to be unable to remove the load of lymph. The remaining lymph collectors become dilated and overloaded, and their valves become incompetent, preventing the lymphatics from performing their function. This failure spreads distally until even the most peripheral lymph vessels, draining into the affected system, also become dilated.[7]

In a parallel process, the cells of the mononuclear phagocytic system of the mesenchymal tissues begin to lose their capability to remove the protein that accumulates. The accumulated interstitial proteins, as osmotically active molecules, attract fluid to the area. This accumulation of protein and fluid is usually a transitory phase, lasting between 1 and 3 weeks.[7]

In the latent phase, there may still be no clinical signs initially of any discernable lymphedema. The latent phase normally varies from about 4 months to 10 years. At the end of the latent phase, pitting of the edematous arm on pressure can be observed. This can be objectively measured by plethysmography and by decreased tissue compressibility using a tissue tonometer.[7,8]

The enlargement of the arm leads to discomfort and complaints in the form of heaviness, weakness, pain, tension, and a sensory deficit of the limb, as well as anxiety, psychological morbidity, maladjustment and social isolation, and increasing hardness of the limb.[9,10] Adipose tissue deposition starts already within the first year after lymphedema onset.[11,12] In time, there is also an increase in the adipose tissue content of the swollen arm. The author has observed this clinically since 1987, when the first lymphedema patient was operated on.[13,14] This phenomenon led to further research as presented in this chapter.[11,12,15,16]

There are various possible explanations for the adipose tissue hypertrophy. There is a physiological imbalance of blood flow and lymphatic drainage, resulting in the impaired clearance of lipids and their uptake by macrophages.[17,18] There is increasing support, however, for the view that the fat cell is not simply a container of fat, but it behaves like an endocrine organ and a cytokine-activated cell,[19,20] and chronic inflammation plays a role here.[21,22] The same pathophysiology goes for primary and secondary leg lymphedema.

For more detailed information about investigational advances and the relationship between slow lymph flow and adiposity, as well as that between structural changes in the lymphatic system and adiposity, see data from studies published by Harvey et al.[23] and Schneider et al.[24]

Other research regarding adipose tissue deposition includes the following:

- The findings of increased adipose tissue in intestinal segments in patients with Crohn disease, known as "fat wrapping," have clearly shown that inflammation plays an important role.[21,25]
- Tonometry can distinguish if a lymphedematous arm is harder or softer than a contralateral arm (if unaffected). If a lower tissue tonicity value is recorded in the

edematous arm, it indicates that there is accumulated lymph fluid in the tissue, and these patients are candidates for conservative treatment methods. In contrast, patients with a harder arm, compared with the healthy one, have an adipose tissue excess that can successfully be removed by liposuction.[8]

- In Graves ophthalmopathy, a major problem is an increase in the intraorbital adipose tissue volume leading to exophthalmos. Adipocyte-related immediate early genes (IEGs) are overexpressed in active ophthalmopathy and cysteine-rich, angiogenic inducer 61 (CYR61) may have a role in both orbital inflammation and adipogenesis and serve as a marker of disease activity.[26]
- Preoperative investigation with volume-rendered computer tomography (VRCT) images showed a significant preoperative increase of adipose tissue in the swollen arm, the excess volume consisting of 81% (range 68%–96%) fat.[11]
- Analyses with dual x-ray absorptiometry (DXA) that was compared to plethysmography in 18 women with arm lymphedema following a mastectomy showed a significant increase of adipose tissue, 73% (range, 43%–111%), in the nonpitting swollen arm before surgery.[12]
- Adipogenesis in response to lymphatic fluid stasis is associated with a marked mononuclear cell inflammatory response.[27]
- Lymphatic fluid stasis potently upregulates the expression of fat differentiation markers both spatially and temporally.[28]
- The underlying pathophysiology of lymphedema drives adipose-derived stem cells toward adipogenic differentiation.[29]
- Consecutive analyses of the content of the aspirate removed under bloodless conditions using a tourniquet, showed a very high content of adipose tissue in 105 women with postmastectomy arm lymphedema (mean 94%, range 58%–100%).[3]

A common misunderstanding among clinicians is that the swelling of a lymphedematous extremity, whether it is primary or secondary, is due purely to the accumulation of lymph and/or fibrosis. Lymph can be removed by the use of noninvasive conservative regimens such as complex decongestive therapy (CDT) and controlled compression therapy (CCT). These therapies work well when the excess swelling consists of accumulated lymph but do not work when the excess volume is dominated by adipose tissue.[14] The same may go for microsurgical procedures using lymphovenous shunts,[30] lymph vessel transplantation,[31] and lymph node transfer.[32]

HOW TO ASSESS THE EFFICACY OF LIPOSUCTION

Today, chronic nonpitting arm lymphedema of more than 4 L in excess can be effectively removed by use of liposuction without any further reduction in lymph transport. Long-term results have not shown any recurrence of the

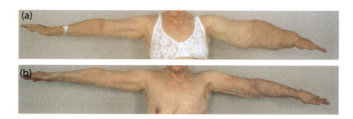

Figure 67.1 (a) A 74-year-old woman with a nonpitting arm lymphedema for 15 years. Preoperative excess volume was 3090 mL. (b) Postoperative result.

arm swelling (Figures 67.1 and 67.2).[2,3,13,14] Promising results can also be achieved for primary and secondary leg lymphedema, where over 6 L in excess volume can be completely reduced (Figures 67.3 and 67.4).[1,33]

Preoperative planning

Made-to-measure compression garments (three sleeves and two gloves) are ordered 2 weeks before surgery. One garment, to be put on the arm at the time of surgery, is sterilized and used for only 2 days since it loses some of its pressure by sterilization. The size of the garments is measured according to the size of the unaffected arm and hand. In stock we always have standard interim gloves and gauntlets (a glove without fingers but with a thumb), used as described later. One interim glove is sterilized to be put on at the time of surgery. Liposuction is executed circumferentially, step-by-step from hand to shoulder, and the hypertrophied fat is removed as much as possible (Figures 67.5 through 67.8).

Surgical technique

The surgical technique for primary and secondary lymphedema has previously been described in detail.[2,3,13,14,34] The technique (Figures 67.3 and 67.4) is similar to that for the arm (Figures 67.5 through 67.8).

Postoperative care

Two days postoperatively, the garments are removed by the patient under supervision so that the patient can take a shower. The arm is lubricated with lotion. Then, the other set of garments is put on and the used set is washed and dried. Change of garments is repeated by the patient after another 2 days before a hospital discharge. The standard glove and gauntlet are usually changed to the made-to-measure glove at the end of the stay.

The patient alternates between the two sets of garments (two sleeves and two gloves) during the first week at home, changing them every other day so that a clean set is always put on after showering and lubricating the arm. Then garments are changed daily. Washing "activates" the garment by increasing the compression due to shrinkage. It also removes products of perspiration that can cause dry and irritated skin.

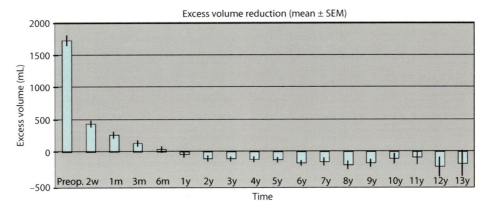

Figure 67.2 Mean postoperative excess volume reduction in 95 women with arm lymphedema following breast cancer.[39]

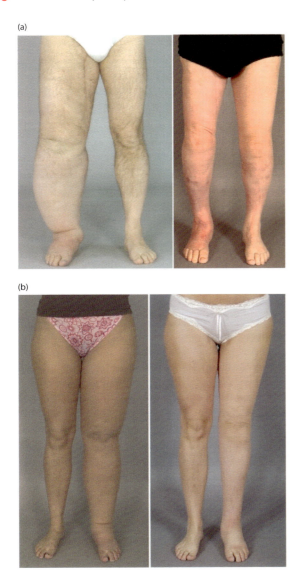

Figure 67.3 (a) Preoperative excess volume 5380 mL (left). Postoperative result after 3 years where excess volume is −255 mL, i.e., the treated leg is somewhat smaller than the normal one (right). (b) Preoperative excess volume 6630 mL (left). Postoperative result after 2 years with complete reduction (right). (Reproduced from Brorson H, Ohlin K, Svensson B. *J Lymphoedema* 2008;1:38−47.)

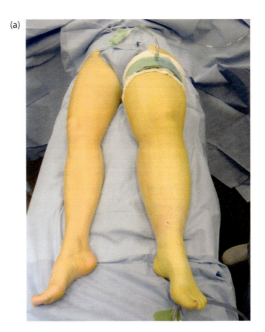

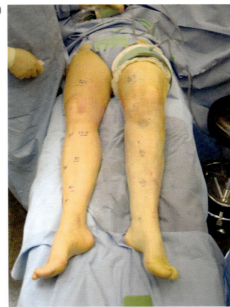

Figure 67.4 (a) Primary lymphedema of 4940 mL before liposuction. (b) After liposuction up to the tourniquet.

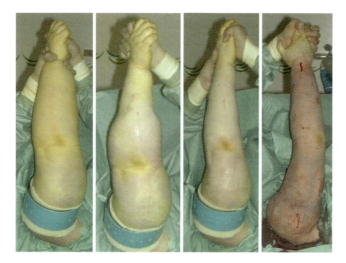

Figure 67.5 Liposuction of arm lymphedema. The procedure takes about 2 hours. From preoperative to postoperative state (left to right). Note the tourniquet, which has been removed at the right, and the concomitant reactive hyperemia.

During the subsequent course, this rigorous compression regime, referred to as controlled compression therapy (CCT), is maintained exactly as described in the next section.

CONTROLLED COMPRESSION THERAPY

A prerequisite to maintaining the effect of liposuction, and, for that matter, conservative treatment, is the life-long, continuous (24 h/day) use of a compression garment.[3,13,14] If the patient has any doubts about continued CCT, the patient is not accepted for treatment.

After initiating compression therapy, the custom-made garment may be taken in at each visit using a sewing machine, to compensate for reduced elasticity and reduced arm volume. This is most important during the first 3 months when the

(a) (b)

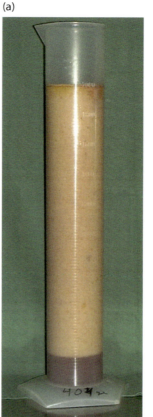
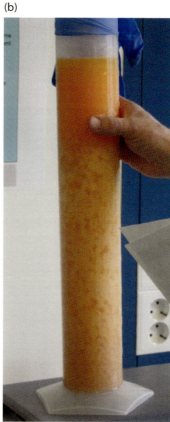

Figure 67.7 The aspirate contains 90%–100% adipose tissue in general. This picture shows the aspirate collected from the lymphedematous arm of the patient shown in Figures 67.5, 67.6, and 67.8 before removal of the tourniquet. The aspirate sediments into an upper adipose fraction (90%) and a lower fluid (lymph) fraction (10%).

most notable changes in volume occur. At the 1- and 3-month visits, the arm is measured for new custom-made garments. This procedure is repeated at 6, 9, and 12 months. If complete reduction has been achieved at 6 months, the 9-month

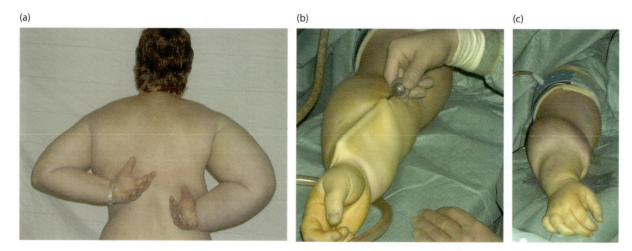

Figure 67.6 (a) Preoperative picture showing a patient with a large lymphedema (2865 mL) and decreased mobility of the right arm. **(b)** The cannula lifts the loose skin of the treated forearm. **(c)** The distal half of the forearm has been treated. Note the sharp border between treated (distal forearm) and untreated (proximal arm) areas.

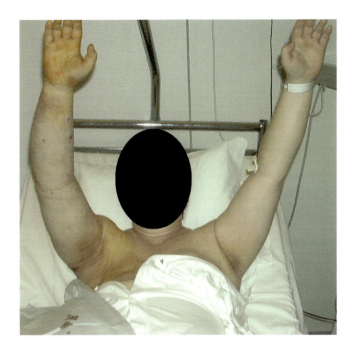

Figure 67.8 The compression garment is removed 2 days after surgery to take measurements for a custom-made compression garment. A significant reduction of the right arm has been achieved, as compared with the preoperative condition seen in Figure 67.5a.

control may be omitted. If this is the case, it is important to remember to prescribe garments for 6 months.

When the excess volume has decreased as much as possible and a steady state is achieved, new garments can be prescribed using the latest measurements. In this way, the garments (two sets of sleeve and glove garments) are renewed three or four times during the first year. The patient is informed about the importance of hygiene (daily shower with soap and water) and skin care (moisturizing the skin with lotion), as all patients with lymphedema are susceptible to infections.[3,13,14]

The life span of two garments worn alternately is usually 4–6 months. After complete reduction has been achieved, the patient is seen once a year when new garments are prescribed for the coming year, usually four garments and four gloves (or four gauntlets). In active patients, six to eight garments and the same amount of gauntlets/gloves a year are needed.

For legs it is often necessary to use up to two to three compression garments on top of each other, depending on what is needed to keep pitting away. The larger the diameter of the leg, the more compression is needed according to the law of Laplace. A typical example is Elvarex compression class 3, Elvarex compression class 2, and Jobst Bellavar compression class 2. The Elvarex class 2 garment can be a leg-length or a below-the-knee garment. Thus, such a patient needs two sets of two to three garments. It is important to take loose measurements at the ankle since the diameter here is small, giving more compression than needed. An

alternative is to order a leg-length garment without the foot part of one of the garments. The follow-up regimen is the same as for arms.

CCT can also be used primarily to effectively treat a pitting edema as an alternative to CDT, which, in contrast to CCT, comprises daily interventions.[13,14]

VOLUME MEASUREMENTS

Volumes are recorded for each patient using the water displacement technique. The displaced water is weighed on a balance to the nearest 5 g, corresponding to 5 mL. Both extremities are always measured at each visit, and the difference in volumes is designated as the edema volume, or more correctly the excess volume. The decrease in the excess volume is calculated in a percentage of the preoperative value.[3,13,14]

LYMPHEDEMA TEAM

To investigate and treat patients with lymphedema, a team comprising a plastic surgeon, an occupational therapist, and a physiotherapist is needed. An hour is reserved for each scheduled visit to the team when arm volumes are measured, garments are adjusted or renewed, the social circumstances are assessed, and other matters of concern are discussed. The patient is also encouraged to contact the team whenever any unexpected problems arise, so that these can be tackled without delay. The team also monitors the long-term outcome, and a visit once a year is necessary, in most cases, to maintain a good functional and cosmetic result after complete reduction.

This regimen omits any repeated "maintenance treatment," since if the excess volume increases, it depends on less patient compliance or worn out garments. Also, one visit a year is economical as compared to conservative treatment, where patients are prescribed massage once a week and repeated maintenance therapies lasting 1–2 weeks.

HOW LIPOSUCTION HELPS

For many patients, conservative treatment does not work well or come up to their expectations, and no matter what therapy they receive, neither conservative treatment nor microsurgical procedures can remove excess adipose tissue.[30–32,35] Subcutaneous tissue debulking is the only option to completely reduce the limb excess volume leading to an improvement in the patient's quality of life.[9,10] In addition, data from a prospective study that evaluated 130 patients with postmastectomy lymphedema treated with liposuction showed that the incidence of erysipelas was reduced by 87%.[36] Mean incidence for pre-liposuction and post-liposuction erysipelas were 0.47 attacks/year (±0.8 standard deviation) and 0.06 attacks/year (±0.3 standard deviation), respectively.

LYMPH TRANSPORT SYSTEM AND LIPOSUCTION

To investigate the effect of liposuction on lymph transport, the author conducted an investigation using indirect lymphoscintigraphy in 20 patients with postmastectomy arm lymphedema. Scintigraphies were performed before liposuction, with and without wearing a garment. This was repeated after 3 and 12 months. In conclusion, it was found that the already decreased lymph transport was not further reduced after liposuction.[37]

WHEN TO USE LIPOSUCTION TO TREAT LYMPHEDEMA

A surgical approach, with the intention of removing the hypertrophied adipose tissue, seems logical when conservative treatment has not achieved satisfactory excess volume reduction and the patient has subjective discomfort of a heavy arm.

Initially, lymphedema starts as a swelling that shows pits on pressure. If treated immediately by conservative regimens, the swelling can disappear. If not, or improperly treated, the swelling increases in time and can end up in an even larger pitting edema with concomitant adipose tissue formation.

The first and most important goal is to transform a pitting edema into a nonpitting one by conservative regimens like CDT or CCT. "Pitting" means that a depression is formed after pressure on the edematous tissue by the fingertip, resulting in lymph being squeezed into the surroundings (Figure 67.9a). To standardize the pitting test, an examiner should press as hard as tolerable by a patient with the thumb on the region to be investigated for 1 minute for arms and up to 3 minutes in legs. Following this the amount of depression is estimated in millimeters. A swelling, which is dominated by hypertrophied adipose tissue, shows little or no pitting[38] (Figure 67.9b).

When a patient has been treated conservatively and shows no or minimal pitting, liposuction can be performed. If quality of life is low, this can be especially effective. The cancer itself is a worry, but the swollen and heavy arm introduces an additional handicap for the patient from a physical, psychosocial, and psychological point of view. Physical problems include pain, limited limb movement and physical mobility, and problems with clothing, thus interfering with everyday activities. Also, the heavy and swollen arm is impractical and cosmetically unappealing, all of which contribute to emotional distress.[9,10]

WHEN LIPOSUCTION SHOULD NEVER BE USED

Liposuction should not be performed in a patient who shows pits on pressure (Figure 67.9a) (see earlier), as it is dominated by accumulated lymph, which can be removed by conservative treatment. In a patient with an arm lymphedema, the authors accept around 4–5 mm of pitting, and

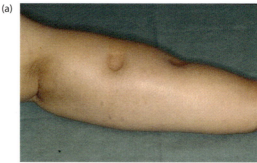

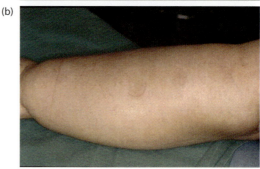

Figure 67.9 **(a)** Marked lymphedema of the arm after breast cancer treatment, showing pitting several centimeters in depth (grade I edema). The arm swelling is dominated by the presence of fluid, i.e., the accumulation of lymph. **(b)** Pronounced arm lymphedema after breast cancer treatment (grade II edema). There is no pitting in spite of hard pressure by the thumb for 1 minute. A slight reddening is seen at the two spots where pressure has been exerted. The "edema" is completely dominated by adipose tissue. The term *edema* is improper at this stage since the swelling is dominated by hypertrophied adipose tissue and not by lymph. At this stage, the aspirate contains either no or a minimal amount of lymph.

in a leg lymphedema 5–6 mm. Patients with more pitting should be treated conservatively until the pitting has been reduced. The reason for not doing liposuction in a pitting edema is that liposuction is a method to remove fat, not fluid, even if theoretically it could remove all the accumulated fluid in a pitting lymphedema without excess adipose tissue formation. Another reason is that a patient without pitting is a compliant patient, who can tolerate continuous compression.

WHEN TO PERFORM LIPOSUCTION

In short, there is no age limit for performing surgery. Any patient with a nonpitting swelling that causes a considerable decreased quality of life can be a candidate for surgery. Surgery should not be performed if the patient has active cancer or wounds.

KEY POINTS

- Excess arm or leg volume without pitting implies that excess adipose tissue is present.

- Excess adipose tissue can be removed by the use of liposuction. Conservative treatment and microsurgical reconstructions cannot remove adipose tissue.
- As in conservative treatment, the lifelong use (24 hours a day) of compression garments is mandatory for maintaining the effect of surgery.
- Clinically there is no difference in performing liposuction in primary or secondary lymphedema.
- There is no age limit for performing surgery.
- Any patient with a nonpitting swelling that causes a considerable decreased quality of life can be a candidate for surgery.
- Surgery should not be performed if the patient has active cancer or wounds.

REFERENCES

1. Brorson H. Liposuction normalizes lymphedema induced adipose tissue hypertrophy in elephantiasis of the leg—A prospective study with a ten-year follow-up. *Plast Reconstr Surg.* 2015;136:133–134.
2. Brorson H. Complete reduction of arm lymphedema following breast cancer—A prospective twenty-one years' study. *Plast Reconstr Surg.* 2015;136:134–135.
3. Hoffner M, Ohlin K, Svensson B et al. Liposuction gives complete reduction of arm lymphedema following breast cancer treatment—A 5-year prospective study in 105 patients without recurrence. *Plast Reconstr Surg Glob Open.* 2018;6:e1912.
4. Kissin MW, Querci della Rovere G, Easton D, Westbury G. Risk of lymphoedema following the treatment of breast cancer. *Br J Surg.* 1986;73:580–584.
5. Segerstrom K, Bjerle P, Graffman S, Nystrom A. Factors that influence the incidence of brachial oedema after treatment of breast cancer. *Scand J Plast Reconstr Surg Hand Surg.* 1992;26:223–227.
6. Gebruers N, Verbelen H, De Vrieze T, Coeck D, Tjalma W. Incidence and time path of lymphedema in sentinel node negative breast cancer patients: A systematic review. *Arch Phys Med Rehabil.* 2015;96:1131–1139.
7. Olszewski WL. *Lymph Stasis: Pathophysiology, Diagnosis and Treatment.* Boca Raton, FL: CRC Press; 1991:648.
8. Bagheri S, Ohlin K, Olsson G, Brorson H. Tissue tonometry before and after liposuction of arm lymphedema following breast cancer. *Lymphat Res Biol.* 2005;3:66–80.
9. Brorson H, Ohlin K, Olsson G, Långström G, Wiklund I, Svensson H. Quality of life following liposuction and conservative treatment of arm lymphedema. *Lymphology.* 2006;39:8–25.
10. Hoffner M, Bagheri S, Hansson E, Manjer J, Troeng T, Brorson H. SF-36 shows increased quality of life following complete reduction of postmastectomy lymphedema with liposuction. *Lymphat Res Biol.* 2017;15:87–98.
11. Brorson H, Ohlin K, Olsson G, Nilsson M. Adipose tissue dominates chronic arm lymphedema following breast cancer: An analysis using volume rendered CT images. *Lymphat Res Biol.* 2006;4:199–210.
12. Brorson H, Ohlin K, Olsson G, Karlsson MK. Breast cancer-related chronic arm lymphedema is associated with excess adipose and muscle tissue. *Lymphat Res Biol.* 2009;7:3–10.
13. Brorson H, Svensson H. Complete reduction of lymphoedema of the arm by liposuction after breast cancer. *Scand J Plast Reconstr Surg Hand Surg.* 1997;31:137–143.
14. Brorson H, Svensson H. Liposuction combined with controlled compression therapy reduces arm lymphedema more effectively than controlled compression therapy alone. *Plast Reconstr Surg.* 1998;102:1058–1067; discussion 1068.
15. Hoffner M, Peterson P, Månsson S, Brorson H. Lymphedema leads to fat deposition in muscle and decreased muscle/water volume after liposuction: A magnetic resonance imaging study. *Lymphat Res Biol.* 2018;16(2):174–181.
16. Trinh L, Peterson P, Brorson H, Mansson S. Assessment of subfascial muscle/water and fat accumulation in lymphedema patients using magnetic resonance imaging. *Lymphat Res Biol.* 2019;17(3):340–346.
17. Vague J, Fenasse R. Comparative anatomy of adipose tissue. In: Renold AE, Cahill GF, eds. *American Handbook of Physiology.* Washington DC: American Physiology Society; 1965:25–36.
18. Ryan TJ. Lymphatics and adipose tissue. *Clin Dermatol.* 1995;13:493–498.
19. Mattacks CA, Sadler D, Pond CM. The control of lipolysis in perinodal and other adipocytes by lymph node and adipose tissue-derived dendritic cells in rats. *Adipocytes.* 2005;1:43–56.
20. Pond CM. Adipose tissue and the immune system. *Prostaglandins Leukot Essent Fatty Acids.* 2005;73:17–30.
21. Borley NR, Mortensen NJ, Jewell DP, Warren BF. The relationship between inflammatory and serosal connective tissue changes in ileal Crohn's disease: Evidence for a possible causative link. *J Pathol.* 2000;190:196–202.
22. Sadler D, Mattacks CA, Pond CM. Changes in adipocytes and dendritic cells in lymph node containing adipose depots during and after many weeks of mild inflammation. *J Anat.* 2005;207:769–781.
23. Harvey NL, Srinivasan RS, Dillard ME et al. Lymphatic vascular defects promoted by Prox1 haploinsufficiency cause adult-onset obesity. *Nat Genet.* 2005;37:1072–1081.
24. Schneider M, Conway EM, Carmeliet P. Lymph makes you fat. *Nat Genet.* 2005;37:1023–1024.
25. Jones B, Fishman EK, Hamilton SR et al. Submucosal accumulation of fat in inflammatory bowel disease: CT/pathologic correlation. *J Comput Assist Tomogr.* 1986;10:759–763.

26. Lantz M, Vondrichova T, Parikh H et al. Overexpression of immediate early genes in active Graves' ophthalmopathy. *J Clin Endocrinol Metab.* 2005; 90:4784–4791.

27. Zampell JC, Aschen S, Weitman ES et al. Regulation of adipogenesis by lymphatic fluid stasis: Part I. Adipogenesis, fibrosis, and inflammation. *Plast Reconstr Surg.* 2012;129:825–834.

28. Aschen S, Zampell JC, Elhadad S, Weitman E, De Brot M, Mehrara BJ. Regulation of adipogenesis by lymphatic fluid stasis: Part II. Expression of adipose differentiation genes. *Plast Reconstr Surg.* 2012; 129:838–847.

29. Levi B, Glotzbach JP, Sorkin M et al. Molecular analysis and differentiation capacity of adipose-derived stem cells from lymphedema tissue. *Plast Reconstr Surg.* 2013;132:580–589.

30. Campisi C, Bellini C, Campisi C, Accogli S, Bonioli E, Boccardo F. Microsurgery for lymphedema: Clinical research and long-term results. *Microsurgery.* 2010; 30:256–260.

31. Baumeister RG, Mayo W, Notohamiprodjo M, Wallmichrath J, Springer S, Frick A. Microsurgical lymphatic vessel transplantation. *J Reconstr Microsurg.* 2016;32:34–41.

32. Cheng MH, Loh CYY, Lin CY. Outcomes of vascularized lymph node transfer and lymphovenous anastomosis for treatment of primary lymphedema. *Plast Reconstr Surg Glob Open.* 2018;6:e2056.

33. Brorson H, Ohlin K, Olsson G, Svensson B, Svensson H. Controlled compression and liposuction treatment for lower extremity lymphedema. *Lymphology.* 2008;41:52–63.

34. Wojnikow S, Malm J, Brorson H. Use of a tourniquet with and without adrenaline reduces blood loss during liposuction for lymphoedema of the arm. *Scand J Plast Reconstr Surg Hand Surg.* 2007;41: 243–249.

35. Tambour M, Holt M, Speyer A, Christensen R, Gram B. Manual lymphatic drainage adds no further volume reduction to complete decongestive therapy on breast cancer-related lymphoedema: A multicentre, randomised, single-blind trial. *Br J Cancer.* 2018;119:1215–1222.

36. Lee D, Piller N, Hoffner M, Manjer J, Brorson H. Liposuction of postmastectomy arm lymphedema decreases the incidence of erysipelas. *Lymphology.* 2016;49:85–92.

37. Brorson H, Svensson H, Norrgren K, Thorsson O. Liposuction reduces arm lymphedema without significantly altering the already impaired lymph transport. *Lymphology.* 1998;31:156–172.

38. Brorson H. Liposuction in arm lymphedema treatment. *Scand J Surg.* 2003;92:287–295.

39. Brorson H, Ohlin K, Olsson G, Svensson B. Liposuction of postmastectomy arm lymphedema completely removes excess volume: A thirteen year study (Quad erat demonstrandum). *Eur J Lymphol.* 2007;17:9.

40. Brorson H, Ohlin K, Svensson B. The facts about liposuction as a treatment for lymphoedema. *J Lymphoedema.* 2008;1:38–47.

68

Liposuction: Can it be applied to management of lipedema?

ROBERT J. DAMSTRA AND TOBIAS BERTSCH

INTRODUCTION

Lipedema is a chronic disorder of unknown etiology that mostly affects women. Clinically, there is a bilateral and symmetrical increase in the fat tissue of the legs, hips, and sometimes arms. Additionally, patients with lipedema suffer from pain with pressure or spontaneous pain of the soft tissue in affected areas. Many patients complain about a feeling of "heavy legs." Whether edema plays a significant role in this disease is the subject of an ongoing discussion at present. It is important to note that there is no scientific evidence for fluid accumulation in patients with pure lipedema. The actual term *lipedema* is a misnomer term, as it evokes the idea of swelling due to fluid accumulation. However, the term refers to swelling—in the sense of an increase in volume—due to the increase in fat tissue.[1]

In most cases, the disproportional fat distribution starts around puberty and continues into the third decade of life. Often, there is a positive family history with an occurrence rate that ranges from 16% to 64%.[2] Complaints, as mentioned earlier, usually start many years later, in most cases after experiencing weight gain.

The diagnosis of lipedema is challenging and based on various criteria that vary between clinical signs and symptoms, as suggested by Wold et al.[3] Currently, there is a more integrated approach that profiles a patient with a more biomedical and psychosocial model to provide better insight into the influence of the disorder on daily life and functioning[1] and not just focus on biomedical signs and symptoms.

Lipedema is often misdiagnosed (as obesity of lymphedema), and it is sometimes under- or overdiagnosed. It is very often seen in combination with progressive obesity. If a patient with lipedema is also morbidly obese, concomitant lymphedema can occur. It should be emphasized that the cause of lymphedema is not lipedema but progressive obesity. The term *lipolymphedema* should be avoided, because it mistakenly suggests that lipedema leads to lymphedema.

Comorbidities can occur, but the majority of chronic edema in more extensive cases is related to the increase in interstitial filtration by gained weight and the reduction of mobility. Some call this disorder "obesity-induced lymphedema with inflammation."[4] However, the primary lymphatics are not affected by lipedema, and edema is not a pathognomonic aspect in the diagnosis of lipedema; in fact, edema discriminates from the diagnosis of lymphedema.[5] Often, patients suffer from psychological vulnerability, low self-esteem and self-acceptance.[6,7]

According to the Dutch guidelines for lipedema,[1] the chronic care model (CCM)[8] and the biomedical psychosocial model from the World Health Organization (WHO) (*International Classification of Functioning, Disability, and Health* [ICF])[9] are helpful in making a health profile of the patient that enables the health-care provider (HCP) to make a dedicated treatment program for this chronic condition. The CCM enables the patient to become self-effective during the maintenance phase of treatment and to become independent from a HCP as much as possible.

In contrast, the Germany guidelines focus on decongestion of the soft tissue including the use of manual lymph drainage (MLD). It has to be emphasized that MLD has never been shown effective for lipedema, although patients and therapists sometimes claim subjective improvements to the overall well-being. When we take the psychological factors into account, the question remains: is it truly the procedure that is helpful, or do other factors play an important role?

LIPEDEMA, LIPOSUCTION, AND OBESITY

There are many beliefs, myths, and nonscientific statements about the lipedema disorder. One of the beliefs is that liposuction is the ultimate operative solution to treat (and cure) lipedema with a long-lasting effect.[10,11] Some authors claim that there are long-lasting improvements to pain, and reductions in bruising, swelling, and even edema; additionally, some even claim that conservative treatments are no longer necessary.[12]

The following three aspects are discussed more intensely:

- How effective is liposuction: is it a cosmetic improvement for the figure or a medical treatment of the disease?
- How long do the effects of liposuction last?
- How does liposuction affect obesity, the major concomitant disease in lipedema?

EFFECTIVENESS OF LIPOSUCTION

The German guidelines for lipedema[13] state that lipedema include edema as an essential clinical symptom and focus on a clinical approach toward lipedema without proper clinimetrics. Essential aspects of this disease like obesity, psychological, lifestyle, and social-cultural issues were not included. The scientific basis of the diagnosis is lacking and based on expert opinions.

Cornely, Rapprich,[14] Schmeller,[15] and Baumgartner[11] claim there are long-lasting results in 97% (after 15 years), 84% (after 6 months), 23% (after 4 years), and 30% (8 years of follow-up) of cases, respectively. These data appear promising but are very heterogeneous. The diagnoses and patient cohorts cannot be compared between studies; the studies have various forms of postoperative treatment and often lack objective clinimetrics, such as range of motion, physical condition, muscle strength, and body mass index (BMI). Second, the questionnaires used in the studies are not validated for the operative treatment of lipedema.[16]

Finally, there is an important bias in all of these studies. In most cases, the treatment was not reimbursed by insurance, and patients had to pay for the expensive treatment. Obviously, this unpredictably influences the motivation, outcomes, and concordance in a positive way.

LONG-LASTING EFFECTS OF LIPOSUCTION

Some doctors who perform liposuction for lipedema claim that "once lipedematous fat is removed, there is no buildup of fat anymore."[13] This statement is applicable in practice if the weight of the patient remains stable. However, this statement contradicts the findings from our clinical experiences where patients regain their weight in many cases.

In general, lipedema is often mentioned as a progressive disease. However, Bertsch et al.[17] showed that there is no scientific basis for a progressive course of lipedema. Rather, weight gain and obesity are very often progressive in combination with secondary complications such as immobility, edema formation, inflammation, psychological disorders, and inaccurate beliefs about the illness.

WHAT ABOUT OBESITY, A MAJOR CONCOMITANT DISEASE IN LIPEDEMA?

The vast majority of lipedema patients are obese. A study from 2015 in the Földi clinic showed that 88% of the lipedema patients had a BMI > 30 kg/m^2.[17] Other centers that treat lipedema patients presented similar data.[18] Recently, the first report of a rare case of a Japanese lipedema patient was presented with a 42-year-old female (BMI 42).[19] Interestingly, the clinical figure in the article clearly showed concomitant obesity, which is also not frequent in Japan. The baseline BMI for women varies between 21.5 and 26.9 at an age of 20 years old,[20] and the Japanese defined obesity to the national definition of obesity as BMI more than 25.[21]

Therefore, weight gain and perhaps ethnic and genetic cofactors play a role in the development of lipedematous tissue to obtain a phenotype of lipedema.

The German Lipedema guidelines recommend a BMI threshold of not more than 32 kg/m^2 for liposuction. This threshold makes sense because lipedema should be classified as a disease and not as obesity. However, the majority of surgeons do not care about this recommendation. This disregard for the threshold becomes visible when reviewing the population of patients who have already undergone liposuction. In the patient population of the study from Wollina and Heinig,[22] 12 (out of 26) patients had a BMI greater than 35 kg/m^2, and the heaviest patient had a BMI of 61.8 kg/m^2. In the studies with the German Lipedema guidelines, the BMI threshold for the patients who underwent liposuction was precautionary and was not mentioned by the surgeons.

If the lipedema patient is morbidly obese (BMI more than 40 kg/m^2), bariatric surgery is more appropriate and should be considered. Bertsch et al. presented a case of a lipedema patient with clinical signs of lipedema who was also majorly obese (BMI 54 kg/m^2).[14] She improved enormously after gastric bypass surgery and reduced her BMI to 28.6 kg/m^2 within 1 year (Figures 68.1a,b and 68.2a,b). The circumference of her legs improved drastically along with her pain in the soft tissue. However, some disfiguration persisted, which can be seen as the effects of the lipedema component of her health issues. The patient kept on wearing garments.

In general, liposuction is not indicated to treat obesity. Therefore, from this perspective, intensive diagnostic tools and clinimetrics are essential to evaluate the health profile of a patient and decide which dedicated therapeutic program should be offered.

CONCLUSIONS

Liposuction is a generally accepted procedure to remove fat from the body. As lipedema is a fat disorder, the technique can be suitable to remove fat in these patients. The question remains: is liposuction the treatment of choice for lipedema? In 2018, the German Federal Joint Committee (G-BA) concluded that in general, "the proof of the effectiveness of liposuction in lipedema was not indisputable."[23]

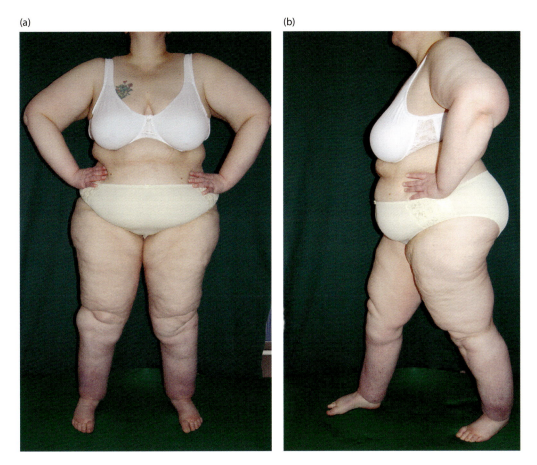

Figure 68.1 **(a,b)** A 42-year-old patient referred with lipedema and obesity (BMI 54) before bariatric surgery with gastric bypass.

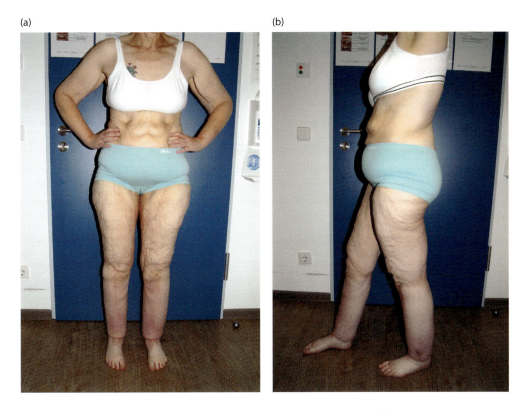

Figure 68.2 **(a,b)** Same patient 14 months postoperatively (55 kg weight loss; BMI 28).

According to the Dutch guidelines,[1] liposuction in lipedema is considered a way to reduce fat in very specific cases. Liposuction has to be performed as super tumescent liposuction in an ambulatory setting as part of an integrated therapeutic armamentarium. Before using liposuction, the associated deteriorating components, such as edema, obesity, unhealthy lifestyle, lack of physical activity, lack of knowledge about the disease, and psychosocial distress, should be addressed using the CCM and the ICF method.

A good patient selection process with clinimetrics and the integration of liposuction as a multidisciplinary therapeutic concept is essential for long-lasting effects. The aspects like physical functionality, psychological factors, and weight gain should be taken into account.

REFERENCES

1. Halk AB, Damstra RJ. First Dutch guidelines on lipedema using the international classification of functioning, disability and health. *Phlebology.* 2017; 32(3):152–159.
2. Langendoen SI, Habbema L, Nijsten TEC, Neumann HAM. Lipoedema: From clinical presentation to therapy. A review of the literature. *Br J Dermatol.* 2009;161(5):980–986.
3. Wold LE, Hines EA, Allen EV. Lipedema of the legs; a syndrome characterized by fat legs and edema. *Ann Intern Med.* 1951;34(5):1243–1250.
4. Greene AK, Grant FD, Maclellan RA. Obesity-induced lymphedema nonreversible following massive weight loss. *Plast Reconstr Surg Glob Open.* 2015;3(6): e426–e423.
5. Birkballe S, Jensen MR, Noerregaard S, Gottrup F, Karlsmark T. Can tissue dielectric constant measurement aid in differentiating lymphoedema from lipoedema in women with swollen legs? *Br J Dermatol.* 2014;170(1):96–102.
6. Dudek JE, Białaszek W, Ostaszewski P. Quality of life in women with lipoedema: A contextual behavioral approach. *Qual Life Res.* 2015;25(2):401–408.
7. Dudek JE, Białaszek W, Ostaszewski P, Smidt T. Depression and appearance-related distress in functioning with lipedema. *Psychol Health Med.* 2018;79(4): 1–8.
8. Wagner EH. Chronic disease management: What will it take to improve care for chronic illness? effective clinical practice. 1998;1:2–4.
9. Stucki G, Grimby G. Applying the ICF in medicine. *J Rehabil Med.* 2004;36(44 Suppl):5–6.
10. Schmeller W et al. Langzeitveränderungen nach Liposuktion bei Lipödem. *Lymphforsch.* 2010;14(2):1–12.
11. Baumgartner A, Hueppe M, Schmeller W. Long-term benefit of liposuction in patients with lipoedema: A follow-up study after an average of 4 and 8 years. *Br J Dermatol.* 2016;174(5):1061–1067.
12. S 1 Leitlinie Lipödem. Verfügbar unter http://www.awmf.org/uploads/tx_szleitlinien/037–012I_S1_Lipoedem_2016–01.pdf.
13. Reich-Schupke S et al. S1 guidelines: Lipedema. *J Dtsch Dermatol Ges.* 2017;15(7):758–767.
14. Rapprich S, Dingler A, Podda M. Liposuction is an effective treatment for lipedema-results of a study with 25 patients. *J Dtsch Dermatol Ges.* 2011;9(1):33–40.
15. Schmeller W, Hueppe M, Meier-Vollrath I. Tumescent liposuction in lipoedema yields good long-term results. *Br J Dermatol.* 2011;166(1):161–168.
16. Bertsch T, Erbacher G, Torio-Padron N. Lipödem – Mythen und Fakten Teil 4. *Phlebologie.* 2019;48(01):47–56.
17. Bertsch T, Erbacher G. Lipödem – Mythen und Fakten Teil 1. *Phlebologie.* 2018;47(02):84–92.
18. Child AH et al. Lipedema: An inherited condition. *Am J Med Genet A.* 2010;152A(4):970–976.
19. Koyama H, Tanaka T, Imaeda K. Suspected case of lipoedema in Japanese woman with a characteristic histology in skin biopsy. *BMJ Case Rep.* 2017; 2017:bcr–2017–221049.
20. Wakamatsu M, Sugawara Y, Zhang S, Tanji F, Tomata Y, Tsuji I. Weight change since age 20 and incident risk of obesity-related cancer in Japan: A pooled analysis of the Miyagi Cohort Study and the Ohsaki Cohort Study. *Int J Cancer.* 2019;144(5):967–980.
21. Funatogawa I, Funatogawa T, Yano E. Do overweight children necessarily make overweight adults? Repeated cross sectional annual nationwide survey of Japanese girls and women over nearly six decades. *BMJ.* 2008;337:a802.
22. Wollina U, Heinig B, Nowak A. Treatment of elderly patients with advanced lipedema: A combination of laser-assisted liposuction, medial thigh lift, and lower partial abdominoplasty. *CCID.* 2014;7:35–42.
23. Gemeinsamer Bundesausschuss vom 20. 2017. Tragende Gründe zum Beschluss des Gemeinsamen Bundesausschusses über eine Änderung der Richtlinie Methoden Krankenhausbehandlung: Liposuktion bei Lipödem. Abrufbar unter: https://www.g-ba.de/downloads/40–268-4488/2017–07-20_KHMe-RL_Liposuktion_TrG.pdf.

Management: 2—Lymphangioma

69

How to manage lymphatic leakage involved in lymphangioma?

XI YANG, XIAOXI LIN, AND NINGFEI LIU

Lymphatic leakage is a common complication secondary to the skin involvement of microcystic lymphangioma, which is also called *lymphangioma circumscriptum* (LC).[1] It is characterized by the appearance of clusters of thin-walled vesicles of varying size (commonly 2–5 mm) that appear as "zosteriform" or "frogspawn." These vesicles are usually filled with colorless fluid and occasionally with blood cells. The proximal limbs, chest wall, abdominal wall, and buccal mucosa are common sites of occurrence.[2] Spontaneous lymphatic leakage from the skin commonly occurs, which can lead to or be associated with cellulitis. Recurrent cellulitis, which causes pain and cosmetic disfigurement, can also occur and may lead to serious infection. Bacteria may readily enter through open vesicles and quickly spread through tissues affected by these lesions. When this occurs, aggressive antibiotic therapy is essential.

Lymphangioma circumscriptum has two components: the clinically obvious dermal vesicular component and a deeper subcutaneous cisternal element. The pathology of these two components shows the large dilated lymphatics on the skin surface and a deeper contractile lymphatic cistern, respectively. The malformed lymphatic cistern lies just above the deep fascia and is not in continuity with the normal lymphatic system around the tissues. The malformed lymphatic cistern produces continuous or intermittent pressure on the contained fluid, which results in saccular dilatation of the subepidermal lymphatics and the clinically visible vesicles[3] (Figure 69.1).

The therapeutic interventions for LC are difficult and frustrating because of the high recurrence rate due to multifocal distribution of lesions and a failure to address the deeper component. The various modalities that have been used in the management of LC are surgical excision, sclerotherapy,[4] electrocautery,[5] radiofrequency,[6,7] radiotherapy,[8] carbon dioxide laser,[9] imiquimod 5% cream,[10] pulsed-dye laser,[11] electrocoagulation,[12] therapeutic lymphangiography,[13] and sirolimus.[14] Radical surgery remains as the definite treatment. However, this treatment may not be practical for many patients because complete resection is rarely achieved.

Carbon dioxide (CO_2) laser can achieve good cosmetic results and resolution of the symptoms with minor and infrequent side effects such as dyspigmentation and mild scarring. The 10,600 nm wavelength of the CO_2 laser is highly absorbed by water, thus, vaporizing underlying skin tissue and sealing the communication channels that connect the superficial vesicles to the deeper components of LC. Although full-field CO_2 laser ablation is very effective in treating LC, it can involve significant downtime and adverse events such as persistent erythema, delayed and permanent hypopigmentation, and scarring.[9] Fractional ablative lasers also result in tissue ablation; however, they do so by creating microthermal zones that promote new collagen production, while the areas of untreated skin promote rapid healing, with less risk of complications compared to fully ablative lasers.[15] But the recurrence rate was significantly high. In the latest review, in 28 patients with LC treated by carbon dioxide laser, only 8 patients remained disease free from 4 months to 3 years, 10 experienced partial recurrences, and 2 experienced complete recurrence.[16]

Sclerotherapy is a useful method for the treatment of LC. Sclerotherapy refers to the introduction of sclerosing agents into the lumen of lymphatic malformation, causing inflammation/thrombosis and subsequent fibrosis (Figure 69.2). Picibanil (OK-432), bleomycin, sodium tetradecyl sulfate, polidocanol, ethanol, and hypertonic saline are the commonly used sclerosants, but the side effects, such as pain, inflammation, hyperpigmentation, ecchymosis, localized urticaria, and skin necrosis, are considerable.[17] Radiofrequency ablation is an alternative method for treating LC. It destroys tissue at low temperatures (40°C–70°C) with minimal damage to adjacent tissues. Theoretically, the reduced thermal energy and destruction of tissue may diminish regrowth of residual malformation and may also improve wound healing. A combination of radiofrequency ablation and sclerotherapy was often used, with

311

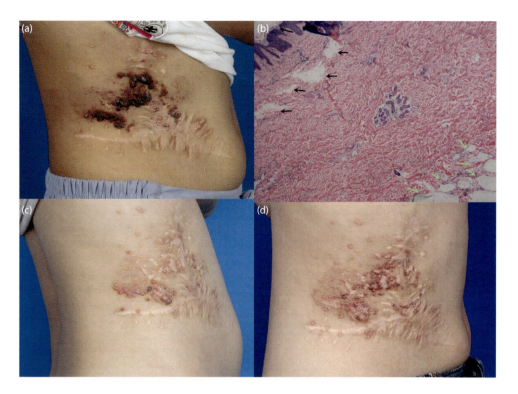

Figure 69.1 (a) A 14-year-old female patient with lymphangioma circumscriptum (LC) and lymphatic leakage on her right abdomen. (b) Histological examination showed dilated thin-walled lymphatic vessels in both the superficial dermis (black arrow) and deep layer (green arrow). (H&E stain, original magnification ×40). (c) 4-year follow-up after selective electrocoagulation therapy. LC and lymphatic leakage showed great improvement. (d) 6-year follow-up showed slight recurrence of the lesion, but the lymphatic leakage did not recur.

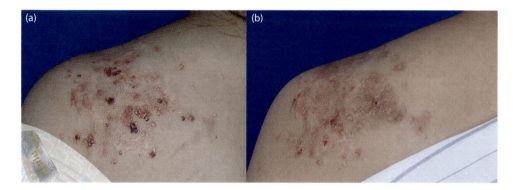

Figure 69.2 (a) A 20-year-old girl with lymphatic leakage and bleeding caused by LC on her left shoulder. (b) LC and lymphatic leakage showed great improvement 12 months after bleomycin sclerotherapy.

radiofrequency ablation targeting the superficial component and sclerotherapy targeting the deeper one, which appears to lead to an early and complete resolution as reported.[18]

Selective electrocoagulation therapy uses an isolated needle with a conductive tip, which can eliminate the deep lymphatic malformation and the superficial vesicles, and an isolated part to reduce the damage to the skin.[12] The goal of the treatment is to obtain faster clearance of both the deep and superficial lesions with minimal scarring. In a study that evaluated 12 patients who were treated with the selective electrocoagulation therapy, all 12 patients achieved near-complete clearance with a mean 8.25-month follow-up

period (Figure 69.3). The local complications included mild pain ($n = 9$), proliferous scarring ($n = 1$), and ulceration ($n = 1$) with no systemic side effects.[12]

Topical imiquimod provides another potential noninvasive treatment for localized LC. Imiquimod can induce cellular production of endogenous interferons and interleukins (IL) through activation of toll-like receptor-7 (TLR-7).[20] Some interferons can decrease cellular production of several proangiogenic factors, inhibit vascular motility and invasion, and induce apoptosis of endothelial cells. The curative efficacy of imiquimod may be related to its capacity for preventing lymphatic vessel formation and inducting

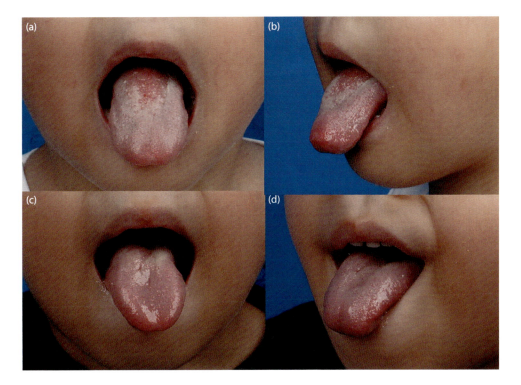

Figure 69.3 **(a,b)** A 4-year-old boy with lymphatic leakage and infection caused by LC on his tongue. **(c,d)** The lesion disappeared and the symptoms were cleared 3 months after treatment.

lymphatic endothelial cell apoptosis. The advantages of this treatment are good cosmetic results and tolerable local irritation; a disadvantage of this treatment is incomplete resolution of the lesion.[10]

Sirolimus, also known as rapamycin, is a macrocyclic compound that exhibits potent immunosuppressive effects and is used in organ transplants to prevent rejection reactions. It inhibits the signaling pathway *mammalian target of rapamycin* (mTOR) involved in important cellular functions including cellular proliferation and angiogenesis.[21] As the abnormal mTOR activity is associated with hamartomatous tumors and vascular proliferations, sirolimus has been used in lymphatic malformations. Both oral and topical sirolimus proved to be effective in the treatment of LC. Rössler et al. reported two cases where oral sirolimus was highly effective in alleviating lymph leakage and other symptoms.[14] Çalışkan and García-Montero reported one and two cases, respectively, of LC treated by topical sirolimus that also showed significant improvement and no side effects.[19,22] Oral sirolimus treatment is associated with side effects including headache, oral ulcers, neutropenia, gastrointestinal problems, and elevations in liver function tests and serum lipids. The side effects of topical sirolimus are much less. The most common side effects of topical sirolimus have been reported as irritation and a burning sensation at the site of application. However, as the penetration capacity of topical sirolimus is weak, probably the deeper lesions will not benefit from the therapy. Additionally, the recurrence of lesions after the discontinuation of the drug suggests that long-term use is mandatory for control of the disease.

In conclusion, lymphatic leakage is a refractory complication of LC. For localized lesions, complete excision is the first choice. But in many cases, the lesions are extensive, and complete excision can hardly be achieved. Multiple treatment modalities are utilized for the extensive lesions, and some treatments can achieve excellent short-term results. But there is still a high recurrence rate due to the difficulty to remove all the deeper components. Sirolimus was recently reported to treat lymphatic leakage in LC and showed remarkable improvement. It is a very promising first-line treatment for LC. Further studies with a larger number of patients are needed for a more accurate assessment of sirolimus efficacy and safety in LC management.

REFERENCES

1. Patel GA, Schwartz RA. Cutaneous lymphangioma circumscriptum: Frog spawn on the skin. *Int J Dermatol.* 2009;48:1290–1295.
2. Latifoglu O, Yavuzer R, Demir Y et al. Surgical management of penoscrotal lymphangioma circumscriptum. *Plast Reconstr Surg.* 1999;103:175–178.
3. Short S, Peacock C. A newly described possible complication of lymphangioma circumscriptum. *Clin Oncol (R Coll Radiol).* 1995;7:136–137.
4. Bikowski JB, Dumont AM. Lymphangioma circumscriptum: Treatment with hypertonic saline sclerotherapy. *J Am Acad Dermatol.* 2005;53:442–444.
5. Noyes AW. A case of lymphangioma circumscriptum. *Br Med J.* 1893;1:1159–1160.

6. Niti K, Manish P. Microcystic lymphatic malformation (lymphangioma circumscriptum) treated using a minimally invasive technique of radiofrequency ablation and sclerotherapy. *Dermatol Surg.* 2010;36: 1711–1717.

7. Sachdeva S. Lymphangioma circumscriptum treated with radiofrequency ablation. *Indian J Dermatol.* 2011;56:77–78.

8. Denton AS, Baker-Hines R, Spittle MF. Radiotherapy is a useful treatment for lymphangioma circumscriptum: A report of two patients. *Clin Oncol (R Coll Radiol).* 1996;8:400–401.

9. Eliezri YD, Sklar JA. Lymphangioma circumscriptum: Review and evaluation of carbon dioxide laser vaporization. *J Dermatol Surg Oncol.* 1988;14:357–364.

10. Wang JY, Liu LF, Mao XH. Treatment of lymphangioma circumscriptum with topical imiquimod 5% cream. *Dermatol Surg.* 2012;38:1566–1569.

11. Lai C, Hanson SG, Mallory S. Lymphangioma circumscriptum treatment with pulsed dye laser. *Pediatr Dermatol.* 2001;18:509–510.

12. Yang X, Jin Y, Chen H et al. Highly selective electrocoagulation therapy: An innovative treatment for lymphangioma circumscriptum. *Dermatol Surg.* 2014;40:899–905.

13. Lee EW, Shin JH, Ko HK et al. Lymphangiography to treat postoperative lymphatic leakage: A technical review. *Korean J Radiol.* 2014;15:724–732.

14. Rössler J, Geiger J, Földi E et al. Sirolimus is highly effective for lymph leakage in microcystic lymphatic malformations with skin involvement. *Int J Dermatol.* 2017;56:e72–e75.

15. Manstein D, Herron GS, Sink RK, Tanner H, Anderson RR. Fractional photothermolysis: A new concept for cutaneous remodeling using microscopic patterns of thermal injury. *Lasers Surg Med.* 2004;34:426–438.

16. Savas JA, Ledon J, Franca K et al. Carbon dioxide laser for the treatment of microcystic lymphatic malformations (lymphangioma circumscriptum): A systematic review. *Dermatol Surg.* 2013;39:1147–1157.

17. Park CO, Lee MJ, Chung KY. Treatment of unusual vascular lesions: Usefulness of sclerotherapy in lymphangioma circumscriptum and acquired digital arteriovenous malformation. *Dermatol Surg.* 2005;31:1451–1453.

18. Khurana A, Gupta A, Ahuja A et al. Lymphangioma circumscriptum treated with combination of Bleomycin sclerotherapy and Radiofrequency ablation. *J Cosmet Laser Ther* 2018;20(6): 326–329.

19. Çalışkan E, Altunel CT, Özkan CK et al. A case of microcystic lymphatic malformation successfully treated with topical sirolimus. *Dermatol Ther.* 2018;31: e12673.

20. Stanley MA. Imiquimod and the imidazoquinolones: Mechanism of action and therapeutic potential. *Clin Exp Dermatol.* 2002;27:571–577.

21. Kobayashi S, Kishimoto T, Kamata S et al. Rapamycin, a specific inhibitor of the mammalian target of rapamycin, suppresses lymphangiogenesis and lymphatic metastasis. *Cancer Sci.* 2007;98:726–733.

22. García-Montero P, Del Boz J, Sanchez-Martínez M et al. Microcystic lymphatic malformation successfully treated with topical rapamycin. *Pediatrics.* 2017; 139(5):e20162105.

70

How to manage recurrent infections involved with lymphangioma?

XI YANG, XIAOXI LIN, AND NINGFEI LIU

Infection is a common complication in lymphatic malformations (LMs)/lymphangiomas, which can have a significant impact on health and quality of life. Bacterial infection of the skin (cellulitis) in LMs has been reported to occur in as high as 30%–70% of patients.[1,2] The mechanism for recurrent infections associated with LMs is still unclear. One of the explanations is that LMs contain protein-rich fluid areas that are poorly vascularized, and the slow flow rate leads to stagnation, which provides microorganisms an environment in which to remain and proliferate, as they cannot be cleared by the abnormally formed lymphatic system.[3] Another possibility is a generalized, rather than a localized, immunologic disorder. Blood counts in 21 children with LMs have shown that 6 of the 21 patients had an absolute lymphocytopenia. Analysis of lymphocytic subtypes revealed T-, B-, and natural killer (NK)-cell deficiency. Lymphocytopenia correlated with extensive, bilateral, and microcystic LM; however, histological analysis did not demonstrate increased lymphocytes in any LM specimens, which rejected the hypothesis that peripheral blood lymphocytopenia is secondary to the accumulation of lymphocytes within the LM.[2] Although the relationship between lymphocytopenia and infection was not addressed in this study, the recognition of lymphocytopenia may have important clinical and prognostic implications. When comparing lymphocytopenic patients (absolute lymphocyte count less than 1500 cells/cm^3) with patients without lymphocytopenia (absolute lymphocyte count greater than 1500 cells/cm^3), patients with LM-associated lymphocytopenia have increased hospitalization requirements, have increased rates of infection, and receive more intensive antibiotic therapy.[4] Moreover, they were more likely to have central line placement, central line infection, bacteremia, prophylactic antibiotics, admission at birth, infections distant from the LM, and treatment complication compared to nonlymphocytopenic patients.

Acute swelling due to intralesional bleeding is a relatively common event in LM and can elicit a low-grade inflammatory response, making them at times difficult to distinguish from acute infection. An infected LM is typically tense, warm, erythematous, and painful, and there may be systemic signs of toxicity (Figures 70.1 and 70.2). Enlarged cervical lymph nodes are often found adjacent to and within an infectious LM. Acute infection within a diffuse lymphatic abnormality of the tongue and/or floor of the mouth can cause rapid enlargement and consequent obstruction of the upper airway and/or interference with swallowing. There are also reports of alarming respiratory distress secondary to extrinsic compression of the trachea and pulmonary parenchyma by infected LM.[5] Recurrent cycles of infection can also cause fibrosis that lead to further expansion of the LM.[6]

Prevention of recurrent infection reduces the morbidity associated with low-flow malformations by minimizing deformity, the rate of hospitalizations, and complications from acute swelling such as airway obstruction. Elevated C-reactive protein (CRP) is not LM specific but was reported as the most consistent and highly sensitive abnormal laboratory finding in infective episodes among LM together with venous malformation (VM), occurring in 37 (93%) episodes of infection.[7] The range of elevated CRP level was 18 mg/L to >270 mg/L (normal <15 mg/L).[7] The white cell count was of less utility in diagnosing infection, as has been previously reported being elevated in less than half of cases with confirmed infection.[7,8] Also previously reported and confirmed here is that it is difficult to culture infective organisms from infected LMs.[9] When cultured, the most common organisms were *Staphylococcus aureus* and *Streptococcus* species that colonize the skin. Less commonly, infections were caused by *Enterococcus faecalis* and *Escherichia coli*.[7]

Episodes of swelling should be promptly treated with appropriate antibiotic(s)—on the presumption that there is bacterial cellulitis.[6] Such an approach carries a risk of treating the wrong bacteria and would contribute to increasing antibiotic resistance. Another uncertainty in the management of infected LMs is the optimal antibiotic and duration of treatment. Penicillin is the first choice for infection

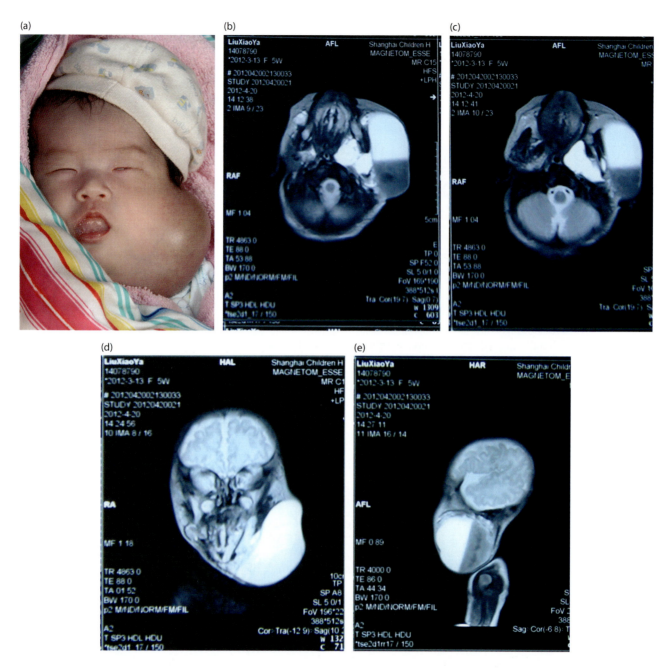

Figure 70.1 (a) A 4-day-old baby girl with a large tense, warm, erythematous mass on the left side of the face, diagnosed as macrocystic lymphatic malformation with hemorrhage and infection. **(b,c,d,e)** The T2W sequence on the magnetic resonance imaging showed cystic high signal area, low signal area after bleeding.

in LMs. For the patient who is unable to tolerate penicillin, clindamycin or erythromycin are alternatives. For patients with recurrent infection, broad-spectrum antibiotics may be chosen for first-line treatment. Often these infections cannot be controlled by oral antibiotics; the patients always need to be hospitalized for intravenous therapy. Intravenous antibiotics can be discontinued after the leukocyte count and blood CRP return to normal and the swelling has diminished. There is a high rate of recurrence of infection in LMs. Short courses of 7–10 days followed by intravenous antibiotics if oral therapy fails have been recommended for LMs,[10] as well as longer antibiotic courses of several weeks to

prevent recurrent infection.[6] Routine prophylactic antibiotic therapy is generally not recommended,[11] with the exception of postsurgical prophylaxis to prevent wound infections.[12] After the acute infection, the involved area often remains firm and edematous for a long time. Lymphatic malformations can also become swollen in the setting of nearby, unrelated infections. Carious primary teeth/dental caries and periodontal disease can be a source for bacterial contamination of a LM. Regularly scheduled dental prophylaxis is mandatory to minimize gingival inflammation and intra-oral bacterial levels. If the tonsils are suspected as the origin of repeated infection, tonsillectomy may be indicated.[6]

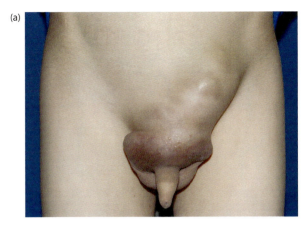

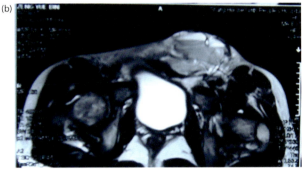

Figure 70.2 **(a)** A 10-year-old boy with lower abdomen giant cystic lymphatic malformation with hemorrhage and infection. **(b)** Mixed signal can be seen in the lymphatic cyst on magnetic resonance imaging.

To prevent infection recurrence in LMs, it is very important to manage the LM lesion after the infection is controlled. Current treatment options include nonoperative management, surgery, sclerotherapy, radiofrequency ablation, and laser therapy. New therapies are emerging, such as sirolimus. Although surgery can be a treatment of choice in certain cases based on the extent of the lesion, location, and relation to important anatomical structures, sclerotherapy is now considered the first line of treatment for LMs in general. Multiple agents are available as sclerosants when performing percutaneous sclerotherapy, and there is wide variation in their use among clinical practices. Bleomycin, doxycycline, OK-432, hypertonic saline, and absolute ethanol are the most common sclerosing agents together with sodium tetradecyl sulfate and polidocanol. Bleomycin is effective in treating both macrocystic and microcystic LMs[13] and is used more often in China. Intralesional bleomycin injection was also effective in treating the remaining or recurrent lesions after surgery (Figure 70.3).[14] More recently, oral sirolimus has been reported to be an efficacious and safe treatment for patients with complicated or refractory vascular anomalies.[15] But this oral medication can reduce immunity and cause infections, and it may not be suitable for LMs with infection.

In conclusion, infection is a common complication in LMs. For patients with recurrent infection, broad-spectrum antibiotics may be chosen as first-line treatment. Often these infections cannot be controlled by oral antibiotics; the patients always need to be hospitalized for intravenous therapy. Longer antibiotic courses of several weeks to prevent recurrent infection are recommended. It is also very important to manage the LM lesion after the infection is controlled. Sclerotherapy would be the first choice to treat the LM lesion in general, except for specific lesions that require surgical excision.

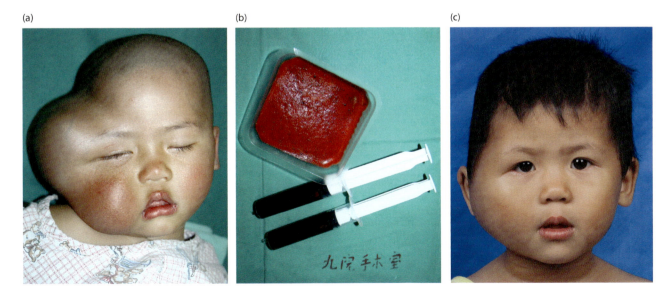

Figure 70.3 **(a)** A 4-year-old patient with a large tense, erythematous mass on the right side of the face, diagnosed as macrocystic lymphatic malformation with hemorrhage and infection. **(b)** A large amount of blood caused by previous bleeding was extracted during the operation. **(c)** Sclerotherapy using ethanol and bleomycin was used to treat the lesion. After one sclerotherapy treatment, the lesions were significantly reduced.

REFERENCES

1. Dasgupta R, Adams D, Elluru R et al. Noninterventional treatment of selected head and neck lymphatic malformations. *J Pediatr Surg.* 2008;43:869–873.
2. Tempero RM, Hannibal M, Finn LS et al. Lymphocytopenia in children with lymphatic malformation. *Arch Otolaryngol Head Neck Surg.* 2006;132:93–97.
3. Manning SC, Perkins J. Lymphatic malformations. *Curr Opin Otolaryngol Head Neck Surg.* 2013;21:571–574.
4. Perkins JA, Tempero RM, Hannibal MC et al. Clinical outcomes in lymphocytopenic lymphatic malformation patients. *Lymphat Res Biol.* 2007;5:169–174.
5. Segado Arenas A, Flores González J-C, Rubio Quiñones F et al. [Severe iatrogenic airway obstruction due to lingual lymphangioma]. *Arch Pediatr.* 2011;18:983–986.
6. Mulliken JB, Burrows PE, Fishman SJ. *Mulliken and Young's Vascular Anomalies: Hemangiomas and Malformations.* Oxford, UK: Oxford University Press; 2013.
7. Wagner KM, Lokmic Z, Penington AJ. Prolonged antibiotic treatment for infected low flow vascular malformations. *J Pediatr Surg.* 2018;53:798–801.
8. Dowling M, Ellis T. A sudden pain in the neck: An atypical presentation of cystic lymphangioma. *BMJ Case Rep.* 2015;2015:bcr2015209505.
9. Garzon MC, Huang JT, Enjolras O et al. Vascular malformations: Part I. *J Am Acad Dermatol.* 2007;56: 353–370; quiz 371–354.
10. Wiegand S, Eivazi B, Zimmermann AP et al. Microcystic lymphatic malformations of the tongue: Diagnosis, classification, and treatment. *Arch Otolaryngol Head Neck Surg.* 2009;135:976–983.
11. Marler JJ, Mulliken JB. Current management of hemangiomas and vascular malformations. *Clin Plast Surg.* 2005;32:99–116, ix.
12. Arneja JS, Gosain AK. An approach to the management of common vascular malformations of the trunk. *J Craniofac Surg.* 2006;17:761–766.
13. Chaudry G, Guevara CJ, Rialon KL et al. Safety and efficacy of bleomycin sclerotherapy for microcystic lymphatic malformation. *Cardiovasc Intervent Radiol.* 2014;37:1476–1481.
14. Yang X, Jin Y, Lin X et al. Management of periorbital microcystic lymphatic malformation with blepharoptosis: Surgical treatment combined with intralesional bleomycin injection. *J Pediatr Surg.* 2015;50:1393–1397.
15. Hammer J, Seront E, Duez S et al. Sirolimus is efficacious in treatment for extensive and/or complex slow-flow vascular malformations: A monocentric prospective phase II study. *Orphanet J Rare Dis.* 2018;13:191.

71

How should aggressive chyloreflux (e.g., chyluria, chyloascites, chylothorax, chyle leakage) be handled?

CRISTOBAL M. PAPENDIECK AND MIGUEL A. AMORE

Chyle is a milky appearing fluid formed exclusively through the jejunoileal epithelium during food digestion as a part of normal fatty acid metabolism. Daily chyle volume depends exclusively on intake, and on epithelial jejunoileum competence.

The chyle is transported by two transit segments, one between the intestine and the cisterna chyli (Pequet), and another from the cisterna chyli through the thoracic duct to the left subclavian-internal jugular vein confluence shared with the systemic interstitial lymph. The lymph in transit through the thoracic duct represents only 20% of chyle lymph and depends on the amount of the intake.

Chyle is rich with triglycerides, long-chain amino acids, lipoproteins, and liposolubile vitamins as well as white blood cells, especially T lymphocytes. Therefore, chylorrhea will deplete serum levels of protein, lymphocytes, and fat-soluble vitamins, resulting in immune dysfunction through loss of immunoglobulins and lymphocytes besides a metabolic acidosis by the electrolyte imbalances. Chylous leaks always means malnutrition or undernutrition. This is the reason for a need for medical treatment with the first therapeutic step being a diet.[1]

The term *chylous reflux* represents the abnormal direction of the chyle flow, either backward (backflow) or forward through other directions (diverted flow), thus appearing in various conditions of chylorrhea (chyle leakage) through the fistulas (lymphangiectasia), through capillary microcystic malformations (lymphangiomatosis), or through mesothelium (pleura, peritoneum) or epithelium (intestinal mucosa, skin), or as a collection in cavities. Most commonly, chyle leakage is into the peritoneal cavity (chylous ascites) or pleural space (chyloperitoneum). But the leakage also results in chyluria (chyle in the urine), chyloptysis (chyle in the sputum), chylopericardium, or cutaneous chyle leakage[1,2] (Figures 71.1 through 71.4).

Chyle leakage can occur in the prenatal as well as postnatal, pediatric, and adult populations with age-related etiological correlation. For example, in adults, chyle leaks are more commonly related to underlying malignancy.

Pleural effusion of the lymph at the prenatal age may cause pulmonary hypoplasia, while postnatal pleural effusion may precipitate respiratory failure, as well as chylous ascites. Bronchopulmonary lymph/chylous effusion always cause some degree of respiratory failure (e.g., lymphangioleiomyomatosis). It may present as malnutrition if it occurs at the intestinal mucosa level as in the case of primary intestinal lymphangiectasia (Waldmann disease).[1–3]

Furthermore, percutaneous or transmucosal leaks can cause a severe psychosocial disability, especially if they occur at the genital or perineal area, mediastinum, or bones (phantom bone disease: Gorham–Stout syndrome), or they can be part of malignant disease when associated with angiosarcoma (Gorham–Stout–Haferkamp disease).

Lymph leakage through the intestinal mucosa leads to exudative enteropathy. It can be local, regional, or systemic, and the severity of the disease depends on its extension. Chyle leak into the intestinal lumen means the presence of a single or multiple fistulas.

Chyle collection always means a functional disorder of the compromised area. For this reason, it also requires treatment in pediatric patients according to its functional implications (e.g., elevation of the diaphragm due to chylous ascites and respiratory compromise, joint disability) as well as compromise of the general and psychosocial conditions (e.g., mega-genitals; periungual, genital, lingual chylorrhea; etc.). The specific diet does not prevent malnutrition. Therefore, it is temporary treatment with a limited role. It does not correct the functional alteration, among other aspects, which is why it must be complemented with other treatments (e.g., octreotide). Diagnostic steps lead, in

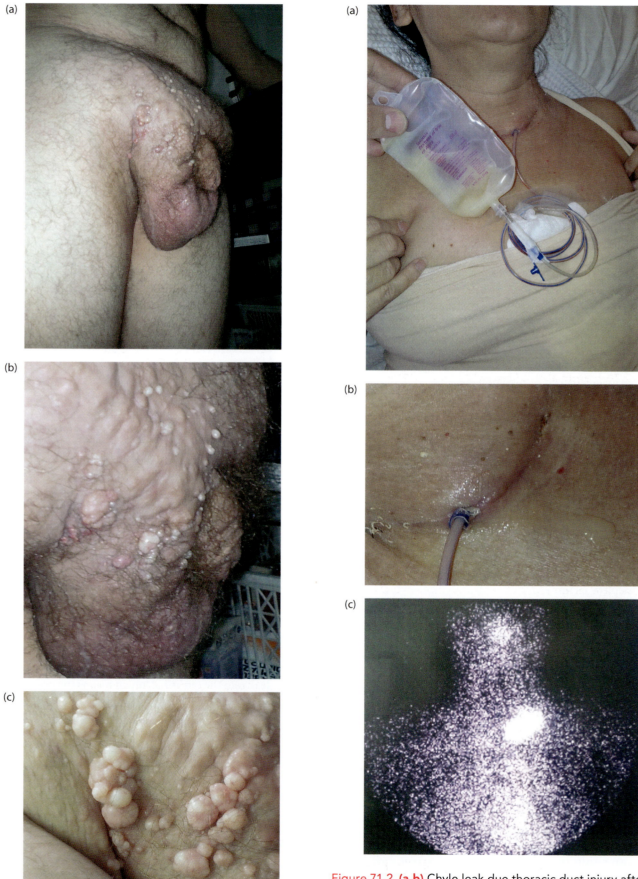

(a)

(b)

(c)

(a)

(b)

(c)

Figure 71.1 **(a,b,c)** Genital chylous fistulas.

Figure 71.2 **(a,b)** Chyle leak due thoracic duct injury after cervical lymphadenectomy. **(c)** Lymphoscintigraphy. Tracer accumulation on left the cervical region.

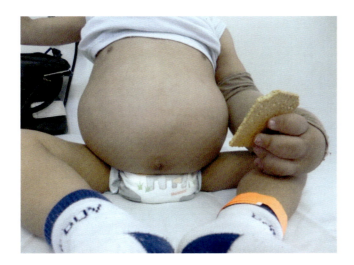

Figure 71.3 Chylous ascites. Upper and lower limb primary lymphedema.

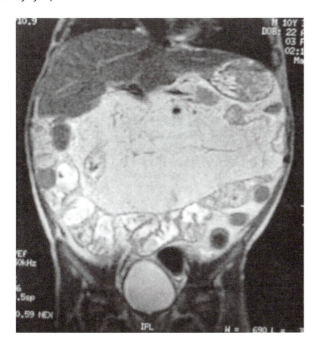

Figure 71.4 Computed tomography (CT) scan demonstrates chylous ascites—chylo-scrotum.

the majority of pediatric patients, to the diagnosis of the level of chyle lymph loss, which generally leads to a surgical treatment.[1]

TREATMENT STRATEGY

The general treatment strategy for chylous reflux/chylorrhea should be based on a dietary regimen to reduce the fatty acid metabolism with appropriate modification of enteral nutrition with either a nonfat or a low-fat diet and medium-chain triglycerides. Total parenteral nutrition with bowel rest may be considered as an additional option for chyle leaks when indicated. As mentioned earlier, if such nutritional measures alone are not sufficient, additional medical

(e.g., octreotide, sirolimus) or surgical interventions should be considered.[1]

The drainage of accumulated chylous fluid is an adjunctive management to surgical treatment. Thoracentesis and paracentesis can relieve symptoms of respiratory failure, but tube thoracostomy is often indicated to obtain continuous drainage. Video-assisted thoracic surgery (VATS) is a technique to allow necessary intervention to manage chylous leakage based on the amount and location of output of the

(a)
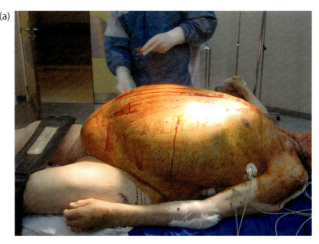

(b)
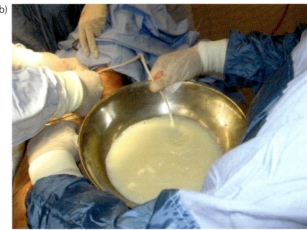

(c)
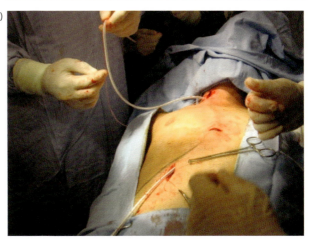

Figure 71.5 (a) Chylous ascites. (b) Chylous ascites drainage. (c) Peritoneo-venous shunt (Denver).

(a)

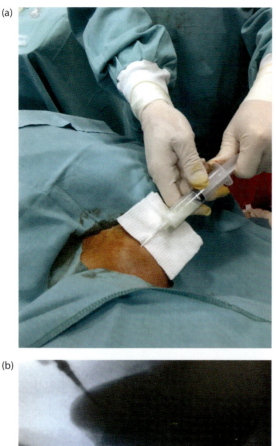

(b)

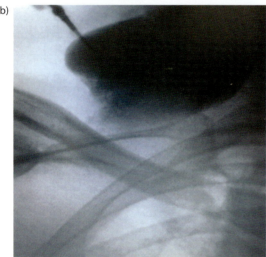

Figure 71.6 **(a)** Cervical chylous cyst—drainage. **(b)** Cervical chylous cyst—sclerotherapy with bleomycin.

chylous leak. Pleural abrasion and pleurodesis with talc or other agents are effective when output measured through a chest tube is less than 500 mL/day. Fibrin glue can be used when no focal drainage point can be determined with diffuse drainage. Partial pleurectomy is another option to resolve symptoms. However, the ligation of the thoracic duct is often indicated for high-output chylous drainage exceeding 1 L/day, either by VATS or thoracotomy. Alternatively, coil embolization of the thoracic duct may be performed through the cannulation of the cisterna chyli. The Denver pleuroperitoneal shunt has also been used for extreme cases of chylothorax.[1,3]

Chylous ascites is also indicated for percutaneous embolization of retroperitoneal lymphatics, which is preferred as the first-line therapy for symptomatic chylous ascites.

(a)

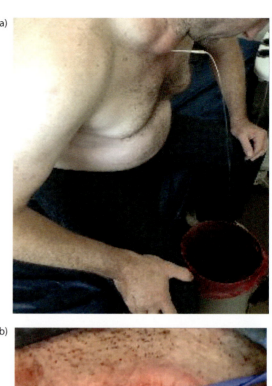

(b)

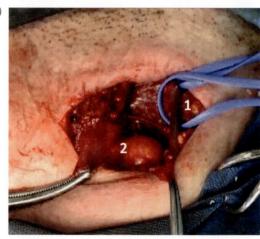

(c)

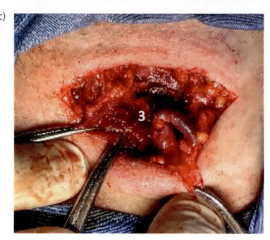

Figure 71.7 **(a)** Right cervical chylous cyst drainage. **(b)** Right cervical chylous cyst. Surgery (1) external jugular vein (2) chylous cyst. **(c)** Chylous cyst—venous anastomosis (3).

However, it requires various combinations of the treatment, following the diagnostic puncture, with intermittent drainage by serial paracentesis, a specific diet with MCT, and octreotide. But if it persists, it requires surgical intervention; a complementary option is a peritoneal-venous shunt (e.g., Degni and Le Veen bypass valves and Denver shunt), shunting the fluid from the peritoneal cavity to the internal or external jugular vein. They should not be used before the age of 7–10 years, and the possible coagulation alteration should be controlled judiciously. They give only an interim temporary solution but do not solve the pathology[1,4] (Figure 71.5).

The cutaneous manifestation of chyle reflux in the external genitalia, thigh, or trunk can be managed first with various sclerosing agents directly injecting to precipitate obliterative lymphangitis: tetracycline, doxycycline, alcohol, polidocanol, OK-432, and bleomycin. The excision of a lymphatic malformation lesion is often the most ideal way to relieve the symptoms caused by cutaneous chylorrhea, including the skin, bowel, thorax, and abdomen (Figure 71.6).

The ideal surgical solution is to reconstruct damaged lymphatics with microsurgical techniques to restore the lymphatic flow by microsurgical anastomoses between lymphatics and veins bypassing disrupted or malformed lymphatics. Therefore, primary chyle leak to pleura, peritoneum, or pericardium, due to dysplasia of the chyle circuit, requires a lymphovenous bypass (e.g., VATS). If the leak is secondary to the surgery (e.g., cardiovascular surgery for the coarctation of the aorta or tricuspid atresia; Fontan operation), the collection must be drained first, and if it persists, a ligation of the thoracic duct or its bypass to the venous system (e.g., azygos vein) should be considered in addition to the pleurodesis with talc and the use of octreotide.[1]

Collections of chyle lymph in preexisting cysts or as an associated anomaly can be sclerosed (Bleomycin, OK431), diverted to the venous system (cysto-venous anastomosis: Amore-Papendieck operation) (Figure 71.7), or resected if possible. In multiple or extensive septated lesions, the indication is currently systemic rapamycin or possibly sildenafil. This consideration is especially valid for Gorham–Stout syndrome, Waldmann disease, and lymphangioleiomyomatosis.[5]

REFERENCES

1. Papendieck CM, Amore MA. Treatment strategy on chylolymphatic/lymphatic reflux. In: Young Wook K, Byung Boong L, Wayne Y, Young SD, eds. *Congenital Vascular Malformations*. New York, NY: Springer; 2017:355–362.
2. Papendieck CM, Amore MA. Treatment strategy on neonatal and infant CVMs. In: Young Wook K, Byung Boong L, Wayne Y, Young SD, eds. *Congenital Vascular Malformations*. New York, NY: Springer; 2017:349–367.
3. Bellini C, Cabano R, De Angelis LC et al. Octreotide for congenital and acquired chylothorax in newborns. A systemic review. *J Paediatr Child Health*. 2018;54:840–847.
4. O'Brien B, Kesby BG, Ogle R et al. Treatment of primary fetal hydrothorax with OK 431(Picibanil) outcome in 14 fetuses and a review of the literature. *Fetal Diagn Ther*. 2015;37:259–266.
5. Amore MA, Papendieck CM. Cyst-Venous anastomosis for the treatment of recurrent cervical chylous cyst. Oral communication presented at: European Congress of Lymphology; September 20–22, 2018; Prague, Czech Republic.

72

Pharmacological considerations for lymphatic malformation management

STANLEY G. ROCKSON

The often inexorable growth and expansion of lymphatic vascular malformations results in substantial morbidity and, in some cases, premature death of these patients. The clinical course is punctuated by infection and dysfunction of various organ systems. In some of these syndromes, severe coagulopathy and hemorrhage are typical, recurrent features. Meaningful therapeutic interventions have been avidly sought; in recent years, these desperately needed advances have derived both from *in vitro* insights[1] and from human clinical trial experience.[2]

Vascular endothelial growth factors (VEGFs) exert the major regulatory influence on lymphatic endothelial cell function and the process of lymphangiogenesis. *In vitro* investigation of the VEGFC/VEGFR3 signaling pathway in lymphatic endothelial cells has disclosed the fact that VEGFC induces activation of PI3K/Akt and MEK/Erk. The PIK3CA/ AKT/mTOR and RAS/MAPK/MEK pathways interact and exert mutual regulation through cross-inhibition and cross-activation. The importance of PI3K in VEGF-C/VEGFR-3– mediated lymphangiogenesis provides a potential therapeutic target for lymphatic overgrowth and, coupled with additional vital *in vivo* human observations, has led to a new era of pharmacological intervention for such patients.

Overactivation of the PI3K/AKT/mTOR or the RAS/ MAPK/MEK pathway leads to dysregulation of normal cellular functions, resulting in cellular proliferation, survival advantage, and angiogenesis, and is thought to be the driver for the development and/or progression of lymphatic and other vascular anomalies.[3] Somatic mutations that lead to inappropriate activation of the PI3K/AKT/mTOR pathway have been shown to result in tissue overgrowth in association with vascular anomalies.

Sirolimus is a specific and potent inhibitor of mTOR, a serine/threonine kinase in the PI3K/AKT pathway that regulates cellular catabolism and anabolism, cell motility, angiogenesis, and cell growth.[4] Initial compassionate use of this mTOR inhibition in the setting of vascular malformation led to the organization of a prospective phase 2 clinical trial to assess the safety and efficacy of orally administered sirolimus in the treatment of complicated vascular anomalies.[2] Using pharmacokinetically guided dosing, sirolimus trough levels were maintained between 10 and 15 ng/mL. The primary outcome measure was the efficacy of sirolimus by the end of course (EOC) six defined by complete or partial response (CR/PR) and the incidence of toxicities and/or infection-related death.

In this paradigm-setting clinical trial, 85% of the patients who completed 12 courses of treatment had a partial response at EOC 12. The trial participants comprised several categories of lymphatic malformation, including microcystic lymphatic malformation ($n=5$); generalized lymphatic anomaly (GLA) ($n=7$); Gorham–Stout disease (GSD) ($n=3$); kaposiform lymphangiomatosis (KLA) ($n=7$); capillary lymphatico/venous malformation ($n=13$); and abnormalities of the central conducting lymphatic channels ($n=3$).[2] Many of these patients experienced improvement in clinical symptoms and quality of life whether or not improvement was noted radiologically.[2] A systematic review of 20 published studies of the treatment of lymphatic malformations with sirolimus has recently been published, supporting drug responsiveness in the majority of treated patients.[5] More recent experience with the drug suggests that low-to-intermediate dose sirolimus (levels <8 ng/mL) can be used for symptomatic relief, with high-dose sirolimus interventions (levels >8 ng/mL) to be employed for patients with aggressive or life-threatening vascular malformations.[3] Topical sirolimus has also been successfully employed to control lymphorrhea and bleeding in those patients with lymphatic malformation who experience cutaneous manifestations.[6–8]

Complex lymphatic malformations also appear to respond favorably to mTOR inhibition. In GLA and GSD, sirolimus has been shown to improve, or at least stabilize, the major manifestations of the disease, with reduction in pleural and pericardial effusions, and bone involvement and with resultant improvement in mobility.[2,9–11]

Sirolimus has also been successfully employed in KLA, either as monotherapy or in combination with steroids and/or vincristine. Here, in addition to its general salutary effects on the lymphatic malformations, it helps to stabilize the coagulopathy and reduce hemorrhage.[2,12,13]

Therapeutic inhibition of mTOR expression has utility in the *PIK3CA*-related overgrowth spectrum (PROS) as well. A recent publication details a postnatal murine model of PROS/CLOVES (congenital, lipomatous, overgrowth, vascular malformations, epidermal nevi, and spinal/skeletal anomalies and/or scoliosis) that partially recapitulates the human disease.[14] The model was useful to demonstrate the efficacy of *PIK3CA* inhibition, in this case with BYL719/alpelisib, in preventing and improving organ dysfunction. On the basis of the model's prediction, 19 patients with PROS (8 with PROS/CLOVES) were treated with the drug, with symptomatic improvement in all patients.

By extension, this treatment approach also has merit for Klippel–Trenaunay syndrome (KTS), now known as capillary lymphatic venous malformation. KTS is thought to belong functionally to PROS, as it is characterized by vascular malformation accompanied by variable overgrowth of soft tissue and bone. Somatic *PIK3CA* mutations have been identified in these patients. In KTS, sirolimus has been observed to have salutary effects on pain, function, and quality of life[2,5,15]; of particular note here is observation that the greatest benefits seem to be enjoyed by those patients who have a significant lymphatic component.[3]

One hypothetical consideration in the context of the therapeutic use of sirolimus, a potent immunosuppressive agent, is the risk of new neoplastic events. Overgrowth syndromes are known, in general, to predispose to embryonal cancers and therefore merit surveillance.[16] However, based on a recent evaluation of self-reports from affected families, along with review of the extant literature, the risk of embryonal cancer, other than Wilms tumor, in children with KTS does not appear to be higher than in the general population.[17]

REFERENCES

1. Coso S, Zeng Y, Opeskin K, Williams ED. Vascular endothelial growth factor receptor-3 directly interacts with phosphatidylinositol 3-kinase to regulate lymphangiogenesis. *PLOS ONE.* 2012;7:e39558.
2. Adams DM, Trenor CC, 3rd, Hammill AM et al. Efficacy and safety of sirolimus in the treatment of complicated vascular anomalies. *Pediatrics.* 2016;137:e20153257.
3. Adams DM, Ricci KW. Vascular anomalies: Diagnosis of complicated anomalies and new medical treatment options. *Hematol Oncol Clin North Am.* 2019; 33:455–470.
4. Huber S, Bruns CJ, Schmid G et al. Inhibition of the mammalian target of rapamycin impedes lymphangiogenesis. *Kidney Int.* 2007;71:771–777.
5. Wiegand S, Wichmann G, Dietz A. Treatment of lymphatic malformations with the mTOR inhibitor sirolimus: A systematic review. *Lymphat Res Biol.* 2018;16:330–339.
6. Ivars M, Redondo P. Efficacy of topical sirolimus (rapamycin) for the treatment of microcystic lymphatic malformations. *JAMA Dermatol.* 2017;153:103–105.
7. Garcia-Montero P, Del Boz J, Sanchez-Martinez M, Escudero Santos IM, Baselga E. Microcystic lymphatic malformation successfully treated with topical rapamycin. *Pediatrics.* 2017;139(5). doi: 10.1542/peds.2016-2105
8. Le Sage S, David M, Dubois J et al. Efficacy and absorption of topical sirolimus for the treatment of vascular anomalies in children: A case series. *Pediatr Dermatol.* 2018;35:472–477.
9. Cramer SL, Wei S, Merrow AC, Pressey JG. Gorham–Stout disease successfully treated with sirolimus and zoledronic acid therapy. *J Pediatr Hematol Oncol.* 2016;38:e129–e132.
10. Dvorakova V, Rea D, O'Regan GM, Irvine AD. Generalized lymphatic anomaly successfully treated with long-term, low-dose sirolimus. *Pediatr Dermatol.* 2018;35:533–534.
11. Ricci KW, Hammill AM, Mobberley-Schuman P et al. Efficacy of systemic sirolimus in the treatment of generalized lymphatic anomaly and Gorham–Stout disease. *Pediatr Blood Cancer.* 2019;66:e27614.
12. Fernandes VM, Fargo JH, Saini S et al. Kaposiform lymphangiomatosis: Unifying features of a heterogeneous disorder. *Pediatr Blood Cancer.* 2015;62:901–904.
13. Safi F, Gupta A, Adams D, Anandan V, McCormack FX, Assaly R. Kaposiform lymphangiomatosis, a newly characterized vascular anomaly presenting with hemoptysis in an adult woman. *Ann Am Thorac Soc.* 2014;11:92–95.
14. Venot Q, Blanc T, Rabia SH et al. Targeted therapy in patients with PIK3CA-related overgrowth syndrome. *Nature.* 2018;558:540–546.
15. Vlahovic AM, Vlahovic NS, Haxhija EQ. Sirolimus for the treatment of a massive capillary-lymphaticovenous malformation: A case report. *Pediatrics.* 2015;136:e513–e516.
16. Rao A, Rothman J, Nichols KE. Genetic testing and tumor surveillance for children with cancer predisposition syndromes. *Curr Opin Pediatr.* 2008;20:1–7.
17. Blatt J, Finger M, Price V, Crary SE, Pandya A, Adams DM. Cancer risk in Klippel–Trenaunay syndrome. *Lymphat Res Biol.* 2019. doi: 10.1089/lrb.2018.0049 [ePub ahead of print]

73

How much different should the management of lymphangioma among the pediatric/neonatal age group be?

CRISTOBAL M. PAPENDIECK AND MIGUEL A. AMORE

Lymphangioma is a benign cystic vascular lymphatic malformation that can present as a single or multiple, micro or macro, uni- or multilocular, simple or mixed (hemo-lymphangioma) lesion. If it is multiple, it can be called *lymphangiomatosis* (Figure 73.1).

Macro-, uni-, or multilocular, cystic lesions are most frequently in the neck, supraclavicular, submaxillary, parathyroid, and nuchal regions. The most frequently affected sites are in the following order: armpits, chest, mediastinum, and intra-abdominal. They can be in all solid organs. The least frequent one is intramuscular, and it is rare in bone, where it must be assessed as a part of Gorham–Stout syndrome and other bone cystic lesions (Figure 73.2).

In all primary lymphedema, a bone cystic lesion should be ruled out as well as an eventual reflux of chyle. In overgrowth syndromes, lymphangiomas should always be ruled out in all different forms of presentation (e.g., CLOVES syndrome, Klippel–Trenaunay syndrome, etc.).

Lymphangiomas in pediatrics mean a risk for a variety of conditions due to their location, and it can present as various disorders, functional mechanical disorders, infection, intracystic hemorrhage (Kasabach–Merritt syndrome), and/or can be characterized by progressive expansion.

Lymphangioma is a disease of the pediatric age, being congenital and generally easy to diagnose. Its prenatal diagnosis and eventual treatment are also possible.[1–4]

TREATMENTS

In macrocystic lymphangiomas, the first therapeutic option is percutaneous sclerotherapy with

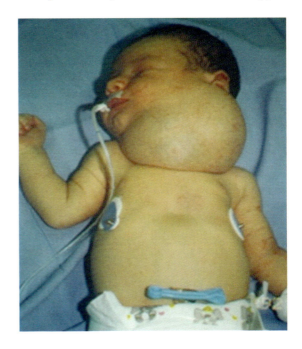

Figure 73.2 Newborn. Cervical macro multicystic lymphangioma.

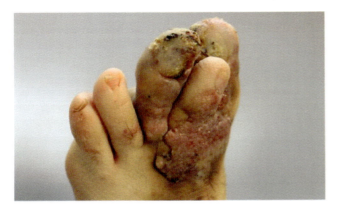

Figure 73.1 Lymphangiomatosis on toes.

bleomycin. Other sclerosing agents have also been proposed: ethanol, polidocanol, picibanil-OK 432, and doxycycline.[1,2,5]

In case of a single localized lymphangioma, surgical resection is possible, and in cases when sclerotheraphy cannot be used, other procedures like laser, lymphovenous shunt, or decompression can be considered as options[1,2,6] (Figure 73.3).

For lymphangiomas that are multicystic, microcystic, or macrocystic, and having the option of sclerosing treatment being contraindicated or exhausted, the use of systemic rapamycin or sildenafil as a second treatment option should be considered. Surgical treatment can be added along with the rapamycin as a viable option, especially in macrocystic lesions (Figure 73.4).[7] Skin lesions, if they are not surgical, can be treated with topical rapamycin.

Patients with single intraosseous lymphangiomas are good surgical candidates, and for multiple ones, rapamycin should be considered as the first option.[1,7]

Greater omentum lymphangiomas are always surgically treated; for mesentery ones, sclerotherapy and/or lymphovenous bypass can be considered (Figure 73.5).

For intestinal lymphangiomatosis, the first option is treatment with rapamycin, and as complementary treatment, if the lesion is segmental, partial surgical resection of jejunum or ileum can be considered.[7]

For retroperitoneal lymphangioma, a lymphovenous shunt should be considered first, to prevent blockage of the retroperitoneal systemic lymphatic transit.[6]

Tongue lymphangiomas can benefit from tongue-based sclerotherapy, with eventual resection and/or systemic rapamycin.[5,7]

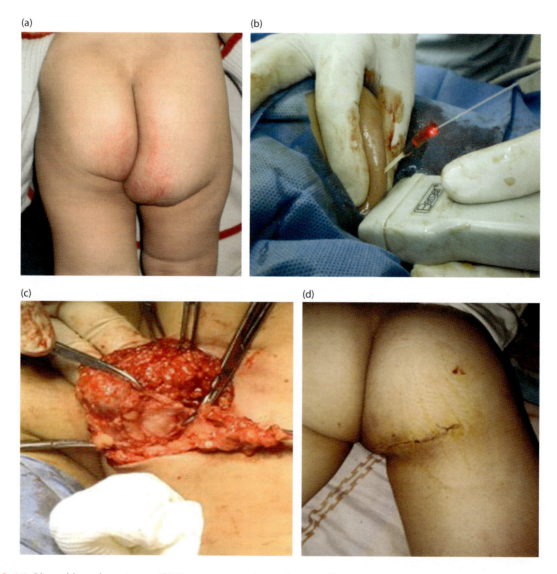

Figure 73.3 (a) Gluteal lymphangioma. (b) Percutaneous laser therapy (first step). (c) Surgery resection (second step). (d) 3 weeks' post-op.

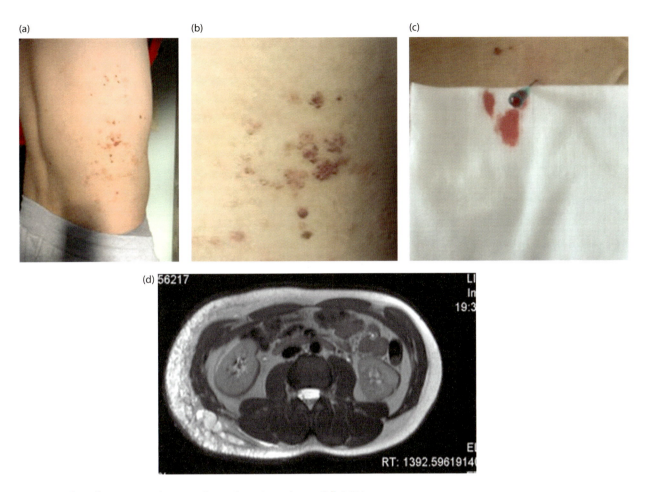

Figure 73.4 **(a,b,c,d)** Micro multicystic hemolymphangioma. **(d)** MR1.

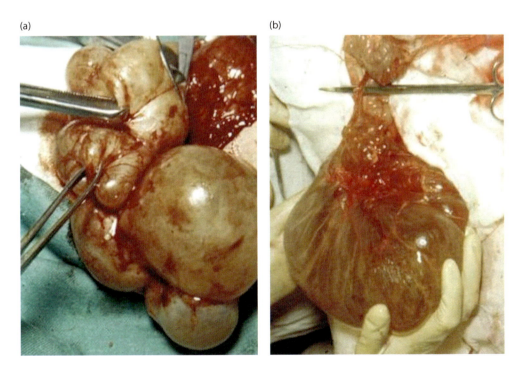

Figure 73.5 **(a,b)** Mesenteric macro multicystic lymphangioma.

REFERENCES

1. Papendieck CM, Amore MA. Treatment strategy on neonatal and infant CVMs. In: Young Wook K, Byung Boong L, Wayne Y, Young SD, eds. *Congenital Vascular Malformations*. New York, NY: Springer; 2017:349–367.
2. Papendieck CM. *Angiodysplasias in Pediatrics. Atlas Color*. Ed. Med. Bogota, Colombia: Panamericana; 1989:123–149.
3. Jones KA, Witte MH. Hereditary and familial lymphedema syndromes. In Lee BB, Bergan J, Rockson SG, eds. *Lymphedema: A Concise Compendium of Theory and Practice*. New York, NY: Springer; 2017: 29–30.
4. Alomari AL, Thiex R, Mulliken JB. Hermann Friedbergs case report and early description of CLOVEs syndrome. *Clin Genet*. 2011;78(4):342–447.
5. Cuervo JL, Galli E, Eisele G et al. Malformaciones linfáticas. Tratamiento precutaneo con bleomicina. *Arch Argent Pediatr*. 2011;1095:417–422.
6. Papendieck CM, Amore MA. Lymphovenous shunts in pediatrics. *ESL XXXV Brussels*, 2019 Abstr.
7. Wiegand S, Wichmnann G, Dietz A. Treatment of lymphatic malformations with the TOR inhibitor sirolimus. A systemic review. *Lymphatic Res Biol*. 2018;16:330–339.

74

Peculiarities in surgical treatment in childhood: Can we ignore?

JUAN CARLOS LÓPEZ GUTIÉRREZ

Nonsurgical treatment, with rapamycin and/or sclerosis, of large lymphatic malformations (LMs) in childhood is often ineffective and fails to eradicate the most important symptoms: functional impairment, deformity, intralesional bleeding, and pain. Additionally, upper airway involvement can be a life-threatening condition in neonates. In these situations, the surgical treatment of LMs should be considered with priority. Three factors are of paramount importance for treatment planning: anatomical area involved, size of the lesion, and age of the patient. However, the surgical treatment can generate important sequelae that must be considered before indicating the procedure. These complications are more common if surgery is performed in low-weight newborns (less than 2500 g) so that any procedure will be safer if performed at a later age.

Massive malformations are the candidates for early surgery. In our 35 years of experience, large debulking procedures have been more effective than repeated sclerosis or long-term sirolimus treatment (Figures 74.1 and 74.2). Each anatomical area involved deserves specific considerations.

NECK AND FLOOR OF THE MOUTH

Oral rapamycin is currently the preferred therapeutic option for LM management in the first months of life, even in premature patients, as it will eventually avoid the need for ventilatory support and tracheostomy if the response is effective.[1–3] Response to rapamycin can take up to 6 weeks. If not, the surgeon must consider that surgery in low-weight patients is indicated. Radical procedures are not recommended. Subtotal excisions of 70%–80% of the estimated malformation volume can be safely performed avoiding the need for ventilatory support and the injury of IX, X, XI, and XII cranial nerves (CNs). Sclerosis of the residual malformation will be performed several months later. Bronchoscopy is mandatory in order to evaluate tracheal mucosal involvement, as it is an indication for tracheostomy and CO_2 laser fulguration.

Facial palsy (due to CN VII injury) is a common complication if neck dissection is not performed under close nerve monitoring. Techniques for facial reanimation in patients with nerve injury are much more complex than LM treatment, so the surgeon should avoid creating a devastating problem where there was a moderate one.[4]

Malformations in the posterior aspect of the neck usually respond to sclerosis. Bleomycin is preferred in smaller lesions and doxycycline in the larger ones. If surgical resection is indicated, the spinal nerve must be preserved as shoulder motion can be severely impaired at long-term follow-up when damaged.

The tongue is frequently involved. Macroglossia with associated mucosal bleeding vesicles, halitosis, pain, and dental malocclusion must be treated early. Radiofrequency ablation, CO_2 laser fulguration, and glossectomy can be safely performed in the first years of life in order to prevent mandibular distortion and speech disorders.

ORBIT

Bleomycin sclerosis is recommended as the first therapeutic option for symptomatic orbital LMs.[5] Severe intralesional bleeding of intraconal malformations is an emergency requiring immediate decompression in order to avoid irreversible visual loss. An expert craniofacial surgery team will decide on an extra- or intracranial approach for such a procedure.

AXILLA AND TRUNK

Surgical excision can be safely performed in the first months of life in noncritical locations such as axilla, thoracic or abdominal wall, and limbs. Excision should be performed maintaining well-vascularized skin flaps. Brachial plexus dissection is unnecessary. Bleomycin sclerosis is a safer procedure for those residual cysts. The breast and nipple areola complex must be carefully preserved in order to avoid

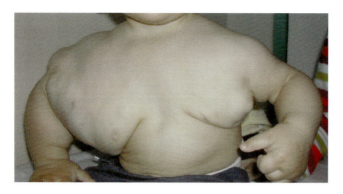

Figure 74.1 Clinical photograph *before* surgical debulking of an extensive lymphatic malformation.

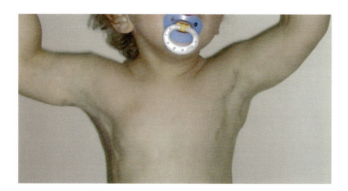

Figure 74.2 Clinical photograph *after* surgical debulking of an extensive lymphatic malformation.

future breast asymmetry and the need for reconstruction in adolescence.

Postoperative lymphatic leaks are common and must be treated by weekly percutaneous evacuation. Cosmetic scar revisions are indicated at long-term follow-up as progressive cutaneous shrinking is frequently noticed.

Capillary malformations are frequently seen in association with large LMs of the thoracic wall as a sign of *PIK3CA*-related overgrowth spectrum (PROS).[6] They never cross the anterior or the posterior midline, which is opposite the random distribution of sporadic capillary malformations of the trunk and should be included in the resection when possible as they are the origin/source of intralesional hemorrhage.

THORAX AND MEDIASTINUM

Surgery for intrathoracic LMs is rarely indicated, as respiratory distress due to airway compression is uncommon. If present, computed tomography–guided sclerosis with doxycycline can be performed. Anomalies of the thoracic duct are often associated, and chylothorax is a potential complication after surgical resection of thoracic malformation lesions needing lympho-magnetic resonance imaging (MRI) and intranodal dynamic lymphography evaluation first and thoracic duct embolization later. Symptomatic pulmonary involvement is rare and easily managed by thoracoscopic segmentectomy or lobectomy. Superior vena cava territory must be examined by ultrasound and MRI as phlebectasias and aberrant dilatations of the innominate, subclavian, and jugular veins are frequently involved as well.

ABDOMINAL CAVITY

LMs are frequently found involving the gastrointestinal tract, the retroperitoneum, and the spleen. Young children present with chronic pain due to large cysts that are better managed by ultrasound-guided sclerosis than surgically.[7,8]

Intussusception or volvulus will need urgent laparotomy. Radical resections should be avoided. The potential risks of extended procedures include severe vascular damage. Four young patients who underwent multivisceral transplants at our institution suffered mesenteric artery and celiac trunk injuries in the context of intestinal LMs excisions.

Preventive splenectomy is not indicated in young children with spleen involvement, as pain or thrombocytopenia is rarely seen. If present, the procedure should be delayed until the second decade of life.

Retroperitoneal and pelvic involvement can be associated with chyluria, uterine chylous leaks, and protein-loss enteropathy. Endovascular management is preferred, but surgical closure of abnormal leaks can be done either laparoscopically or by laparotomy.

EXTERNAL GENITALIA

Lymphedema or chylous reflux are more common than macrocystic lesions in this anatomical area. Differential diagnosis is mandatory in order to avoid mismanagement. Surgical excision and scrotal debulking can be performed in order to improve cosmetic appearance, pain, and discomfort.

Infants with severe perianal involvement develop recurrent infections and chronic constipation. Their surgical management needs a temporary sigmoidostomy. CO_2 laser fulguration of external vesicles is not effective unless deeper tissues with LM involvement are surgically excised.

UPPER LIMB

Treatment of LMs of the arm, forearm, and hand in the pediatric population is challenging. For unknown reasons, they are always located in the postaxial aspect of the limb and never in the preaxial area. Sclerosis is frequently ineffective, and intramuscular involvement is common. Surgical excision cannot be radical as function must be preserved. Staged procedures are always preferred. If the presence of veins, arteries, fat, and aberrant tissue is noticed, diagnosis of *PTEN*-hamartoma syndrome has to be considered. Phlebectasias of the basilic and cephalic veins are common; therefore, the risk of pulmonary embolism must be carefully evaluated. Preventive ligation of progressively dilated veins is recommended.

LOWER LIMB

LMs of the thigh, leg, and foot are differently managed than lymphedema. They belong in most cases to the PROS group of disorders. Asymmetry is common deserving careful follow-up in young children. Phlebectasias are nearly always present in both aberrant and normal veins. Deep venous system patency examination and endovascular closure of large dilated veins should be performed. Staged debulking procedures can help to achieve a normal limb contour.

In summary, surgical management of LMs when indicated must be performed early in life. The mortality rate of fetal diagnosed large LMs is still unacceptable and as high as 87%.[9] Prenatal treatment with sirolimus is indicated for most severe cases. In the neonatal period, there is no advantage for a "wait-and-see" policy until older age. If life-threatening conditions occur in premature babies, surgical management can be safely performed.

REFERENCES

1. Laforgia N, Schettini F, De Mattia D, Martinelli D, Ladisa G, Favia V. Lymphatic malformation in newborns as the first sign of diffuse lymphangiomatosis: Successful treatment with sirolimus. *Neonatology.* 2016;109:52–55.
2. Triana P, Miguel M, Díaz M, Cabrera M, López Gutiérrez JC. Oral sirolimus: An option in the management of neonates with life-threatening upper airway lymphatic malformations. *Lymphat Res Biol* 2019. https://doi.org/10.1089/lrb.2018.0068
3. Strychowsky JE, Rahbar R, O'Hare MJ, Irace AL, Padua H, Trenor CC 3rd. Sirolimus as treatment for 19 patients with refractory cervicofacial lymphatic malformation. *Laryngoscope.* 2018;128:269–276.
4. Balakrishnan K, Bauman N, Chun RH. Standardized outcome and reporting measures in pediatric head and neck lymphatic malformations. *Otolaryngol Head Neck Surg.* 2015;152:948–953.
5. Lagreze WA, Joachimsen L, Gross N et al. Sirolimus-induced regression of a large orbital lymphangioma. *Orbit.* 2019;38(1):79–80.
6. Luks VL, Kamitaki N, Vivero MP et al. Lymphatic and other vascular malformative/overgrowth disorders are caused by somatic mutations in *PIK3CA. J Pediatr.* 2015;166:1048–1054.
7. Madsen HJ, Annam A, Harned R et al. Symptom resolution and volumetric reduction of abdominal lymphatic malformations with sclerotherapy. *J Surg Res.* 2019;233:256–261.
8. Churchill P, Otal D, Pemberton J, Ali A, Flageole H, Walton JM. Sclerotherapy for lymphatic malformations in children: A scoping review. *J Pediatr Surg.* 2011;46:912–922.
9. Noia G, Pellegrino M, Masini L, Visconti D, Chiaradia G, Caruso A. Fetal cystic hygroma: The importance of natural history. *Eur J Obstet Gynecol Reprod Biol.* 2013;170(2):407–413.

PART 5

Combined vascular malformations: Hemolymphatic malformations/ Klippel–Trenaunay syndrome

Diagnosis

75

To what extent should diagnostic study be extended for assessment of arteriovenous malformation involvement in Klippel–Trenaunay syndrome?

MASSIMO VAGHI

Klippel–Trenaunay syndrome (KTS) represents various combinations of three different types of vascular malformations—venous malformation, lymphatic malformation, and/or capillary malformation—accompanied by variable overgrowth of soft tissue and bone as one of a combined form of vascular malformations together with Parkes Weber syndrome (PWS).

The diagnostic approach to KTS, in general, therefore, should be carried out and based on the following scheme to deal with all the vascular malformations involved with this unique condition.

The persistence of a lateral embryonal vein is one of the most common truncular venous malformations of the lower limbs according to the Hamburg classification.[1] This "forgotten" vein by Vollmar[2] may be a component of the KTS or an isolated manifestation of a vascular anomaly.

In both cases, the first diagnostic goal is to understand if it represents a pathological vein itself or a collateral circulation of a deep venous system that could be aplastic or hypoplastic. The presence and the functionality of the deep venous system represent the key for a possible treatment of the superficial vein. The marginal vein is also called the embryonal vein in the case of aplasia of the deep venous system. There is sometimes difficulty in making a differential diagnosis between KTS and PWS on clinical evaluation of the patient since the clinical picture might be similar.

Stephan Belov recommended a complete study of the venous system and in case of the presence of a embryonal vein (marginal vein with aplasia of the deep venous system) to search for the presence of a peripheral AV shunt that had to be ligated.[3] This procedure was termed a "skeletonization of the embryonal vein" (Figure 75.1) in order to reduce the blood volume in the pathological vein.[6]

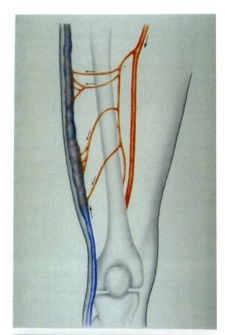
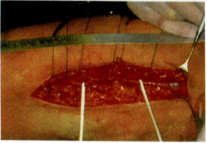

Figure 75.1 Belov technique of skeletonization of the marginal vein. (Taken from Loose D, Weber J. *Angeborene Gefaessmissbildungen*. NordlandDruck Verlag; 1997:217.)

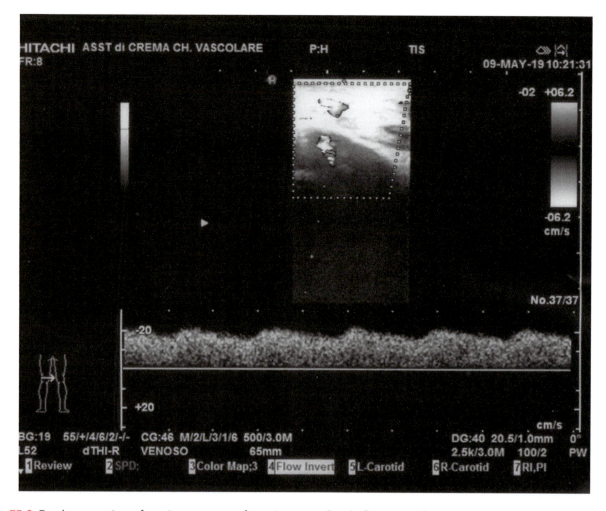

Figure 75.2 Duplex scanning of a vein: presence of continuous pulsatile flow sign of active arteriovenous shunt.

How can the presence of AV shunts be detected and their presence be localized? The presence and hemodynamical importance of AV shunts in the embryonal vein were long debated between specialists. According to Weber's arteriographic studies on 97 patients suffering from persistence of the marginal vein, AV shunts are present in 49% of patients. Of these, AV shunts were clearly demonstrated in 21% of patients and suspected in 48%.[4] In half of the cases, these shunts are hemodynamically relevant and were treated by embolization. Ultrasound examination may highlight the presence of a pulsatile venous flow, which is a clear sign of an AV shunt.[5]

On the basis of the recommendations for the study of the venous malformation, ultrasound (Figure 75.2) investigation completed with magnetic resonance imaging (MRI) and magnetic resonance angiography (MRA) is able to detect the presence and the localization of AV shunts in order to disconnect them before the marginal vein treatment. Time-resolved sequences as used in dynamic contrast-enhanced MRI (dceMRI) may allow visualization of both the arterial and venous vessels, differentiating them according to the acquisition time and the contrast

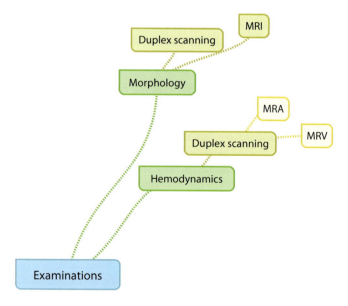

Figure 75.3 Diagnostic flowchart for the detection of arteriovenous shunts in the presence of the marginal vein of the lower limbs.

density (MIP reconstruction), and detection of the AV shunts together with the anatomy of the venous system. Angiography will be reserved for those cases in which a significant AV shunt to the marginal vein is present, with the aim to close it endovascularly (Figure 75.3).

Arteriographic studies are indicated only when we have demonstrated the presence of these shunts and we have planned a transcatheter embolization or in cases of inconclusive dceMRI. Another interesting diagnostic tool is transarterial lung scintigraphy, which has a high sensitivity in detecting AV shunts and in quantification of the shunt itself. This diagnostic method is not diffuse on the territory; it is a functional examination that can give good physiological results but no information about the localization of the pathology; as mentioned previously, it has a very high sensitivity but lack of specificity. This diagnostic modality has some value in the detection of a micro AV shunt.

The presence of significant, active, nontreated AV shunts may cause significant bleeding during marginal vein resection and a reduction of effectiveness of endovascular procedures.

REFERENCES

1. Belov St. Classification, terminology, and nosology of congenital vascular defects. In: Belov S, Loose DA, Weber J, eds. *Vascular Malformations*. Reinbek, Germany: Einhorn-Presse; 1989:25–30.
2. Vollmar J, Voss E. Vena marginalis lateralis persistens—Die vergessene Vene der Angiologen. *VASA*. 1979;8:192–202.
3. Belov St. Congenital agenesia of the deep vein of the lower extremities: Surgical treatment. *J Cardiovasc Surg*. 1972;13:594–598.
4. Weber J, Daffinger N. Congenital vascular malformations: The persistence of marginal and embryonal veins. *VASA*. 2006;35:67–77.
5. Lee BB, Antignani PL, Baraldini V et al. ISVI-IUA consensus document—Diagnostic guidelines on vascular anomalies: Vascular malformations and hemangiomas. *Int Angiol*. 2015;34:333–374.
6. Loose D, Weber J. *Angeborene Gefaessmissbildungen*. NordlandDruck Verlag; 1997:217.

76

How much should diagnostic investigations incorporate visceral involvement for Klippel–Trenaunay syndrome?

MASSIMO VAGHI

Klippel–Trenaunay syndrome is a complex vascular malformation characterized by the presence of capillary malformation, venous-truncular and extra-truncular malformation, and lymphatic malformation frequently accompanied by variable overgrowth of soft tissue and bone. Visceral involvement in Klippel–Trenaunay syndrome is not so rare, and it is known to involve almost exclusively the pelvic organs/parts (Figure 76.1) of the gastrointestinal or genitourinary system.[1–4] Usually this involvement is associated with the extension of the capillary malformation of the skin to the abdominal and thoracic wall. Therefore, when capillary malformations are present, further diagnostic workup is needed for evaluation of the visceral involvement, as mentioned earlier.

The investigations should be driven by clinical symptomatology: pain, bleeding, pleural and/or abdominal effusion, and chylous or lymphatic leakage. The hematologic involvement is often represented by anemia, which could be acute or chronic, and alteration of the clotting system characterized by elevated values of D-dimer (e.g., localized intravascular coagulation [LIC]), which represents a risk of thromboembolic or hemorrhagic complications. Therefore, a diagnostic workup including complete blood count (CBC) with coagulation labs (D-dimer and fibrinogen) should be performed in these patients (Figure 76.2).

The real incidence of the visceral pathology is variable or perhaps unknown and underestimated because the presence of the visceral pathology is evaluated only in symptomatic patients. Hematochezia is the most frequent sign and usually is related to mucosal involvement of colon segments. The lesion may be single or multiple. The extension of the colic lesion may be variable. Involvement of the bladder is also infrequently described, which can be presented as hematuria.[5] Bleeding from luminal organs is investigated by endoscopic techniques and/or imaging techniques like contrast computed tomography (CT) scan and further with magnetic resonance imaging (MRI) for the evaluation of parenchymal organs, the presence of pleural or abdominal effusion, the thickening of the intestinal mucosa, and the evaluation of the abdominal vascular system.

There is an association between the distal colic involvement by venous malformation and ectasia of the inferior mesenteric vein which may cause portal thrombosis. The intestinal symptomatology may be chronic or acute. In the chronic cases, the symptomatology is often sideropenic/iron deficiency anemia, due to occult bleeding. These patients will have positive occult blood test in the stool. In these cases, endoscopic examinations are indicated.

In case of negative examination results, the small bowel should be investigated with the aid of a microcapsule. The examination with the greatest sensitivity for intestinal bleeding is radioisotope-tagged red blood cell scintigraphy (e.g., whole-body blood pool scintigraphy), but it is not able to give the precise information of the location of the bleeding site. In case of acute bleeding, endoscopic investigations are required, because in addition to diagnostics, they allow a therapeutic approach. If the origin of the bleeding is cannot be defined with these tools, a contrast CT scan can be added for further verification of the bleeding sites, and it can be used to make a decision with regard to whether surgical intervention or endovascular therapy is indicated.[6]

The diagnostic investigation of visceral involvement of the lymphatic component of Klippel–Trenaunay syndrome is more complex. In these patients, genital involvement may be detected using lymphoscintigraphic studies. Ultrasound, CT, and MRI are useful in the diagnosis and evaluation of thoracic as well as abdominal effusion and also for detecting the presence of lymphatic or chylous cysts[7] (Figure 76.3).

Pathology and leakage from the thoracic duct may be recognized with the aid of transnodal lymphography or

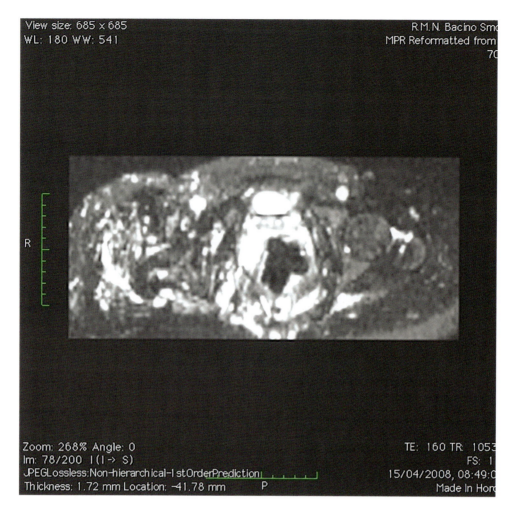

Figure 76.1 Magnetic resonance imaging demonstrating rectal involvement in patients suffering from Klippel–Trenaunay syndrome.

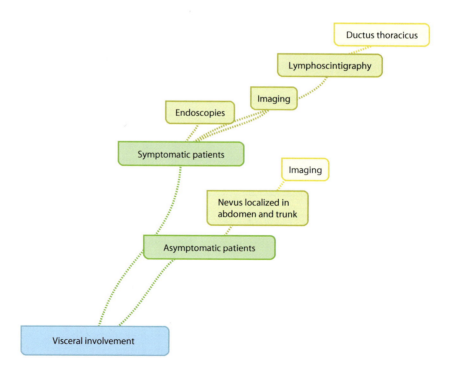

Figure 76.2 Diagnostic flowchart according to the urgency of symptomatology.

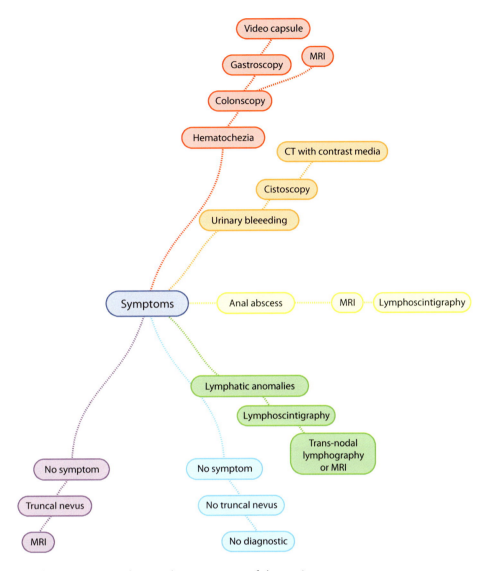

Figure 76.3 Diagnostic flowchart according to the symptoms of the patient.

transnodal MRI. The contrast medium is lipiodol for the radiographic investigation and gadolinium for MRI, which can be acquired with the angiographic sequences.

For both imaging modalities, contrast is injected into the lymph nodes at the groin bilaterally, which can be identified by ultrasound examination. Such studies are generally indicated for the cases of lymph or chylous leakage from the skin and also recurrent cellulitis in the genital area, severe dyspnea, abdominal distension, and malabsorption syndrome.

The approach to diagnose "hidden" visceral vascular anomalies should be symptoms oriented, although the presence of cutaneous capillary malformation on the trunk is often associated with an increased risk for involvement of visceral organs. However, one exception to such an approach is women in childbearing age who will get some advice based on pelvic MRI findings for the plan of pregnancy or type of delivery depending on the location of malformed vessels and their proximity to genital organs.[8]

REFERENCES

1. Thosani N, Ghouri Y, Shah S, Reddy S, Arora G, Scott LD. Life-threatening gastrointestinal bleeding in Klippel–Trenaunay syndrome. *Endoscopy.* 2013;45(Suppl 2UCTN):E206.

2. Kocaman O, Alponat A, Aygun C et al. Lower gastrointestinal bleeding, hematuria and splenic hemangiomas in Klippel–Trenaunay syndrome: A case report and literature review. *Turk J Gastroenterol.* 2009;20(1):62–66.

3. Li T, Hu SY, Chen ZT, Chen ZQ, Zhi XT. Colorectal cavernous hemangioma in Klippel–Trenaunay syndrome: A rare cause of abdominal pain and hematochezia. *Surgery.* 2015;157(2):402–404.

4. Wilson CL, Song LM, Chua H et al. Bleeding from cavernous angiomatosis of the rectum in Klippel–Trenaunay syndrome: Report of three cases and literature review. *Am J Gastroenterol.* 2001;96:2783–2788.

5. Hockley NM, Bihrle R, Bennet RM 3rd, Curry JM. Congenital genitourinary hemangiomas in a patient with Klippel–Trenaunay syndrome: Management with the neodymium:YAG laser. *J Urol*. 1989;141:940–941.

6. Strate LL, Gralnek IM. ACG clinical guideline: Management of patients with acute lower gastrointestinal bleeding. *Am J Gastroenterol*. 2016;111(4):459–474.

7. Dasgupta R, Fishman SJ. Management of visceral vascular anomalies. *Semin Pediatr Surg*. 2014;23(4):216–220.

8. Horbach SE, Lokhorst MM, Oduber CE, Middeldorp S, van der Post JA, van der Horst CM. Complications of pregnancy and labour in women with Klippel–Trénaunay syndrome: A nationwide cross-sectional study. *BJOG*. 2017;124(11):1780–1788.

Management: 1

77

How to decide priority for treatment among congenital vascular malformation components

JAMES LAREDO AND BYUNG-BOONG LEE

Optimal treatment of congenital vascular malformations (CVMs) utilizes both traditional excisional surgical therapy and minimally invasive endovascular therapy.[1,2] Endovascular therapy employing both embolization therapy and sclerotherapy is the treatment of choice for unresectable CVM lesions.[3–5] Surgical excision of CVM lesions has been shown to be more effective when combined with endovascular treatments.[1–6] The indications for treatment of CVMs are listed in Table 77.1.

TREATMENT GUIDELINES

The treatment strategy should initially focus on the primary vascular malformation, followed by treatment of secondary disorders affecting other organ systems such as the musculoskeletal and integumentary systems (e.g., limb length discrepancy).[4,5]

Correction of hemodynamic sequelae produced by the primary lesion should be given priority and often requires excisional surgery. After addressing the primary CVM, adjunctive surgery to treat the secondary disorders associated with the CVM lesion may then proceed. Examples of corrective surgery include Achilles tendon lengthening, and reconstructive surgery to correct cosmetic facial or limb deformities.[5–8]

The optimal combination of the various treatment modalities should be selected based on precise characterization of the embryological, morphological, and hemodynamic nature of the CVM lesion. When treatment is indicated, eradication of the lesion nidus is essential to prevent recurrence.[5,7–9] A controlled aggressive approach must be tempered with a realistic assessment of the long-term results of the treatment regimen.

The traditional conservative approach is recommended for the majority of CVM lesions, where most of these are venous malformations (VMs).[7–10] A typical VM lesion without bone involvement can safely be monitored until the age of 2 or more years, when the child is mature enough to tolerate the various procedures required for diagnosis and treatment.[6–8]

Earlier intervention may be required when a VM lesion produces the vascular bone syndrome, resulting in discrepancy of long bone growth, or when the lesion is located at an anatomical area threatening life, limb, or vital functions.[7–10]

SURGICAL TREATMENT

Surgical excision has long been the treatment of choice in eliminating the CVM nidus and remains the gold standard for the treatment of CVMs. Complete eradication of the nidus of CVM is required to achieve an effective cure and may often require extensive resection with significant morbidity.[1–5] Incomplete excision of the lesion nidus may be unavoidable in cases due to the prohibitively high morbidity associated with radical surgical therapy and may result in a higher likelihood of recurrence.

The traditional role of surgical excision as the first line of treatment has been replaced by endovascular therapies.[11–19] Associated with fewer complications, endovascular treatments have become the preferred approach in the treatment of patients with unresectable CVM lesions and/or patients who are high surgical risk. Combination therapy of endovascular treatments with surgical resection has resulted in significantly improved outcomes compared with surgical excision alone.[20,21] The most commonly performed endovascular procedures, embolization therapy and sclerotherapy, both enhance the safety and effectiveness of surgical excision.[11–14] Preoperative embolization and sclerotherapy of the CVM lesion can reduce the morbidity and likelihood of complications (e.g., intraoperative bleeding) associated with surgical resection.[6–8]

Table 77.1 Indications for treatment of congenital venous malformations

- Hemorrhage
- High-output heart failure (arteriovenous [AV] shunting malformation)
- Secondary ischemic complications (AV shunting malformation)
- Secondary complications of chronic venous hypertension (venous malformation)
- Lesions located at life-threatening region (e.g., proximity to the airway), or located at the region threatening vital functions (e.g., seeing, eating, hearing, or breathing)
- Disabling pain
- Functional impairment
- Cosmetically severe deformity
- Vascular-bone syndrome
- Lesions located at the region with potentially high risk of complication (e.g., hemarthrosis, deep vein thrombosis and/or pulmonary embolism)
- Lymph leak with/without infection (lymphatic malformation)
- Recurrent sepsis, local and/or general

ENDOVASCULAR TREATMENT

As mentioned earlier, endovascular treatment with embolization and/or sclerotherapy is the treatment of choice for surgically unresectable CVM lesions.[10-14] This approach is especially useful in the treatment of diffuse infiltrating extra-truncular CVM lesions and in extensive lesions that extend beyond the deep fascia with involvement of muscle, tendon, and/or bone.

Multisession endovascular therapy is the preferred approach utilizing the minimally effective volume of embolization/sclerotherapy agents during each session in order to minimize morbidity. The most commonly utilized endovascular treatment agents include sclerosants such as absolute ethanol, sodium tetradecyl sulfate (Sotradecol), and polidocanol, and embolization agents such as Onyx, N-butyl cyanoacrylate (NBCA), polyvinyl alcohol (Ivalon), and coils. These agents are often utilized in various combinations, simultaneously or in multiple stages.[11-16]

Absolute ethanol remains the sclerosing agent of choice in the treatment of extra-truncular CVM lesions, especially in situations where the lesion is surgically unresectable, such as in the diffuse infiltrating type.[11,13,14] Ethanol is the most powerful sclerotherapy agent with excellent long-term results and outcomes. It also carries the highest risk of complication and morbidity among the various sclerosing agents.[11,14]

The risk of cardiopulmonary complications during the ethanol sclerotherapy is significant, as direct ethanol exposure may produce pulmonary artery spasm and vasoconstriction with subsequent cardiopulmonary arrest. Pulmonary hypertension is potentially fatal and occurs when a significant dose of ethanol reaches the pulmonary circulation. Ethanol sclerotherapy should be performed under general anesthesia with continuous cardiopulmonary monitoring.

To minimize injury to adjacent tissues, the minimally effective dose of ethanol should be administered in divided doses over multiple treatment sessions. Ethanol can be diluted to 60% when used to treat superficial CVMs or lesions in close proximity to nerves. During sclerotherapy, residual ethanol may be drained prior to removal of needles. Direct compression of the vein draining the CVM during treatment may prevent early drainage during ethanol injection. The maximal dose of ethanol should not exceed 1 mg/kg of body weight per treatment session.[11-16]

Sotradecol is a detergent sclerosing agent that was approved for clinical use in the treatment of varicose veins by the U.S. Food and Drug Administration in 2005. It is mainly used for the treatment of varicose veins and can be administered in liquid form or as a foam preparation. Sotradecol has been shown to be efficacious in the treatment of low-flow CVMs such as VMs and lymphatic malformations (LMs).[15,17-19] Compared to ethanol, Sotradecol is equally effective in the treatment of VMs and can be safely administered without general anesthesia and does not have the deleterious effects on the pulmonary vasculature. Sotradecol is considered first-line therapy in the treatment of VMs.

NBCA glue is an embolization agent primarily used preoperatively in the treatment of surgically resectable CVM lesions. Embolization of the lesion with NBCA glue facilitates surgical dissection and helps minimize intraoperative blood loss. The glue-filled lesion can be safely identified and dissected to minimize injury to adjacent tissues.[10,12,14]

The major disadvantage of coil and/or glue embolization is that its mechanism of action is artery/vein occlusion with subsequent thrombosis without any permanent injury to the blood vessel endothelium. Recanalization of an extra-truncular CVM nidus may result in lesion recurrence.

TREATMENT OF VENOUS MALFORMATIONS

Compared to the arteriovenous malformation (AVM), VMs exhibit a relatively benign clinical course and often do not require aggressive treatment. Furthermore, the risks associated with the administration of ethanol are prohibitive in the majority of patients with symptomatic VMs. In this group of patients, sclerotherapy with Sotradecol and/or polidocanol is usually first-line therapy, leaving ethanol as the last option.[17-19]

Foam sclerotherapy[15] has gained popularity over traditional liquid sclerotherapy in the treatment of VM lesions with excellent treatment outcomes. It is especially useful in the treatment of palmar and plantar lesions with transdermal extension and in VM lesions involving the skin and mucous membranes.

TREATMENT OF ARTERIOVENOUS MALFORMATIONS

Most AVM lesions will eventually require treatment. Preoperative endovascular embolization and sclerotherapy have been shown to improve the safety and efficacy of subsequent surgical resection, resulting in significantly reduced morbidity and mortality (e.g., intraoperative bleeding).[2,3,12,13] Postoperative supplemental endovascular therapy has also been shown to be of benefit in the surgical treatment of AVMs. Precise delivery of the embolization and sclerosing agents directly into the nidus of the lesion is required for successful endovascular therapy. A combination endovascular approach where all three routes of delivery (transarterial, transvenous, and direct puncture) are utilized to obliterate the AVM lesion nidus is most efficacious.

The high-flow nature of AVM lesions makes treatment extremely challenging. It is worth emphasizing that treatment of extensive lesions is palliative and goal oriented, rather than curative. Treatment goals should be set for each patient prior to treatment. A high-flow fistulous AVM lesion should be approached with the goal to control the inflow artery and draining vein with endovascular embolization agents, followed by treatment of the lesion nidus with ethanol. Alternatively, the lesion nidus can be embolized with NBCA glue, followed by surgical excision.

REFERENCES

1. Lee BB, Villavicencio L. Chapter 68. General Considerations. Congenital Vascular Malformations. Section 9. Arteriovenous Anomalies. In: Cronenwett JL, Johnston KW, eds. *Rutherford's Vascular Surgery*. 7th ed. Philadelphia, PA: Saunders Elsevier; 2010:1046–1064.
2. Lee BB. Chapter 76. Arteriovenous malformation. In: Zelenock GB, Huber TS, Messina LM, Lumsden AB, Moneta GL, eds. *Mastery of Vascular and Endovascular Surgery*. Philadelphia, PA: Lippincott, Williams and Wilkins; 2006:597–607.
3. Lee, BB, Laredo J, Deaton DH, Neville RF. Chapter 53. Arteriovenous malformations: Evaluation and treatment. In: Gloviczki P, ed. *Handbook of Venous Disorders: Guidelines of the American Venous Forum*. 3rd ed. London, UK: A Hodder Arnold; 2009: 583–593.
4. Lee BB, Bergan J, Gloviczki P et al. Diagnosis and treatment of venous malformations—Consensus document of the International Union of Phlebology (IUP)-2009. *Int Angiol*. 2009;28(6):434–451.
5. Lee BB, Laredo J, Kim YW, Neville R. Congenital vascular malformations: General treatment principles. *Phlebology*. 2007;22(6):258–263.
6. Loose DA. Surgical management of venous malformations. *Phlebology*. 2007;22:276–282.
7. Lee BB, Bergan JJ. Advanced management of congenital vascular malformations: A multidisciplinary approach. *J Cardiovasc Surg*. 2002;10(6):523–533.
8. Lee BB. Critical issues on the management of congenital vascular malformation. *Annals Vasc Surg*. 2004;18(3):380–392.
9. Lee BB, Laredo J, Seo JM, Neville R. Chapter 29. Hemangiomas and vascular malformations. In: Mattassi R, Loose DA, Vaghi M, eds. *Treatment of Lymphatic Malformations*. Milan, Italy: Springer-Verlag Italia; 2009:231–250.
10. Lee BB. Changing concept on vascular malformation: No longer enigma. *Ann Vasc Dis*. 2008;1(1):11–19.
11. Lee BB, Kim DI, Huh S et al. New experiences with absolute ethanol sclerotherapy in the management of a complex form of congenital venous malformation. *J Vasc Surg*. 2001;33(4):764–772.
12. Lee BB, Do YS, Yakes W et al. Management of arterial-venous shunting malformations (AVM) by surgery and embolosclerotherapy. A multidisciplinary approach. *J Vasc Surg*. 2004;3:596–600.
13. Lee BB, Laredo J, Neville R. Arterio-venous malformation: How much do we know? *Phlebology*. 2009; 24:193–200.
14. Rosenblatt M. Endovascular management of venous malformations. *Phlebology*. 2007;22:264–275.
15. Lee BB, Bergan J. Chapter 12. Transition from alcohol to foam sclerotherapy for localized venous malformation with high risk. In: Bergan J, Van Le Cheng, eds. *A Textbook—Foam Sclerotherapy*. London, UK: The Royal Society of Medicine Press Ltd; 2008: 129–139.
16. Lee BB, Do YS, Byun HS, Choo IW, Kim DI, Huh SH. Advanced management of venous malformation (VM) with ethanol sclerotherapy: Mid-term results. *J Vasc Surg*. 2003;37(3):533–538.
17. Van der Vleuten CJ, Kater A, Wijnen MH, Schultze Kool LJ, Rovers MM. Effectiveness of sclerotherapy, surgery, and laser therapy in patients with venous malformations: A systematic review. *Cardiovasc Intervent Radiol*. 2014;37(4):977–989.
18. Qiu Y, Chen H, Lin X, Hu X, Jin Y, Ma G. Outcomes and complications of sclerotherapy for venous malformations. *Vasc Endovascular Surg*. 2013;47(6): 454–461.
19. Horbach SE, Lokhorst MM, Saeed P, de Goüyon Matignon de Pontouraude CM, Rothová A, van der Horst CM. Sclerotherapy for low-flow vascular malformations of the head and neck: A systematic review of sclerosing agents. *J Plast Reconstr Aesthet Surg*. 2016;69(3):295–304.
20. Lee BB. Advanced management of congenital vascular malformation (CVM). *Int Angiol*. 2002;21:209–213.
21. Mattassi R. Individual indications for surgical and combined treatment in so-called inoperable cases of congenital vascular defects. In: Balas P, ed. *Progress in Angiology*. Turin, Italy: Edizioni Minerva Medica; 1992:383–390.

78

Management of vascular bone syndrome: How aggressive and when?

JONG SUP SHIM AND YOUNG-WOOK KIM

DEFINITION

A congenital vascular malformation (CVM) affecting the lower extremity (LE) can cause bone and/or joint abnormality that can cause joint pain, early development of osteoarthritis, joint contracture, bone deformity, or leg length discrepancy (LLD), particularly in patients of growing age (Figure 78.1). Congenital vascular bone syndrome (CVBS) is defined as a LLD due to abnormal bone growth in patients with CVM.[1]

Development of LLD is attributed to either overgrowth or undergrowth of the affected limb. In clinical practice, CVBS is often diagnosed by the presence of a LLD greater than 2 cm in CVM patients.

PATHOPHYSIOLOGY

There have been case reports of LLD in patients with CVM since the nineteenth century. Among them, in 1900, Klippel and Trenaunay described cases of CVM patients with limb elongation, skin nevus (due to capillary malformation), and varicose veins (due to venous malformation).[2] Parkes Weber also described cases of patients with CVM showing limb hypertrophy and clinical signs of arteriovenous malformation (AVM).[3,4]

The earlier described conditions (Klippel–Trenaunay syndromes and Parkes Weber syndrome) have been well-known causes of limb overgrowth and hypertrophy. However, the pathology of the limb overgrowth has not yet been well explained.

In order to explain the mechanism of limb overgrowth in patients with CVM, many hypotheses have been proposed, including increased vascularity of the growth plate of the long bone, increased intramedullary small vessels, high oxygen tension, and elevated temperature.[5]

A possible relationship between CVM and bone undergrowth was also noticed much later. In 1948, Servelle and Trinquecoste[6] described two cases of patients with CVM with limb undergrowth with phleboliths and hamartomas,

and in 1949, Martorell[7] reported a case of arm undergrowth with severe bone destruction. In 1986, Belov et al.[8] described undergrowth of bone attributed to blood flow reduction in a limb.

Mechanical or hemodynamic causes may explain the undergrowth of long bones in patients with CVMs: a pressure effect on the metaphysis of long bone and decreased perfusion to the bone that can occur in an AVM lesion owing to the steal phenomenon.[9,10]

In the past, there were many animal studies attempting to explain the causes of CVBS. An overgrowth of long bones was observed in animal study when deep veins were ligated. The authors concluded that the etiology of an overgrowth of the long bone may be venous stasis rather than hyperemia at the growth plate.[11] Others performed angiography after deep vein ligation and noticed the development of multiple small areteriovenous (AV) shunts.[12,13] Based on these experiments, it was concluded that bone hypertrophy was always induced only by AV shunts, either large (macrofistula) or small (microfistula) AV fistula.

The effect of AV shunts on osteoblasts is controversial, as bone growth may be induced by high oxygen tension or by hypoxia secondary to a steal phenomenon. Recently, a relationship among the bone vasculature, bone growth, and molecules with both angiogenic and osteogenic activity has been discovered. Vascular endothelial growth factor (VEGF) can act directly on osteoblasts.[14,15]

Other known factors that influence skeletal development are growth factors such as fibroblast growth factor (FGF), transforming growth factor (TGF), bone morphogenic protein (BMP), insulin-like growth factor (IGF), and platelet-derived growth factor (PDGF).[16] The role of these molecules in the development of CVBS needs to be investigated.

CLINICAL FEATURES

CVBS can develop in all types of CVM patients.[17] It is frequently associated with clinical features of other types of

353

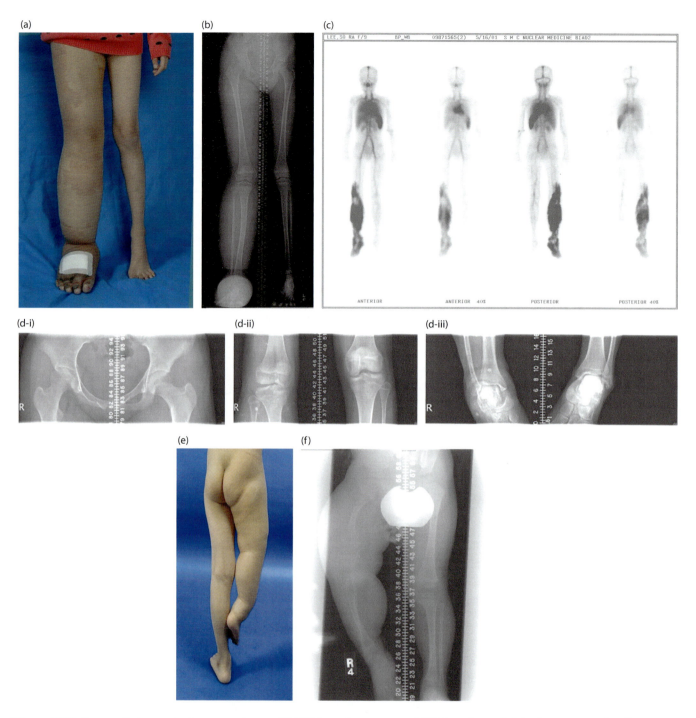

Figure 78.1 Congenital vascular bone syndrome (CVBS) in various types of CVM patients. **(a)** A photogram of a 15-year-old girl who shows right leg hypertrophy and port-wine skin spot due to mixed-type CVM syndrome combining AVM, capillary malformation (CM), and lymphatic malformation (LM). **(b)** Spot scanogram of lower extremity shows 4.8 cm of leg length discrepancy (LLD) due to overgrowth of the affected limb. **(c)** Whole-body blood pool radioscintigraphy in a 12-year-old girl with right lower leg venous malformation. **(d)** Spot scanogram shows 2.7 cm LLD due to overgrowth of the affected right leg. **(e)** A photogram of a 4-year-old boy with LM affecting the right leg. **(f)** Long bone x-ray shows 9.5 cm LLD due to undergrowth of the affected right leg.

CVM such as port-wine stain, nevus, varicosity, limb hypertrophy, intermittent episodes of leg pain, leg heaviness, joint pain or joint contracture, pathological long bone fracture, lateral scoliosis of the spine, etc. (Figure 78.2).

CVBS can cause not only physical deformity but also functional and psychosocial problems. Many studies[18–23] examining the effects of LLD have shown that minor LLDs are usually inconsequential, while discrepancies more than 2 cm (as mentioned earlier) may result in gait problems, scoliosis and pelvic tilting, consequent low back and knee contracture and pain, in addition to cosmetic dissatisfaction.

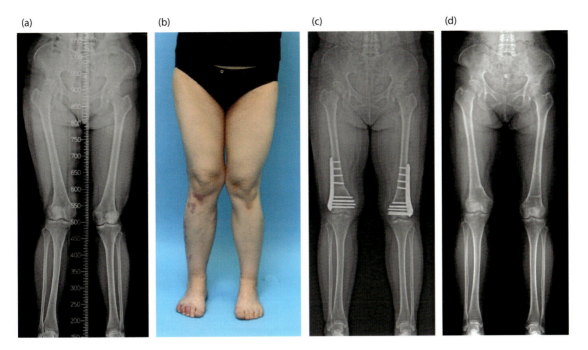

Figure 78.2 Angular deformity and leg length discrepancy (LLD) in a patient with CVM. **(a)** A long bone x-ray in a 45-year-old female patient with genu valgum deformity due to overgrowth of the right femur, both knee pain and LLD of 3 cm. **(b)** Photogram of the patient shows genu valgum deformity, pelvic tilting, and port-wine skin lesion on the right lower leg. **(c)** A long bone x-ray in the patient after corrective osteotomies at the distal femur of the both legs. **(d)** A long bone x-ray after removal of bone plates and screws shows improved genu valgum deformity and LLD at 2 years after the surgery.

TREATMENT OF LEG LENGTH DISCREPANCY IN VASCULAR BONE SYNDROME

Generally, when proper intervention to treat the vascular malformation lesions is not effective or not applicable to precipitate abnormal long bone growth, a direct intervention to the bone to modify the growth may be considered preferably as the last option to correct the length discrepancy. Simple guidelines on the major treatment options, expressed in terms of the magnitude of the predicted discrepancy, can assist in treatment decision-making (Table 78.1).

In growing pediatric patients, the goal of treatment is to prevent immobility, which occurs after the completion of growth rather than in the growing limb. The above principles should be emphasized with the flexibility to adapt to the needs of patients, the environment, motivation, and understanding of the patients, as well as the etiology of LLD. For example, such operation as "leg-lengthening operation" is too risky to imply to the patient with mental defects (e.g., intellectual disability), and we offer less complex and less time-consuming operations to this subgroup of patients.

There are generally four types of treatments available for patients with LLD that include (1) shoe-lift or brace fitting, (2) long-side epiphysiodesis, (3) long-side bone shortening, and (4) short-side bone lengthening.[24,25] In case of severe LLD, the contralateral lower extremity epiphysiodesis may be performed simultaneously to reduce the amount of LLD. The indications for the treatment differ according to the LLD. Generally, patients with LLD less than 2 cm can be

Table 78.1 General guideline for treatment of patients with limb length discrepancy

Limb length discrepancy	Recommended treatment
0–2 cm	No treatment
2–6 cm	Orthotic use, epiphysiodesis, skeletal shortening
6–20 cm	Limb reconstruction (limb lengthening with or without adjunctive procedures)
>20 cm	Prosthetic fitting (with or without surgical optimization)

Source: Helanski MA, Noonan KJ. In: Weinstein SL, Flynn JM, eds. *Lovell and Winter's Pediatric Orthopaedics.* 7th ed. Philadelphia, PA: Wolters Kluwer; 2014:1341–1387.

treated nonsurgically, and shoe lift can be used as needed. When LLD is between 2 and 6 cm in length, epiphysiodesis is a good option for patients in their growing age. However, a bone shortening or bone lengthening operation can also be considered in adult patients. The bone lengthening operation is a good option for patients with LLD of greater than 6 cm. For patients with LLD greater than 20 cm, prosthetic treatment is usually considered. In addition to these general rules, age, height of the patient, and soft tissue condition of the affected limb should be considered in choosing an optimal treatment strategy for those patients with CVBS. For example, the bone lengthening procedure can be performed for patients with short stature even though LLD is less than 3–4 cm. Also, a soft tissue condition in the affected limb is another important factor to determine which treatment to perform for patients with CVBS. A soft tissue condition should include the vessels, nerves, muscle, and skin altogether, so that if there is any doubt of the elasticity of the muscle and skin in particular, and if it is not sufficient enough to afford such a leg-lengthening operation, we offer different types of surgery to correct LLD:

1. Shoe correction is usually indicated for patients who are not indicated for surgical treatment and can calibrate the shoe by inserting a 1 cm-high insole. However, LLD of 2–4 cm should be corrected by raising the heel outside of the shoe.

2. Epiphysiodesis is performed only for patients who are at growing age. This operation is usually indicated when final LLD is expected to be 2–6 cm after completion of the long bone growth. For the epiphysiodesis, it is critical to determine an optimal timing of the operation by calculating the expected bone growth (growth calculation).[26,27] Several methods of growth calculation have been reported by various authors. The most widely used methods are the Anderson and Green growth remaining method,[28] the Mosley straight-line graph method,[29] and the multiplier method.[30] After determining the optimal time for surgery, surgical methods of epiphysiodesis should be considered. The epiphysiodesis can usually be performed at the proximal tibial epiphyseal plate, distal femoral epiphyseal plate, or at both sites of the growth plates. The selection of epiphysiodesis procedure depends on the soft tissue condition (e.g., vascular malformation, etc.) around the knee, the remaining growth, and the

expected final LLD.[31] When there is a serious CVM lesion around the knee area of the affected limb, epiphysiodesis should be avoided due to risk of vascular injury. The advantages of the epiphysiodesis include more cosmetic than other type of surgery due to small scars, short hospital stay, fast recovery time, and low cost.[32] However, this operation can be performed based on the future prediction of remaining bone growth, which may be inaccurate.[24] And this operation aims to reduce the growth of the longer leg, so the final height of the patient will be shorter. Open permanent fusion of the epiphyseal plate was developed by Phemister.[33] Several methods using small skin incisions were introduced recently. The percutaneous epiphysiodesis is an effective method to stop the long bone growth by drilling and curettage of the epiphyseal plate through a small skin incision (Figure 78.3).[34–36] A temporary stopping of the long bone growth can be achieved by percutaneous epiphysiodesis using transphyseal screws (Figures 78.4 and 78.5), metal staple fixation (Figure 78.6), or growth inhibition using an 8-plate.[37,38] When it is uncertain to determine an optimal timing of epiphysiodesis with growth calculation, temporarily stopping the growth plate can be performed, expecting its advantage to avoid overcorrection. However, this requires a skin incision and a secondary procedure to remove the implant. Additionally, it may be followed by abnormally accelerated (rebound phenomenon) or delayed bone growth after removal of the internal fixation apparatus. Therefore, the growth suppression procedure that temporarily stops the growth plate is more often used in an angular deformity correction.

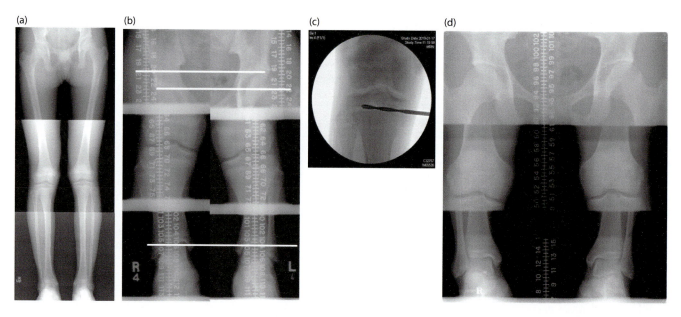

(a)   (b)   (c)   (d)

Figure 78.3 Percutaneous epiphysiodesis for a 12-year-old girl with congenital vascular bone syndrome (CVBS). **(a)** A long bone x-ray of the lower extremity in a 12-year-old female patient with CVM affecting the left leg that resulted in the overgrowth of the femur and the tibia. An expected final leg length discrepancy (LLD) was calculated to be 3.5 cm between the two legs. **(b)** Lower extremity scanogram shows LLD of 2 cm due to an overgrowth of the left leg. **(c)** Percutaneous epiphysiodesis of the left distal femur and the proximal tibia was performed. **(d)** At 4 years after the operation, lower extremity scanogram showed that LLD was completely corrected at her age of 16 years.

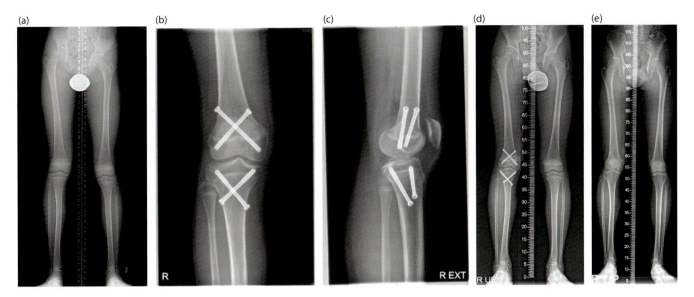

Figure 78.4 Epiphysiodesis by percutaneous epiphysiodesis using transphyseal screws (PETS) for a patient with Klippel–Trenaunay syndrome (KTS). **(a)** On a long bone x-ray of a 12-year-old girl with KTS showed 3 cm overgrowth of the right femur. The expected final leg length discrepancy (LLD) was calculated to be 4.7 cm. **(b,c)** PETS was performed at the distal femoral and the proximal tibial epiphyseal plates. **(d)** At 1 year after the operation, LLD was decreased to 2 cm. **(e)** At 3 years after the operation, lower extremity long bone scanogram showed no LLD in her age of 16 years.

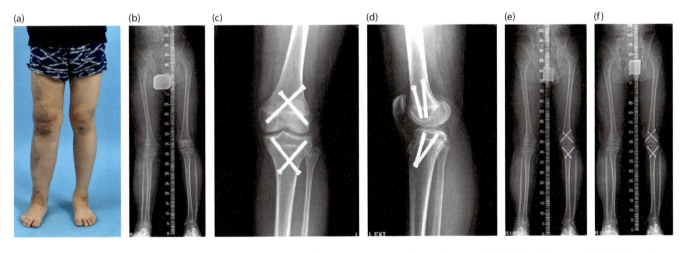

Figure 78.5 Epiphysiodesis by percutaneous epiphysiodesis using transphyseal screws (PETS) (undergrowth in Klippel–Trenaunay syndrome [KTS]). **(a)** A photogram of 12-year-old boy with KTS showing right leg hypertrophy and brown-colored skin spots at the lateral aspect of the right lower extremity. **(b)** A long bone x-ray of the patient showed undergrowth of the affected limb by 3.5 cm and an expected final LLD was calculated to be 5.5 cm. **(c,d)** PETS was performed in the epiphyseal plate of the distal femur and the proximal tibia of the left side. **(e)** On a long bone x-ray at 1 year after the operation, LLD decreased to 3.2 cm. **(f)** On a long bone x-ray at 2 years after the operation, LLD decreased to 2.3 cm. The patient is still growing, so we expect that the LLD will be further reduced until the time when long bone growth is finished.

If reduction of the tibial length of 2 cm or more is required, a concomitant proximal fibular epiphysiodesis should be performed.[24]

3. Bone shortening is usually indicted for adult patients who have missed an optimal operation time for epiphysiodesis and have already completed bone growth.[39] It has a relatively simple, short duration of treatment, and is a relatively safe procedure compared to the bone lengthening operation. However, when there is a severe vascular malformation lesion around the operation site of the bone surgery, the bone shortening operation is not the preferred method.[39] In that situation, a bone lengthening operation of the normal leg (shorter leg) is recommended. Approximately 5–6 cm length of the femur or 3–4 cm length of the tibia can be shortened without leaving loss of muscle function (Figure 78.7).[24] Femur shortening is technically easier to perform than tibial shortening. When major tibial shortening is required, it is recommended to shorten the tibia to maintain the same level of both knee joints. When bone shortening is performed in patients with KTS, soft tissue management should be done very carefully to avoid excessive bleeding, infection,

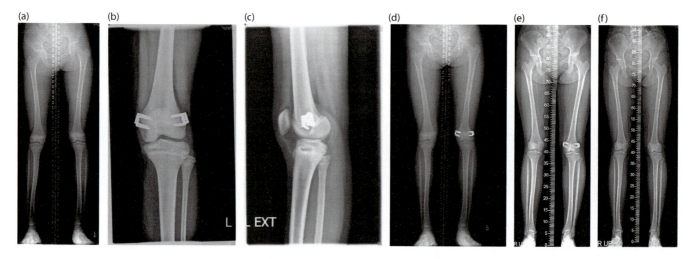

Figure 78.6 Epiphysiodesis by staples. **(a)** A long bone x-ray in a 11-year-old female patient with left leg congenital vascular malformation (CVM) showed overgrowth of left femur by 4 cm. An expected final leg length discrepancy (LLD) was calculated to be 5.7 cm. **(b,c)** Epiphysiodesis by staples was performed in the distal femur, and percutaneous epiphysiodesis was performed in the proximal tibia of the affected leg. **(d)** Long bone x-ray at 1 year after the operation shows LLD decreased to 2.7 cm. **(e)** Long bone x-ray at 3 years after the operation shows no LLD in her age of 14 years. **(f)** The staples were removed at the age of 15 years. No LLD is shown on final x-ray of the patient.

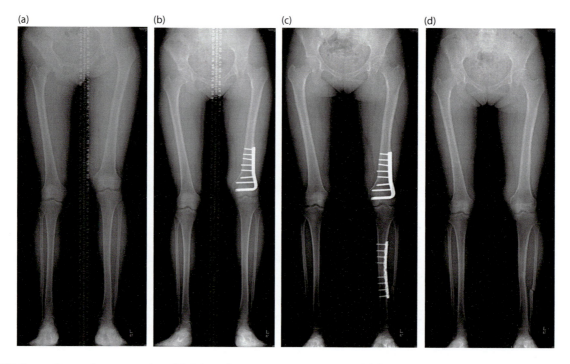

Figure 78.7 Bone shortening operation. **(a)** A long bone x-ray in a 22-year-old female patient revealed left leg hypertrophy and overgrowth by 7 cm due to CVM. **(b)** At the first-stage operation, femoral shortening of 4 cm was performed at the left distal femur. **(c)** At 6 months after the first operation, left tibio-fibular shortening of 3 cm was performed as the second-stage operation. **(d)** At 1 year after the second-stage operation, the bone plate and the screws were removed as the third-stage operation. The patient recovered without complication. A long bone x-ray showed no leg length discrepancy.

or impaired wound healing. At the femur, the bone shortening procedure is usually performed at the distal part of the osteotomy to promote healing of the osteotomy site, which gives little effect on the strength of the quadriceps muscle or range of motion of the knee joint.[40]

4. A bone lengthening operation is an operation to adjust the lengths of both legs by lengthening the normal leg.

The gradual bone lengthening by distraction osteogenesis is possible after an operation with application of a special instrument (Ilizarov apparatus, etc.).[41] The advantage of this method is an increase of height. However, many complications may develop following this procedure, including infection and deformation of the pin, large scar, inconvenience due to the attached

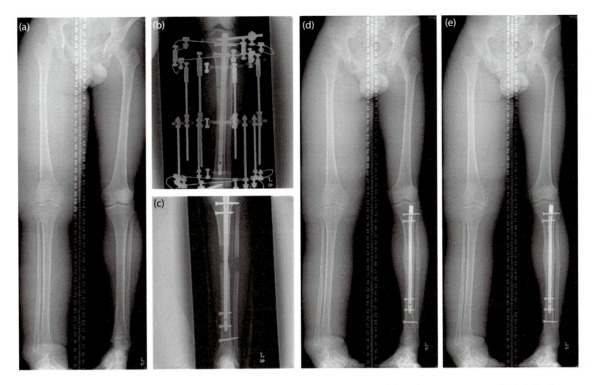

Figure 78.8 Bone lengthening operation. **(a)** A long bone x-ray in a 25-year-old male patient revealed right lower extremity hypertrophy and 6 cm of leg length discrepancy (LLD) due to KTS (venolymphatic malformation). **(b,c)** Bone lengthening operation at the left tibia was performed by lengthening over intramedullary (IM) nailing (LON) technique. **(d)** Five-centimeter lengthening of the tibia and fibula were available without complication. **(e)** At 1 year after the operation, the IM nail was removed. On a long bone x-ray, LLD was reduced from 6 to 1 cm.

apparatus, and long duration of the treatment.[41,42] Additionally, the bone lengthening operation cannot be performed on the pathological site of the leg due to the risk of serious complications, such as bleeding, infection, and delayed bone formation, which can result in delayed bone healing or bone defect catastrophe.[24,42] Therefore, the bone lengthening operation should be performed on the normal leg. Though it is theoretically possible to lengthen the leg 10 cm or more, this carries a higher risk of complication when the bone lengthening is greater than 20% of the original length.[42]

Considering the advantages and disadvantages of each procedure, surgeons should thoroughly discuss with a patient and/or parents/guardians regarding all treatment options and expected complications of each surgical procedure.

Recently, a modified, gradual bone lengthening procedure using a new surgical technique and instruments has been introduced to shorten the treatment duration and reduce the complication rate (Figure 78.8).[43–46]

REFERENCES

1. Mattassi R, Vaghi M. Vascular bone syndrome—Angio-osteodystrophy: Current concepts. *Phlebology*. 2007;22(6):287–290.
2. Klippel M, Trenaunay P. Du naevus variqueux et osteo-hypertrophique. *Arch Gen Med*. 1900;3:641–672.
3. Weber FP. Haemangiectasic hypertrophies of the foot and lower extremity. Congenital or acquired. *Presse Med*. 1908;15:261–266.
4. Weber FP. Haemagiectasis hypertrophy of limbs. Congenital phlebarteriectasis and so called congenital "varicose veins." *Br J Child Dis*. 1918;15:13–17.
5. Kelly PJ, Janes JM, Peterson LFA. The effect of arteriovenous fistulae on the vascular pattern of the femora of immature dogs, a microangiographic study. *J Bone Joint Surg Am*. 1959;41:1101–1108.
6. Servelle M, Trinquecoste P. Des angiomes veineux (about venous angiomas). *Arch Mal Couer*. 1948;41:436–438.
7. Martorell F. Hemangiomatosis braquial osteolítica. *Angiologia*. 1949;1:219.
8. Belov St, Loose DA, Müller E. *Angeborene GefäXfehler (Congenital vascular defects)*. Reinbeck, Germany: Einhorn Presse Verlag; 1986:35–37.
9. Janes JM, Musgrove JE. Effect of arteriovenous fistula on growth of bone; an experimental study. *Surg Clin North Am*. 1950;30(4):1191–1200.
10. Mattassi R. Differential diagnosis in congenital vascular-bone syndromes. *Semin Vasc Surg*. 1993;6(4):233–244.
11. Servelle M. Stase veineuse et croissance osseuse (venous stasis and bone growth). *Bull Acad Natl Med*. 1948;132:471–474.
12. Soltesz L. Contribution of clinical and experimental studies of the hypertrophy of the extremities in congenital arteriovenous fistulae. *J Cardiovasc Surg*. 1965;260.

13. Brookes M, Singh M. Venous shunt in bone after ligation of the femoral vein. *Surg Gynecol Obstet.* 1972;135(1):85–88.

14. Zelzer E, McLean W, Ng YS et al. Skeletal defects in VEGF(120/120) mice reveal multiple roles for VEGF in skeletogenesis. *Development.* 2002;129(8):1893–1904.

15. Deckers MM, van Bezooijen RL, van der Horst G et al. Bone morphogenetic proteins stimulate angiogenesis through osteoblast-derived vascular endothelial growth factor A. *Endocrinology.* 2002;143(4):1545–1553.

16. Carano RA, Filvaroff EH. Angiogenesis and bone repair. *Drug Discov Today.* 2003;8(21):980–989.

17. Kim YW, Lee SH, Kim DI, Do YS, Lee BB. Risk factors for leg length discrepancy in patients with congenital vascular malformation. *J Vasc Surg.* 2006;44(3):545–553.

18. Gofton JP. Persistent low back pain and leg length disparity. *J Rheumatol.* 1985;12(4):747–750.

19. Grundy PF, Roberts CJ. Does unequal leg length cause back pain? A case-control study. *Lancet.* 1984;2(8397):256–258.

20. Soukka A, Alaranta H, Tallroth K et al. Leg-length inequality in people of working age. The association between mild inequality and low-back pain is questionable. *Spine.* 1991;16(4):429–431.

21. Gross RH. Leg length discrepancy: How much is too much? *Orthopedics.* 1978;1(4):307–310.

22. Vitale MA, Choe JC, Sesko AM et al. The effect of limb length discrepancy on health-related quality of life: Is the "2 cm rule" appropriate? *J Ped Orthop-B.* 2006;15(1):1–5.

23. DiMeglio A, Canavese F, Charles YP. Growth and adolescent idiopathic scoliosis: When and how much? *J Ped Orthop.* 2011;31(1 Suppl):S28–S36.

24. Helanski MA, Noonan KJ. Leg-length discrepancy. In: Weinstein SL, Flynn JM, eds. *Lovell and Winter's Pediatric Orthopaedics.* 7th ed. Philadelphia, PA: Wolters Kluwer; 2014:1341–1387.

25. Stanitski DF. Limb-length inequality: Assessment and treatment options. *J Am Acad Orthop Surg.* 1999;7(3):143–153.

26. Shapiro F. Developmental patterns in lower-extremity length discrepancies. *J Bone Joint Surg Am.* 1982;64(5):639–651.

27. Lee SC, Shim JS, Seo SW et al. The accuracy of current methods in determining the timing of epiphysiodesis. *Bone Joint J.* 2013;95-B(7):993–1000.

28. Anderson M, Green WT, Messner MB. Growth and predictions of growth in the lower extremities. *J Bone Joint Surg Am.* 1963;45:1–14.

29. Moseley CF. A straight-line graph for leg-length discrepancies. *J Bone Joint Surg Am.* 1977;59(2):174–179.

30. Paley D, Bhave A, Herzenberg JE et al. Multiplier method for predicting limb-length discrepancy. *J Bone Joint Surg Am.* 2000;82(10):1432–1446.

31. Menelaus MB. Correction of leg length discrepancy by epiphyseal arrest. *J Bone Joint Surg Br.* 1966;48(2):336–339.

32. Canale ST, Christian CA. Techniques for epiphysiodesis about the knee. *Clin Orthop Relat Res.* 1990;255:81–85.

33. Phemister DB. Operative arrestment of longitudinal growth of bones in the treatment of deformities. *J Bone Joint Surg.* 1933;15(1):1–15.

34. Borowski A, Bajelidze G, Bowen JR. Hypertrophy associated with vascular malformations: Analysis of growth and results of epiphysiodesis. *Orthopedics.* 2018;41(4):e574–e579.

35. Ghanem I, Karam JA, Widmann RF. Surgical epiphysiodesis indications and techniques: Update. *Curr Opin Pediatr.* 2011;23(1):53–59.

36. Edmonds EW, Stasikelis PJ. Percutaneous epiphysiodesis of the lower extremity: A comparison of single-versus double-portal techniques. *J Pediatr Orthop.* 2007;27(6):618–622.

37. Metaizeau JP, Wong-Chung J, Bertrand H et al. Percutaneous epiphysiodesis using transepiphyseal screws(PETS). *J Pediatr Orthop.* 1998;18(3):363–369.

38. Sinha R, Weigl D, Mercado E et al. Eight-plate epiphysiodesis. *Bone Joint J.* 2018;100-B(8):1112–1116.

39. Kenwright J, Albinana J. Problems encountered in leg shortening. *J Bone Joint Surg Br.* 1991;73(4):671–675.

40. Barker KL, Simpson AH. Recovery of function after closed femoral shortening. *J Bone Joint Surg Br.* 2004;86(8):1182–1186.

41. Ilizarov GA. The tension-stress effect on the genesis and growth of tissues. Part I. The influence of stability of fixation and soft-tissue preservation. *Clin Orthop Relat Res.* 1989;238:249–281.

42. Paley D. Problems, obstacles, and complications of limb lengthening by the Ilizarov technique. *Clin Orthop Relat Res.* 1990;(250):81–104.

43. Park HW, Yang KH, Lee KS et al. Tibial lengthening over intramedullary nail with use of the Ilizarov external fixator for idiopathic short stature. *J Bone Joint Surg Am.* 2008;90(8):1970–1978.

44. Oh CW, Song HR, Kim JW et al. Limb lengthening with submuscular locking plate. *J Bone Joint Surg Br.* 2009;91(10):1394–1399.

45. Schiedel FM, Pip S, Wacker S et al. Intramedullary limb lengthening with the intramedullary skeletal kinetic distractor in the lower limb. *J Bone Joint Surg Br.* 2011;93(6):788–792.

46. Horn J, Hvid I, Huhnstock S et al. Limb lengthening and deformity correction with externally controlled motorized intramedullary nails: Evaluation of 50 consecutive lengthenings. *Acta Orthop.* 2019;90(1):81–87.

79

How aggressively should varicose veins be managed in Klippel–Trenaunay syndrome?

SERGIO GIANESINI AND ERICA MENEGATTI

KLIPPEL–TRENAUNAY SYNDROME VENOUS HEMODYNAMIC IMPAIRMENT

Lower limb varicose veins represent one of the venous malformation components of the Klippel–Trenaunay syndrome (KTS), together with lymphatic as well as capillary malformations (port-wine stains) and soft-tissue/bone hypertrophy.[1]

In this context, abnormal venous structures, often described as "varicosities," are usually located on the lateral aspect of the limb and can be associated with deep venous system abnormalities, such as hypoplasia, aplasia, or aneurysmal dilation.[2]

Typically, these varicose vessels are directly connected with the iliofemoral tract, potentially representing alternative drainage routes in case of deep venous system hypoplasia or aplasia.

Up to 68% of these cases are represented by remnants of the lateral marginal vein, also known as "persistent sciatic vein" or "lateral marginal vein."[3]

In patients with KTS, Yamaki et al. reported the great saphenous vein reflux in 20% of cases, while small saphenous vein and marginal vein reflux were found in 7% and 15% of subjects, respectively. In this study population, a venous dysplasia, aplasia, and hypoplasia was identified in 20% of cases.[4]

In addition to atypical leg veins, identified in up to two-thirds of patients with KTS,[2] superficial and deep veins can also undergo aneurysmal dilation because of congenital wall weakness and/or persistently increased ambulatory venous pressure.[5]

Venous involvement in KTS affects the superficial, deep, and perforating system simultaneously in up to 64.7% of cases.[3]

Lower limb venous impairment is a common cause of symptomatology and, in particular, pain for KTS patients. The symptoms are associated with venous reflux, thrombosis, and calcification caused by localized intravascular coagulation (LIC) among the venous malformations.[6]

STRATEGIC MANAGEMENT OF KLIPPEL–TRENAUNAY SYNDROME VENOUS DISORDERS

Considering the KTS pathophysiological complexity, a multidisciplinary diagnostic and therapeutic approach is necessary and needs to be developed in centers with expertise and experience for vascular malformations treatment.

Each patient has his or her own unique reflux pattern and disease expression so that a custom-made therapeutic plan should be made considering the patient's compliance. In this context, a typical situation is represented by the ablation of a superficial vein actually representing a bypassing drainage route in compensation of a deep system hypoplasia or aplasia (Figures 79.1 and 79.2).

Assessing the deep venous abnormality and patency before performing any procedure on the superficial system is of paramount importance. While in the past this was obtained by contrast venography, nowadays ultrasound scanning and magnetic resonance (MR) venography can easily provide the needed anatomical and hemodynamic details. Moreover, this noninvasive imaging must describe the extension and severity of the venous involvement and exclude the presence of significant arteriovenous malformations.[7]

The high sensitivity and specificity of lower extremity duplex imaging makes it the best initial diagnostic study.[8]

Magnetic resonance imaging (MRI) offers more details, including the description of soft tissues and more detailed vascular analysis by means of gadolinium contrast.[7]

A preoperative compression test of the superficial veins with ultrasonography is a fundamental test for all the potential candidates to analyze the effects of ablation on the deep system to exclude a postoperative hemodynamic overload.

If the superficial system compression leads to a mild dilation of the deep vessels on ultrasonography, but also to an increase in their flow velocity, further considerations are recommended

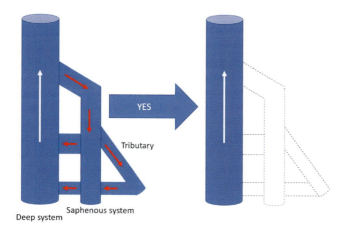

Figure 79.1 Correct indication/requirement for the incompetent great saphenous vein and/or tributary veins ablation is deep venous system patency with normally developed deep venous system.

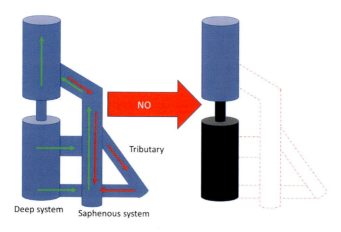

Figure 79.2 Incorrect or rather contraindication to ablate the incompetent saphenous and tributary system is "hypoplasia, aplasia, and deep vein thrombosis of deep veins." In these patients, refluxing saphenous and/or tributary veins serve as collaterals for bypassing a deep venous obstruction and provide a pathway for venous drainage of the affected extremity.

before indicating superficial vein ablation, since venous congestion of a hypoplastic deep system could occur.[9]

Before proceeding with a vein ablation in a patient with KTS, assessing the coagulation status is also fundamental. Malformed vessels are prone to develop local intravascular coagulation (LIC) as well as systemic disseminated intravascular coagulopathy (DIC) in the presence of stimulating factors such as trauma.[10]

At the same time, vascular malformation can easily bleed significantly, mostly due to an abnormal venous wall structure as an embryonic tissue remnant, so making the venous thromboembolism prophylaxis in the patients with high risk of hemorrhage is a delicate step in KTS management.[11]

In terms of timing of the venous procedure, an early correction of venous hypertension has been indicated as favorable in reducing lower limb length discrepancy and venous hemodynamic alterations.[12,13]

Early treatment of venous malformations in KTS has been reported even at 2 weeks after birth, with successful outcomes at 7 years follow-up.[14] Yet, evidence regarding the impact of venous disorders on bone growth has not been reported.

A special condition that requires even more clinical attention in KTS management is pregnancy, which is indeed usually discouraged because of the complication risk.[15]

KTS-related symptoms have been reported to worsen in 43% of pregnant women, with a deep venous thrombosis and pulmonary incidence of 5.8% and 2.3%, respectively, which is significantly higher than in healthy pregnant females.[16]

Whenever planning an eventual venous procedure on patients with KTS, the choice of anesthesia type requires special attention. In the case of a neuroaxial anesthesia, excluding spinal vascular malformations by MRI is fundamental. At the same time, general anesthesia requires exclusion of airways vascular malformations as well.[17]

In this contest, a laryngeal mask airway can be taken into consideration so as to minimize airway intubation trauma.

KLIPPEL–TRENAUNAY SYNDROME VARICOSE VEINS MANAGEMENT OPTIONS

Both medical and procedural approaches can be taken into consideration in patients with KTS who have symptoms and signs attributed to superficial varicose veins. The procedural option should be pursued in case of significant symptomatology and/or in advanced stages of the disease, carefully assessing the functionality of both the deep and superficial venous systems as discussed earlier, and the potential hemodynamic alterations following that the incompetent vein ablation should be prepared to manage.

MEDICAL MANAGEMENT

Considering the complexity and still not full pathophysiological comprehension of KTS, conservative management is the gold standard for the initial approach to superficial venous incompetence in the context of this malformed vessel disease.

The validity of this strategy has been demonstrated by Sung et al. with only four venous insufficiency cases out of 19 patients with KTS—17 patients with low extremity and 2 patients with upper extremity involvement—requiring an operative intervention: at 4.1 years mean follow-up, no significant adverse outcomes were reported in any of the 19 patients.[18]

A lifestyle favoring proper physical activity and graduated compression stockings use represents first-line chronic venous disease management in these patients.

Specific protocols of calf pump activation in the aquatic environment and intermittent pneumatic compression can be taken into consideration for edema control.[19]

It should be noted that diuretics should not be prescribed for lower limb edema management, and the need for anticoagulation has to be assessed for each patient, individually taking into account the coagulopathy status of each patient as determined by labs (D-dimer, fibrinogen, thrombocyte count). Patients with pain and palpable phleboliths respond well to anticoagulation therapy with low molecular weight heparin. But these patients can develop a higher postprocedural (or even intraprocedural) thrombotic risk, so making proper perioperative thrombo-prophylaxis evaluation is mandatory.[20]

Thrombotic risk in KTS should be considered in every patient, particularly in females, with regard to contraindicating the use of oral contraceptives.[2]

Plantar venous return has been identified as a major contributor in leg drainage, even representing a risk factor for venous insufficiency development.[21] Consequently, correction of limb discrepancies is helpful also in venous return optimization. While minor defects can be managed by custom-made plantar soles, major discrepancies (leg length discrepancy greater than 2 cm) require evaluation for orthopedic surgery. For more details, see Chapter 78.

INTERVENTIONAL MANAGEMENT

If there is failure to control the venous disease by conservative measures, interventional management by surgery or endovenous procedures can be considered.

In general, recurrent bleeding episodes, nonhealing venous ulcers, repeated venous thrombosis, and severe venous symptomatology represent strong indications to evaluate the feasibility of the vein ablation.

The authors' opinion is that cosmetic aims should not represent an indication to the procedure in KTS patients, considering that up to one-third of interventions can lead to complications.[11] Considering the risk of bleeding, open surgical approaches have become indicated mainly for patients not eligible for minimally invasive techniques such as endovenous thermal ablation or foam sclerotherapy. The Mayo Clinic Group, one of the most experienced in the topic, reported pain relief in 50% of patients after surgical, ligation, and stripping venous treatment, yet also reported the need for reintervention in 13 of the 49 assessed cases.[2] It is fundamental to remember that pain in KTS can be not just of venous origin, but also neuropathic; therefore, a proper clinical evaluation before proceeding with an indication to venous procedures is required.[22]

Eventual inferior vena cava filter positioning should be considered for patients at a significantly higher risk of thromboembolic perioperative complications, especially in case of extensive venous malformations representing a risk factor.[10] Even giant embryonic veins have been demonstrated to be treated successfully by proper therapeutic strategies, yet evaluating accurately the risk/benefit and including all the safety measures such as the previously mentioned filter positioning and eventual tourniquet use for bleeding risk minimization.[23] In the last 20 years, endovenous thermal

devices and foam embolization have offered the chance for a less invasive approach compared to surgery, resulting in an equally satisfying anatomical outcome.[24,25]

Transdermal lasers have also demonstrated successful results in capillary malformations associated with KTS. In particular, it should be remembered that lighter lesions in the pediatric age group respond better than darker lesions of the adult population. In this latter case, nontraditional Krypton and copper lasers can be taken into consideration.[18] Foam sclerotherapy represents a valid alternative for malformative varicose veins in close proximity with neural structures that potentially can be damaged by thermal energy or surgical resection.[26]

In conclusion, as reported in the dedicated International Union of Phlebology (IUP) consensus document, proper varicose vein treatment in KTS is feasible and associated with satisfying results, provided that a careful evaluation and selection of every specific case are previously performed.[27]

REFERENCES

1. Baskerville PA, Ackroyd JS, Lea Thomas M et al. The Klippel–Trenaunay syndrome: Clinical, radiological and haemodynamic features and management. *Br J Surg.* 1985;72:232–236.
2. Jacob AG, Driscoll DJ, Shaughnessy WJ et al. Klippel–Trénaunay syndrome: Spectrum and management. *Mayo Clin Proc.* 1998;73(1):28–36.
3. Delis KT, Gloviczki P, Wennberg PW et al. Hemodynamic impairment, venous segmental disease, and clinical severity scoring in limbs with Klippel–Trenaunay syndrome. *J Vasc Surg.* 2007;45(3):561–567.
4. Yamaki T, Konoeda H, Fujisawa D et al. Prevalence of various congenital vascular malformations in patients with Klippel–Trenaunay syndrome. *J Vasc Surg Venous Lymphat Disord.* 2013;1(2):187–193.
5. Paes EH, Vollmar JF. Aneurysm transformation in congenital venous angiodysplasias in lower extremities. *Int Angiol.* 1990;9(2):90–96.
6. Lee A, Driscoll D, Gloviczki P et al. Evaluation and management of pain in patients with Klippel–Trenaunay syndrome: A review. *Pediatrics.* 2005;115:744–749.
7. Gloviczki P, Driscoll DJ. Klippel–Trenaunay syndrome: Current management. *Phlebology.* 2007;22(6):291–298.
8. Howlett DC, Roebuck DJ, Frazer CK et al. The use of ultrasound in the venous assessment of lower limb Klippel–Trenaunay syndrome. *Eur J Radiol.* 1994;18(3):224–226.
9. Kim YW, Lee BB, Cho JH et al. Haemodynamic and clinical assessment of lateral marginal vein excision in patients with a predominantly venous malformation of the lower extremity. *Eur J Vasc Endovasc Surg.* 2007;33(1):122–127.

10. Oduber CE, van Beers EJ, Bresser P et al. Venous thromboembolism and prothrombotic parameters in Klippel–Trenaunay syndrome. *Neth J Med.* 2013; 71(5):246–252.

11. Malgor RD, Gloviczki P, Fahrni J et al. Surgical treatment of varicose veins and venous malformations in Klippel–Trenaunay syndrome. *Phlebology.* 2016; 31(3):209–215.

12. Belov S. Correction of lower limbs length discrepancy in congenital vascular-bone diseases by vascular surgery performed during childhood. *Semin Vasc Surg.* 1993;6:245–251.

13. Baraldini V, Coletti M, Cipolat L et al. Early surgical management of Klippel–Trenaunay syndrome in childhood can prevent long-term haemodynamic effects of distal venous hypertension. *J Pediatr Surg.* 2002;37:232–235.

14. Rahimi H, Hassannejad H, Moravvej H. Successful treatment of unilateral Klippel–Trenaunay syndrome with pulsed-dye laser in a 2-week old infant. *J Lasers Med Sci.* 2017;8(2):98–100.

15. Horbach SE, Lokhorst MM, Oduber CE et al. Complications of pregnancy and labour in women with Klippel–Trénaunay syndrome: A nationwide cross-sectional study. *BJOG, Int J Obstet Gynaecol.* 2017; 124(11):1780–1788.

16. Horbach SE, Lokhorst MM, Oduber CE, Middeldorp S, van der Post JA, van der Horst CM. Complications of pregnancy and labour in women with Klippel–Trénaunay syndrome: A nationwide cross-sectional study. *BJOG, Int J Obstet Gynaecol.* 2017;124(11):1780–1788.

17. Sivaprakasam MJ, Dolak JA. Anesthetic and obstetric considerations in a parturient with Klippel–Trenaunay syndrome. *Can J Anesthesia.* 2006; 53(5):487–491.

18. Sung HM, Chung HY, Lee SJ et al. Clinical experience of the Klippel–Trenaunay syndrome. *Arch Plast Surg.* 2015;42(5):552–558.

19. Gianesini S, Tessari M, Bacciglieri P et al. A specifically designed aquatic exercise protocol to reduce chronic lower limb edema. *Phlebology.* 2017;32(9): 594–600.

20. Kihiczak GG, Meine JG, Schwartz RA et al. Klippel–Trenaunay syndrome: A multisystem disorder possibly resulting from a pathogenic gene for vascular and tissue overgrowth. *Int J Dermatol.* 2006;45(8):883–890.

21. Uhl JF, Gillot C. Anatomy of the foot venous pump: Physiology and influence on chronic venous disease. *Phlebology.* 2012;27(5):219–230.

22. Meijer-Jorna LB, Breugem CC, de Boer OJ et al. Presence of a distinct neural component in congenital vascular malformations relates to the histological type and location of the lesion. *Human Pathol.* 2009; 40:1467–1473.

23. Rathore A, Gloviczki P, Bjarnason H. Management of giant embryonic vein in Klippel–Trénaunay syndrome. *J Vasc Surg Venous Lymphat Disord.* 2018;6(4):523–525.

24. Clinical Practice Guidelines for Klippel–Trenaunay syndrome. Boston Children's Hospital [Internet]. 2016. Available from https://k-t.org/assets/images/content/BCH-Klippel–Trenaunay-Syndrome-Management-Guidelines-1-6-2016.pdf

25. Frasier K, Giangola G, Rosen R et al. Endovascular radiofrequency ablation: A novel treatment of venous insufficiency in Klippel–Trenaunay patients. *J Vasc Surg.* 2008;47(6):1339–1345.

26. Gianesini S, Menegatti E, Tacconi G et al. Echo-guided foam sclerotherapy treatment of venous malformation involving the sciatic nerve. *Phlebology.* 2009;24(1):46–47.

27. Lee BB, Baumgartner I, Berlien P et al. Diagnosis and treatment of venous malformations. Consensus document of the International Union of Phlebology (IUP): Updated 2013. *Int Angiol.* 2015;34(2):97–149.

80

How aggressive should management be of indolent stasis ulcer in Klippel–Trenaunay syndrome?

SERGIO GIANESINI AND ERICA MENEGATTI

GENERAL CONSIDERATIONS

An extended analysis of chronic venous disease management in Klippel–Trenaunay syndrome (KTS) is reported in the Chapter 85. Herein, the focus is on the challenging KTS cases of indolent stasis ulcer management.

Leg ulceration remains an absolute indication for the treatment despite the fact that treatment results show variable degrees of efficacy. Approximately 20% of the population older than 80 years of age is affected either by a healed or an active venous ulceration.[1] Even more frustrating, data show approximately up to 69% recurrence rates in patients who receive the treatment. Patients' compliance with the treatment protocol and compression stockings was identified as the primary factor relating to healing and recurrent ulcerations.[2]

Despite the significant advancement in wound care, a factor that is usually underestimated in the diagnostic and therapeutic strategies is that 20% of ulcerations are actually multifactorial in their etiology.[3,4]

KTS usually involves at least both the superficial and deep venous system, eventually interesting also the perforating veins.[5]

A particularly accurate assessment of the lesion and of the underlying hemodynamic impairment is mandatory in KTS, together with an equally mindful therapeutic approach. By the definition of KTS, the venous malformation (VM) as a major vascular malformation component will combine with the lymphatic malformation (LM) together with capillary malformation (CM) to make the local hemodynamic condition more complicated.

Hence, the stasis ulcer among the KTS will often represent the combined outcome/condition of hemodynamic impact of two, VM and LM, if not three lesions, including CM, so that the stasis ulcer among the KTS warrants a thorough assessment on these three vascular malformation components altogether for appropriate management of the involved vascular malformation as well.

INDOLENT STASIS ULCERATION IN KLIPPEL–TRENAUNAY SYNDROME

Stasis ulceration of venous origin is related to the lack of calf pump ejection of the venous blood. In patients with KTS, it is first of all mandatory to verify the satisfying calf pump functionality.[6]

This aspect is crucial also for edema management, easily accumulated in case of significant VM. Moreover, avoiding the stasis of the metabolic products leads also to a more efficient wound healing process, which is usually impaired in patients with KTS.[7]

The soft tissue/bony malformations can impair the posture and the related calf pump function, thus limiting even more the healing process. An accurate evaluation should include a weight-bearing analysis and an eventual correction of significant postural defects as well.

A case report has recently showed the possibility of deep venous system reconstruction in a patient with KTS who is affected by a nonhealing leg ulcer. Despite the success of the single case, the same authors point out the need for carefully evaluating the KTS candidates for surgical procedures; indeed, a risk/benefit analysis cannot be done at the moment based on the paucity of the available literature on the topic.[8]

In 2008, Nguyen et al. reported the successful treatment of a KTS ulcer by means of antiangiogenic therapy based on an oral inhibitor of multiple receptor tyrosine kinases. The rationale is to be found in the demonstrated role in

KTS pathogenesis of VG5Q mutations for angiogenic factors, leading to VM proliferation. The case was successfully treated by the drug and showed ulcer recurrence when the drug was interrupted. Nevertheless, the same authors highlighted that the therapeutic choice was taken once all the other options failed (compression, elevation, photodynamic therapy, laser skin surgery, vein resection). No other publications were found on this topic in the following years, leaving once again the risk/benefit analysis for this therapeutic approach unanswered.[9]

In 2012, Dixit et al. reported the single case experience of a nonhealing KTS ulcer treated by helium-neon and light-emitting diode lasers.[10] The rationale is based on the possibility of stimulating the energy process of the mitochondria by targeting specific chromophores with laser wavelengths. This type of laser emission has been demonstrated to be beneficial in animal studies for ulcer healing.[11]

Nevertheless, apart from these few references, no other significant data can be found in the literature in support of such a therapeutic approach in KTS. Particular attention should be paid to the KTS patient's ulcer treatment modality of choice—to whatever surgical or laser or chemical injury could potentially trigger an angiogenic response complicating the initial condition. Until more evidence is produced on the topic, it should be reminded that angiogenesis plays a crucial role in wound healing, and the balance of this process is still unclear even in non-KTS patients.[12]

CONCLUSIONS

Complications following invasive procedure can be significant and are not rare in KTS patients. Major surgery and debulking procedures are not currently supported by strong evidence in the long term.[13]

Currently, based on limited data, a conservative approach remains preferable in KTS ulcer management. The use of appropriate graduated compression, limb elevation, and adequate lifestyle remain the pillar of this condition treatment, as already written back in 1965 by Lindenauer et al.[14]

Innovative drugs and devices can potentially offer benefits in KTS ulcer healing, but the current lack of evidence-based data urge further proper investigations before allowing a proper risk/benefit analysis.

REFERENCES

1. Cornwall JV, Doré CJ, Lewis JD. Leg ulcers: Epidemiology and aetiology. *Br J Surg.* 1986;73:693–696.
2. Langer V. Preventing leg ulcer recurrence. *Indian Dermatol Online J.* 2014;5(4):534–535.
3. Bumpus K, Maier MA. ABC of wound care. *Curr Cardiol Rep.* 2013;15(4):346.
4. Marston W. Evaluation and treatment of leg ulcers associated with chronic venous insufficiency. *Clin Plastic Surg.* 2007;34(4):717–730.
5. Volz K, Kanner C, Evans J et al. Klippel–Trenaunay Syndrome. *J Ultrasound Med.* 2016;35:2057–2065.
6. Araki CT, Back TL, Padberg FT et al. The significance of calf muscle pump function in venous ulceration. *J Vasc Surg.* 1994;20:872–879.
7. Gates PE, Drvaric DM, Kruger L. Wound healing in orthopaedic procedures for Klippel–Trenaunay syndrome. *J Pediatr Orthop.* 1996;16(6):723–726.
8. Shahbahrami K, Resnikoff M, Shah A et al. Chronic lower extremity wounds in a patient with Klippel–Trenaunay syndrome. *J Vasc Surg Cases Innov Tech.* 2019;5:45–48.
9. Nguyen S, Franklin M, Dudek A. Skin ulcers in Klippel–Trenaunay syndrome respond to sunitinib. *Transl Res.* 2008;151(4):194–196.
10. Dixit S, Maiya AG, Umakanth S et al. Closure of non-healing chronic ulcer in Klippel–Trenaunay syndrome using low-level laser therapy. *BMJ Case Rep.* 2012;2012. doi: 10.1136/bcr-2012-006226.
11. Whelan HT, Buchmann EV, Dhokalia A et al. Effect of NASA light emitting diode irradiation on molecular changes for wound healing in diabetic mice. *J Clin Laser Med Surg.* 2003;21:67–74.
12. Honnegowda TM, Kumar P, Udupa EG et al. Role of angiogenesis and angiogenic factors in acute and chronic wound healing. *Plast Aesthet Res.* 2015;2:243–249.
13. Noel AA, Gloviczki P, Cherry KJ Jr et al. Surgical treatment of venous malformations in Klippel–Trénaunay syndrome. *J Vasc Surg.* 2000;32:840–847.
14. Lindenauer SM. The Klippel–Trenaunay-Weber syndrome: Varicosity, hypertrophy and hemangioma with no arteriovenous fistula. *Ann Surg.* 1965;162:303–314.

Management: 2

81

How should aggressive gastrointestinal bleeding in Klippel–Trenaunay syndrome be handled?

MASSIMO VAGHI

The incidence of colorectal venous malformations in patients with Klippel–Trenaunay syndrome (KTS) is unknown, and it is presumed that between 1% and 12% of patients are affected.[1,2] Bleeding in patients suffering from KTS is usually located in the colon and rectum. The type of bleeding varies from occasional, chronic, acute, to life threatening. The bleeding may be associated with consumptive coagulopathy, which is related to the dimensions of the venous malformation and adds to the severity of symptoms and complexity of treatment (Figure 81.1).

In case of occasional bleeding, there is no need for therapy. The therapy may remain conservative with iron supplements and antifibrinolytic drugs as long as iron supplementation is sufficient to maintain physiological levels of hemoglobin (Hb). Interventional therapy has to be considered in cases where frequent blood transfusion is necessary and/or in case of acute, life-threatening hemorrhage.

Treatment options are substantially different between the two modalities used: one is endoscopic and another is surgical. There are also reports that demonstrated the possibility of using endovascular techniques (embolization) in the treatment of these malformations (Figure 81.2).[3–6]

Endoscopic treatment allows submucosal access to the malformation to inject sclerosants, including ethanol, or to deliver thermal energy through laser fibers in case of localized malformation lesions. Submucosal injection of sodium tetradecyl sulfate or ethanol causes fibrosis of dilated vessels and resolution of the symptomatology.[6,7]

Recently, an innovative approach with embolization of the superior hemorrhoidal arteries (similar to the treatment of hemorrhoids) achieved good results in a patient with chronic bleeding from rectal venous malformations in KTS. The bilateral coil embolization should diminish the blood flow in the ectatic veins and prevent further bleeding among the patients who were treated before with local intramucosal sclerotherapy without any clinical effects.[6]

In case of repetitive bleeding and/or acute bleeding without any response to the local therapeutic approach and/or embolization, a surgical approach should be considered. The approach should be related to the extent of vascular pathology in the bowel. The aim of the intervention is usually to treat the involved bowel segment. Usually the malformation lesion is localized in the submucosa, and submucosal sclerosing or submucosal suture should be considered. In case of multifocal involvement, a long sleeve resection of the bowel should be kept as the last option and used only as the last resort. For distal extension, mucosectomy or pull-through techniques should be considered. More extensive involvement may need complete colectomy. Anterior rectal resections may be performed laparoscopically or with open laparotomy.

All of these patients are at risk of thromboembolism by the nature of venous malformation. Therefore, adequate monitoring of vein patency by ultrasonography is mandatory as thromboembolic prophylaxis measurement. In case of deep venous thrombosis in the settings of contraindications for anticoagulation, a prophylactic inferior vena cava filter is indicated.

The aim of the therapy should be to improve quality of life. In less severe and chronic cases, iron and vitamin supplementation is necessary. In more complex cases, submucosal sclerotherapy represents the first choice of intervention. More invasive interventions are reserved for patients who do not respond to conventional sclerotherapy and also these techniques should be directed to the mucosa and submucosa in order to spare intestinal and rectal resection.

Although the transarterial embolization is not useful or indicated and brings no clinical benefit to pure venous malformation, it could be justified for consideration as an additional option for the management of rectal bleeding among patients with KTS.[8]

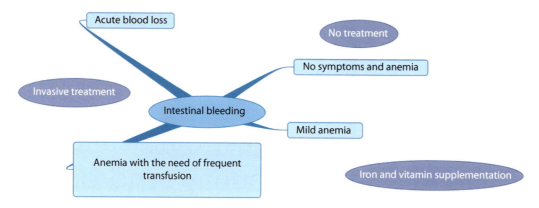

Figure 81.1 Mind mapping for the approach to intestinal bleeding in Klippel–Trenaunay syndrome.

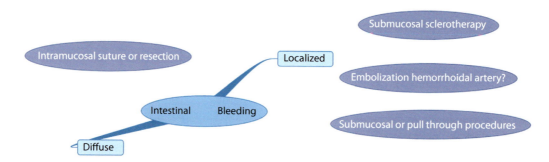

Figure 81.2 Mind mapping regarding the operative approach to intestinal bleeding in Klippel–Trenaunay syndrome.

REFERENCES

1. Morelli J. In: Kliegman RM, Behrman RE, Jenson HB, Stanton BF, eds. *Vascular Disorders. Kliegman: Nelson Textbook of Pediatrics*, 18th ed. St. Louis, MO: Saunders; 2007:2269–2270.
2. Servelle M, Bastin R, Loygue J et al. Hematuria and rectal bleeding in the child with Klippel and Trenaunay syndrome. *Ann Surg.* 1976;183:418–428.
3. Fishman SJ, Shamberger RC, Fox VL. Endorectal pull-through abates gastrointestinal hemorrhage from the colorectal venous malformations. *J Pediatr Surg.* 2000;35:982–984.
4. Natterer J, Joseph JM, Denys A. Life threatening rectal bleeding with Klippel–Trenaunay syndrome controlled by angiographic embolization and rectal clips. *J Pediatr Gastroenterol.* 2006;42(5):581–584.
5. Herman R, Kunisaki S, Molitor M, Gadepalli S, Dillman JR, Geiger J. Rectal bleeding, deep venous thrombosis, and coagulopathy in a patient with Klippel–Trénaunay syndrome. *J Pediatr Surg.* 2012; 47:598–600.
6. Kulungowski AM, Fox VL, Burrows PE et al. Porto mesenteric venous thrombosis associated with rectal venous malformations. *J Pediatr Surg.* 2010; 45:1221–1227.
7. Dasgupta R, Fishman SJ. Management of visceral vascular anomalies. *Semin Pediatr Surg.* 2014;23(4): 216–220.
8. El-Sheikha J, Little MW, Bratby M. Rectal venous malformation treated by superior rectal artery embolization. *Cardiovasc Intervent Radiol.* 2019;42: 154–157.

82

Therapeutic considerations for infection, sepsis, and lymphatic leak management in patients with Klippel–Trenaunay syndrome

JOVAN N. MARKOVIC AND CYNTHIA K. SHORTELL

Congenital vascular malformations (CVMs) associated with patients with Klippel–Trenaunay syndrome (KTS) vary in size, extent, and morbidity.[1-3] The clinical consequences and treatments of these lesions vary accordingly. In patients with KTS, vascular malformations can be prone to hemorrhage, infection, sepsis, and/or lymphatic leak.[4]

In patients with KTS who have infected malformations, it is important to recognize signs of infection early to minimize the risk of sepsis.[4] These patients should be promptly evaluated with early initiation of oral antibiotic therapy. Some KTS patients who are acutely ill may require admission to the hospital for treatment with intravenous antibiotics, which can be converted to the oral route of administration following exclusion of the risk for sepsis. Frequently, KTS patients require a prolonged course of treatment for a minimum of 3 weeks of antibiotic therapy. Infected superficial vascular lesions can be percutaneously drained followed by antibiotic treatment, which can often facilitate recovery from the infection. If feasible, cultures should be obtained prior to initiation of antibiotics to help in directing antibiotic therapy, although cultures can be negative despite signs and symptoms of infection.

In the most severe cases, infected superficial lesions can progress to bacteremia and sepsis. Therefore, KTS patients with suspected signs of cellulitis and/or phlebitis should receive early empiric antibiotic treatment with coverage effective against β-hemolytic streptococci and methicillin-sensitive *Staphylococcus aureus* (penicillin, amoxicillin, or first-generation cephalosporins).[5] In patients who do not respond to the previously mentioned antibiotic therapy, empiric coverage for methicillin-resistant *S. aureus* (MRSA) should be initiated.[6] Every effort should be taken to obtain cultures to accordingly direct antibiotic treatment, as in rare cases, atypical pathogens can be the source of infection. Gionis et al. described a case of *Escherichia coli* infection in

the lower extremity of a pediatric patient with KTS.[7] The antibiotic treatment should be guided according to the consult with infectious disease specialists.

In patients with recurrent skin infection, some practitioners recommend the use of prophylactic antibiotic therapy, although there are no data to support this treatment regimen. Others also suggest the use of hyperbaric oxygen delivery. However, data to support this treatment modality in patients with KTS still remain limited. In patients with KTS who are febrile and acutely ill but do not have signs and symptoms of superficial infection, it is important to determine the source of infection by obtaining a contrast-enhanced computed tomography (CT) scan. CT scan imaging should be carefully examined for any intra-abdominal and/or deep tissue abscess formation(s). It is important to emphasize that these patients should be immediately empirically treated with broad-spectrum antibiotic coverage (including the coverage for gram-negative bacteria) as described earlier, while waiting for determination of the source of infection to avoid time delay and to reduce the risk of progression to sepsis. Ultrasonography should be avoided in these cases, as ultrasonography is not highly sensitive for intra-abdominal and deep tissue lesions, and the lesions may not be apparent on ultrasonography until after the severe bacteremia develops. In addition, performing ultrasonography as a nonnecessary step may delay diagnosis. These patients should be admitted to the intensive care with continuous monitoring of vital signs and scheduled blood labs appropriate for sepsis workup. Well-localized and accessible intra-abdominal and/or deep tissue abscesses can be percutaneously drained by interventional radiology once the patient is hemodynamically stable. At this time, cultures should be obtained and the initial empirical antibiotic treatment should be substituted with an antibiotic regimen determined by culture sensitivity. Huskins et al. described four patients with KTS with gram-negative enteric bacteremia who presented acutely ill without signs of superficial infection.[8] One of these patients had a persistent, recurrent *E. coli* infection suggestive of persistent focal abscess as a source of infection.[8]

In the experience from the Mayo Group that included 252 patients with KTS (116 male patients [46%] and 136 female patients [54%]) ranging in age from birth to 83.4 years (median age 11.9), data showed that patients who had recurrent infection of digits were successfully treated with amputation.[3] In this study, 13% of patients with KTS had cellulitis. Amputation of affected digits or limbs was performed in 19 patients.[3] Debulking procedures were recommended only for focal and small lesions, as debulking procedures carry significant risk for damage of venous and lymphatic structures and can lead to increased edema of the affected extremity. In addition debulking is associated with scar formation, recurrence, chronic wound infection, and chronic lymphatic leak.[3]

Lymphatic leak is another complication associated with patients with KTS.[9] It is morphologically characterized by disruption of the lymphatic system architecture and is clinically characterized by the presence of leaking lymphatic fluid, superficial vascular blebs, and/or lymphedema. Lymphatic components associated with KTS are at risk for chronic leakage either due to a triggering factor or the disruption of lymphatic architecture. The treatment of lymphatic leak should be initiated to reduce the risk of complications (most commonly, decrease in functional capability, lymphangiectasia, infection, and/or lymphadenitis). Initial management of chronic lymphatic leak consists of conservative management including compression stockings and elevation of the affected extremity, along with meticulous wound care (if present). When conservative measures are inadequate, endovenous ablation with laser, radiofrequency, and sclerotherapy are indicated. Superficial, chronically leaking lymphatic blebs may be treated with ablative CO_2 laser therapy.[10] Reconstructive surgery has been described as an efficient treatment modality when performed in the "early" clinical stages. This is due to the fact that the residual lymph transporting system remains functionally salvageable, and surgical restoration and relief of lymphatic obstruction and stasis can result in revitalization of transiently paralyzed lymphatic vessels to resume normal function. It is worth emphasizing that lymphatic surgery is frequently complicated with postoperative infection that could potentially worsen an already complex clinical condition associated with patients with KTS. In addition, given that vascular malformations associated with KTS are present since birth, it is challenging to determine the "early" clinical stage, and reconstructive surgery is reserved for cases with new-onset lymphatic lymphedema caused by a triggering factor (i.e., injury, infection, another procedure). Despite the promising initial results, the role of reconstructive lymphatic surgery is confined only to the highly specialized medical centers, and it remains to be further elucidated before it can be considered as a standard of care for lymphatic disorders associated with patients with KTS. Any invasive intervention (i.e., surgical debulking, excision of the marginal vein) can be complicated by lymphatic leak in patients with KTS, especially if a malformation is extra-truncular. These patients should be carefully monitored after the procedure, as lymphatic leak may be complicated by superimposed infection that can progress to sepsis.[10]

REFERENCES

1. Gloviczki P, Driscoll DJ. Klippel–Trenaunay syndrome: Current management. *Phlebology*. 2007; 22(6):291–298. Review.
2. Baskerville PA, Ackroyd JS, Browse NL. The etiology of the Klippel–Trenaunay syndrome. *Ann Surg*. 1985;202:624–627.
3. Jacob AG, Driscoll DJ, Shaughnessy WJ et al. Klippel–Trénaunay syndrome: Spectrum and management. *Mayo Clin Proc*. 1998;73:28.
4. Gloviczki P, Stanson AW, Stickler GB et al. Klippel–Trenaunay syndrome: The risks and benefits of vascular interventions. *Surgery*. 1991;110:469–479.
5. Stevens DL, Bisno AL, Chambers HF et al. Practice guidelines for the diagnosis and management of skin and soft tissue infections: 2014 update by the Infectious Diseases Society of America. *Clin Infect Dis*. 2014;59(2):147–159.
6. Liu C, Bayer A, Cosgrove SE et al. Infectious Diseases Society of America. Clinical practice guidelines by the Infectious Diseases Society of America for the treatment of methicillin-resistant *Staphylococcus aureus* infections in adults and children. *Clin Infect Dis*. 2011;52(3):e18–e55.
7. Gionis D, Kalabalikis P, Zachariadis B et al. Hyperbaric oxygen delivery in treatment of a child with Klippel–Trenaunay syndrome complicated with a limb threatening *Escherichia coli* infection. *Intensive Care Med*. 2000;26(3):35.
8. Bird LM, Jones MC, Kuppermann N, Huskins WC. Gram-negative bacteremia in four patients with Klippel–Trenaunay–Weber syndrome. *Pediatrics*. 1996;97(5):739–741.
9. Maari C, Frieden IJ. Klippel–Trénaunay syndrome: The importance of "geographic stains" in identifying lymphatic disease and risk of complications. *J Am Acad Dermatol*. 2004;51:391.
10. Lee BB, Laredo J, Neville R. Current status of lymphatic reconstructive surgery for chronic lymphedema: It is still an uphill battle! *Int J Angiol*. 2011; 20(2):73–80.

83

How to manage coagulopathy in Klippel–Trenaunay syndrome?

ALFONSO TAFUR, EVI KALODIKI, AND JAWED FAREED

INTRODUCTION

Klippel–Trenaunay syndrome (KTS), "a capillary-lymphatic-venous malformation associated with soft tissue/skeletal hypertrophy," is a complex congenital low-flow vascular malformation frequently associated with thrombosis.[1] This propensity toward thrombotic complications anchors in the presence of venous dilatations, vessel injury, and inflammation, which is often triggered by the treatments, including sclerotherapy, surgical resection, or amputations. Moreover, a procoagulant status is recognized and described with a signature decreased protein C, protein S, and a D-dimer elevation. Thus, as expected, patients with KTS are at risk to develop venous thromboembolism (VTE), including deep vein thrombosis and pulmonary embolism. Despite the absence of data with regard to the incidence rates of thrombosis among these patients, in part due to the relative rarity of the disease, VTE is suspected to occur in between 8% and 20% of the patients with this syndrome.[2] Moreover, sequelae complications of VTE, including chronic thromboembolic pulmonary hypertension and worsening of post-thrombotic syndrome, have been described. Chronic thromboembolic pulmonary hypertension is presumed to be a consequence of recurrent pulmonary embolism secondary to the number and extent of low-flow vascular malformations. A late diagnosis of chronic thromboembolic pulmonary hypertension is believed to be a pervasive oversight among patients with KTS.[3,4] Similarly, peripheral thrombosis and phleboliths correlate with increased venous pressure and may be associated with progression of the disease. These phleboliths are attributed to the consumptive coagulopathy by localized intravascular coagulation (LIC) due to the low flow in the vascular malformation.[5,6]

Treatment guidelines for this potentially lethal complication are missing due to a paucity of evidence-based literature and clinical trials that could provide better insights into treatment and prevention strategies for VTE among patients with KTS. In this chapter, we describe pathophysiological mechanisms, describe diagnostic workup, and summarize treatment strategies.

PATHOPHYSIOLOGY

The Virchow triad, named after the eminent German physician Rudolf Virchow, is characterized by hypercoagulability, hemodynamic changes, and endothelial injury or dysfunction (Figure 83.1).[7] In a review of 75 patients, including 54 adults and 21 children, with history of KTS, Oduber and collaborators encountered that 39% of the patients had clear signs of prior VTE. These patients had elevated plasma levels of D-dimer and a tendency toward lower protein C and free protein S levels when compared to controls.[8] The presence of D-dimer, two crosslinked D fragments of fibrin, is a product of fibrin degradation and is interpreted as a sign of persistent fibrinolysis among any patients with coagulopathy. Moreover, the extent of the vascular malformation, assessed by magnetic resonance imaging (MRI), is related to the levels of these coagulopathy markers. Specifically, among 40 patients with MRI, the D-dimer levels were highest among those with extensive disease. Similarly, the extent of the disease was also correlated with elevated D-dimers in a cohort of 118 patients with venous malformation evaluated over 2 years.[9] A coagulation abnormality was detected in 58% of the patients in this cohort. In addition, higher levels of D-dimer were correlated with both the severity score and the anatomical extension of the disease. In a study by Hung et al., D-dimer levels among 24 pediatric patients with vascular malformation positively correlated with the presence of palpable phleboliths.[10] Thus, clinicians should be alert for potential coagulopathy in patients with extensive disease and those with palpable, often painful, phleboliths.

Blood stasis is reasonably speculated to be part of the mechanism of the hypercoagulability among patients with KTS. A decrease in the calf venous pump function is linked to patients with this syndrome. Stasis due

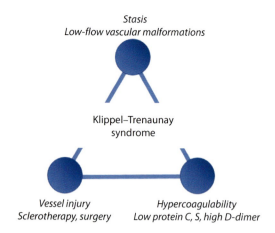

Stasis
Low-flow vascular malformations

Klippel–Trenaunay
syndrome

Vessel injury
Sclerotherapy, surgery

Hypercoagulability
Low protein C, S, high D-dimer

Figure 83.1 Virchow triad in the patient with KTS.

to pelvic veins is also attributed to be a distinguishing reason for the higher likelihood of coagulopathy among patients with KTS relative to other vascular malformations. Injury is also a trigger for VTE; the development of thrombosis is higher in frequency postoperatively. Associated triggers prevalent in patients with KTS may include sclerotherapy, surgical resection, fractures, and prolonged immobilization, which are also capable of transforming a localized intravascular coagulopathy to disseminated disease.[11]

DIAGNOSIS

While a diagnosis of superficial venous thrombosis and deep vein thrombosis will have high diagnostic accuracy with compression ultrasound of the extremities, contrast computed tomography (CT) remains recommended for diagnosis of pulmonary embolism. The definition of a coagulopathy without VTE is more complicated. There is distinction of the extent of the vascular malformation associated with the levels of D-dimer. Indeed, levels of D-dimer seem to be highly specific to the extent of venous malformations with low flow such as KTS relative to patients with high-flow disease including Parkes Weber syndrome. In a study including 280 patients with cutaneous and subcutaneous congenital vascular anomalies, there were 26 patients with high-flow lesions including arteriovenous malformation, capillary malformation, and Parkes Weber syndrome. Eight of 11 patients with KTS had marked elevation of D-dimer. The sensitivity of D-dimer levels to detect venous anomaly was estimated between 36.4% and 50.5%, 95% confidence interval (CI).[12] Note, however, that although a D-dimer may guide the distinction of the type of vascular malformation, it should not be used in lieu of comprehensive evaluation. Similarly, although there is a correlation between the D-dimer level response after sclerotherapy and the likelihood of success after sclerotherapy treatment in patients with venous malformations, these levels should not be interpreted as a license to decrease cautious surveillance of patients with KTS.[13]

It is important to distinguish localized intravascular coagulopathy versus disseminated disease. Severe disease will often have lower fibrinogen levels and a variable platelet count. One must distinguish these phenomena from the Kasabach–Merritt phenomenon, which will have a signature of thrombocytopenia secondary to platelet trapping within a vascular tumor.[14] Patients who progress to disseminated intravascular coagulopathy will have an increase in bleeding likelihood as well as depletion of platelets and coagulation factors.[12] A failure to distinguish localized intravascular coagulation among patients with KTS may lead to catastrophic complications.[15,16] Although some cases with localized intravascular coagulation do go undiagnosed and remain asymptomatic for several years, the majority will experience painful intralesional thrombosis. The clinician should suspect worsening of the limited intravascular coagulopathy in patients who have new pain, thrombosis, or bleeding over lesion sites. Hemarthrosis on large hematomas has been observed among patients with progressive localized intravascular coagulopathy.

MANAGEMENT

The main opportunity for management resides in VTE prevention. Patients with KTS who need surgery or hospitalization carry risk factors that will be exacerbated in these high-risk scenarios. Thus, anticoagulation for primary prevention should be considered and provided for the expected period at risk, which implies that depending on the reason for admission and bleeding risk, the anticoagulant should be continued for at least 2 weeks after discharge. The duration of anticoagulation should be personalized according to the VTE risk stratification specific to the patient and reason for admission. For the medically ill population, one may consider direct oral anticoagulants or low-molecular-weight heparin (LMWH) for this indication.[17]

Although there is no clear definition of the ideal agent to treat the coagulopathy among these patients, several agents have been considered. In a study by Nguyen et al., aspirin was evaluated as an alternative in the treatment of venous malformation coagulopathy.[5] The authors did a survey among patients with venous malformations. There were 38 patients who agreed to participate out of 65 approached. There were benefits described, including less aching or shooting pain or fullness and swelling as described by 17 patients. Moreover, discontinuation of aspirin was actually associated with exacerbation of symptoms in five out of six patients who took aspirin. Although this was a retrospective evaluation, it suggests there might be a group of patients who can benefit from this simple strategy. Reye syndrome, however, remains a potential complication that should be discussed with pediatric patients. A dose of 5 mg/kg/day up to 83 mg/day of aspirin is recommended by some authors for pediatric patients with extensive KTS.

In patients with coagulopathy, several authors have advocated the use of LMWH over the use of warfarin. In concordance with this suggestion, the use of warfarin will be more complicated among patients of young age, as the consumptive coagulopathy is likely to make international normalized ratio (INR) monitoring cumbersome and often unreliable given the alterations in baseline coagulation measurements. If warfarin needs to be used in patients with an underlying coagulopathy, one should consider confirming the factor level target for these patients.[18] To accept or negate the adequacy of the INR target, a chromogenic factor X of 43–17% should match the INR level between 2 and 3.5.[19] For LMWH, one specific regime that has been proposed among patients who will go for a procedure and have low levels of fibrinogen, is to use LMWH for a period of 10 days before procedures followed by extended prophylaxis. There is no consensus regarding the adequate level of fibrinogen to trigger periprocedural transfusion; however, there is growing evidence for using a target of 1.5–2 g/L.[20] LMWH has also been noted to decrease pain and bleeding in patients with vascular malformations who have palpable phleboliths and an elevated D-dimer.[17]

Direct oral anticoagulants have been used to treat patients with VTE and vascular malformations including KTS.[21–23] The data on its use are limited to small case series and case reports; however, they do represent an interesting alternative for patients who need extended prevention. A promising option is the use of low-dose anticoagulation for extended recurrence prevention in patients with history of thrombosis. In adults with history of VTE, a low dose of apixaban (2.5 mg twice a day) or a low dose of rivaroxaban (10 mg daily) had comparable efficacy in the prevention of thrombosis recurrence with a very low likelihood of bleeding.[24,25] However, the safety of these options remains unproven in patients with KTS.

REFERENCES

1. Lee BB. Klippel–Trenaunay syndrome: Is this term still worthy to use? *Acta Phlebologica.* 2012;13(2):83–85.
2. Baskerville PA, Ackroyd JS, Lea Thomas M et al. The Klippel–Trenaunay syndrome: Clinical, radiological and haemodynamic features and management. *Br J Surg.* 1985;72(3):232–236.
3. Ulrich S, Fischler M, Walder B et al. Klippel–Trenaunay syndrome with small vessel pulmonary arterial hypertension. *Thorax.* 2005;60(11):971–973.
4. Johnson JN, Driscoll DJ, McGregor CG. Pulmonary thromboendarterectomy in Klippel–Trenaunay syndrome. *J Thorac Cardiovasc Surg.* 2010;140(3):e41–e43.
5. Nguyen JT, Koerper MA, Hess CP et al. Aspirin therapy in venous malformation: A retrospective cohort study of benefits, side effects, and patient experiences. *Pediatr Dermatol.* 2014;31(5):556–560.
6. Lee B, Laredo J. Venous malformation: Treatment needs a bird's-eye view. *Phlebology.* 2013;28(2):62–63.
7. Bagot CN, Arya R. Virchow and his triad: A question of attribution. *Br J Haematol.* 2008;143(2):180–190.
8. Oduber CE, van Beers EJ, Bresser P et al. Venous thromboembolism and prothrombotic parameters in Klippel–Trenaunay syndrome. *Neth J Med.* 2013;71(5):246–252.
9. Mazoyer E, Enjolras O, Bisdorff A et al. Coagulation disorders in patients with venous malformation of the limbs and trunk: A case series of 118 patients. *Arch Dermatol.* 2008;144(7):861–867.
10. Hung JW, Leung MW, Liu CS et al. Venous malformation and localized intravascular coagulopathy in children. *Eur J Pediatr Surg.* 2017;27(2):181–184.
11. Beier UH, Schmidt ML, Hast H et al. Control of disseminated intravascular coagulation in Klippel–Trenaunay-Weber syndrome using enoxaparin and recombinant activated factor VIIa: A case report. *J Med Case Rep.* 2010;4:92.
12. Dompmartin A, Acher A, Thibon P et al. Association of localized intravascular coagulopathy with venous malformations. *Arch Dermatol.* 2008;144(7):873–877.
13. Leung YC, Leung MW, Yam SD et al. D-dimer level correlation with treatment response in children with venous malformations. *J Pediatr Surg.* 2018;53(2):289–292.
14. Mazoyer E, Enjolras O, Laurian C et al. Coagulation abnormalities associated with extensive venous malformations of the limbs: Differentiation from Kasabach–Merritt syndrome. *Clin Lab Haematol.* 2002;24(4):243–251.
15. Muluk SC, Ginns LC, Semigran MJ et al. Klippel–Trenaunay syndrome with multiple pulmonary emboli—An unusual cause of progressive pulmonary dysfunction. *J Vasc Surg.* 1995;21(4):686–690.
16. Oishi SN, Ezaki M. Venous thrombosis and pulmonary embolus in pediatric patients with large upper extremity venous malformations. *J Hand Surg Am.* 2010;35(8):1330–1333.
17. Maguiness S, Koerper M, Frieden I. Relevance of D-dimer testing in patients with venous malformations. *Arch Dermatol.* 2009;145(11):1321–1324.
18. Baumann Kreuziger LM, Datta YH, Johnson AD et al. Monitoring anticoagulation in patients with an unreliable prothrombin time/international normalized ratio: Factor II versus chromogenic factor X testing. *Blood Coagul Fibrinolysis.* 2014;25(3):232–236.
19. Sanfelippo MJ, Sennet J, McMahon EJ. Falsely elevated INRs in warfarin-treated patients with the lupus anticoagulant. *WMJ.* 2000;99(3):62–64, 43.
20. Levy JH, Goodnough LT. How I use fibrinogen replacement therapy in acquired bleeding. *Blood.* 2015;125(9):1387–1393.
21. Vandenbriele C, Vanassche T, Peetermans M et al. Rivaroxaban for the treatment of consumptive coagulopathy associated with a vascular malformation. *J Thromb Thrombolysis.* 2014;38(1):121–123.
22. Yasumoto A, Ishiura R, Narushima M et al. Successful treatment with dabigatran for consumptive coagulopathy associated with extensive vascular malformations. *Blood Coagul Fibrinolysis.* 2017;28(8):670–674.

23. Ardillon L, Lambert C, Eeckhoudt S et al. Dabigatran etexilate versus low-molecular weight heparin to control consumptive coagulopathy secondary to diffuse venous vascular malformations. *Blood Coagul Fibrinolysis.* 2016;27(2):216–219.

24. Agnelli G, Buller HR, Cohen A et al. Apixaban for extended treatment of venous thromboembolism. *N Engl J Med.* 2013;368(8):699–708.

25. Weitz JI, Lensing AWA, Prins MH et al. Rivaroxaban or aspirin for extended treatment of venous thromboembolism. *N Engl J Med.* 2017;376(13):1211–1222.

84

Klippel–Trenaunay syndrome: Pain and psychosocial considerations

JAMISON HARVEY, MEGHA M. TOLLEFSON, PETER GLOVICZKI, AND DAVID J. DRISCOLL

Klippel–Trenaunay syndrome (KTS) is a congenital disorder characterized by capillary malformation (CM), venous malformation (VM) with or without lymphatic malformation, and limb length and/or circumference discrepancy that is linked to mutations in the *PIK3CA* gene (Figure 84.1).[1-3] In addition to the physical manifestations of KTS, many patients experience acute, subacute, or chronic pain. In addition, a significant number of patients are burdened with psychiatric and psychosocial issues. Pain has been reported to occur in 38%–88% of patients with KTS, and psychiatric conditions have been reported in 23%.[4-6]

PAIN

Nearly two-thirds of patients with KTS experience pain (Figure 84.2).[5] In one study, it was more common in adults 18–50 years of age (80.1%), and least common in patients less than 5 years of age (11.9%). Patients who had any KTS complication were more likely to have pain than those without complications. Those who had VMs of the buttocks, lower extremities, and feet were more likely to have pain than those with VMs in other locations.[5]

Chronic venous insufficiency

One of the most frequent causes of pain in patients with KTS is chronic venous insufficiency. Venous abnormalities are a hallmark of KTS. Varicose veins become more prominent and problematic with increasing age. The discomfort associated with venous valvular incompetence of the frequently large, mostly lateral superficial persistent embryonic venous system usually is described as a "dull, achy" sensation and typically is more noticeable as the day progresses because of venous blood pooling.

The mainstay of treatment of this type of pain and discomfort is external compression of the venous system with elastic or nonelastic garments or bandages. In selected cases among symptomatic KTS patients who do not respond to compression therapy, surgical intervention, sclerotherapy, endovascular laser, or radiofrequency ablation is indicated.

Cellulitis and lymphangitis

Patients with KTS are prone to cellulitis. Chronic lymphedema is a major cause of cellulitis and lymphangitis, with 13% of patients experiencing infections due to cellulitis.[4] These patients are more susceptible to infection because of poor skin integrity associated with impaired venous and lymphatic drainage. Thus, it is imperative for patients to maintain excellent skin hygiene and wash the affected body parts thoroughly with soap and water at least twice daily. For patients with recurrent cellulitis, dilute bleach baths or soaks can be helpful. The preparation includes 0.5 cups of household bleach to a full bathtub (approximately 40 gallons) of lukewarm water. It is important that they wear clean stockings every day and allow their shoes and feet to dry between shoe changes. In addition to the above-mentioned supportive measures, the mainstay of treating pain associated with cellulitis and/or lymphangitis is treatment of underlying infection.

Growing pains

Growing pains are a common cause of pain even in healthy children. Children with KTS are just as likely to have growing pains as are healthy children, and reassurance is generally sufficient.

Thrombophlebitis

Superficial thrombophlebitis is common in KTS, and in one series, it occurred in 15% of patients.[4] Aseptic inflammation probably results from venous stasis, sometimes associated with coagulopathy, localized intravascular coagulopathy (LIC), for example, in the abnormal veins.

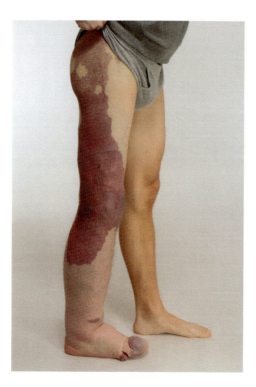

Figure 84.1 A 22-year-old male patient with Klippel–Trenaunay syndrome, with a painful right leg that was longer and larger than the left. The patient had the full spectrum of the syndrome with venous, capillary, and lymphatic malformations. Note the extensive lateral capillary and venous malformation, chronic lymphedema, and digital anomalies of the right foot.

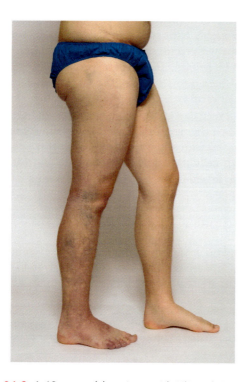

Figure 84.2 A 19-year-old patient with Klippel–Trenaunay syndrome with extensive capillary and venous malformation and chronic, throbbing pain of the longer right leg and the foot.

This type of pain is best treated with simple analgesics and nonsteroidal anti-inflammatory agents along with compression and elevation. If pain recurs, vein stripping or endovenous ablation, phlebectomy, or injection sclerotherapy are helpful.

Deep vein thrombosis and pulmonary embolism

Deep vein thrombosis (DVT) and pulmonary embolism (PE) are more common in patients with KTS than in those without KTS and varicose veins.[7] In a Mayo Clinic series of 252 patients, 11 (4%) had DVT, and 9 (4%) had PE, which was fatal in one patient.[4] Pain is a usual presentation of DVT, in addition to swelling and cyanotic discoloration of the leg. It is important to diagnose and treat immediately any DVT with anticoagulation, or selectively, with pharmacomechanical thrombectomy, if the DVT involves the iliofemoral veins. Given the high risk of DVT and PE, female patients with KTS are cautioned to avoid estrogen-containing contraceptives and heed precautionary measures to prevent thrombosis during long periods of immobilization.

Intraosseous vascular malformations

Rarely, patients with KTS present with intraosseous vascular malformations that can cause intense pain.[8] When VMs involve long bones, there is an increased risk of fracture. A variety of analgesics can be tried, but in most cases, surgical removal of the malformation may be necessary. If the lesions cannot be removed, management of the pain can be quite challenging.

Calcified or scarred vascular malformations

Calcified vascular malformations can be a source of pain if located around structures that are mobile, such as the ankle joint. This can occur in natural calcification of a vascular malformation or as a result of a previous sclerotherapy of the malformation. If well localized, surgical removal may relieve this type of pain.

Arthritis

Arthritis occurs in a small number of patients with KTS, but in those patients, it is a major problem. Usually it involves the knee but can also involve the ankle. Destruction of cartilage occurs likely from recurrent hemarthrosis when the vascular malformation is within a joint. The presence of the vascular malformation may create a chronic synovitis. Patients typically try to limit pain by flexing the knee and can develop a flexion contracture (Figure 84.3). Treatment includes analgesics and maneuvers to prevent the flexion contracture. This may involve physical therapy, passive stretching, and bracing. Synovectomy may be useful. If the

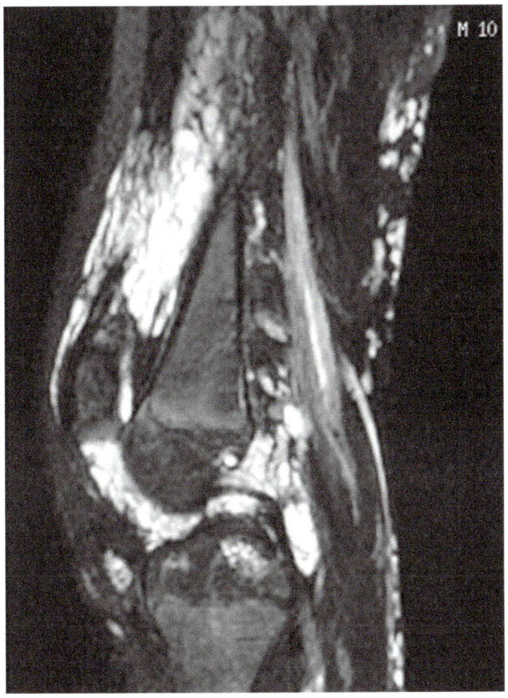

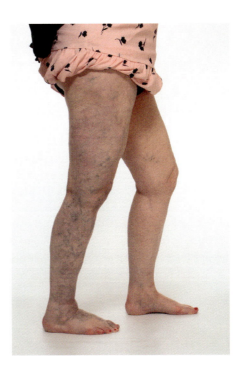

Figure 84.3 Painful synovial and cartilage damage in a patient with Klippel–Trenaunay syndrome and diffuse, infiltrating extra-truncular venous malformation.

flexion contracture is severe enough to prevent walking and the leg cannot be straightened, amputation may be necessary to control the pain and allow the patient to walk with a prosthesis.

Neuropathic pain

Neuropathic pain results from damage or dysfunction of neuronal pathways and is a shooting, burning, aching (or a combination) pain that is poorly responsive to conventional analgesics. The pain may be quite disabling and associated with hyperesthesia. Neuropathic pain can result from damage to nerves at the time of operation but can also result from effects of the venous abnormality on the nerve that shares the neurovascular bundle (e.g., pain associated with persistent sciatic vein). It may result from direct compression of the nerve and/or abnormal venous pressure of the nutrient vascular system of the nerve. The management of neuropathic pain is difficult, as such pain responds poorly to conventional analgesics and less well to opioids. Gabapentin or pregabalin are sometimes of benefit to neuropathic pain.

PSYCHIATRIC AND PSYCHOSOCIAL ISSUES

KTS can be a disfiguring condition, but there is limited information regarding the psychiatric and psychosocial effects of this disfigurement. There is also limited data

Table 84.1 Psychiatric diagnoses in 410 patients with Klippel–Trenaunay syndrome

Psychiatric diagnosis	Number of patients (%)
Depression	62 (15.1%)
Anxiety	21 (5.1%)
Substance abuse disorder	15 (3.7%)
Sleep disorder	9 (2.2%)
ADHD[a]	9 (2.2%)
Developmental delay	5 (1.2%)
Bipolar disorder	3 (0.7%)
Other	10 (2.4%)

Source: From Harvey JA, Nguyen H, Anderson KR et al. *J Am Acad Dermatol.* 2018;79(5):899–903.
[a] Attention-deficit/hyperactivity disorder.

regarding the psychiatric burden of patients with KTS. In a retrospective cohort of 410 patients who fulfilled strict KTS diagnostic criteria, 95 patients had a diagnosed psychiatric condition (23.2%), and 62 patients had psychiatric symptoms, with the most abundant being difficulty sleeping ($n = 41$, 10%) (Table 84.1).[5] Pain ($p = 0.0134$), CM of the hand ($p = 0.0057$), and deep venous thrombotic/embolic events ($p = 0.0094$) were all associated with a psychiatric diagnosis (Figure 84.4). Increasing age was associated with lower rates of a psychiatric diagnosis ($p = 0.0002$). Twenty-seven patients had general psychiatric symptoms but did not have a diagnosed psychiatric illness in the medical record.[5] One case report highlighted a patient with KTS and concomitant bipolar affective disorder.[9]

Figure 84.4 A 25-year-old female patient with Klippel–Trenaunay syndrome, with a larger and longer right leg, with capillary and venous malformations and lateral persistent embryonic veins. She had major depression.

Psychosocial stressors

The most apparent psychosocial stressors were related to financial stress, work difficulty, and relationships based on a retrospective cohort.[5] The most common general symptoms reported were difficulty sleeping, anxiety, depression, (Figure 84.5), sexual dysfunction, suicidal ideation, abuse, and relationship instability. In the pediatric cohort, there were problems with school for either too many absences or school not accommodating for disability, difficulty with friendships, and severe bullying from other students.[5] Given the retrospective nature of the study, it is likely this prevalence is much higher.

A different prospective study of 55 adults and 33 children with KTS reported limitations of daily activities (88%), social consequences (20%), sexual problems (13%), relational problems (11%), and impact of disease on the family (9%).[10] Another survey conducted on KTS patients found that their baseline quality of life was significantly lower than that of the general population, and these patients had more bodily pain.[11]

In conclusion, patients with KTS should be routinely screened for symptoms of pain and psychiatric and psychosocial burden. Multidisciplinary clinics are of help, and the patient should be referred to psychiatrists, psychologists, and support groups if needed.

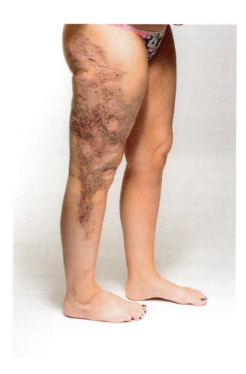

Figure 84.5 A 54-year-old woman with Klippel–Trenaunay syndrome, with chronic pain and major depressive disorder.

REFERENCES

1. Wassef M, Blei F, Adams D et al. Vascular anomalies classification: Recommendations from the International Society for the Study of Vascular Anomalies. *Pediatrics* 2015;136(1):e203–e214.
2. Kurek KC, Luks VL, Ayturk UM et al. Somatic mosaic activating mutations in *PIK3CA* cause CLOVES syndrome. *Am J Hum Genet.* 2012;90(6):1108–1115.
3. Luks VL, Kamitaki N, Vivero MP et al. Lymphatic and other vascular malformative/overgrowth disorders are caused by somatic mutations in *PIK3CA*. *J Pediatr.* 2015;166(4):1048–1054.
4. Jacob AG, Driscoll DJ, Shaughnessy WJ, Stanson AW, Clay RP, Gloviczki P. Klippel–Trenaunay syndrome: Spectrum and management. *Mayo Clin Proc.* 1998; 73(1):28–36.
5. Harvey JA, Nguyen H, Anderson KR et al. Pain and psychosocial comorbidities associated with Klippel–Trenaunay Syndrome. *J Am Acad Dermatol.* 2018; 79(5):899–903.
6. Baskerville PA, Ackroyd JS, Thomas ML, Browse NL. The Klippel–Trenaunay syndrome: Clinical, radiological and hemodynamic features and management. *Br J Surg.* 1985;72:232–236.
7. Fowkes FJ, Price JF, Fowkes FG. Incidence of diagnosed deep vein thrombosis in the general population: Systematic review. *Eur J Vasc Endovasc Surg.* 2003;25:1–5.
8. Enjolras O, Ciabrini D, Mazoyer E, Laurian C, Herbereteau D. Extensive pure venous malformation in the upper or lower limb: A review of 27 cases. *J Am Acad Dermatol.* 1997;36:219–225.
9. Velayudhan L, Gangadhar B. Bipolar affective disorder with Klippel–Trenaunay syndrome. *Aust N Z J Psychiatry.* 2007;41(11):937–938.
10. Van der Ploeg HM, van der Ploeg MNS, van der Ploeg-Stapert JD. Psychological aspects of Klippel–Trenaunay syndrome. *J Psychosom Res.* 1995;39(2):183–191.
11. Oduber CE, Khemlani K, Silevis Smitt JH, Hennekam RC, van der Horst CM. Baseline quality of life in patients with Klippel–Trenaunay syndrome. *J Plast Reconstr Aesthet Surg.* 2010;63(4):603–609.

85

Klippel–Trenaunay syndrome and complex venous malformations: Should multimodality approach be standard of care?

KUROSH PARSI AND MINA KANG

INTRODUCTION

Klippel–Trenaunay syndrome (KTS) is a congenital vascular disorder composed of an extensive network of diffuse and infiltrative dysplastic veins and venules that can involve the dermis, subcutaneous fat, subfascial space, muscle, joints, and bones of lower limbs (Figure 85.1), frequently accompanied by variable degrees of discrepancy in the growth of soft tissue and/or bone of affected lower extremities. Capillary (CM) and lymphatic malformations (LM) may coexist. When an arteriovenous malformation (AVM) is present, the condition is termed *Parkes Weber syndrome* (PWS). The venous malformation (VM) component of KTS can involve the labia and extend into the pelvis involving the vulvar and pelvic veins (Figure 85.2).

KTS is typically unilateral involving one of the lower limbs but may be bilateral. The vascular changes are usually associated with fat hypertrophy, muscle atrophy, and bony hypertrophy or atrophy of the affected limb. The limb length asymmetry can result in a limp and secondary scoliosis (Figure 85.3). The tissue hypertrophy is more prominent in PWS.

An important venous anomaly in KTS is the persistent embryonic marginal vein (Figure 85.4). This vein is a superficial vein located on the lateral aspect of the leg extending from the lateral calf to the lateral thigh. Patients may also present with a persistent embryonic sciatic vein that travels along the length of the sciatic nerve and can closely mimic the symptoms of sciatica.

INVESTIGATIONS

Prior to any intervention, all patients with KTS should undergo the following investigations.[1]

Duplex ultrasound

A comprehensive duplex ultrasound (DUS) assessment should be performed to include the following:

- B-mode and Doppler flow assessment of all vascular components of the condition.
- Venous incompetence mapping of both the superficial and deep venous systems to determine the presence or absence of the named veins, reflux, and thrombosis. Absence of valves or hypoplastic valves should be identified and documented.

Magnetic resonance imaging

Magnetic resonance imaging (MRI) in combination with venography (MRV) and/or arteriography (MRA) is required in most patients with complex malformations to determine the extent of the condition, to determine involvement of other structures, and to guide intervention.

D-dimer, coagulation, and thrombophilia screening

Patients with extensive VMs and in particular KTS have elevated D-dimer levels due to ongoing thrombus formation within the lesions and subsequent fibrinolysis. The localized thrombus formation is termed *localized intravascular coagulopathy* (LIC). An elevated D-dimer is expected in these patients and does not indicate a venous thromboembolic (VTE) event. A baseline D-dimer level is important to obtain before interventions. This will allow monitoring of the thrombotic activity in the long term. Reduction of D-dimer following interventions is another indicator of success in treating patent VMs. Other measurements should include fibrinogen, platelet

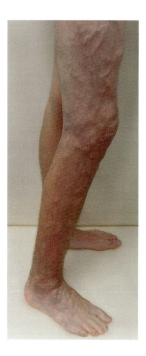

Figure 85.1 Klippel–Trenaunay syndrome (KTS) affecting the right lower limb. The lateral distribution of the venous anomalies is typical for this condition.

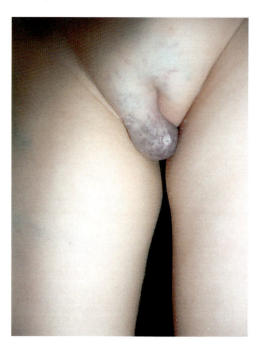

Figure 85.2 Labial involvement in Klippel–Trenaunay syndrome (KTS) affecting the right lower limb.

count, and clotting times. Fibrinogen and platelet count will be reduced in LIC, whereas clotting times will be prolonged.

We obtain a thrombophilia screening in patients at high risk of VTE or when treating high-risk lesions where extension of thrombosis or pulmonary embolism can have catastrophic outcomes. Examples include neck VMs where lesions drain into major neck veins, and eyelid lesions where there is a risk of orbital vein or cavernous sinus thrombosis. Patients with KTS who have other comorbidities and an

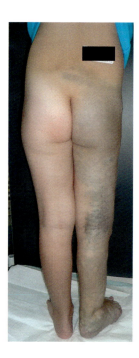

Figure 85.3 Limb asymmetry and scoliosis in a patient with Klippel–Trenaunay syndrome (KTS).

increased risk of deep vein thrombosis (DVT), or those with a personal or family history of VTE may require screening. Currently, there is no consensus for prophylactic insertion of inferior vena cava (IVC) filters in this cohort of patients, despite the fact that patients with KTS can become severely coagulopathic during interventions.

Orthopedic assessment

All patients with KTS should receive a comprehensive orthopedic assessment. Limb length and circumference measurements will be required and should be repeated periodically. The spine needs to be assessed for scoliosis.

TREATMENT

Treatment of KTS, PWS, and similar complex vascular malformations is not simple and requires careful planning, staging, and a specific treatment plan for each individual component of the condition.[2] Different vascular components of KTS differ in their architecture, distribution, and flow dynamics. The treatment for an intramuscular VM is vastly different than that of a LM with no flow. The same type of malformation may require a different approach to treatment depending on the lesion size, morphology (e.g., septation, segmentation), location, distribution, thickness of the lesion wall, and involvement of the surrounding structures. For instance, an extensive subfascial VM involving muscles, tendons, joints, and adjacent to nerves would require a carefully planned treatment approach like all other congenital vascular malformations.

Given the variable nature of each KTS component (VM, LM, and CM), the variable size and distribution of each component and the diffuse distribution, KTS and similar

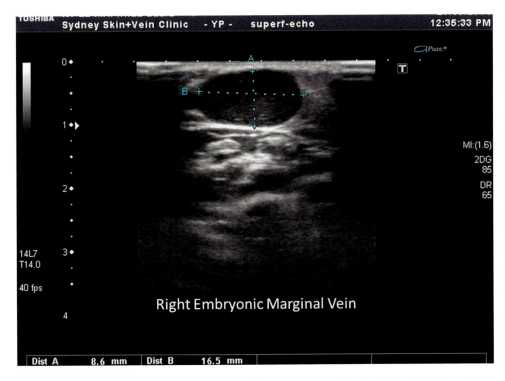

Figure 85.4 B-mode ultrasound image demonstrating an embryonic marginal vein of the right lateral leg measuring 16.5 mm in diameter.

complex malformations should only be treated using a multi-modal approach through a combination of all modern interventional and surgical methods in multidisciplinary settings.

Capillary component of Klippel–Trenaunay syndrome

This component of KTS is primarily of cosmetic significance. Treatment may be attempted using vascular lasers such as the pulsed-dye laser (585 nm), the yellow laser (570 nm), or light devices. In general, CMs of lower limbs do not respond very well to any of these modalities, especially in older adults.

Lymphatic component of Klippel–Trenaunay syndrome

The lymphatic component of KTS can be macrocystic, microcystic, or a combination of both (Figure 85.5). Secondary complications include infections and bleeding. The macrocystic component presents with large lymphatic cysts with thin walls containing lymphatic fluid. The lesions can be subcutaneous or subfascial and very infiltrative.

Treatment of the macrocystic LMs is aided by ultrasound guidance. Individual cysts need to be accessed first and drained while maintaining the access. The authors routinely use perilesional tumescent anesthesia to provide and maintain internal compression around the drained cysts. This is followed by intralesional injection of an irritant sclerosing agent such as doxycycline, bleomycin, ethanol, or picibanil (OK-432). Detergent sclerosants such as sodium tetradecyl sulfate (STS) and polidocanol (POL) are less effective than irritant sclerosants in treating LMs. The authors prefer

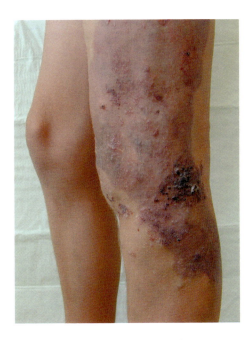

Figure 85.5 Microcystic lymphatic malformation (LM) presenting as small blood-filled vesicles in a patient with Klippel–Trenaunay syndrome (KTS). Note the extensive capillary malformation (CM). (Photograph courtesy of Professor Hugo Partsch.)

intralesional doxycycline given its lower potential for complications compared with other embolic agents used for LMs.

Alternatively, larger cysts can be ablated with endovenous laser ablation (EVLA). Diffuse and infiltrative LMs of the neck (cystic hygromas) are often best treated surgically by careful dissection. Microcystic LMs can be treated by subcutaneous injection of bleomycin. Radiofrequency ablation can also be used to treat larger lymphatic cysts, and specialized hand pieces can be used to treat microcystic LMs.

New emerging therapies include sildenafil, propranolol, sirolimus, and vascularized lymph node transfer.

Venous component of KTS

VMs can involve multiple tissue compartments in KTS. The vessel size, distribution, and wall thickness may be vastly different; hence, the treatment modality should be selected based on the lesion characteristics.

STRATEGY

When faced with extensive venous anomalies spread across multiple tissue compartments, the physician may wonder where to start. In such circumstances, a strategy should be devised where one limb segment is treated at a time, and as comprehensively as possible. For instance, a limb can be divided into several regions such as the foot and ankle, the lateral calf, the knee, the popliteal area, and the lateral thigh. Each region is then treated separately but comprehensively.

Within each region, all tissue compartments (e.g., intraosseous, subfascial, intramuscular, subcutaneous, and dermal) should be treated individually using the appropriate modalities for that tissue compartment. In general, deeper and larger lesions should be treated first to control flow and prevent recanalization. The aim of the treatment should be to achieve maximal elimination of intralesional blood flow where the vessels of the network are ablated or occluded, while flow from adjoining vessels is eliminated or minimized. Ongoing flow into the treated segments will result in recanalization. By treating the larger, high-pressure, deeper vessels and minimizing flow from adjoining segments, recanalization can be controlled, and treatment efficacy can improve. The interventions should be scheduled in a timely fashion and not more than 2–3 weeks apart. Large time gaps in between procedures will result in recanalization and a lack of progress.

SUBFASCIAL AND INTRAMUSCULAR COMPARTMENT

This is usually the deepest compartment affected by VMs in KTS. Subfascial lesions should be approached with caution due to the presence of delicate structures in this compartment, including nerves, tendons, and ligaments (Figure 85.6). EVLA and n-butyl cyanoacrylate (n-BCA) should be used with caution due to the increased risk of adhesions, burn injury to sensitive structures, and nerve damage. Tumescent-assisted ultrasound-guided sclerotherapy (TUGS) using foam sclerosants is a flexible treatment option that can perfectly complement the other modalities. Multiple access points using short cannulas and catheters will be required to access all lesions or to ablate larger lesions. Embolic agents, foam sclerosants, or laser fibers are then introduced sequentially via each access point to ablate the target lesions.

SUBCUTANEOUS COMPARTMENT

Selection of the treatment modality would depend on the wall thickness, size, and location of the lesion. In our experience, TUGS is suitable for small to medium-sized vessels of up to 2 mm in diameter. Our choice of sclerosant for TUGS to treat subcutaneous VMs is STS 1.5% foam.

EVLA achieves better results when treating larger lesions or those with thicker walls. While foam sclerosants induce endothelial surface injury, EVLA achieves transmural damage and is therefore more suitable for lesions with thick walls. If present, the embryonic marginal vein should be ablated first before other subcutaneous lesions are treated. The embryonic marginal vein can be readily treated with a combination of EVLA and TUGS and would not require surgical excision as long as the hemodynamic condition (e.g., blood flow and volume) and local condition (e.g., collaterals with the perforators) are amenable with minimal risk of surrounding tissue damage (e.g., skin necrosis due to the proximity to the skin/epidermis).

n-BCA glue is a locally occlusive agent that should be reserved for extensive and infiltrative lesions, and to complement EVLA and TUGS. Subdermal injection of n-BCA can result in formation of palpable nodules, granuloma formation, glue extrusion, and perforation.[3] There is also a risk of skin tattooing if the n-BCA used is colored.

EVLA should be performed with caution when treating subcutaneous VMs that completely replace the fat layer and extend up to the dermis (Figure 85.6). The subdermal location with no intervening tissue plane would make the perilesional infiltration of tumescent anesthesia very difficult, hence increasing the risk of burn injuries to the dermis.

Power phlebectomy can be used in the subcutaneous layer to remove VMs, especially postembolization. It is a very useful debulking tool and can help with the treatment of large surface areas.[4,5]

DERMAL COMPARTMENT

Dermal VMs are best treated with foam sclerotherapy (Figure 85.7). We prefer using polidocanol (POL) 0.5% foam for this purpose. POL foam is injected into the target vessels either under ultrasound guidance or by direct visualization. POL is less likely to cause pigmentation or ulceration when used to treat intradermal vessels. The treatment can be optimized and potentiated when tumescent fluid is infiltrated in the perivenous space.[6] This provides an internal compression that helps with better closure of target veins. Vascular lasers cannot achieve resolution of dermal VMs and should only be reserved for CMs.

OTHER CONSIDERATIONS

Orthopedic complications such as limb length and girth discrepancy and scoliosis need to be managed by orthopedic surgeons. For leg length discrepancy (LLD), orthopedic treatment (e.g., epiphyseal ablation) will be required when LLD exceeds 2–3 cm (for more details, please see Chapter 78). Hematologic complications such as hypercoagulability

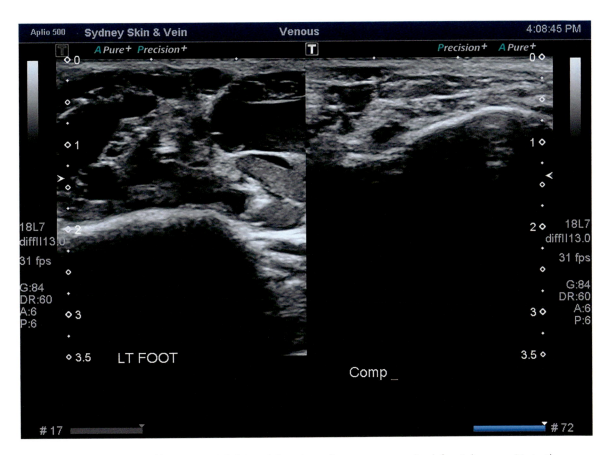

Figure 85.6 Extensive venous malformation (VM) involving the subcutaneous and subfascial space. Note the venous anomaly has completely replaced other tissues and extends from the underlying bone to skin.

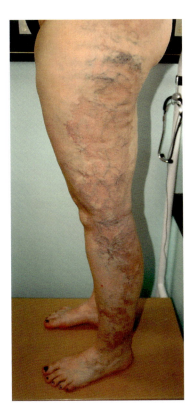

Figure 85.7 Prominent dermal veins in a patient with Klippel–Trenaunay syndrome (KTS) affecting the left leg.

and symptomatic or silent pulmonary embolism can occur. High-risk patients will require long-term and even indefinite anticoagulation therapy.

CONCLUSION

In conclusion, KTS is a complex vascular anomaly where the treatment can be challenging and frustrating. The affected limb should be divided into regions and each region treated separately and comprehensively. Within each region, VMs involving each tissue compartment may require different treatment modalities. Maximal elimination of intralesional blood flow within the vascular network should be aimed for where not only the lesion is ablated but also the flow from adjoining compartments is minimized.

REFERENCES

1. Lee BB, Antignani PL, Baraldini V et al. ISVI-IUA consensus document diagnostic guidelines of vascular anomalies: Vascular malformations and hemangiomas. *Int Angiol.* 2015;34:333–374.
2. Lee BB, Bergan J, Gloviczki P et al. Diagnosis and treatment of venous malformations. Consensus document of the International Union of Phlebology (IUP)-2009. *Int Angiol.* 2009;28:434–451.

3. Parsi K, Kang M, Yang A et al. Granuloma formation following cyanoacrylate glue injection in peripheral veins and arteriovenous malformation. *Phlebology*. 2019. doi: 10.1177/0268355519856756.

4. Parsi K, Kang M, Trimboli A. Ultrasound-guided TriVex-powered phlebectomy for debulking of peripheral vascular anomalies—A novel treatment technique. *Phlebology*. 2019;34(8):523–529.

5. Duan SJ, Jiang RZ, Zhang YX et al. Removal of benign superficial masses using the TriVex system: Preliminary clinical results. *Surg Innov*. 2018;25:230–235.

6. Thibault P. Perivenous tumescent compression to enhance sclerotherapy results and reduce adverse effects. In: *XVIth World Meeting of the Union Internationale de Phlebologie*. Monaco, September 20, 2009, pp. 38–39.

Capillary Malformations (CMs)

Diagnosis

86

Is this capillary malformation? Differential diagnosis and other dermal vascular lesions

KUROSH PARSI AND MINA KANG

INTRODUCTION

Capillary malformations (CMs) are common congenital vascular malformations, historically known as port-wine stains (Figure 86.1). CMs are dysplastic dermal vessels that are present at birth and grow proportionate to the child's growth. CMs never involute and in time get thicker and darker. Later in life, CMs may adopt a nodular morphology, especially on the face, referred to as a "cavernous hemangioma" (Figure 86.2). This is a misnomer given that CMs are malformations and not tumors or hemangiomas.

CMs can present as a component of a complex vascular malformation such as a CM-arteriovenous malformation (CM-AVM), associated with a RASA-1 mutation.[1] Often CM is the only visible component of the lesion, and the underlying AVM may only present as a pale halo or patch surrounding the CM due to cutaneous steal syndrome (Figure 86.3). It is important to diagnose the underlying AVM in a CM-AVM and distinguish it from a simple CM due to the significant hemodynamic sequelae that are associated with AVMs.

CMs can coexist with venolymphatic malformations (capillary venous lymphatic malformation [CVLM]) (Figure 86.4). The lymphatic component can become hyperkeratotic and verrucous (Figure 86.5a and b).

DIFFERENTIAL DIAGNOSES

Capillary malformations and hemangiomas

It is important to elicit the congenital nature of the lesion while taking the patient's history. This will help distinguish CMs from the more common hemangiomas of infancy (HOI; Figure 86.6). CMs, similar to all other vascular malformations, are present at birth, while HOI are not present at birth and arise later during infancy. Congenital hemangiomas can cause confusion given their presence at birth.[2,3] Both rapidly involuting congenital hemangiomas (RICHs; Figure 86.7) and noninvoluting congenital hemangiomas (NICHs; Figure 86.8) are present at birth and need to be differentiated from CMs. Tissue biopsy may be required to differentiate between these conditions if clinical signs and imaging are insufficient. The most important implication is the treatment modality, given that a NICH enlarges in time and may require excision or embolization or a combination of these treatments, whereas a CM does not require significant intervention and may be treated with vascular laser therapy.

Tufted angioma

This vascular tumor can appear as a flat vascular patch and be confused with a CM. Tufted angioma can result in a consumption coagulopathy termed *Kasabach–Merritt syndrome* that may require emergency treatment. Tissue biopsy will be required to make the diagnosis.[4]

Sturge–Weber and PHACES syndromes

Two conditions that deserve a special mention are Sturge–Weber syndrome and the PHACES syndrome. In Sturge–Weber syndrome, the CM is typically on a trigeminal cranial nerve V (branches V1-V2) distribution of the face, which can be confused with flat hemangiomas observed in PHACES syndrome. The implications and treatment are significantly different. The hemangioma in PHACES syndrome is typically a large plaque-like hemangioma involving the V1-V2 and even V3 distribution. It is commonly unilateral, although it can be bilateral. Patients with PHACES syndrome may also have other anomalies including a posterior fossa brain malformation (P), hemangioma as described earlier (H), arterial anomalies typically

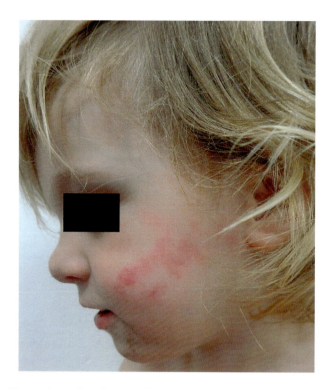

Figure 86.1 Capillary malformation on the left cheek of a 2-year-old female.

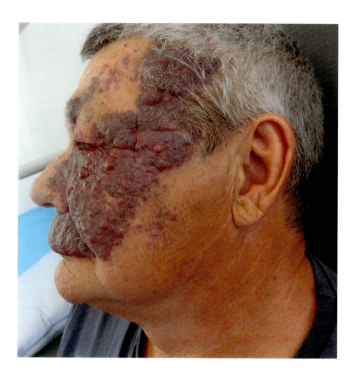

Figure 86.2 Hyperplastic capillary malformation (CM) previously referred to as a "cavernous hemangioma" involving the left cheek.

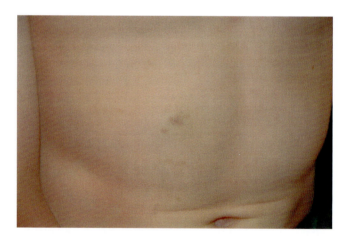

Figure 86.3 Capillary malformation-arteriovenous malformation (CM-AVM). Note the pale patch surrounding the CM due to cutaneous steal syndrome.

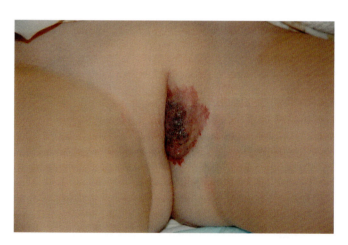

Figure 86.4 Segmental capillary-venolymphatic malformation (CVLM) involving the left labia. Note hemorrhage in the microcystic lymphatic component.

involving the ascending aorta and brachiocephalic arteries (A), cardiac anomalies including atrial and ventricular septal defects and a patent ductus arteriosus (C), eye abnormalities (E), and sternal defects (S). The importance of PHACES syndrome and the large facial hemangioma is to alert the physicians of the potential structural anomalies involving the heart, eyes, central nervous system (CNS), and arterial vascular system. In contrast, patients with Sturge–Weber syndrome need to be screened for brain AVMs as well as CNS abnormalities and, in particular, vascular malformations ipsilateral to the CM. It is worth emphasizing that patients with Sturge–Weber syndrome are at high risk for secondary complications due to episodes of seizures and glaucoma. The absence of seizures and/or glaucoma within the first 4 years of life is used as exclusion criteria for Sturge–Weber syndrome. For more details, see Chapter 90.

(a)

(b)

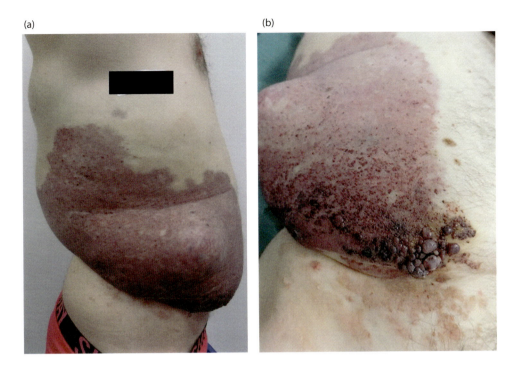

Figure 86.5 **(a)** Mosaic capillary-venolymphatic malformation (CVLM) affecting the right flank. **(b)** Note the verrucous nature of the lymphatic component of the CVLM.

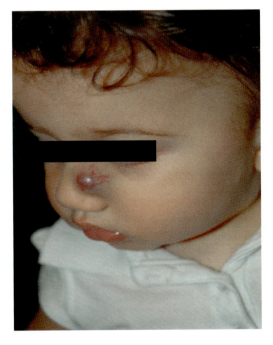

Figure 86.6 Hemangioma of infancy (HOI) with radiating vessels arising from the central vascular tumor.

Proteus and Cobb syndromes

CMs can be a component of other congenital syndromes, in particular Cobb and Proteus syndromes.[5] CMs and other vascular anomalies overlying the spine should prompt the physician to look for abnormality of the underlying spinal

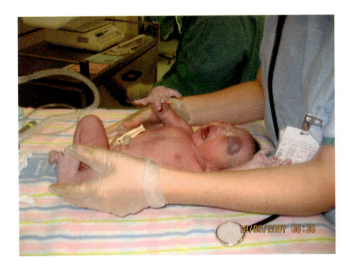

Figure 86.7 Rapidly involuting congenital hemangioma of infancy (RICH) of the left upper eyelid present at birth.

cord. This is especially the case in Cobb syndrome, where the CM is a manifestation of the underlying cutaneo-meningospinal angiomatosis. Patients with isolated CMs or hemangiomas overlying the spinal cord require magnetic resonance imaging (MRI) and spinal angiography to elicit pathology in the underlying spine. Computed tomography (CT) imaging may detect intramedullary or epidural hemorrhage. Plain CT with bone windows will determine

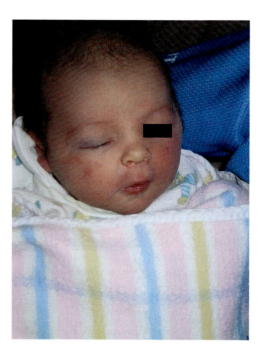

Figure 86.8 Noninvoluting congenital hemangioma of infancy (NICH) of the right upper eyelid present at birth.

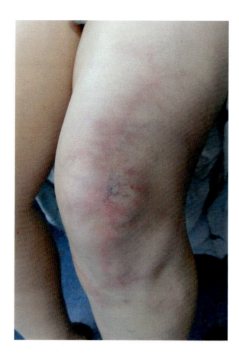

Figure 86.9 Cutis marmorata telangiectatica congenita (CMTC) of the left lower leg, demonstrating skin atrophy and livedo racemosa.

whether the lesion originates from the spinal canal or from the vertebral body. Duplex ultrasound, while useful in some cases, is not adequately sensitive and will not provide adequate detail of the extent of infiltration.

Cutis marmorata telangiectatica congenita

Cutis marmorata telangiectatica congenita (CMTC) is a congenital multisystemic disorder with features including livedo racemosa, phlebectasias, and cutaneous and subcutaneous atrophy. The most important cutaneous manifestation of CMTC is livedo racemosa. This is a reticulate vascular eruption that should not be confused with a CM. While livedo racemosa has reticulate morphology, CM presents as a continuous telangiectatic patch or plaque. CMTC primarily involves the extremities and less commonly the trunk and face (Figure 86.9). It is associated with limb length and circumference discrepancy, glaucoma, intellectual disability, patent ductus arteriosus, and arterial stenosis.

Telangiectatic conditions

Some telangiectatic conditions can be morphologically similar to CMs and be misdiagnosed. Generalized essential telangiectasia (GET) is a syndrome of widespread primary telangiectasias of unknown etiology (Figure 86.10). GET can cover large areas of skin and be confused with a CM.

Localized essential telangiectasia (ET) can be confused with a segmental or mosaic CM (Figure 86.11a and b). Spider angiomas (nevi) are dilated ascending arterioles that

present with a central arteriole and plethora of radiating thin-walled vessels (Figure 86.12). When spider angiomas are large, they acquire a patch morphology that may be confused with a CM. Despite the patch morphology, the central arteriole(s) remain a prominent feature of spider angiomas. Dermoscopy, and if not available the application of a

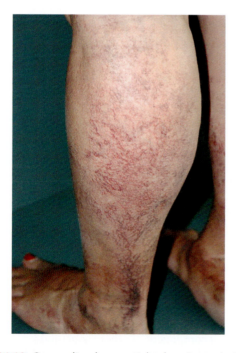

Figure 86.10 Generalized essential telangiectasia (GET) affecting the left lower limb.

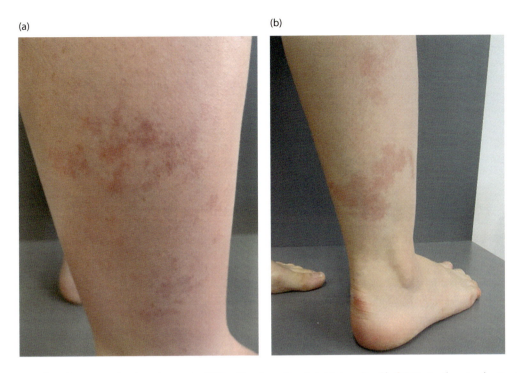

Figure 86.11 **(a)** Localized essential telangiectasia (ET) affecting the right lateral calf. **(b)** Note the similarity to a segmental capillary malformation (CM) of the same distribution.

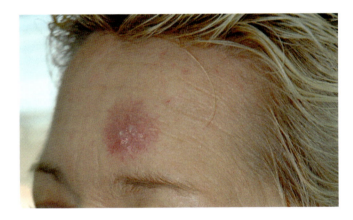

Figure 86.12 Large spider angioma with radiating arterioles arising from a central ascending arteriole.

glass slide to the lesion, would reveal the central arteriole(s) that will continue to appear pulsatile despite the pressure applied by the glass slide.

CONCLUSION

In conclusion, CMs are relatively common vascular anomalies that can be found in isolation or as a component of a complex vascular anomaly. An underlying genetic condition may be present. Similar conditions include hemangiomas, flat vascular tumors, and telangiectatic conditions.

REFERENCES

1. Lee BB, Antignani PL, Baraldini V et al. ISVI-IUA consensus document diagnostic guidelines of vascular anomalies: Vascular malformations and hemangiomas. *Int Angiol*. 2015;34:333–374.
2. Mulliken JB, Glowacki J. Hemangiomas and vascular malformations in infants and children: A classification based on endothelial characteristics. *Plast Reconstr Surg*. 1982;69:412–422.
3. Lee BB, Laredo J. Hemangioma and venous/vascular malformation are different as an apple and orange! Editorial. *Acta Phlebol*. 2012;13:1–3.
4. Enjolras O, Wassef M, Mazoyer E et al. Infants with Kasabach–Merritt syndrome do not have "true" hemangiomas. *J Pediatr*. 1997;130(4):631–640.
5. Turner JT, Cohen MM Jr, Biesecker LG. Reassessment of the Proteus syndrome literature: Application of diagnostic criteria to published cases. *Am J Med Genet A*. 2004;130:111–122.

87

How much diagnostic assessment for port-wine stains should be extended for other vascular malformations to exist together?

PETER BERLIEN

The English term for the most common capillary malformation, *port-wine stain*, is completely wrong and describes perhaps exclusively the situation in an adult, untreated patient. But in childhood one can say: A lesion that has the color of port wine is never a "simple" capillary malformation according to the International Society for the Study of Vascular Anomalies (ISSVA) classification.

This means that a capillary malformation is often the tip of an iceberg of a mixed vascular malformation, where at birth or at the first sign of it, not all parts are fully marked.[2] So like in all other congenital vascular anomalies, even in capillary malformations, not only the question of "what" has to be answered but even the "where" and the "how" (Figure 87.1). Only the nevus simplex or salmon patch has a tendency for spontaneous regression because this is an immature vascular regulation. All other forms of capillary malformation have the tendency to progress. This is caused by several conditions. One is that even in pure capillary malformation due to permanent hyperperfusion, a secondary hypertrophy of the affected tissue results in tuberous transformations. The other is the effects on other vascular structures in the malformation. So the most important diagnostic procedure in the newborn is the repeated clinical investigation of any changes of the capillary malformation. In perioral findings, an inspection of the mouth floor is obligatory. If there are enoral any findings even an endoscopy of the esophageal and tracheal tract has to be performed to detect mucosal infiltration.[1] The similar situation is in anogenital findings. Here in case of anal effects, a proctoscopy in boys with penile findings cyst-urethroscopy and in girls with vulvar findings additional vaginoscopy.

Another consideration for diagnosis is as follows: Is the capillary malformation limited to the dermal plexus or are other structures and/or other vascular systems affected (Figure 87.2)? Primary darker lesions and/or hypertrophic lesions are never a "port-wine stain" but a mixed vascular malformation.

The basic investigation is the high-resolution ultrasound with color-coded duplex mode (CCDS). In the B-scan mode, one can investigate the thickness of the dermis, the subcutaneous structure, and possibly musculature as a sign of deeper extension. Sponge structures are a symptom for mixed lymphatic malformations.[2] High fluid signals in the Doppler mode are a sign of an arterial malformation. In this case, thermography is the next step. A "simple" capillary malformation is ever normotherm. Any hyperthermia or hot spot is a sign of an arteriovenous (AV) shunt (Figure 87.3). Especially in centrofacial lesions, this is the differential diagnosis for Wyborn–Mason syndrome. In case of Sturge–Weber syndrome or Klippel–Trenaunay syndrome, thermography can detect early AV connections before they cause complications. This means that this investigation must be repeated throughout childhood to detect later formation.

In cases of cutis marmorata telangiectatica congenita (CMTC), there are two different pathophysiological processes: First, in contrast to port wine stain with soft tissue hypertrophy [please see author's note], here exists a hypoplasia of the capillary plexus. Second, shunts from the precapillary part drain directly to the postcapillary veins with a steal effect that reduced the microcirculation followed by a hypotrophy of the affected regions.[3]

[Author's note: The author prefers the term *hyperplasia* to *hypertrophy* on this unique condition, because *hypertrophy* generally represents a result of any tissue enlargement either by tumor proliferation even in benign or malignant tumors or any cell enlargement even by hypernutrition or metabolic disorders. At the same time, *hyperplasia* represents the process of enlargement of cells and/or collagen with normal cell numbers in normal mitosis in contrast to *neoplasia*, where we have a greater number of cells. But by definition, the congenital vascular malformations (CVMs) are differentiated from the vascular tumor based on this cellular/mitotic

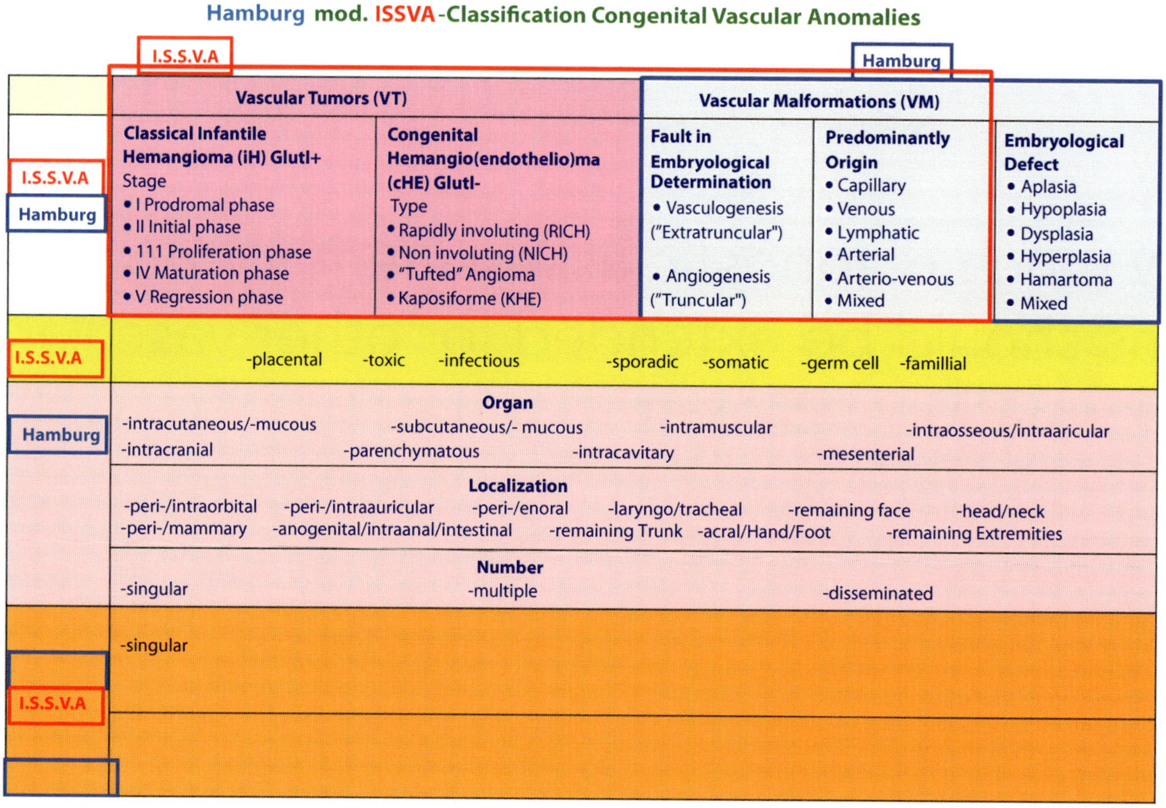

Hamburg mod. ISSVA-Classification Congenital Vascular Anomalies

I.S.S.V.A			Hamburg		
	Vascular Tumors (VT)		**Vascular Malformations (VM)**		
	Classical Infantile Hemangioma (iH) GlutI+	**Congenital Hemangio(endothelio)ma (cHE) GlutI-**	**Fault in Embryological Determination**	**Predominantly Origin**	**Embryological Defect**
I.S.S.V.A / Hamburg	Stage • I Prodromal phase • II Initial phase • 111 Proliferation phase • IV Maturation phase • V Regression phase	Type • Rapidly involuting (RICH) • Non involuting (NICH) • "Tufted" Angioma • Kaposiforme (KHE)	• Vasculogenesis ("Extratruncular") • Angiogenesis ("Truncular")	• Capillary • Venous • Lymphatic • Arterial • Arterio-venous • Mixed	• Aplasia • Hypoplasia • Dysplasia • Hyperplasia • Hamartoma • Mixed
I.S.S.V.A	-placental -toxic -infectious -sporadic -somatic -germ cell -famillial				
Hamburg	**Organ** -intracutaneous/-mucous -subcutaneous/- mucous -intramuscular -intraosseous/intraaricular -intracranial -parenchymatous -intracavitary -mesenterial				
	Localization -peri-/intraorbital -peri-/intraauricular -peri-/enoral -laryngo/tracheal -remaining face -head/neck -peri-/mammary -anogenital/intraanal/intestinal -remaining Trunk -acral/Hand/Foot -remaining Extremities				
	Number -singular -multiple -disseminated				
	-singular				
I.S.S.V.A					

Figure 87.1 Overlapping schema of the International Society for the Study of Vascular Anomalies and Hamburg classifications. It shows that there are no contradictions but different aspects. The Hamburg classification incorporates the embryological origin and provides a tool for indication, in general, and kind of therapy.

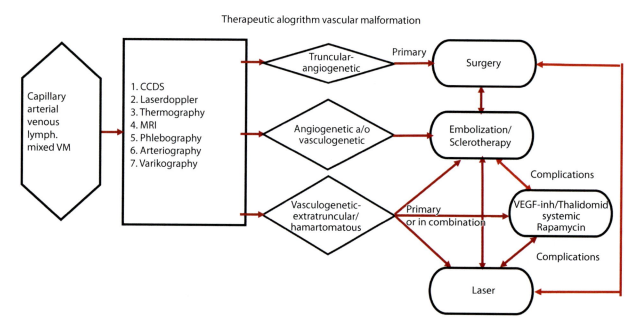

Therapeutic alogrithm vascular malformation

Figure 87.2 Diagnostic and therapeutic algorithm of congenital vascular malformation. The more angiogenetic truncular, the more surgery; the more vasculogenetic extra-truncular, the more interventional procedures.

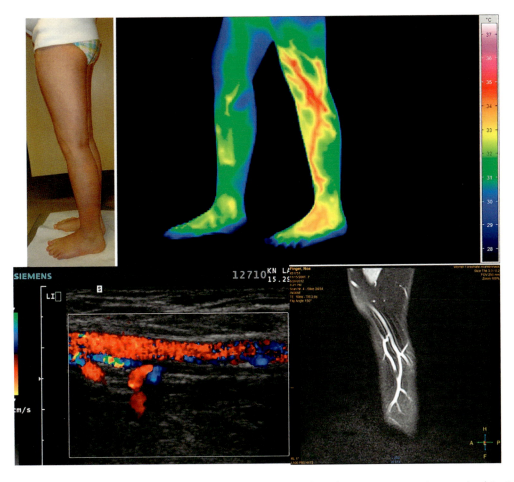

Figure 87.3 Secondary arterialization of a persistent marginal vein in Klippel–Trenaunay syndrome. At this time, there are no clinical symptoms, but the thermography is able to detect early hyperperfusion. The color-coded duplex mode and angiography show the arteriovenous fistula.

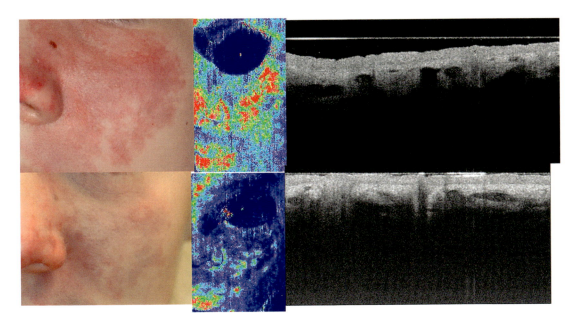

Figure 87.4 Even after several flashlamp-pumped pulsed-dye laser sessions remaining port wine stain. The laser-Doppler shows furthermore an increased microcirculation; the optical coherence tomography (OCT) is able to detect the cause: dilated subdermal vessels. After three sessions with pulsed alexandrite occlusion of these vessels, reduction of microcirculation and clinical clearance of the Parkes Weber syndrome.

activity, so the author chose the term *hypertrophy* for the majority of the readers for proper understanding.]

Because the resolution of ultrasound or magnetic resonance imaging (MRI) is not sufficient here, optical coherence tomography (OCT) and laser-Doppler-tomography are necessary (Figure 87.4). With these techniques, one can detect the shunts and can perform laser occlusion to enhance the microcirculation under control with OCT and laser Doppler.

In the case of hereditary hemorrhagic telangiectasia, in addition to the endoscopic examination, laser-Doppler-tomography is important to detect the micro-AV-shunts to prevent bleeding.[4]

If there is any sign that the soft tissue or body cavities or pelvic region are affected, this is an indication for MRI. An angiography is only helpful if AV malformation is suspected.

A biopsy with histological examination is only necessary in cases of difficult differential diagnosis to exclude malignant tumors, e.g., a mixed capillary/lymphatic malformation can look like a rhabdomyosarcoma.

REFERENCES

1. Berlien H-P. Laser therapy for venous malformations. In: Richter G, Suen J, eds. *Head and Neck Vascular Anomalies—A Practical Case-Based Approach.* San Diego, CA: Plural Publishing; 2015:224–228.
2. Diagnosis and treatment of venous malformations. Consensus document of the International Union of Phlebology (IUP): Updated 2013. *Int Angiol.* 2015; 34(2):97–149.
3. Mulliken JB. Capillary malformations, hyperceratotic stains, telangiectasias and miscellaneous vascular blots. In: Mulliken JB, Burrows PE, Fishman SJ, eds. *Mulliken and Youngs Vascular Anomalies: Hemangiomas and Malformations.* 2nd ed. New York, NY: Oxford University Press; 2013.
4. Poetke M, Philipp C, Großewinkelmann A et al. Die Behandlung von Naevi flammei bei Säuglingen und Kleinkindern mit dem blitzlampengepumpten Farbstofflaser. *Monatsschrift Kinderheilkunde.* 2001;32:405–415.

Management

88

Port-wine stains/capillary malformation among patients with Klippel–Trenaunay syndrome: How to select candidate for laser therapy and when

PETER BERLIEN

Klippel–Trenaunay syndrome (KTS) or "angio-osteohypertrophy syndrome," named in the Hamburg classification and also listed in the upcoming *International Classification of Diseases, 11th Revision* (*ICD-11*), is a typical example of the triad of vasculogenic extra-truncular malformation, angiogenetic truncular malformation, and general mesodermal affection (Figure 88.1). But, in contrast to CLOVES (congenital, lipomatous, overgrowth, vascular malformations, epidermal nevi, and spinal/skeletal anomalies and/or scoliosis) or Proteus syndrome,[4] the soft tissue, lipomatous tissue, and also osteo-hypertrophy among KTS is not primarily present but develops over the years as secondary conditions.

One more pathophysiological mechanism that underlines KTS (besides the embryological defect) is chronic hyperperfusion, which induces hypertrophy. Therefore, the destruction of this pathological vasculature network can reduce this hypernutrition and subsequently prevent development of the secondary complications, including the secondary effects on the skin with formation of tuberous transformation as a secondary venous complication and also dermal hypertrophy.

This normalization attempt further affects the other vascular problem of KTS—the "marginal vein" as the truncular venous malformation. The persistent marginal vein is not primarily insufficient at the beginning but will be affected by the extended venous backflow from the capillary beds and by additional loading by the transmuscular arteriovenous (AV) fistulas, which are not in functional status at birth but become more active over the years and drain into the marginal vein. As described in Chapter 87, thermography is the key diagnostic procedure.

It is important to emphasize that due to the fact that this truncular part of this venous malformation remains as the persistent marginal vein on one hand, while hypoplasia or aplasia of the deep and/or saphenous veins coexists on the other hand, this marginal vein fulfills a very important function in venous blood return and cannot simply be removed—the conservation of this marginal vein is essential. This assessment needs to be included in the treatment planning, since venous blood flow from the affected extremity may depend on the marginal vein patency, and obliteration or exclusion of the marginal vein from the circulation carries the risk of impairment of venous return from the affected extremity.

Nevertheless, there are various approaches based on laser therapy (Figure 88.2). First, for the capillary malformation of the dermis, the flashlamp-pumped pulsed-dye laser (FPDL) remains a treatment of choice. But, for larger venules, deeper capillaries, and/or dilated lymphatic spaces, which cannot be treated with the FPDL due to the limited penetration depth of the wavelength and the limited volume due to the short pulses, transcutaneous treatment with the long pulse alexandrite, Nd:YAG, or suitable diode laser under sufficient surface cooling is the treatment of choice.

However, taking into account that this capillary malformation is a vasculogenic extra-truncular defect, it can never be healed and will recur. In other words, this procedure has to be repeated throughout life as new capillary malformation lesions form.

An optimal protocol is to begin the therapy after the first year with sessions under general anesthesia in approximately 3-month intervals until a sufficient symptom resolution is achieved. There are two reasons to support this strategy: one is the reduction of pathological hyperperfusion, and another is the lightening of the "port-wine stain" before the children realize their malformation can have psychological and/or social adverse effects. We strongly advocate against using/considering the term "cosmetic," as these lesions are a part of a much more severe hemodynamic pathology.

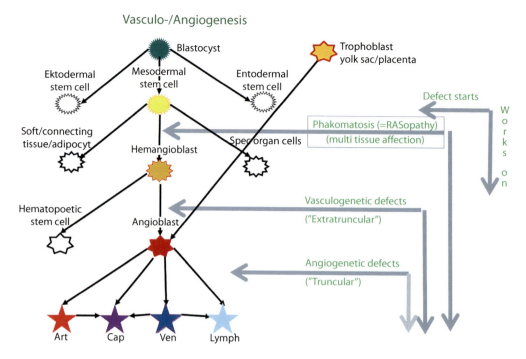

Figure 88.1 The embryological origin of the vascular system explains the different kinds of defects. The earlier in the mesodermal differentiation the defect happens, the more all tissues of mesodermal origin are involved; when the defect happens in the late angiogenesis, truncular malformation of *differentiated* vessels occurs. But when it happens in the vasculogenesis before differentiation to the different vessel types, extra-truncular malformations occur. A typical truncular malformation is congenital heart defects, while a typical extra-truncular malformation is represented by CLOVES or Klippel–Trenaunay syndrome with truncular malformation as a persistent marginal vein and extra-truncular capillary malformation.

Principles of treatment

Superficial cutaneous:
Flat findings:	*Flash/amp pumped Dye laser*
Teleangiectatic findings:	*KTPLaser*
Tuberous findings:	*pulsed Nd:YAG Laser*
Hyperceratotic findings:	*CO_2-Laser*

Intra- and subcutaneous,
up to a depth of 1–15 mm:
Transcutaneous Nd:YAG(1064) Laser with Ice-Cube Cooling Bare fiber impression-technique

Subcutaneous, voluminous,
> depth/thickness of 10 mm:
Nd:YAG (1064/1320) Laser interstitial or intraluminal

Hollow Organs,
Body Cavities:
Nd:YAG(1064/1320) Laser endoscopic in Air/Water,

Figure 88.2 Algorithm to choose the right laser system for each kind of vascular malformation.

These children have a disease that causes several impairments that require planning and proper treatment. Therefore, it is important to include psychosocial assessment and adequate management in the treatment algorithm for these patients. In most cases, this could be achieved until the age of 3–4 years. Then, if any recurrence should occur, it is recommended to start the next treatment cycle before the children reach school age to reduce the risk of having a difficult situation due to missing school.

Another treatment modality is the management of transmuscular AV fistulas. In adult patients with enlarged fistulas, angiographic embolization is the first procedure. But sometimes the arterial origin is difficult to find for catherization. In this case, a percutaneous coagulation with a cw Nd:YAG or near-infrared diode laser (Figure 88.3), similar to the treatment of perforator varicose veins or in larger fistulas an intraluminal occlusion, is indicated.[2]

The optimal time frame for this protocol is applicable to the second FLPDL (Pulsed Dye Laser) cycle, even in the same session. This procedure is even further applicable to the third secondary complication, the dilated insufficient marginal vein (Figure 88.4). But in contrast to the previous procedure for the other conditions, here instead, a naked bare fiber special applicator, e.g., a ring system or diffusor, allows for the treatment of even larger dilated veins.[1,3]

Another option is foam sclerotherapy of the marginal vein. But in contrast to the treatment of conventional varicose veins, here we have the risk of undetected communication to the deep venous system with the risk of uncontrolled washing out of the foam to the circulation. Especially in childhood, this can cause systemic complications. When the marginal vein is massively dilated and/or after thrombophlebitis, only surgical resection can be performed.

In conclusion, early laser therapy of the port-wine stain itself and early occlusion of the AV fistulas is warranted to prevent the need for surgical operations.

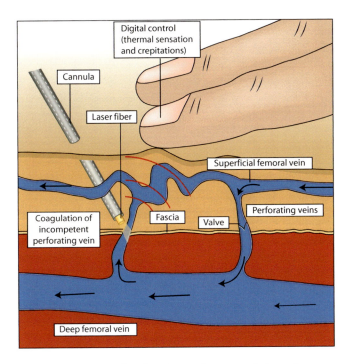

Figure 88.3 Principle of perivascular coagulation of transmuscular arteriovenous shunts to the marginal vein, similar to the treatment principle of perforator varices.

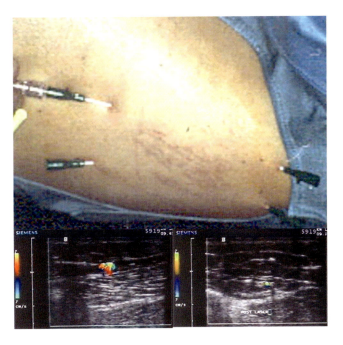

Figure 88.4 Intraluminal coagulation of a dilated marginal vein and perivascular coagulation of arteriovenous shunts at the same session. Sonography shows the exact position of the laser fiber tip in the lumen of the vein; the color-coded duplex mode signal detects the CO_2 production during the coagulation as a "color bruit signal" at the end when the vein is occluded.

REFERENCES

1. Berlien HP, Waldschmidt J, Müller G. Laser treatment of cutaneous and deep vessel anomalies. In: Waidelich W, ed. *Laser Optoelectronics in Medicine*. Berlin, Germany: Springer Verlag; 1988:526–528.
2. Fuchs B, Philipp C, Engel-Murke F, Shaltout J, Berlien H-P. Techniques for endoscopic and non-endoscopic intracorporeal laser applications. *Endosc Surg Allied Technol*. 1993;1:217–223.
3. Urban P, Poetke M, Müller U, Philipp C, Berlien H-P. Interstitial Nd:YAG laser treatment of vascular malformations controlled by color-coded duplex sonography (CCDS). *Med Laser Appl*. 2011;26:85.
4. Urban P, Berlien HP, Tinschert S. Vascular malformations in particular syndromes with regional overgrowth. *Eur J Vasc Med*. 2013;42:35–26.

89

To what extent should surgical excision be implemented to port-wine stains, and when?

PETER BERLIEN

The aim of *early* laser therapy of capillary malformations is to avoid the need for surgical excision by preventing its secondary complications.[1,4] But in adult patients with a long history of port-wine stains that were either never treated or not treated for an extended period of time (regardless of the reasons), the secondary changes of soft tissues and bone structures can be so significant that even with successful laser therapy, they will remain unchanged. For example, in patients with facial port-wine stain cutis laxa, lipomatous overgrowth and bone extension remain despite laser treatment. This represents an indication for surgical resection.

For patients where surgical resection is indicated (as described earlier), precise treatment planning is important. Due to the vasculogenic defect in capillary malformations, the formation of pathological vascularization is an inborn error of this region, so that even after the radical resection with free flaps, pathological vessels may occur. Therefore, a coordinated procedure has to be planned. This procedure should include several laser sessions, not only with flash-lamp-pumped pulsed-dye laser (FPDL) but even with near-infrared lasers (described in Chapter 88).[2,3] As much of a reduction of the pathological vessel should be achieved as is possible (Figure 89.1). Then, in the interval, surgical resection of the cutis laxa and other excessive tissue can be performed. In case of deformity of denture, proper surgery for mandibular bone correction can be added to reconstitute the function.

If there is any sign of early recurrence after the healing, laser therapy can be started immediately under thermographic and laser Doppler surveillance. In such cases, an additional pharmacological therapy could be indicated, as described in Chapter 90.

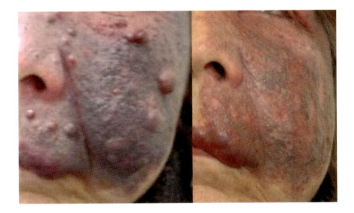

Figure 89.1 Untreated port-wine stain in an adult woman. In addition to the soft tissue hypertrophy, massive tuberous transformations, not "angiomas," are developed, which have the risk of bleeding from their central artery. After several laser sessions with flashlamp-pumped pulsed-dye laser, and alexandrite for skin clearance, soft tissue hypertrophy on the lip and cheek remains. This is an indication for surgical excision.

REFERENCES

1. Berlien HP. Laser treatment of vascular malformations. In: Mattassi R, Loose DA, Vaghi M, eds. *Hemangiomas and Vascular Malformations*. Berlin, Germany: Springer; 2015:291–305.
2. Lee BB, Baumgartner I, Berlien HP et al.; International Union of Angiology. Consensus Document of the International Union of Angiology (IUA)-2013. Current concepts on the management of arteriovenous malformations. *Int Angiol*. 2013;32(1):9–36.
3. Poetke M, Urban P, Berlien P. Vascular lesions: Hemangiomas In: Raulin C, Karsai S, eds. *Laser and IPL Technology in Dermatology and Aesthetic Medicine*. New York, NY: Springer; 2011.
4. Poetke M, Philipp C, Großewinkelmann A et al. Die Behandlung von Naevi flammei bei Säuglingen und Kleinkindern mit dem blitzlampengepumpten Farbstofflaser. *Monatsschrift Kinderheilkunde*. 2001;32: 405–415.

90

To what extent could laser therapy and surgical excision be combined for port-wine stain management?

PETER BERLIEN

First and foremost, for any indication for any therapy, a clear and accurate diagnosis is required. Not every facial red macula is a "port-wine stain" (PWS), as it can be a clinical finding associated with a similar or a quite different diagnosis. If it changes rapidly after birth, especially if it is characterized by fast growth, it is never a capillary malformation but a highly aggressive infantile hemangioma that requires immediate therapy specific for this subtype of hemangioma.

If the lesion is midfacially located and pale, without changes of dermal structure, and without a thrill, there is a high level of confidence it is a nevus simplex Unna. But, if the lesion is midfacially located and has a pasty structure with bruit and/or thrill, it is suggestive of Wyburn-Mason syndrome.[1] If the skin has a rough structure with hyperkeratotic segments, it seems to be a mixed capillary lymphatic malformation (Figure 90.1), which is even erroneously named a *verrucous angioma*, although it is not a vascular tumor but a vascular malformation.

Location alone cannot be used for definitive diagnosis. If the PWS lesion is located on the face, not all PWSs on the face are Sturge–Weber syndrome. But, at birth not all typical symptoms for a Sturge–Weber syndrome diagnosis are present, e.g., glaucoma and seizure(s).[6] However, there is a high risk for this syndrome if the lesions affect the entire face, including periocular and/or perioral regions. (For further diagnostic assessment, see Chapter 87.)

Clinically suspected Sturge–Weber syndrome represents a challenging situation with regard to the optimal way to discuss treatment planning with the patient's family/guardians. More specifically, if we inform the parents/guardians that diagnosis is most likely Sturge–Weber syndrome, this can be perceived that they have a very ill child. However, clinically it is beneficial, as this provides an opportunity for early intervention to minimize the risks for secondary complications caused by glaucoma and seizure(s). In such

a clinical situation, it makes sense to discuss each clinical scenario (relative to findings) with the parents/guardians and to recommend a management algorithm that should be based on diagnosis for Sturge–Weber syndrome. We should not withhold the diagnosis from the patients/guardians (medico-ethico-legally), and all the clinical findings need to be openly and fully discussed prior to any treatment planning.

The indication for early laser therapy is the same as described in Chapter 88 for Klippel–Trenaunay syndrome. In Sturge–Weber syndrome, but even in "simple" capillary malformation, the secondary soft tissue hypertrophy and bone hypertrophy on the maxilla and midface bone are caused by hyperperfusion. Early elimination of the pathological capillary network can significantly minimize the risk of these complications. Furthermore, the lightening of the vascular birthmark reduces psychosocial impairment, e.g., before the children come to preschool age. This means that an intensive treatment protocol has to be performed before the patient is 4 years old.

The fourth year is not relevant for the treatment algorithm. The treatment of the capillary malformation is life-long. However, the fourth year is relevant for the differential diagnosis for simple capillary malformation or Sturge–Weber syndrome, because in our experience, 80% of seizures occur within the first year, and 60% of cases of glaucoma develop before 24 months of life in these patients. The same is true for mental retardation. This means that if seizures and/or glaucoma do not occur within the first 4 years of life, Sturge–Weber syndrome can be excluded from further diagnostic workup, and we can stop the working diagnosis of "Sturge–Weber syndrome." This is the reason for using general anesthesia for laser treatment of the capillary malformation for additional ophthalmoscopy to detect the early onset of glaucoma.

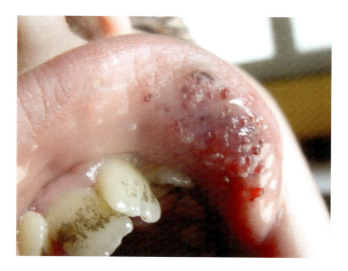

Figure 90.1 Mixed capillary lymphatic hyperkeratotic malformation on the lip. In such a case, a thorough inspection of the entire oral cavity is mandatory, and a risk of additional involvement of pharynx and/or larynx should be assessed for the same findings.

Congenital Vascular Anomalies

- The more late angiogenesis with structured vessels the more surgery

- The more remaining embryonal vessels the more sclerotherapy

- The more fistulas/shunts the more embolization

- The more capillary/disseminated vessels the more Laser

- The more vasculogenetic disseminated findings the more systemic therapy with mToR-inhibitors (Rapamycin)

- The more angiogenetic vessels the more systemic therapy with VEGF-inhibitors/Thalidomid

Figure 90.2 List of keywords to choose the optimal treatment regimen for the different kinds of vascular malformations. One can see the importance of the embryological assessment.

During this time, neurological and regular ophthalmic examination should be repeated. It is worth emphasizing that eye exams need to include not only the eye pressure measurements but also, and much more importantly, ophthalmoscopy (to evaluate the optic papilla) should be included because its pathology progresses very fast with elevated eye pressure. This test can be performed easily during the general anesthesia for laser therapy.[2–4]

In large mixed capillary malformation, the tendency for early recurrence is very high. In these cases, therapy with mTOR inhibitor sirolimus following clearance with laser therapy reduces this process and subsequently extends the interval of therapy. However, data show, as with other experiences with pharmacological therapy (either systemic or topical), that this treatment modality is efficient only during the administration of medication to prevent the development of new pathological vessels.[5] But immediately after stopping the therapy, regrowth of the pathological vasculature occurs. The same clinical course characterizes photodynamic therapy (PDT), either systemic or topical (Figure 90.2).

Therefore, surgical excision in patients with PWS is no longer indicated as a primary treatment option. Only in a few cases of extended mixed lymphatic capillary malformation with primary verrucous formation will a local excision be necessary. But for all surgical procedures, one has to take into account that due to the full dermal involvement of the malformation, a simple shaving with split skin graft is not technically feasible and/or sufficient, and only full skin excision with free flap skin transplantation can be performed. But even this large wound induces a neovascularization during the healing process, which is the outcome of a congenital error, which manifests as malformed vessels.

REFERENCES

1. Berlien HP. Clinical features and evaluation of superficial and deep capillary malformation. In: Kim YW, Lee BB, Yakes W. *Congenital Vascular Malformation.* Berlin, Germany: Springer Verlag; 2017:129–138.
2. Patil B, Sinha G, Nayak B, Sharma R, Kumari S, Dada T. Bilateral Sturge–Weber and phakomatosis pigmentovascularis with glaucoma, an overlap syndrome. *Case Rep Ophthalmol Med.* 2015;2015:106932.
3. Happle R. Phacomatosis pigmentovascularis revisited and reclassified. *Arch Dermatol.* 2005;141(3):385–388.
4. Mandal RK, Ghosh SK, Koley S, Roy AC. Sturge–Weber syndrome in association with Klippel–Trenaunay syndrome and phakomatosis pigmentovascularis type IIb. *Indian J Dermatol Venereol Leprol.* 2014;80(1):51–53.
5. Nelson JS, Jia W, Phyng TL, Mihm MC Jr. Observations on enhanced port wine stain blanching induced by combined pulsed dye laser and rapamycin administration. *Lasers Surg Med.* 2011;43(10):939–942.
6. Neto FXP. Clinical features of Sturge–Weber syndrome. *Int Arch Otorhinol.* 2008;12(4):565–570.

Epilogue

It has taken a long time to complete this extraordinary journey, and I never expected to encounter such difficulty, with so many "unknowns" to my limited "knowns." Indeed, without constant guidance from my mentor, Leonel Villavicencio of the Uniformed Services University of the Health Sciences (USUHS), and the generous, unlimited support of my two coeditors, Peter Gloviczki of the Mayo Clinic and Francine Blei of Lennox Hill Hospital and also Assistant Editor, Jovan Markovic of Duke University, this mission would have remained hopelessly bogged down in eternal confusion.

Indeed, when we began to organize the consensus on venous malformations, along with primary lymphedema/lymphatic malformations, commissioned by the International Union of Phlebology (IUP) in 2007, we were quite surprised and embarrassed to find out there were many issues mired in controversy, with no clear answers to be incorporated into the consensus.

We initially took them lightly, and unintentionally neglected them, until we encountered more hotly debated issues through a subsequently organized consensus for arteriovenous malformations that was commissioned by the International Union of Angiology (IUA). I reluctantly took Leonel's advice to start addressing these issues by collecting and saving them for future review.

Through subsequent updates on these consensuses for venous malformations and lymphatic malformations/primary lymphedema, as well as new additional consensuses for vascular anomaly and chronic lymphedema that we organized for the IUA and IUP, we recognized the serious nature of these controversial ideas for the first time.

They were the tip of the iceberg, which we could not simply ignore.

Leonel gave decisive help through his perspective in sorting out these many contentious topics. We discussed them through numerous communications while organizing the consensuses, and they became a turning point for us to tackle this ever-challenging task with determination.

Leonel, ever the proud Peter Bent Brigham–trained cardiovascular surgeon, dedicated his entire career to venous surgery and remained a beacon to many pupils like me for over three decades until he peacefully passed away last January. Though he could not fulfill his commitment to write the Foreword, his closest friend and colleague, Hugo Partsch of Austria, kindly stepped in to write it for us.

Leonel remained my mentor through all these years, giving me unlimited support for my work on vascular malformations, just as John Bergan had for me with lymphedema. Especially for this project with all of its complex issues, I personally owe Leonel for providing 100% of the inspiration behind this effort, ever since we organized the first IUP consensus for venous malformations in 2007.

So, I personally wish to dedicate this project and book to Leonel. After all, without his constant encouragement, I would have remained a career transplant surgeon without ever having ventured out into the ever-challenging but fertile world of vascular malformations.

Byung-Boong Lee
A proud student of Leonel Villavicencio
Editor

Index